NUTRITION

REVISED FIRST EDITION

NUTRITION

REVISED FIRST EDITION

DAVID C. NIEMAN, DHSC, MPH FACSM
Appalachian State University

DIANE E. BUTTERWORTH, DHSC, MPH, RD
Appalachian State University

CATHERINE N. NIEMAN, MS, RD

 Wm. C. Brown Publishers

Book Team

Editor *Colin H. Wheatley*
Developmental Editor *Jane DeShaw*
Production Editor *Ann Fuerste*
Designer *Mark Elliot Christianson*
Art Editor *Margaret R. Buhr*

Wm. C. Brown Publishers

President *G. Franklin Lewis*
Vice President, Publisher *George Wm. Bergquist*
Vice President, Operations and Production *Beverly Kolz*
National Sales Manager *Virginia S. Moffat*
Group Sales Manager *Vincent R. Di Blasi*
Vice President, Editor in Chief *Edward G. Jaffe*
Marketing Manager *John W. Calhoun*
Advertising Manager *Amy Schmitz*
Managing Editor, Production *Colleen A. Yonda*
Manager of Visuals and Design *Faye M. Schilling*
Production Editorial Manager *Julie A. Kennedy*
Production Editorial Manager *Ann Fuerste*
Publishing Services Manager *Karen J. Slaght*

WCB Group

President and Chief Executive Officer *Mark C. Falb*
Chairman of the Board *Wm. C. Brown*

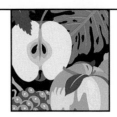

To Professors U. D. Register and Kathleen Zolber, who have patterned excellence in research, teaching, and writing in the nutrition profession.
    David C. Nieman

To my husband, Deacon, and my daughter, Laura, with appreciation for their understanding, love, forbearance, and assistance.
    Diane E. Butterworth

To my late father, Floyd Nixon, who inspired me to serve others in love.
    Catherine N. Nieman

B R I E F   C O N T E N T S

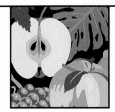

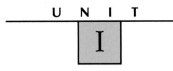
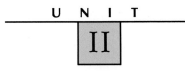
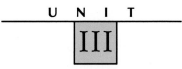
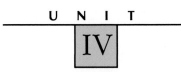

C O N T E N T S

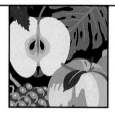

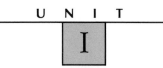

PREFACE

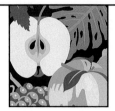

As noted in the 1988 Surgeon General's Report on *Nutrition and Health* (1), our nutritional problems today are no longer related to deficiency but to excess. Diseases related to nutritional deficiency have diminished (for example, scurvy from lack of vitamin C and pellegra from lack of niacin), but diseases related to dietary excess and imbalance have increased. For example, eight of the top ten diseases in the U.S. (including heart disease and cancer), have been related to diet and to excessive alcohol intake. Although many food factors are involved, the Surgeon General states that "chief among them is the disproportionate consumption of foods high in fats, often at the expense of foods high in complex carbohydrates and fiber that may be more conducive to health."

The good news, however, is that a health-promotion revolution is taking place. In magazines and newspapers and on the radio and television, the topics of nutrition, health, and wellness are being widely discoursed. Many Americans are becoming involved in combating the diseases related to life-style, and it is beginning to pay off. Some of the changes that have already occurred include an increase in life expectancy, decreasing death rates from heart disease, a sharp decline in cigarette smoking, a decrease in alcohol consumption, and an improvement in dietary patterns (2).

Nutrition, Revised First Edition, includes a discussion of these changes, with a focus on the role of nutrition in enhancing life and health. Our hope is that reading this text will inspire you to become involved in the health-promotion revolution.

About This Book

Nutrition is a traditional nutrition textbook in that it covers basic and cardinal concepts such as measurement of the diet, the role of nutrients in body function, and nutrition throughout the life cycle. The "health-promotion" perspective of this text, however, makes it unique. Health promotion is the science and art of helping people change their life-style to move toward a state of optimal health (3). Therefore, *Nutrition* emphasizes the positive contributions of nutrition to life and health—not controversy or debate—and is designed to help you improve your understanding of nutrition and the skills of health promotion.

Organization

The fifteen chapters of *Nutrition* are grouped into four units.

Unit I: Nutrition and Health Promotion. Chapter 1 explains the health-promotion concept in detail. Chapter 2 covers trends in the American diet and nutritional recommendations of the U.S. government and various professional organizations. In chapter 3, methods of measuring the diet are discussed, and chapter 4 provides information about the safety of our food supply.

Unit II: Energy in Nutrition. Chapters 5–7 explore the contributions of carbohydrate, lipids, and protein to nutrition, examining the quantity and quality of each that is needed for good health. Chapter 8 provides an overview of the "energy equation" and the factors that influence it. The problem of obesity in this country, and the relationship of diet and exercise to both prevention and treatment, are covered in chapter 9.

Unit III: Vitamins, Minerals, Water, and Your Health. Chapters 10 and 11 explain the role of vitamins and minerals in the diet, and the importance of water to body physiology is discussed in chapter 12.

Unit IV: Nutrition throughout the Life Cycle. The chapters in this unit focus on special nutrition needs during certain time periods. Nutrition for pregnant women and for infants is summarized in chapter 13. Nutrition needs during the years of growth—childhood and adolescence—is discussed in chapter 14. Chapter 15 covers the nutrition requirements of the elderly, an area of increasing concern.

Features

Chapter Outline

Each chapter begins with an overview, in outline form, of the contents of the chapter. Reading this before beginning the chapter will give the student an idea of the material to be covered, and it will be a useful reference when the student is studying for exams.

Illustrations and Tables

The numerous figures and tables in the text will help reinforce the nutrition information presented in the text. All information is up-to-date. Included in this revised edition are the 1989 Recommended Daily Allowances tables. Appendix A: Index of Nutrient Tables, is a handy reference for all tables found in this text.

Sidebars

Boxed inserts called Sidebars appear in some chapters. These highlight nutrition topics of special interest and concern.

Health-Promotion Insights

Most chapters contain a Health-Promotion Insight that focuses on a particular topic of nutrition related to the subject covered in the chapter. Some of the issues discussed include the role of saturated fats and cholesterol in cardiovascular disease, the relationship between diet and behavior, the connection between diet and cancer risk, and the importance of carbohydrate in the diet of the endurance athlete.

Summary

A summary at the end of each chapter highlights all the important chapter information and will be helpful when the student reviews for exams.

References

A complete list of up-to-date references is included at the end of each chapter. This list provides the student with an extensive source of reading for continued study.

Health-Promotion Activities

Each chapter ends with self-assessment inventories and other activities to help the student understand the health-promotion concept. For example, a self-quiz will show the students how their diets compare to that of the average American. Students will have the opportunity to design their own aerobic exercise program, and analyze their sodium consumption.

Appendixes

To make studying easier, we have attempted to include as many nutrient tables as possible within the text, rather than at the end of the book. Therefore, for your convenience, Appendix A provides a list of these tables, as well as some of the figures pertaining to nutrients.

Appendix B is a comprehensive food composition table that is simple and easy to understand. In addition to listing the nutrients in foods, this table lists dietary fiber, sodium, saturated fat, and cholesterol contained in each food.

Appendix C is a concise explanation of the human digestive system and features a color illustration of the digestive system. Appendix D contains tables of weights, measures, and conversions. Appendix E provides a list of organizations that are excellent sources of nutrition information, and Appendix F is a list of recommended cookbooks and magazines related to food and nutrition. Appendix G contains the complete Dietary Guidelines for Americans (Third Edition, 1990), published by the U.S. government. New to this edition is Appendix H, a basic review of nutrition biochemistry.

Glossary

Throughout the text, important terms are set off in boldface type. Concise definitions of these terms can be found in the Glossary.

Supplementary Materials

Supplementary materials accompanying this text are designed to help students in their learning activities and to help instructors plan course-work and presentations. These supplementary materials include:

Instructor's Manual/Test Item File is an excellent teaching supplement that provides a chapter overview, learning objectives, an annotated chapter outline, and teaching strategies for additional in-class and out-of-class learning activities. The Instructor's Manual also has 70 master transparencies and contains the Test Item File, which is a printout of all test questions available in TestPak.

Transparencies include 48 two- and four-color acetates. These are in addition to the 70 master transparencies found in the Instructor's Manual.

TestPak is a computerized test bank that has more than 750 questions organized by chapter. It is page referenced directly to the text.

QuizPak is a computerized self-testing program available for students. QuizPak contains an additional 600 questions not found in the text.

Diet Assessment Software

Diet Assessment Software called *Nutrition Profile* is an easy-to-use dietary assessment, developed by Wellsource, Inc., that determines diet evaluation, ideal weight and energy requirements, and recommendations for dietary as well as life-style changes. *Nutrition Profile* features nutrition scores graphically displayed, diet according to food groups, detailed personal recommendations for diet improvement, and energy balance report.

        Food Processor II Nutrition System Software analyzes food, intakes, menus, and recipes. The program analyzes 45 foods per run; daily intakes can be automatically averaged. Intakes can be compared to a nutrients requirement profile based on the Recommended Dietary Allowances, the Canadian Recommended Nutrient Intake of the U.S. RDA (used in food labeling). These nutrient recommendations are individualized for age, weight, height, activity level, gender, pregnancy, and lactation. Further programming can be done to reflect special dietary needs such as low-sodium or low-cholesterol. Contact your Wm. C. Brown sales representative or Customer Service Wm. C. Brown (1–800–338–5578) for a demonstration diskette.

Acknowledgments

We would like to thank the following reviewers for their assistance:

Maxine Cochran
William Penn College

Edith B. Davis
Our Lady of Holy Cross College

J. H. Garvin
University of Cincinnati

Margarette Harden
Texas Tech University

Edward J. Hart
Bridgewater State College

Gladys Jennings
Washington State University

Judith S. Matheisz
Erie Community College

Mary B. Nelson
Southeastern Louisiana University

Jeanne Polak
Los Angeles Valley College

F. Eric Sills
Eastern College

Glenn P. Town
Wheaton College

In addition, we wish to thank John Gobble of Wellsource, Inc., Clackamas, Oregon, for his assistance with chapters 2, 3, 5, and 6.

References

1. U.S. Department of Health and Human Services. 1988. The Surgeon General's Report on *Nutrition and Health*. DHHS (PHS) Publication no. 88–50211. Washington, D.C.: U.S. Government Printing Office.
2. U.S. Department of Health and Human Services. 1991. *Healthy People 2000: National Health Promotion and Disease Prevention Objectives*. DHHS Publication No. (PHS)91–50212. Washington, D.C.: U.S. Government Printing Office.
3. O'Donnell, M. P. 1986. Definition of Health Promotion: Part II: Levels of Programs. *American Journal of Health*

UNIT
I

Nutrition and Health Promotion

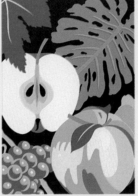

What should we eat to be healthy? Unit I will clarify the association between nutrition and the leading causes of death in the United States. The Public Health Service has developed nutritional objectives to promote the health of Americans. Since individual response is the key to achieving these objectives, strategies for changing eating behavior will be discussed in chapter 1.

The dietary guidelines are presented in chapter 2, along with a discussion of trends in the American diet since 1900. In order to apply the guidelines, the tools and methods for evaluating and planning diets are described in chapter 3. Chapter 4 discusses how to evaluate food safety and quality.

1

The Health-Promotion Concept

INTRODUCTION

*I*n the quest for a long and healthy life, many people fear recent reports of a chronic disease epidemic and look toward nutrition as a cure-all. What should we eat to be healthy? Every day someone tries to tell us what we should or should not eat. Newspapers, magazines, radio, television, and salespeople certainly have enough to say on the topic, but unfortunately much of what they say is confusing. This chapter will clarify the association between life-style (nutrition in particular) and the leading causes of death in the United States.

In response to the alarming rise in chronic disease between 1900 and 1985, the Public Health Service published health objectives for 1990. Nutrition was one of the fifteen areas of greatest importance for improving the health of the public. Although considerable progress has been made toward these objectives, there is still much work to be done. Individual response is the key. Strategies for changing eating behavior are presented in this chapter.

A Chronic Disease Epidemic

The leading causes of death in the United States have changed dramatically since 1900, shifting from infectious to chronic diseases (see table 1.1). For example, pneumonia/influenza was the leading cause of death in 1900, whereas heart disease was the leading cause of death in 1985. Cancer and cerebrovascular disease (stroke), now the second and third leading causes of death, respectively, were the seventh and fourth leading causes of death, respectively, in 1900. In 85 years the proportion of mortality from the chronic diseases has increased 250 percent (1) (see figure 1.1). The severity of the chronic disease epidemic is appalling.

As of 1987, nearly 63,400,000 Americans have some form of heart or blood-vessel disease (2). Cardiovascular diseases account for one million deaths per year, with nearly one in every five of the victims under the age of 65. As many as 1.5 million Americans will have a heart attack this year, and more than one-third of them will die. The economic cost is staggering, totaling $85.2 billion in 1987. Yet the vast majority of heart disease is preventable, especially by controlling cigarette smoking, high blood pressure, blood cholesterol, diet, exercise, and other lifestyle factors.

Cancer is the nation's second leading cause of death, with 452,000 people dying each year (3). Cancer will strike three of every four families during this generation's lifetime, and one in every four people. Most of this cancer is

TABLE 1.1
The ten leading causes of death in the United States — 1900 and 1985

1900	1985
1. Pneumonia and influenza	1. Heart disease
2. Tuberculosis	2. Cancer
3. Diseases of the heart	3. Stroke
4. Stroke	4. Accidents
5. Diarrhea, enteritis, and ulceration of the intestine	5. Chronic obstructive pulmonary diseases
6. Nephritis	6. Pneumonia and influenza
7. Cancer	7. Diabetes mellitus
8. Accidents	8. Suicide
9. Diphtheria	9. Chronic liver disease and cirrhosis
10. Diseases of early infancy	10. Atherosclerosis (hardening of the arteries)

Data from National Center for Health Statistics.

FIGURE 1.1
The proportion of deaths attributable to major causes of death in the United States in 1900 and in 1985. The names of chronic diseases are noted in color.

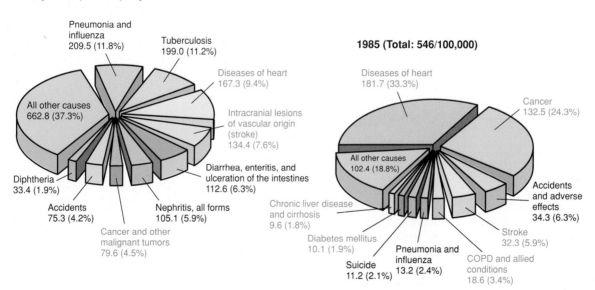

1900 (Total: 1,779/100,000)

Pneumonia and influenza 209.5 (11.8%)
Tuberculosis 199.0 (11.2%)
Diseases of heart 167.3 (9.4%)
All other causes 662.8 (37.3%)
Intracranial lesions of vascular origin (stroke) 134.4 (7.6%)
Diphtheria 33.4 (1.9%)
Diarrhea, enteritis, and ulceration of the intestines 112.6 (6.3%)
Accidents 75.3 (4.2%)
Nephritis, all forms 105.1 (5.9%)
Cancer and other malignant tumors 79.6 (4.5%)

1985 (Total: 546/100,000)

Diseases of heart 181.7 (33.3%)
Cancer 132.5 (24.3%)
All other causes 102.4 (18.8%)
Accidents and adverse effects 34.3 (6.3%)
Chronic liver disease and cirrhosis 9.6 (1.8%)
Stroke 32.3 (5.9%)
Diabetes mellitus 10.1 (1.9%)
Pneumonia and influenza 13.2 (2.4%)
COPD and allied conditions 18.6 (3.4%)
Suicide 11.2 (2.1%)

probably preventable. The National Cancer Institute and the American Cancer Society report that low-fiber, high-fat diets contribute to 35 percent of all cancers, and cigarette smoking causes 30 percent of all cancers (4).

Approximately 11 million Americans have diabetes. Diabetes is a major cause of death, shortening the life expectancy of an individual by one-third. About 250,000 new cases are diagnosed each year. Diabetes is the number-one cause of blindness in the United States, and it also causes cardiovascular diseases, stroke, gangrene, and kidney disease (5,6,7). The economic burden is overwhelming at $18 billion annually. And yet, it is estimated that 75 percent of all individuals with diabetes could control their blood sugar without medication if proper diet and exercise therapy were followed (8).

One of every four adults (about 40 million) is obese (9). Obesity has been linked to a number of problems and diseases, including cardiovascular disease, cancer, hypertension, diabetes, gallbladder disease, respiratory problems, and early death (10). However, obesity can be controlled and prevented largely through long-term nutrition and exercise programs.

After reviewing the chronic disease data, the Institute of Medicine concluded that "the heaviest burdens of illness in the United States today are related to aspects of individual behavior, especially long-term patterns of behavior often referred to as 'life-style' " (11).

The Health-Promotion Concept

The World Health Organization in 1947 defined **health** as "a state of complete physical, mental, and social well-being, and not merely the absence of disease" (12). An individual's health is determined by four major factors:

Environment—physical, economic, prenatal
Heredity—congenital defects, genetic
    predisposition
Health Care Services—technology, facilities,
    availability and accessibility of services
    and personnel
Life-style—diet, exercise, stress, sleep

Health planners estimate that 50 percent or more of the leading causes of death are associated with life-style factors (13). The individual therefore has tremendous potential to prevent disease by changing his or her life-style.

Health promotion is the science and art of helping people change their life-style to move toward optimal health (14). The focus is on behaviors that result in improved life-style, because only when people take action and change their behaviors do they improve their health and prevent disease. Table 1.2 lists the specific controllable life-style risk factors for the leading causes of death in the U.S.

Self-responsibility, therefore, is a central theme in health promotion. A health-promotion program will be most successful when it provides the skills and environment necessary for the participants to take responsibility for making the choices in their lives that are consistent with health. The health-promotion activities in this book are designed to help individuals change their eating behavior to move toward optimal health.

*T*ABLE 1.2
Life-style risk factors associated with the leading causes of death in the United States

Cause of Death	Life-Style Risk Factors
Heart disease	Smoking, high blood pressure, high serum cholesterol, diabetes, obesity, lack of exercise, stress
Cancer	Smoking, alcohol, sun exposure, radiation, worksite hazards, environmental pollution, obesity, diet
Stroke	High blood pressure, high serum cholesterol, smoking, diet, obesity, lack of exercise, stress
Accidents	
Motor vehicle	Alcohol, nonuse of seat belts, speed, automobile design, roadway design
Other than motor vehicle	Alcohol, smoking, product design, home hazards, handgun availability
Chronic obstructive pulmonary diseases	Smoking, environmental pollutants, worksite hazards
Influenza/pneumonia	Vaccination status, smoking, alcohol, diet
Diabetes	Obesity, diet
Suicide	Stress, alcohol and drug misuse, handgun availability
Chronic liver disease and cirrhosis	Alcohol
Atherosclerosis	Smoking, high blood pressure, high serum cholesterol, diabetes, obesity, lack of exercise, stress

From J. E. Fielding, "Health Promotion and Disease Prevention at the Worksite," p. 239. Reproduced, with permission, from the *Annual Review of Public Health*, vol. 5. © 1984 by Annual Reviews Inc.

TABLE 1.3
Nutritional risk factors associated with the leading causes of death in the United States

Cause of Death	Nutritional Risk Factors
Heart disease	High total and saturated fat intake, high dietary cholesterol intake, obesity, excessive salt intake
Cancer	High total fat intake; low fiber intake; high alcohol intake; salt-cured, smoked, and nitrite-cured foods
Stroke	High total and saturated fat intake, high dietary cholesterol intake, obesity, excessive salt intake
Accidents	Alcohol
Chronic obstructive pulmonary diseases	None
Influenza/pneumonia	Malnutrition, alcohol
Diabetes	Obesity
Suicide	Alcohol
Chronic liver disease and cirrhosis	Alcohol, malnutrition
Atherosclerosis	High total and saturated fat intake, high dietary cholesterol intake, obesity, excessive salt intake

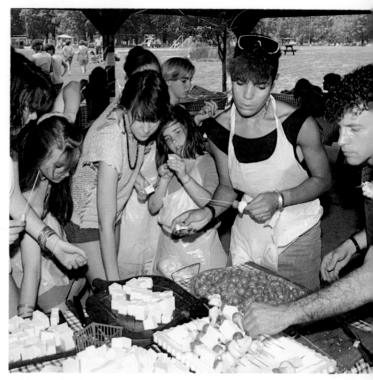
Eating nutritious food affects our lives.

Nutrition: An Integral Component

Since the early 1970s scientific research has consistently associated dietary factors with disease. In February 1977, the U.S. Senate Select Committee on Nutrition and Human Needs issued the **Dietary Goals for the United States** (15). The dietary recommendations were introduced with this statement: "The overconsumption of foods high in fat, generally, and saturated fat in particular, as well as cholesterol, refined and processed sugars, salt and/or alcohol has been associated with the development of one or more of six to ten leading causes of death: heart disease, some cancers, stroke and hypertension, diabetes, arteriosclerosis, and cirrhosis of the liver." The nutritional risk factors associated with the leading causes of death in the U.S. are shown in table 1.3.

Life-style has a significant impact on our immediate as well as long-term functioning, and nutrition is an integral component of our life-style. Following are the results of health-promotion efforts in the U.S. in the last twenty years.

The American Response: A Health Revolution

In 1979, *Healthy People:* The Surgeon General's Report on Health Promotion and Disease Prevention, was published to "encourage a second public health revolution in the history of the United States." (1). Because the first public health revolution against infectious disease was very successful (only two percent of U.S. people now die from infectious disease), efforts were focused on chronic diseases like heart disease, cancer, stroke, and diabetes, which account for more than 70 percent of all deaths in America (16) (see figure 1.1).

Healthy People called for both professionals and lay people to use available knowledge and skills to help reduce preventable death and disease in all age groups in our population by 1990. Measurable goals were established, and specific strategies to meet these goals were developed and implemented both in treatment and, more important, in prevention.

The Public Health Service identified nutrition as one of the fifteen areas of greatest importance for improving the health of the public (17). Recently, new nutrition objectives for the

In 1990, the U.S. Department of Health and Human Services published *Promoting Health/Preventing Disease: Year 2000 Objectives for the Nation.* The goals and objectives in this document, including 24 nutrition objectives, outline an agenda for action, a strategy for improving the health of the nation by the year 2000. These objectives were a continuation of the process started in 1980. Selected year 2000 nutrition objectives are summarized below.

1. Reduce overweight among people ages 20 through 74 to a prevalence of no more than 20 percent. (Baseline: 25.7 percent in 1976-1980.)

2. Increase to at least 50 percent the proportion of overweight people age 12 and older who have adopted sound dietary practices combined with physical activity to achieve weight reduction. (Baseline: 30 percent of overweight women and 25 percent of overweight men for people age 18 and older in 1985.)

3. Reduce average dietary fat intake to no more than 30 percent of calories and average saturated fat intake to no more than ten percent of calories among people age two and older. (Baseline: 36.4 percent of calories from total fat and 13.2 percent from saturated fat in 1985.)

4. Increase to at least 50 percent the proportion of people age 12 and older who consume at least three servings daily of foods rich in calcium. (Baseline: 20 percent in 1985-86.)

5. Increase average intake of dietary fiber and complex carbohydrates in the diets of adults to five or more daily servings for vegetables and fruits and to six or more daily servings for grain products and legumes to provide between 20 and 30 grams of daily dietary fiber. (Baseline: two and one-half servings of vegetables and fruits and three servings of grain products and legumes for women ages 19 through 50 in 1985; data on men available later. Approximately 10 grams of dietary fiber in 1987.)

6. Decrease salt and sodium intake so at least 65 percent of home meal preparers prepare foods without adding salt, at least 80 percent of people avoid using salt at the table, and at least 40 percent of adults regularly purchase foods modified or lower in sodium. (Baseline: 54 percent of women aged 19 through 50 who served as the main meal preparer did not use salt in food preparation, and 68 percent of women aged 19 through 50 did not use salt at the table in 1985; 20 percent of all people aged 18 and older regularly purchased foods with reduced salt and sodium content in 1988.)

7. Increase to at least 75 percent the proportion of mothers who exclusively or partially breastfeed their babies in the early postpartum period and to at least 50 percent the proportion who continue breastfeeding until their babies are five to six months old. (Baseline: 54.3 percent at discharge from birth site and 21.1 percent at five or six months in 1988.)

8. Achieve useful and informative nutrition labeling for virtually all processed foods and at least 40 percent of fresh meats, poultry, fish, fruits, vegetables, baked goods, and ready-to-eat carry away foods. (Baseline: 60 percent of sales of processed foods regulated by FDA had nutrition labeling in 1988; baseline data on fresh and carry-away foods unavailable.)

9. Increase to at least 95 percent the proportion of school lunch and breakfast services with menus that are consistent with the Dietary Guidelines for Americans. (Baseline data available later.)

10. Increase to at least 5,000 brand items the availability of processed food products that are reduced in fat, saturated fat, and cholesterol. (Baseline: 2,500 in 1986.)

11. Increase to at least 75 percent the proportion of the nation's schools that provide nutrition education from preschool through grade 12, preferably as part of comprehensive school health education. (Baseline: available later.)

year 2000 were developed, and they are described in table 1.4.

Since *Healthy People* was published, the second public health revolution has gained strength. Health professionals, hospitals, fitness centers, books, the media, and even the workplace have cooperated to advance the revolution. Let's take a look at the results of this nationwide effort thus far.

The National Center for Health Statistics reports that life expectancy at birth reached a new high of 74.7 years in 1984, an increase of 27.4 years since 1900 (16) (see figure 1.2). They also found that the age adjusted death rate for heart disease, the leading cause of death, decreased by 28 percent between 1970 and 1984 (see figure 1.3). During the same period the age adjusted death rate for stroke, the third leading cause of death in the U.S., decreased by 50 percent. These changes can be partly attributed to positive changes in the life-style of Americans.

The 1985 National Health Promotion and Disease Prevention study was designed to monitor progress toward the health objectives for 1990 (18). Its findings include the following.

55 percent of adults eat breakfast every day
55 percent of women and 42 percent of men consider their weight to be about right
44 percent of women and 25 percent of men are trying to lose weight
86 percent or higher are aware of the three major risk factors of heart disease
40 percent of the adults (43 percent male, 38 percent female) reported that they exercise or play sports regularly

This midcourse review of all fifteen areas and 226 objectives revealed that about half of all the objectives will be achieved by 1990 (19).

Life expectancy at birth, U.S. 1900–1985.

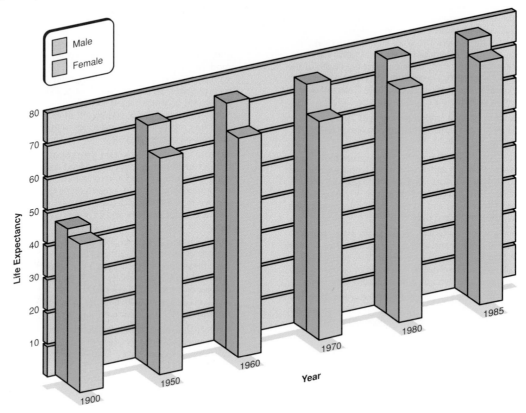

In the first National Survey of Worksite Health Promotion Activities, 66 percent of worksites reported that they had at least one health-promotion activity. Of the sites, 38 percent offer stress-management programs, 36 percent smoking-control programs, 32 percent fitness programs, 16.8 percent nutrition programs, 14.7 percent weight-control programs, and 20 percent off-the-job accident prevention (20).

Consumption studies have also indicated some positive trends in eating behaviors. The use of butter and lard has declined by 74 percent and 81 percent, respectively, since the beginning of the century. Egg use has also declined 28 percent since its peak in 1951. Red meat consumption has declined, and poultry and fish consumption have increased. Fresh fruit and vegetable consumption has also increased by 13 and 24 percent, respectively (21).

A recent survey of Americans showed that 51 to 55 percent watched their consumption of salt, sugar, and fat, and that 42 percent watched their intake of high-cholesterol foods (22).

The evidence suggests that another public health revolution is underway, but statistics indicate that much more remains to be done. Each of us is challenged to apply nutrition principles and behavior-change techniques to further this revolution and our own health.

The Individual Response

As individuals, we can do much to improve our health by establishing eating behaviors that are consistent with disease prevention and health promotion. We can begin to build a commitment to better nutrition for the health of our bodies by examining what influences our eating behaviors, deciding to take responsibility, and making a plan to succeed at desired changes in our eating behavior.

What Shapes Our Eating Behaviors

Before we can take a closer look at how to change our eating behaviors, we must direct our attention toward what shapes our eating behavior (see Health-Promotion Activity 1.1).

FIGURE 1.3
Trends in death rates from selected causes, U.S. 1900–1985.

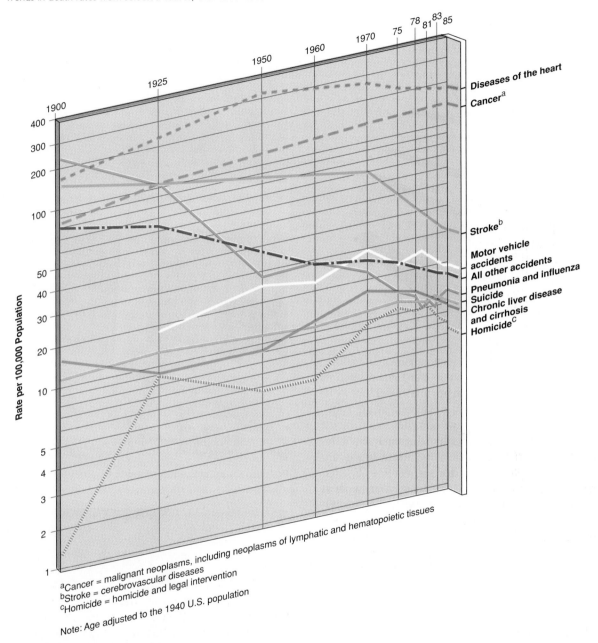

Diseases of the heart
Cancer[a]
Stroke[b]
Motor vehicle accidents
All other accidents
Pneumonia and influenza
Suicide
Chronic liver disease and cirrhosis
Homicide[c]

Rate per 100,000 Population

[a]Cancer = malignant neoplasms, including neoplasms of lymphatic and hematopoietic tissues
[a]Cancer = malignant neoplasms
[b]Stroke = cerebrovascular diseases
[c]Homicide = homicide and legal intervention

Note: Age adjusted to the 1940 U.S. population

Physiologic Influences

One of the reasons that we eat is to fulfill needs. Abraham Maslow depicted this in a triangular model known as the hierarchy of needs (23) (see figure 1.4). The bottom level of the triangle shows basic physiological needs. Certainly hunger is the signal that our body needs fuel for energy, growth, repair, and maintenance. The physiologic need varies with numerous factors such as age, sex, metabolic rate, health status,

level of physical activity, pregnancy, lactation, hormonal secretions, use of drugs, and disabilities. These factors may alter the number of Calories or the specific nutrients that are needed.

Psychological Influences

Foods can also fulfill psychological needs. Moods and emotions, for instance, can affect eating behaviors. Children are told that foods will make them feel better. Still wanting to feel

FIGURE 1.4

Maslow's hierarchy of human needs.

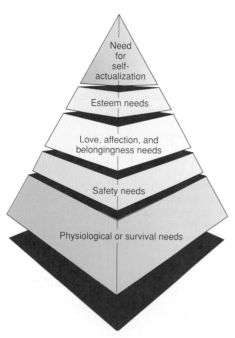

Need for self-actualization

Esteem needs

Love, affection, and belongingness needs

Safety needs

Physiological or survival needs

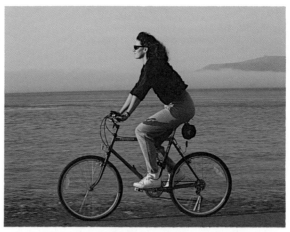

An active life-style increases the need for Calories.

better, adults eat to relieve tension, boredom, and depression. Food is also used as a reward in our society. Children who are quiet or well-behaved may be given a sweet-tasting food. Likewise, adults who have completed a difficult task may be rewarded with a dinner in their favorite restaurant. Additionally, some foods are eaten to fulfill the need for self-esteem. For example, we might order steak, lobster, or snails at restaurants to impress others with our knowledge, money, or good taste. Even serious eating disorders such as anorexia nervosa, bulimia, or obesity can develop from fulfilling psychological needs with the overindulgence or deprivation of food. Eating disorders will be discussed in chapter 9.

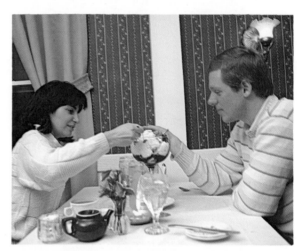

We often reward ourselves with food.

Environmental Influences

Various environmental influences affect our food choices, including exposure to food-related customs and traditions, ethnic factors, religious factors, parental and peer influence, and merchandising and marketing techniques.

Food-Related Customs and Traditions

Each person associates particular foods with customs and traditions. Thanksgiving dinner, for instance, may always include turkey. Christmas

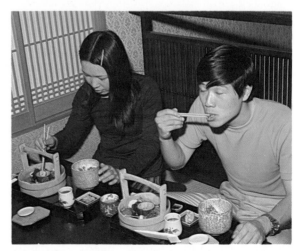

Culture influences our food habits.

dinner, on the other hand, may include turkey, ham, or goose. Birthdays, for some individuals, mean having cake, whereas others might expect pie. Breakfast on the weekends may always involve pancakes and fresh fruit. Food associations based on tradition or custom become integrated into our eating behaviors and are passed from one generation to the next.

Ethnic Factors

Ethnic background strongly shapes our eating behavior. For instance, beans and corn are often associated with Mexico, rice with Asia, tomato sauce and pasta with Italy, beef and potatoes with England, and pastry with France. Individual preferences often result from early exposure to these foods at home. Today, Americans can experience many different ethnic foods through cookbook recipes, international restaurants, food festivals, and friends from different ethnic backgrounds.

Religious Factors

Religious background may also influence what people eat. For instance, individuals who belong to the orthodox Jewish faith abstain from eating pork and shellfish, and members of the Seventh-day Adventist faith observe a vegetarian diet. Similarly, individuals of the Mormon faith do not drink caffeinated hot beverages.

Parental and Peer Influence

Until we leave home, our parents usually influence what we eat, when we eat, and how much we eat. Parents are not only responsible for our early exposure to foods but also for our psychological response to foods. This was discussed in a previous section of this chapter. During adolescence, peers become a powerful influence over our eating behavior. Whether we choose to bring a lunch from home or buy a lunch at school often depends on what our friends do. Certainly our alcohol consumption is directly related to that of our peers. Chapter 14 will further discuss the impact of peers on eating behavior.

Merchandising and Marketing Techniques

The food industry is highly competitive, and billions of dollars are spent each year to market new and old food products. Research may be done to see if a new food product is acceptable to consumers. As a product evolves, consumers test it for taste, smell, texture, and other sensory perceptions. Suggestions are then incorporated into

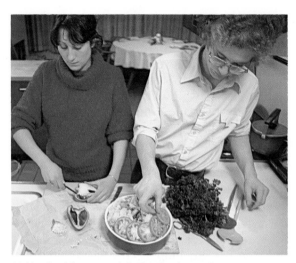
Making food from scratch is cheaper than eating out.

the development of the final product. Once the test market approves, packaging and marketing begin.

Advertising is a powerful tool to influence potential consumers. Consider these advertising budgets for 1986 (24):

Nabisco cookies: $38 million
Mars candy: $140 million
Coca-Cola: $152 million
McDonald's: $592 million

A large portion of the advertising budget for many products is devoted to television. This is not surprising, since the average American watches 25 hours of television per week. In supermarkets also, marketing strategies are at work in the placement and display of products. For example, children's cereals are always placed at their eye level.

Food Accessibility

Both the affordability and the availability of foods affect whether or not the public uses them. The price of food may limit our ability to purchase it. Buying items in the supermarket to make meals from scratch is usually cheaper than buying more convenient, prepackaged items, and eating out may cost between three and ten times as much as preparing the same meal at home. Even so, more than one in every three food dollars is spent eating out. As consumers we must constantly weigh the value of our time against the extra cost of convenience. Furthermore, convenience may also have nutritional costs to consider.

Although the American supermarket is still restricted by season changes, crop failures, and import problems, a tremendous variety of foods is available to us. This is mainly due to improvements in storage and preservation techniques, as well as transport methods. Unfortunately, the wide variety of nutritious foods in the supermarket is not always a reflection of the foods available to the family in its own refrigerator and cupboards.

Food Characteristics

For one reason or another we all have our favorite foods. They appeal to our senses: taste, color, texture, temperature, appearance, flavor, and aroma. A green apple that has a sour taste, cool temperature, and crisp texture may appeal to one person, whereas another might prefer a red apple with a warm temperature, sweet taste, and soft texture.

Changing Your Eating Habits

Self-Responsibility

The last section discussed the fact that many personal and social factors influence our eating behavior. Although these factors must be taken into consideration when we attempt to change our eating behavior, commitment is based first on making ourselves accountable for our food choices. Many times we convince ourselves and others that someone or something beyond our control makes us act the way we do. For example, one student who had a dorm room and food-service contract said that he was gaining weight because most of the cafeteria food was fried. A woman reported that although she wanted to eat lower-fat meals, her family would rebel against any change. She felt defeated before she tried food changes. Although there is no question that these are difficult situations, each of us can take control of what we eat.

A major step in taking responsibility for ourselves is to realize we make choices that have an impact on our physical, mental, social, and spiritual well-being. If you are not moving toward your nutritional goals, you have the power, the right, and the responsibility to choose differently. Realizing that you have a choice can help you plan your strategy for change.

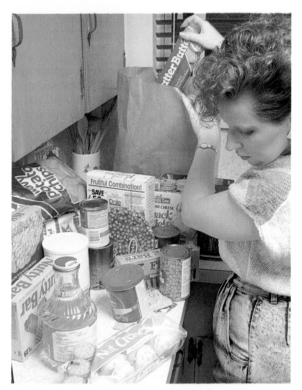
Check for nutritious food selections before you get the grocery bags home.

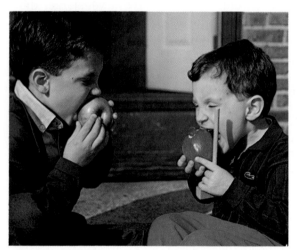
Food characteristics like color, texture, and temperature influence our food choices.

Determinants of Health Behavior

Many studies have been conducted to determine why we do what we do and how to change unhealthy behaviors. One current model of health behavior suggests three major determinants of health behavior: predisposing, enabling, and reinforcing factors (25) (see figure 1.5).

FIGURE 1.5

Three determinants of health behavior. *Note:* Solid lines imply contributing influence, and dotted lines imply secondary effects. Numerals indicate the approximate order in which the actions usually occur.

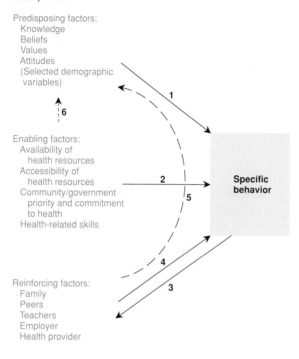

Predisposing Factors

The impetus to change occurs when the predisposing factors underlying a particular health behavior are challenged. These factors include knowledge, beliefs, attitudes, habits, and values. They can be based on accurate information or unreliable sources. Misinformation soon becomes so entangled with the facts that it is difficult to separate them. New information also needs to be incorporated into the existing pool of knowledge so behavior can be adjusted.

Traditionally, health education emphasized knowledge as the key to changing people's eating behavior. Many of us know that eating breakfast is important, and yet we skip it. Most of us know that various types of chips are high in both salt and fat, but we still eat them several times per week. Knowledge is a necessary foundation for change, but is not sufficient by itself (25). Other motivating factors must be stirred in order to move a person to action. One way to motivate is to use a decision-making approach that challenges individuals to examine at least one of the predisposing factors. This approach will be discussed in the next section.

Enabling Factors

Enabling factors are the resources and skills necessary to adopt a change. Resources that support healthy eating habits are becoming more available and may include cookbooks, professionals, special foods, and cooking classes.

Reinforcing Factors

Many people are successful at changing behavior for a while but slowly slide back into old habits. Reinforcing factors are particularly important in maintaining healthy eating behaviors. Parents, family, friends, co-workers, and employers all give us both negative and positive feedback on our efforts to change. We differ in how much support and encouragement we need, and it will vary with circumstances.

All three of the determinants of health work together to help us change our eating behaviors. Predisposing factors give us the motivation to take a closer look at ourselves and evaluate whether we need to change. Enabling factors aid us in making changes by providing the necessary resources and skills. However, after behavior changes have occurred, the hard part begins—maintenance. Reinforcing factors play an important role in this phase, providing positive feedback from friends, family, and employers, as well as monetary incentives and other rewards (see Health-Promotion Activity 1.3).

A Decision-Making Process

Consider the following messages: *Take vitamins. All the nutrients are in a well-balanced diet. Fast foods are convenient. Fast foods are high in fat and salt. Eat more fruit and vegetables. Eat less snack food. Drink your milk. Whole milk is high in fat. Potatoes cause you to gain weight. Potatoes are high in protein.* We receive conflicting messages about nutrition from many different sources. This chapter has already examined the impact that physiologic, psychological, and environmental influences have on our eating behavior. How can we decipher the messages about food selection? By using the same decision-making process that you would apply when purchasing a new car or selecting an apartment. Good decisions are always conscious and deliberate.

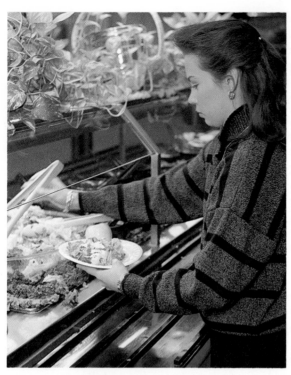
Each person must decide to select nutritious foods.

There are several steps in the decision-making process.

1. Defining the problem, and setting goals and objectives
2. Weighing the cost and benefits of the goals and determining if they are realistic
3. Choosing a plan of action
4. Taking action
5. Prizing the action
6. Reevaluation

Let's look at each step in more detail.

Step 1: Nutritional goals have been set for the American public and are described in detail in chapter 2. These goals, along with a record of food intake, can help individuals identify the problem areas in their eating behavior. In most cases, a plan of action can be developed by consulting a registered dietitian and chapters in this book.

Step 2: Are the goals and objectives realistic, and are they measurable? Small goals that address one area at a time have the greatest likelihood for success. Specific statements that include the number of teaspoons, cups, and/or times per week will allow for comparison when measuring progress.

Step 3: Choosing a plan of action in order to accomplish goals has already begun with steps one and two. Now various chapters in this book that apply will help you in being specific. While establishing the plan, incorporate reinforcing factors. These factors will be built-in motivators to keep you going during difficult periods.

Step 4: Start the plan as soon as possible, and do your best to maintain your specific goals. Flexibility in scheduling is important, however, as well as a willingness to resume the program if you have a setback. It is important to realize that the program could be difficult, but try to stay on it at least 80 percent of the time.

Step 5: Prizing the action involves not only being happy and satisfied with the decision to change but being willing to tell others about your goals. This helps others to be supportive and encourage your efforts. Positive thinking will also give you confidence.

Step 6: Reevaluating the initial plan is necessary for several reasons. Have you succeeded with your goals, and how will you continue? Does the plan need to be adjusted? Are you satisfied with the plan and the results? Can you stick with it? Do you wish to do more? How do these changes affect your health? Do you feel better? What will continue to motivate you? These are some of the answers to seek when evaluating the outcome of decisions.

Certainly the decision-making process must be evaluated, but allow a reasonable length of time to accomplish goals. Many nutritional goals and guidelines today are based on the prevention of disease or on health promotion. Health benefits may not be realized for twenty years. Healthy eating, though, can affect how you feel and behave today. Don't forget to assess such variables as energy level, performance, bowel habits, attention span, and irritability level. Whether or not one makes a permanent behavior change depends most on his or her level of motivation. When evaluating your plan, focus not only on the goal but on the process, making every effort to increase the internal and external motivation to succeed.

SUMMARY

1. Today the leading causes of death in the United States are chronic diseases. Heart disease is the leading killer of adults, followed by cancer and stroke. Although these diseases have many causes, life-style is a major contributing factor.
2. Health promotion is the science and art that helps people change their life-style to move toward optimal health.
3. There is increasing evidence that life-style, particularly nutrition, is associated with the leading causes of death. Since nutritional risk factors for the chronic diseases have been identified, individuals have tremendous potential to prevent disease and promote their own health.
4. In response to the dramatic rise in chronic diseases in the U.S. since 1900, the Public Health Service established nutrition as one of fifteen areas of greatest importance for improving the health of the public. Several objectives were established and implemented for improved nutrition in the U.S. by 1990.
5. Considerable progress has been made toward the 1990 health objectives in each of the fifteen identified areas, including nutrition. A midcourse review reports that half of all objectives will be met by 1990. Still there is much work to be done.
6. Our food habits are shaped by numerous factors: physiologic, psychologic, environmental, food accessibility, and food characteristics. Determining which factors influence our eating behavior can help us change.
7. The three major determinants of health behavior are predisposing, enabling, and reinforcing factors. Predisposing factors help motivate people and include knowledge, beliefs, attitudes, habits, and values. Enabling factors are the resources and skills that are necessary to adopt a change. Reinforcing factors give an individual the support and encouragement needed to maintain new health behaviors.
8. The decision-making process should be used in determining food selections that are consistent with optimal health. The six steps in decision making are defining the problem, setting realistic goals and objectives, choosing a plan of action, taking action, prizing the action, and reevaluation.

REFERENCES

1. Office of the Assistant Secretary for Health and Surgeon General.1979. *Healthy People:* The Surgeon General's Report on Health Promotion and Disease Prevention. DHEW (PHS) Publication No. 79-55071. Washington, D.C.: U.S. Government Printing Office.
2. American Heart Association. 1987 Heart Facts. Dallas: American Heart Association.
3. American Cancer Society. 1985 Cancer Facts and Figures. New York: American Cancer Society.
4. Doll, R., and R. Peto. 1981. *The Causes of Cancer: Quantitative Estimates of Avoidable Risks of Cancer in the U.S. Today.* New York: Oxford University Press.
5. National Diabetes Advisory Board. 1980. The Treatment and Control of Diabetes: A National Plan to Reduce Mortality and Morbidity. NIH Publication No. 81-2284.
6. Anderson, L. A., et al. 1982. *Nutrition in Health and Disease.* Philadelphia: J. B. Lippincott Co.
7. Anderson, J. W., Gustafson, N. J., Tietyen-Clark, J. 1987. Dietary Fiber and Diabetes: A Comprehensive Review and Practical Application. *Journal of the American Dietetic Association* 87(9):1189-97.
8. West, M. W. 1983. "Diabetes Mellitus." In *Nutritional Support of Medical Practice,* H. A. Schneider, C. E. Anderson, and D. B. Coursin, eds. Philadelphia: Harper & Row Publishers, Inc.
9. Wong, F. L., and F. L. Trowbridge. 1984. Nutrition Surveys and Surveillance: Their Application to Clinical Practice. *Clinical Nutrition* 3:94-99.
10. National Institutes of Health. Consensus Development Conference Statement. 1985. *Health Implications of Obesity.* February: 11-13.
11. Division of Mental Health and Behavioral Medicine, Institute of Medicine. 1982. *Health and Behavior: Frontiers of Research in the Biobehavioral Sciences,* by D. A. Hamburg, G. R. Elliott, and D. L. Parron. Washington, D.C.: National Academy Press.
12. World Health Organization. 1947. Constitution of the World Health Organization. Chronicle of the World Health Organization 1: 29-43.
13. Dever, A. 1980. *Community Health Analysis: A Holistic Approach.* Rockville, MD: Aspen Systems Corporation.
14. O'Donnell, M. R. 1986. Definition of Health Promotion. Part II: Levels of Programs. *American Journal of Health Promotion* 1 (2):6-9.
15. U.S. Senate Select Committee on Nutrition and Human Needs. 1977. *Dietary Goals for the United States.* Stock No. 052-070-04376-8. Washington, D.C.: U.S. Government Printing Office.
16. National Center for Health Statistics. 1986. Health, United States, 1986. DHHS (PHS) Publication No. 87-1232. Washington, D.C.: U.S. Government Printing Office.
17. Department of Health and Human Services. 1980. Promoting Health and Preventing Disease: Objectives for the Nation. Washington, D.C.: U.S. Government Printing Office.
18. Department of Health and Human Services, Public Health Service. 1986. Health Promotion Data for the 1990 Objectives: Estimates from the National Health Interview Survey of Health Promotion and Disease Prevention: United States, 1985, by O. T. Thornberry, R. W. Wilson, and P. M. Golden. NCHS Advancedata, Number 126, September 19.

19. U.S. Department of Health and Human Services. Office of Disease Prevention and Health Promotion, Public Health Service. 1986. The 1990 Health Objectives for the Nation: A Midcourse Review. Washington, D.C.: U.S. Government Printing Office.

20. Windom, R. E., J. M. McGinnius, and J. E. Fielding. 1987. Examining Worksite Health Promotion. *Business and Health.* (July): 36–37.

21. U.S. Department of Agriculture, Human Nutrition Information Service. 1985. Nationwide Food Consumption Survey, Continuing Survey of Food Intakes by Individuals: Women 19–50 Years and Their Children 1–5 Years, 1 Day, 1985. U.S. Department of Agriculture, Rept. 85–1. Men 19–50 Years, 1 Day, 1985. U.S. Department of Agriculture, Rept. 85–3.

22. *USA Today.* May 3, 1984.

23. Maslow, Abraham, H. 1968. *Toward a Psychology of Being.* Princeton: Van Nostrand.

24. Liebman, B. 1988. The All-American Junk Food Diet. *Nutrition Action HealthLetter.* (May): 8.

25. Greene, Lawrence, et al. 1980. *Health Education Planning: A Diagnostic Approach.* Palo Alto, CA: Mayfield Publishing Company.

HEALTH-PROMOTION ACTIVITY 1.1
Why Do You Eat?

The following is a list of factors that affect the dietary practices and patterns of individuals. Determine how much each factor influences your eating behaviors by rating these factors as 3 (very important), 2 (somewhat important), 1 (seldom important), and 0 (never important).

Physiologic Influences

1. Weight   _____
2. Physical activity level   _____
3. Pregnancy/lactation   _____
4. Health   _____
5. Hunger   _____

Psychological Influences

1. Safety/security   _____
2. Tension   _____
3. Boredom   _____
4. Depression   _____
5. Other moods or emotions   _____
6. Holidays   _____
7. Special events   _____

Environmental Influences

1. Customs/traditions   _____
2. Ethnic background   _____
3. Family   _____
4. Peers   _____

5. Advertisements   _____
6. Television/radio   _____
7. Beliefs   _____

Food Accessibility

1. Food costs   _____
2. Food availability   _____
3. Convenience   _____
4. Time   _____

Which of the factors affecting your dietary practices scored more than 1?

Are you satisfied with the factors that you use to help you make decisions about what to eat? If not, try the decision-making process.

HEALTH-PROMOTION ACTIVITY 1.2
Nutrition Sources

Look through your cupboards, pantry, and refrigerator. Do you purchase any foods that you believe have special health benefits? List these foods in the left-hand column, and indicate what you hope they will do in the right-hand column.

Foods or Drink	Beliefs of Health Benefit
_____	_____
_____	_____
_____	_____
_____	_____
_____	_____

Circle the sources of information that you use to form your beliefs about food.

parents   local agencies (e.g., American
trainers   Heart Association)
nutrition courses   friends
popular magazines   teachers
health food stores   health courses
coaches   professional journals
health professionals   government bulletins
                       newscasters

Compare the sources you currently use with the list of reliable sources of nutrition information that are found in appendix E. Are you using the best sources? List one source that is unfamiliar to you that you will investigate in the next month.

HEALTH-PROMOTION ACTIVITY 1.3
A Health-Promotion Contract

How healthy will you be one year from today? What changes do you need to make in your dietary habits in order to maintain or improve your present health? In order to achieve a goal, the plan must be conscious and deliberate. The following contract will get you started.

Goals

I will accomplish the following goals by _____ .

Objectives

The following are the specific steps I will take to accomplish the above goals. I will record my progress in a daily journal, which will be used to judge the success of my project.

Plan of Action

This is how I plan to carry out the above objectives on a day-to-day basis.

Enabling Factors

These are the up-to-date, professional sources that I am using as guidelines in developing my objectives and plans. I am including the specific chapter and page numbers in this book. I will also include teachers, health professionals, cookbooks, supermarkets, and health agencies that will help me to accomplish my goals and objectives.

Reinforcing Factors

I will reward myself in the following ways.

I will enlist the following people or groups for support.

_____ _____
My signature   Supporter's signature

This is an initial commitment to change. However, goals and objectives may be modified as your understanding increases.

2

U.S. Dietary Trends and Guidelines

INTRODUCTION

Open nearly any magazine or newspaper today and you will be sure to find at least one article on nutrition. Public interest in nutrition and fitness is at an all-time high. Has this interest, however, translated into improved eating practices by Americans? This chapter will review trends in the American diet from the beginning of this century to the present.

Beginning in 1977, several health agencies of the government and public sectors published dietary guidelines for Americans in response to American dietary trends from 1910 to the 1970s. Concern was expressed over the increasing use of animal fats and the decreasing use of carbohydrate from grains, fruits, and vegetables. The current dietary guidelines will be reviewed in this chapter.

The American food supply is the most abundant, safe, and varied in the world (1). Furthermore, Americans have access to this treasurehouse at a comparatively low cost. The average American spends only fifteen percent of disposable income on food. Two-thirds of this is spent on food eaten at home, and about one-third on food eaten away from home.

In spite of easy access to this bountiful supply of food, Americans have many concerns about their diets. Nutritional factors have been associated with six of the ten leading causes of death in the United States: high blood pressure, coronary heart disease, cancer, cardiovascular disease, chronic liver disease, and non-insulin-dependent diabetes mellitus (2). Public in-

terest in nutrition is at an all-time high, and magazines, newspapers, television, and radio have deluged Americans with detailed information on nutrition and health.

Have Americans responded to the media blitz with improved dietary practices? This chapter will review trends in the American diet from the beginning of this century to the present and will summarize nutrition recommendations from various health organizations. In general, we will discover that despite all the attention and talk, the majority of Americans are not presently consuming "prudent" or recommended diets. However, a growing number are making some improvements in the quality of their diets.

*F*IGURE 2.1

During this century, carbohydrate consumption has fallen, whereas use of fat has increased.

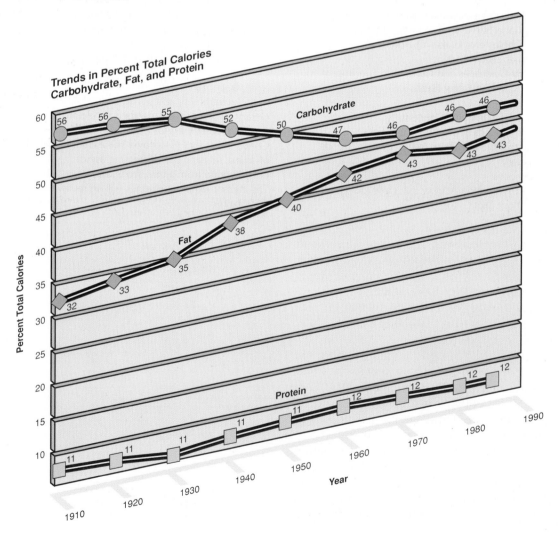

Surveys That Measure What Americans Eat

National food-consumption surveys such as the 1977–78 **Nationwide Food Consumption Survey** (NFCS) from the United States Department of Agriculture (USDA) and the second **National Health and Nutrition Examination Survey** (NHANES II) from the National Center for Health Statistics provide a wealth of information about dietary patterns and practices of representative samples of the U.S. population (3). The **Economic Research Service** of the USDA also supplies "food disappearance" data (quantities of 350 foods that "disappear" into the food distribution system). Other studies providing information on food and nutrient intake include the **Lipid Research Center Program** of the National Heart, Lung, and Blood Institute (NHLBI) of the National Institutes of Health; the **Total Diet Study** of the Food and Drug Administration (FDA); and a long-term dietary study of adults that is conducted by the USDA. Some of these surveys will be discussed in more detail in chapter 3. In this chapter, results from these surveys will be summarized.

U.S. Dietary Trends Since the Turn of the Century

The Economic Research Service food disappearance data reveal several important trends regarding intake of **carbohydrate, fat,** and **protein** during this century (4,5). In the national food supply, carbohydrate during the mid-1980s contributed 46 percent, fat 43 percent, and protein 12 percent of the total Caloric intake, whereas in 1910 the comparable percentages were 56 percent, 32 percent, and 12 percent, respectively (see figure 2.1). As we shall see later in this chapter, the 1910 figures are much closer to the recommended levels.

The decline in carbohydrate as noted in figure 2.1 is due to a decrease in **starch**—from 39 percent in 1909 to 22 percent in 1982 (see figure 2.2). In chapter 5, carbohydrate will be discussed in more detail. Starches are predominantly found in grains, legumes, fruits, and vegetables. In contrast to the decline in starch intake, the percent of Calories provided by processed **sweeteners** (sugar in soft drinks, for example), and also **sugars** occurring naturally in foods (such as in milk and fruits), has increased

from 17 percent to 24 percent. With the decline in starch and increase in processed sweeteners has come a decline in the fiber content of the U.S. diet, measured recently at only 11 grams/day instead of the 25–35 grams/day recommended by the National Cancer Institute (6).

Sweeteners

Much of the increase in use of added sweeteners comes from the tremendous explosion in use of soft drinks. Soft drinks are the number-one source of sugar in the American diet and the number-one beverage used in the United States (see chapter 12). During the mid-1980s, Americans consumed an average of 486 cans of soda pop per person per year, double that of 1970. More than 50 percent of the U.S. population consumes carbonated soft drinks. Children 5–12 years of age average 5.6–7.7 fluid ounces/day of regular soda; adolescents 13–18 years of age, 8.6–12.6 fluid ounces/day; and adults 19–44 years of age, 8.1–13.0 fluid ounces/day (7). (Note: 8 fluid ounces equals one cup, and one can of soda pop has 12 fluid ounces.)

Since 1975, the U.S. per capita consumption of sweeteners has risen sharply, due mainly to the increased use of **high fructose corn syrup.** This is a special sugar that is commercially produced from cornstarch. Certain enzymes are used to convert the starch into

F**IGURE 2.2**

Use of starch has fallen steeply during this century, whereas sugar consumption has increased.

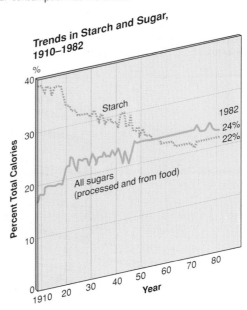

fructose. The high fructose corn syrup (HFCS) can be used in slightly smaller amounts to produce the same sweetness as sugar, and it costs less (8). For every 56-pound bushel of corn, 33 pounds of HFCS can be produced. Most soft-drink companies now use HFCS as the major sweetener in soft drinks. In 1983, the per capita consumption of HFCS was 31 pounds per person, versus just five pounds per person in 1975. Table 2.1 outlines the growing use of sweeteners by Americans, especially in the form of HFCS. Most people are unaware that their sweetener consumption in so high because sugar is "hidden" in so many foods (see chapter 5).

Trends in Food Consumption

Figure 2.3 highlights the percent changes in Calories, fat, carbohydrate, and protein since 1910. The level of fat in the American diet has increased 25 percent, while the content of carbohyrate has decreased 21 percent. Calorie and protein levels have changed little. What food-selection changes by Americans are responsible for these trends?

Figures 2.4 through 2.10 summarize the major changes in individual food groups from 1910–1970 and 1985 (4,5).

1. Figure 2.4 shows that between 1910 and 1985, use of poultry climbed dramatically. In fact, per capita consumption of turkey and chicken now approaches that of beef:

70.1 versus 79.2 pounds per person per year, respectively. Beef consumption peaked in 1975, and then fell six percent during the next decade. Use of pork has remained somewhat stable throughout the century. Fish consumption, however, has increased nearly 23 percent between 1970 and 1985.

2. Use of dairy products decreased nearly 26 percent between 1910 and 1970 (see figure 2.5). This decrease is largely explained by the drop in consumption of fluid milk (mainly whole milk) and cream. However, with the increase in use of cheese, low-fat milk, and yogurt, dairy-product consumption is showing a slight rebound. Cheese consumption has risen from 4.3 to 22.4 pounds per person per year. Use of ice cream has jumped from 7.6 pounds per person per year in 1920 to 18.0 pounds per person per year in 1985.

TABLE 2.1
Per capita U.S. consumption of sweeteners

Year	Pounds/Person	Percent Sucrose	Percent HFCS*
1975	124.2	72%	4%
1983	132.9	53%	23%
1992	148.0	42%	31%

* HFCS = high fructose corn syrup

From E. Zamula, "Basic to Our Food Chain is Plain Old Field Corn." *FDA Consumer*, November 1984, pp. 24–27.

FIGURE 2.3
Calories and protein consumption have changed little during this century, whereas use of carbohydrate has decreased and fat has increased.

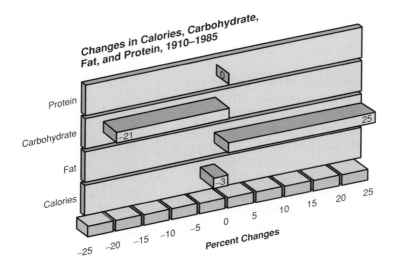

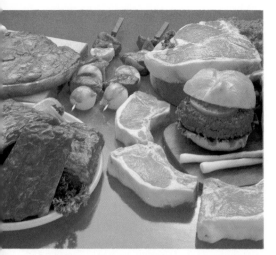

FIGURE 2.4

Use of poultry has climbed dramatically since the turn of the century; beef consumption is falling.

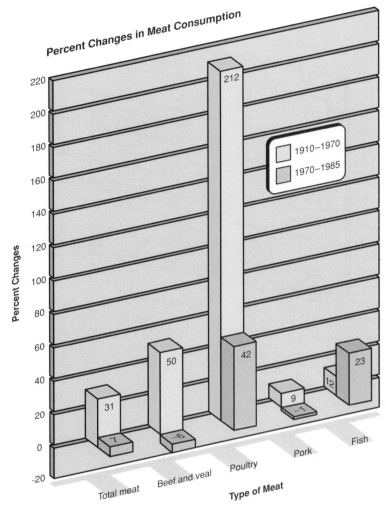

Percent Changes in Meat Consumption

Legend: 1910–1970, 1970–1985

(Total meat: 31, 7; Beef and veal: 50, -6; Poultry: 212, 42; Pork: 9, -1; Fish: 12, 23)

Y-axis: Percent Changes (-20 to 220)
X-axis: Type of Meat

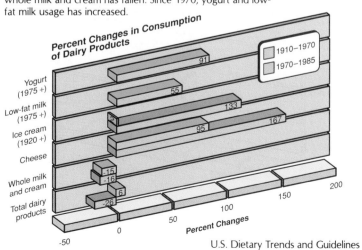

FIGURE 2.5

Use of dairy products has decreased, primarily because use of whole milk and cream has fallen. Since 1970, yogurt and low-fat milk usage has increased.

Percent Changes in Consumption of Dairy Products

Legend: 1910–1970, 1970–1985

Yogurt (1975 +): 91
Low-fat milk (1975 +): 55
Ice cream (1920 +): 133, 167
Cheese: 2, 95
Whole milk and cream: -15, -16
Total dairy products: 6, -26

X-axis: Percent Changes (-50 to 200)

FIGURE 2.6

After falling 41 percent between 1910 and 1970, use of fresh fruit is now climbing.

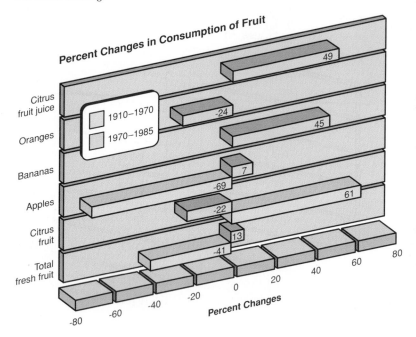

Percent Changes in Consumption of Fruit

Legend:
- 1910–1970
- 1970–1985

- Citrus fruit juice: 49
- Oranges: -24, 45
- Bananas: 7
- Apples: -69, 61
- Citrus fruit: -22, 13
- Total fresh fruit: -41

Percent Changes (axis: -80, -60, -40, -20, 0, 20, 40, 60, 80)

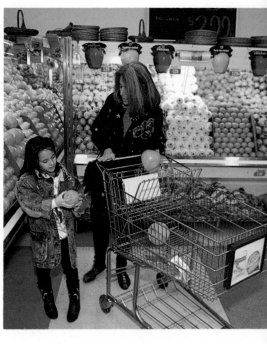

FIGURE 2.7

Use of total fresh vegetables has shown a strong increase since 1970.

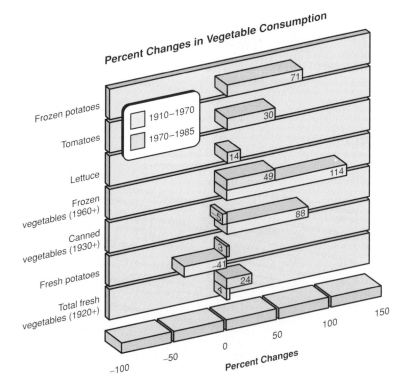

Percent Changes in Vegetable Consumption

Legend:
- 1910–1970
- 1970–1985

- Frozen potatoes: 71
- Tomatoes: 30
- Lettuce: 14
- Frozen vegetables (1960+): 49, 114
- Canned vegetables (1930+): 5, 88
- Fresh potatoes: 3, -41
- Total fresh vegetables (1920+): 4, 24

Percent Changes (axis: -100, -50, 0, 50, 100, 150)

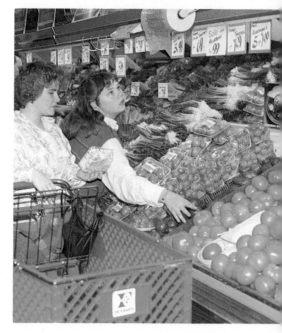

After showing a strong decrease from 1910 to 1970, use of grain products is now increasing.

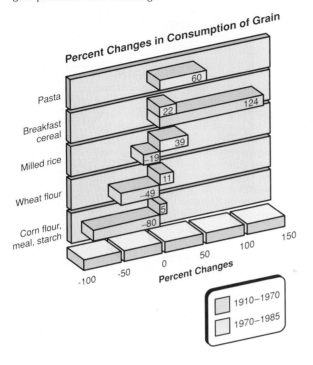

Percent Changes in Consumption of Grain

- Pasta: 60
- Breakfast cereal: 22, 124
- Milled rice: -19, 39
- Wheat flour: -49, 11
- Corn flour, meal, starch: -80, -5

Percent Changes: -100, -50, 0, 50, 100, 150

- 1910–1970
- 1970–1985

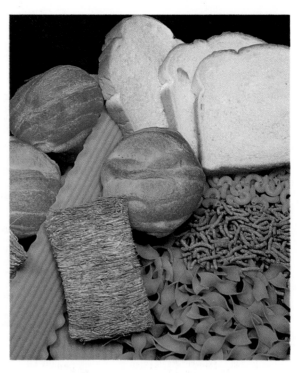

3. Figure 2.6 shows that after falling 41 percent between 1910 and 1970, use of fresh fruit is now climbing. Consumption of apples parallels this pattern and is supported by a strong increase in use of bananas, now America's favorite fruit (26 pounds per person per year in contrast to 17.4 and 12 pounds per person per year for apples and oranges, respectively). Use of citrus juice has jumped nearly 50 percent since 1950, while use of fresh citrus fruit has dropped 22 percent.

4. Use of total fresh vegetables (excluding potatoes) has shown a strong increase since 1970 (see figure 2.7). Fresh potato consumption fell 41 percent between 1910 and 1970 but is now showing a slight increase. Use of frozen potatoes (primarily due to the fast-food industry) has increased 71 percent since 1970. Use of all frozen vegetables has climbed steadily throughout the century, while use of canned vegetables is now decreasing after a strong early increase. After fresh potatoes (120 pounds per person per year), use of lettuce (23.7 pounds per person per year) and tomatoes (13.4 pounds per person per year) ranks at the top of America's vegetable menu.

5. One of the more significant changes in the food supply has been the decline in use of grain products (see figure 2.8). Between 1910 and 1970, use of corn, wheat, and rice decreased sharply. Use of wheat flour and corn products, for example, decreased 49 percent and 80 percent, respectively, during this time period. All grain products are now showing strong increases in consumption.

6. Total fat consumption is now at its highest level, up nearly 40 percent since 1940 (see figure 2.9). However, use of two primary animal fats, lard and butter, dropped dramatically between 1910 and 1985, 86 percent and 73 percent, respectively. Use of plant oils is up sharply, led by margarine at 575 percent (1910 to 1985). Use of shortening has doubled since 1920, and consumption of salad and cooking oil is up 38 percent since 1970.

FIGURE 2.9

Total fat consumption continues to climb, led by plant oils; use of animal fats is falling.

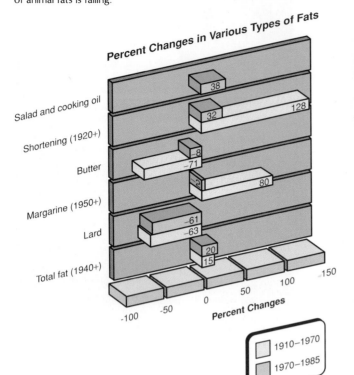

Percent Changes in Various Types of Fats

- Salad and cooking oil: 38
- Shortening (1920+): 32, 128
- Butter: −8, −71
- Margarine (1950+): −2, 80
- Lard: −61, −63
- Total fat (1940+): 20, 15

Percent Changes: −100, −50, 0, 50, 100, 150

1910–1970
1970–1985

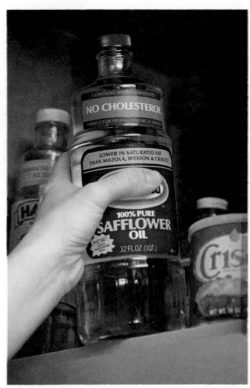

FIGURE 2.10

Refined sugar is being replaced with corn and noncaloric sweeteners. Use of eggs and coffee is falling.

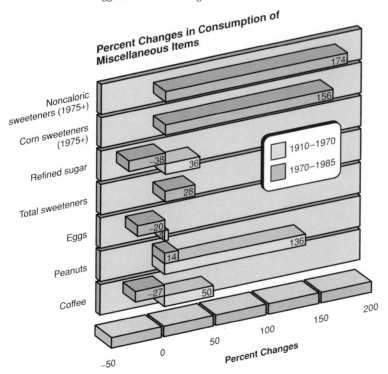

Percent Changes in Consumption of Miscellaneous Items

- Noncaloric sweeteners (1975+): 174
- Corn sweeteners (1975+): 156
- Refined sugar: −38, 36
- Total sweeteners: 28
- Eggs: −20
- Peanuts: 14, 136
- Coffee: −27, 50

1910–1970
1970–1985

Percent Changes: −50, 0, 50, 100, 150, 200

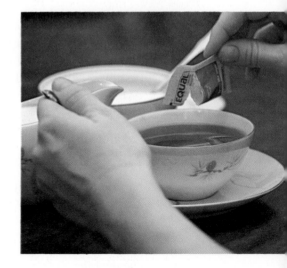

7. Sugar consumption, as already stated, has risen to an all-time high. Although total sweetener intake has increased 28 percent since 1970, use of refined sugar intake has been largely replaced by corn and noncaloric sweeteners (see figure 2.10). Egg usage, after holding steady during the first part of this century, has fallen 20 percent since 1970. Coffee usage, after rising 50 percent between 1910 and 1970, has also fallen (28 percent) since 1970 (see chapter 12).

Table 2.2 outlines the animal and vegetable sources of protein and fat in the U.S. food supply (9). Vegetable sources account for the increase in fat in the food supply, mainly because of greater use of cooking and salad oils and the shift from butter and lard to margarine and shortening. Although the amount of total protein has remained quite stable over the last century, the source of protein has changed considerably. In 1980, animal products provided more than two-thirds of the total protein; in 1909–13, animal and vegetable products contributed about equal amounts of protein. Most of this change can be attributed to increased use of meat, poultry, and fish and to decreased use of grain products.

Trends in Vitamins and Minerals

Despite the lower amounts of carbohydrate and higher amounts of fats being consumed by Americans, the levels of most vitamins and minerals in the food supply were higher in 1980 than in 1909–13 (9). The major factors contributing to this increase were the year-round availability of a great variety of foods and the general acceptance of enriched and fortified foods. Large increases occurred in the levels of niacin, thiamin, and riboflavin in the food supply, along with smaller increases in vitamin C, iron, vitamin B_{12}, calcium, and vitamin A. The levels of phosphorus and zinc were almost unchanged, whereas the levels of vitamin B_6 and magnesium decreased.

Information from national diet surveys show that intakes of protein; vitamins B_{12}, C, and A; thiamin; riboflavin; niacin; and phosphorus are adequate for all age and sex categories (10). Nutrient intakes less than 80 percent of the Recommended Dietary Allowances (RDA) include zinc, copper, manganese, vitamin B_6, iron, magnesium, and calcium. These low intakes were

TABLE 2.2
Types of protein and fat in the U.S. food supply

Year	Protein		Fat	
	Animal	Vegetable	Animal	Vegetable
1910	52%	48%	83%	17%
1950	64%	36%	75%	25%
1980	68%	32%	58%	42%

Data from U.S. Department of Agriculture, Economic Research Service.

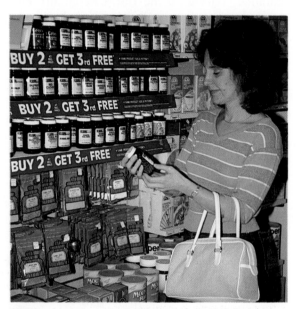

Millions of Americans are regular users of vitamin/mineral supplements.

found mainly in women. Individuals whose diets are most apt to be deficient are young children, teenage girls, women of childbearing age, and the elderly. These issues will be explained in greater detail in chapters 14 and 15.

Despite the fact that most reputable nutritionists state that one will rarely need to take vitamin or mineral supplements if a variety of wholesome foods is consumed, millions of Americans are regular users of **food supplements.** According to a survey conducted by the Food and Drug Administration, 40 percent of adult Americans take some kind of vitamin/mineral supplement (11). Use of supplements is even higher in certain segments of the population. For example, two-thirds of adults in Western states use supplements, with 40 percent consuming one to three supplements per day. A study on elderly people living in a Southern California retirement center showed that 72 percent used supplements (67 percent used vitamin

C pills daily). The most frequently cited reasons for using supplements are "to prevent colds and other illnesses" and "to make up for what is not in food." The three most frequently used food supplements are multiple vitamins, vitamin C, and multiple vitamin plus iron (see chapter 10).

National Surveys on Calorie, Fat, and Cholesterol Intakes of Americans

Figures 2.1 through 2.10 provide "food disappearance" data from the USDA Economic Research Service. As we will discuss in chapter 3, these data are useful for demonstrating changes from year to year, but they tend to overestimate the actual amount of food Americans eat.

Table 2.3 summarizes the information from a number of national studies that have evaluated the precise number of Calories consumed by Americans (12,13,14,15). The total average energy intake, depending on the national study, ranges from 2,300–2,600 Calories per day for men, and 1,500–1,750 Calories per day for

TABLE 2.3
Calories and fat in the American diet

Population Studied	Name of Study	Kcal	Fat
Men 35–59 yrs	LRCP*	2,600	40%
Women 35–59 yrs		1,750	39%
Men 35–57 yrs	MRFIT†	2,500	38%
Men 18–75 yrs	NHANES‡	2,400	37%
Women 18–75 yrs		1,600	37%
Men 19–64 yrs	NFCS§	2,300	42%
Women 19–64 yrs		1,500	41%
Men 19–50 yrs	CSFII‖	2,560	36%
Women 19–50 yrs		1,588	37%

*Lipid Research Clinics Program (1972–1975)
†Multiple Risk Factor Intervention Trial (1973–1975)
‡National Health and Nutrition Examination Survey (1976–1980)
§Nationwide Food Consumption Survey (1977–1978)
‖Nationwide Food Consumption Survey, Continuing Survey of Food Intakes by Individuals (1985)

Data from U.S. Department of Agriculture, Economic Research Service.

FIGURE 2.11
The most frequently consumed foods in America are low in fiber and high in salt, sugar, and fat.

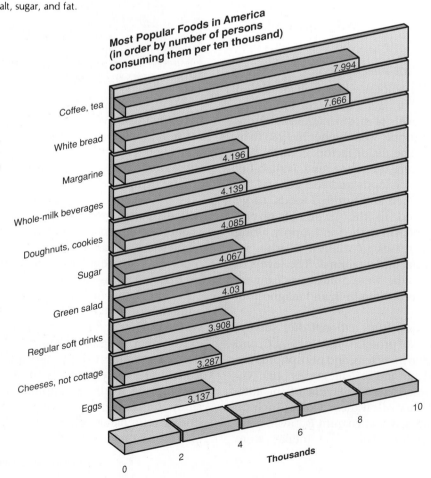

Most Popular Foods in America
(in order by number of persons consuming them per ten thousand)

Food	Thousands
Coffee, tea	7.994
White bread	7.666
Margarine	4.196
Whole-milk beverages	4.139
Doughnuts, cookies	4.085
Sugar	4.067
Green salad	4.03
Regular soft drinks	3.908
Cheeses, not cottage	3.287
Eggs	3.137

women. The number of Calories available to the average American is 3,450 Calories per day, an amount much higher than Americans actually consume. Calories from the food supply are lost due to waste, both at the grocery store and at home (see chapter 3). Calories from dietary fat range from 36–42 percent of total Calories (30 percent is considered optimal) for men and 37–41 percent for women. Notice that these figures are slightly lower than those given in figure 2.1 (food disappearance data overestimates the actual amount of food consumed by Americans).

Dietary data from 11,658 adults in the second National Health and Nutrition Examination Survey (NHANES II) (1976–1980) was recently analyzed to outline which foods in the American diet are most popular and the major contributors of Calories (16). Figures 2.11 and 2.12 summarize this information.

Figure 2.11 shows that the most frequently consumed food items in the U.S. are foods low in fiber and relatively high in salt, sugar, and fat. Nearly 80 percent of Americans consume coffee, tea, and white bread every day. Margarine, whole milk, doughnuts, cookies, sugar, green salad, and regular soft drinks are used daily by approximately 40 percent of Americans. Of these foods, only green salad is recommended for regular and frequent consumption.

Figure 2.12 shows that white bread, rolls, and crackers provide almost ten percent of total Calories consumed by Americans. Cakes and other pastries are the second most important sources of Calories, followed closely by alcoholic beverages. Whole milk, hamburgers and meat loaf, beef steaks, regular soft drinks, hot dogs and lunch meats, eggs, and french fries follow in order.

*F*IGURE 2.12

White breads, doughnuts, and cookies supply fifteen percent of all the Calories Americans consume.

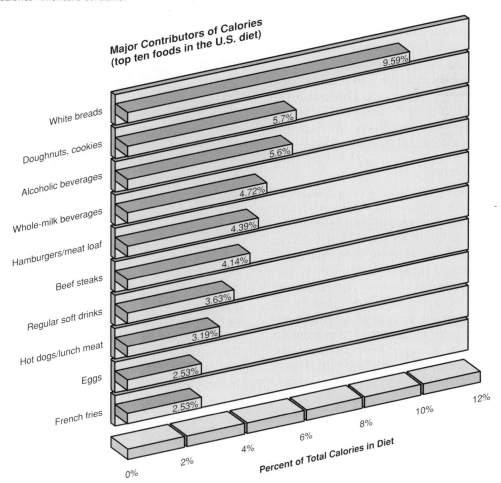

Major Contributors of Calories (top ten foods in the U.S. diet)

White breads	9.59%
Doughnuts, cookies	5.7%
Alcoholic beverages	5.6%
Whole-milk beverages	4.72%
Hamburgers/meat loaf	4.39%
Beef steaks	4.14%
Regular soft drinks	3.63%
Hot dogs/lunch meat	3.19%
Eggs	2.53%
French fries	2.53%

0%   2%   4%   6%   8%   10%   12%

Percent of Total Calories in Diet

*F*IGURE 2.13

Meats are the major source of fat in the American diet.

Sources of Fats in the U.S. Diet

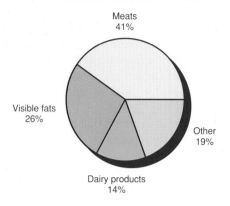

Meats 41%

Visible fats 26%

Other 19%

Dairy products 14%

*F*IGURE 2.14

Slightly more than half of Americans eat breakfast every day.

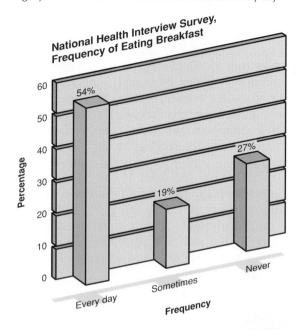

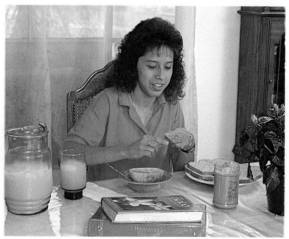

Other data from national dietary surveys are equally revealing (13,14). For the average American, five times as much carbohydrate is obtained from white as from whole-grain, dark breads. Beef provides 15 percent of all fat consumed by Americans. Hot dogs and lunch meats are the second most important source of fat, followed closely by whole milk and pastries. Meat, fish, and poultry combined contribute to 41 percent of the total fat consumption, with fats and oils contributing 26 percent, and milk, cream, and cheese 14 percent (see figure 2.13). Eggs provide 36 percent of the total **cholesterol** in the U.S. diet. Beef is the second most important source of cholesterol, supplying 16 percent of all cholesterol consumed by Americans.

Other Diet Trends

Trends in consumption have been accompanied by changes in eating patterns. Traditional family meals have been replaced, in part, by between-meal snacks and by meals eaten away from the home (17). Snacks now supply 18 percent of the Calories consumed by Americans, with 50 percent of the population snacking regularly more than once a day (25 percent of Americans do not snack) (18). Only 39 percent of Americans eat the traditional three meals a day (28 percent eat four times per day, 15 percent fives times per day, and 8.3 percent two times per day) (10). Figure 2.14 shows that while 54 percent of people report eating breakfast every day, 19 percent report eating breakfast "sometimes," and 27 percent never (19).

The percentage of the food dollar spent on away-from-home food consumption increased from 27 percent in 1960 to more than 33 percent in 1970 and is expected to exceed 40 percent by 1990. The average American now eats out an average of 3.7 times per week, or 192 times a year (20). Seventy-seven million eat out every day at 300,000 restaurants. "Eating out" expenses average $50 per household per week.

These trends are expected to continue for several reasons (21). These include increasing employment among women, decrease in family size, increase in per capita income, change from traditional life-styles, and a general desire and demand for convenience.

Fast-food restaurants now corner 41 percent of the eating-out dollars (versus 25 percent in 1958). Major concerns about fast foods include their tendency to be high in sodium, fat, and Calories while being low in vitamins A and C and in dietary fiber (21). Table 2.4, however, shows that not all fast foods have these traits (22). Some of the fast-food chains are offering such foods as baked fish, reduced-Calorie dressings, roasted chicken breasts, and multigrain buns as well as salad bars.

Overall, it appears that the nutrient intake of many individuals depends in large part on what is served at various restaurants and cafeterias. However, people need not feel helpless. Good nutrition requires that people learn to eat in a rational way, whether snacking, eating at home, or eating away from home. Eating nutritiously on the road is becoming easier with the increase in variety of healthful foods offered at both fast-food restaurants and supermarkets.

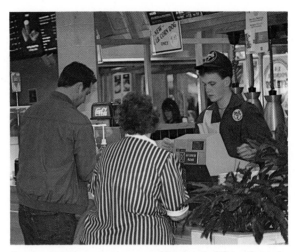
Fast-food restaurants now corner 41 percent of the eating-out dollars.

Dietary Guidelines and Goals Help Fuel Improved American Eating Habits

In response to American dietary trends from 1910 to the 1970s (see figures 2.1 through 2.10), several health agencies of the government and public sectors published dietary guidelines for Americans, beginning in 1977. Many health professionals and nutritionists were concerned about the increasing use of animal fat from meats and dairy products and the decreasing use of carbohydrate from grains, fruits, and vegetables. Research was demonstrating that these dietary trends were associated with the major killer diseases, in particular, cardiovascular disease and cancer. Experts decided that the American public needed to be warned.

U.S. Dietary Goals

In February 1977, the U.S. Senate Select Committee on Nutrition and Human Needs issued the **Dietary Goals for the United States** (23). This was the first of several government reports setting prudent dietary guidelines for Americans as a reaction to the negative changes occurring in the U.S. diet.

The U.S. Senate Select Committee introduced its dietary recommendations with this statement:

> *The overconsumption of foods high in fat, generally, and saturated fat in particular, as well as cholesterol, refined and processed sugars, salt and/or alcohol has been associated with the development of one or more of six to ten leading causes of death: heart disease, some cancers, stroke and hypertension, diabetes, arteriosclerosis and cirrhosis of the liver. (23)*

The committee then submitted seven dietary goals.

1. To avoid overweight, consume only as much energy (Calories) as is expended; if overweight, decrease energy intake and increase energy expenditure.
2. Increase the consumption of complex carbohydrates and "naturally occurring" sugars from about 28 percent of energy intake to about 48 percent of energy intake.
3. Reduce the consumption of refined and processed sugars by about 45 percent to account for about ten percent of total energy intake.

TABLE 2.4
Some fast-food chains are offering healthier foods

	Calories	Fat (pats*)	Fat (percent of Calories)	Sodium (mg)
McDonald's				
Hamburger	255	2.6	35	520
Chicken McNuggets	314	5.0	54	525
Filet-O-Fish	432	6.6	52	781
Big Mac	563	8.7	53	1,010
Sausage Biscuit	582	10.4	61	1,380
Roy Rogers				
Plain Potato	211	0	0	65
Potato w/ oleo	274	1.9	24	161
Roast Beef Sandwich	317	2.7	29	785
Crescent Roll	287	4.7	56	547
Potato w/ Broccoli 'n Cheese	376	4.8	43	523
Crescent Sandwich w/ Sausage	449	7.7	59	1,289
Crescent Sandwich w/ Ham	442	7.5	58	1,192
Wendy's				
Pasta Salad (½ cup)	134	1.6	40	400
Chicken Sandwich on wheat bun	320	2.6	28	500
Taco Salad	390	4.8	40	1,100
Broccoli & Cheese Potato	500	6.6	45	430
Cheese Stuffed Potato	590	9.0	52	450
Hardee's				
Chef's Salad	272	4.2	53	517
Chicken Fillet Sandwich	510	6.9	46	360
Shrimp Salad	362	7.7	72	941
Bacon Cheeseburger	686	11.1	55	1,074
Arby's				
Roasted Chicken Breast (no bun)	254	1.9	25	930
Broccoli & Cheese Potato	540	5.8	37	480
Mushroom & Cheese Potato	510	5.8	39	640
(Fried) Chicken Breast Sandwich	584	7.4	43	1,323
Sausage & Egg Croissant	530	9.3	59	745
Long John Silver's				
Baked Fish w/ sauce	151	0.5	12	361
Mixed Vegetables	54	0.5	33	570
Corn on the Cob	176	1.1	20	0
Coleslaw	182	4.0	74	367
Fish w/ batter (2 pc)	404	6.4	53	1,346
Burger King				
Veal Parmigiana	580	7.1	42	805
Bacon Double Cheeseburger	600	9.3	53	985
Specialty Chicken Sandwich	690	11.1	55	775
Jack in the Box				
Shrimp Salad (no dressing)	115	0.3	8	460
Taco Salad	377	6.3	57	1,436
Chicken Supreme Sandwich	601	9.5	54	1,582
Kentucky Fried Chicken				
Breast (Original Recipe)	199	3.1	53	558
Extra Crispy Dark Dinner**	765	14.2	63	1,480

*Pats-of-butter equivalent. A pat of butter contains 3.8 grams of fat.
**Includes drumstick, thigh, mashed potatoes, gravy, coleslaw, and roll.

From B. Liebman article in *Nutrition Action Healthletter,* June 1985, p. 51. Reprinted from *Nutrition Action Healthletter* which is available from the Center for Science in the Public Interest, 1501 16th Street, N.W., Washington, D.C. 20036, for $19.95 for 10 issues.

4. Reduce overall fat consumption from approximately 40 percent to about 30 percent of energy intake.
5. Reduce saturated-fat consumption to account for about ten percent of total energy intake; balance that with polyunsaturated and monounsaturated fats, which should account for about ten percent of energy intake each.
6. Reduce cholesterol consumption to about 300 milligrams a day.
7. Limit the intake of sodium by reducing the intake of salt to about 5 grams a day.

The goals suggested the following changes in food selection and preparation.

1. Increase consumption of fruits and vegetables and whole grains.
2. Decrease consumption of refined and other processed sugars and foods high in such sugars.
3. Decrease consumption of foods high in total fat, and partially replace saturated fats, whether obtained from animal or vegetable sources, with polyunsaturated fats.
4. Decrease consumption of animal fat, and choose meats, poultry, and fish, which will reduce saturated fat intake.
5. Except for young children, substitute low-fat and nonfat milk for whole milk, and low-fat dairy products for high-fat dairy products.
6. Decrease consumption of butterfat, eggs, and other high-cholesterol sources. Some consideration should be given to easing the cholesterol goal for premenopausal women, young children, and the elderly in order to obtain the nutritional benefits of eggs in the diet.
7. Decrease consumption of salt and foods high in salt content.

These dietary goals caused quite a stir in the United States, prompting discussion and controversy among nutritionists and others. It became clear that Americans would need to alter their diets greatly to conform to the recommendations (24–27) (see figure 2.15).

During the ensuing years, many other organizations and professional groups have submitted their own dietary guidelines, most of them very supportive of the original U.S. Dietary

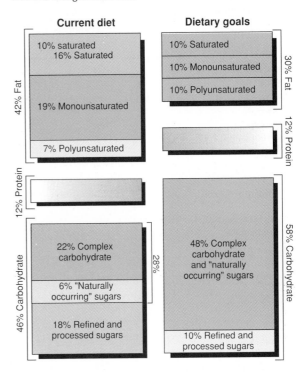

*F*IGURE 2.15
The U.S. Dietary Goals published in 1977 recommended dramatic changes in the diet.

Goals report (28–35). In 1988 the Surgeon General's Report on Nutrition and Health was published (28). This extensive report concluded that overconsumption of foods high in fat and underconsumption of foods high in complex carbohydrate and fiber are responsible for much of the burden of illness and death in the U.S. The 1988 Surgeon General's Report was followed by the 1989 National Research Council's report, Diet and Health, which drew similar conclusions. Dietary recommendations have been made by other government agencies and various heart disease and cancer prevention groups. Other nations around the world have also published dietary guidelines, including Canada, France, Norway, New Zealand, Australia, Denmark, Great Britain, Japan, and Sweden (26).

Table 2.5 summarizes some of the more important of the U.S. guidelines. Notice that the majority of these reports have recommended that Americans reduce their intake of total fat, saturated fat, cholesterol, and salt, while moderating alcohol and Calories and increasing complex carbohydrate and dietary fiber. In practice, Americans are urged to meet these dietary

TABLE 2.5
Dietary recommendations to the American public

Recommendations	U.S. Dietary Goals, 1977 (23)	Surgeon General, 1988 (28)	NIH, NCI 1985	DHHS 1985 (30)	AHA/NCEP 1988 (34, 35)	NAS/DNC 1982 (31)	NRC, 1989 (29)
Limit or reduce total fat (% of cal)	<30%	Yes	<30%	Yes	<30%	<30%	<30%
Reduce saturated fat (% of cal)	To 10%	Yes	NC	Yes	<10%	As total fat only	<10%
Increase polyunsaturated fat (% of cal)	To 10%	NS	No	No	NS	No	NS
Limit cholesterol (mg/day)	<300	Yes	NC	Yes	<300	NC	<300
Limit simple sugars	Yes	Yes, for some people	NC	Yes	NC	NC	NC
Increase complex carbohydrate	>55%	Yes	Yes	Yes	Yes	Through whole grains, fruits, and vegetables	>55%
Increase fiber	Yes	NS	25–35g	Yes	NS	Yes	
Restrict salt (g/day)	<5	Yes	NC	Yes	Yes	Through salt-cured, pickled, smoked foods	<6
Moderate alcohol	Yes	Yes	Yes	Yes	Yes	Yes	Yes
Maintain ideal weight, exercise	Yes	Yes	Yes	Yes	Yes	NS	Yes
Other	Reduce animal foods, increase plant foods	Calcium-, iron-, and fluoride-rich foods/water for some people	Variety in diet	Variety in diet	Fat- and cholesterol-restricted more for high risk	Emphasize fruits and vegetables	Avoid dietary supplements; eat wide variety of plant foods

(Note: NCI = National Cancer Institute; DHHS = Dept. of Health and Human Services; AHA/NCEP = American Heart Association/National Cholesterol Education Program; NAS/DNC = National Academy of Sciences/Comm. on Diet, Nutrition and Cancer; NRC = National Research Council) NS = not specifically; NC = no comment.

guidelines by increasing consumption of whole grains, fruits, and vegetables, and by decreasing use of fatty meats and high-fat dairy products.

The U.S. Dietary Goals drew attention to the need for federal guidelines for the public about diet and health. In 1979, the USDA issued a colorful, visually attractive bulletin entitled "Food." Then in 1980 and 1985, the USDA and U.S. Department of Health and Human Services (HHS) issued the Dietary Guidelines for Americans (30). The USDA has supported Dietary Guidelines with several other consumer bulletins, such as "Ideas for Better Eating," "Food 2: A Dieter's Guide," "Food 3: Eating the Moderate Fat and Cholesterol Way," and "The Sodium Content of Your Food." The USDA is also stressing the importance of food and fitness to health with a half-hour videotape, "Inside/Out." The USDA's Human Nutrition Information Service (HNIS) has cooperated with the American National Red Cross in developing a six-session nutrition course that focuses on implementing the Dietary Guidelines and on other nutrition topics of public interest. The course "Better Eating for Better Health" (ANRD/USDA, 1984) is now offered by local Red Cross chapters across the country.

The **1985 Dietary Guidelines for Americans** focused on seven guidelines. Figure 2.16 summarizes these. Appendix G of this book contains the complete guidelines. Although the thrust of these guidelines is similar to the Dietary Goals (less animal products, more plant food, less sugar, salt, and fat), the USDA avoided being too specific. (Note: Sidebar 2.1 gives some tips for modifying recipes, and Sidebar 2.2 includes recipes that follow the USDA Dietary Guidelines.)

Most attention has focused on the "avoid too much fat, saturated fat, and cholesterol" guideline (26). The amount of dietary fat and cholesterol appropriate for healthy Americans remains a point of considerable controversy (see chapter 6). However, some quantitative guidelines have been proposed, at least since 1970. In that year, the Inter-Society Commission for Heart Disease Resources released a report, "Primary Prevention of the Atherosclerotic Diseases." They proposed the following levels: less than 35 percent of energy from fat, less than ten percent from saturated fat, and less than 300 milligrams of cholesterol per day. In 1988, the National Cholesterol Education Program, National Institutes of Health, released their report, calling for less than 30 percent of energy from fat, less than ten percent from saturated fat, and less than 300 milligrams of cholesterol per day (35). Many other authoritative groups have concurred with one or more of these numbers for prevention of both heart disease and cancer. These groups include the Committee on Diet, Nutrition, and Cancer of the National Academy of Sciences/National Research Council (31); the American Cancer Society (32); the National Institutes of Health (33); and the American Heart Association (34).

Only a short time ago, the question of whether or not the standard American diet promoted cancer was hotly contested. Within the last few years, however, official recognition that diet is related to cancer has continued to increase. Many experts now promote the idea that diet is the most important cancer risk factor, associated with 35 percent of all cancer. This will be discussed in more detail in chapter 10 (Health-Promotion Insight).

One remarkable fact, however, is that the dietary recommendations for prevention of both heart disease and cancer are very similar, with

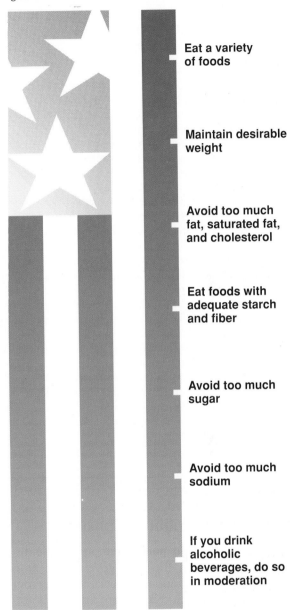

*F*IGURE 2.16

The 1985 Dietary Guidelines for Americans focused on seven guidelines.

Eat a variety of foods

Maintain desirable weight

Avoid too much fat, saturated fat, and cholesterol

Eat foods with adequate starch and fiber

Avoid too much sugar

Avoid too much sodium

If you drink alcoholic beverages, do so in moderation

emphasis on increased fruits, vegetables, and whole grains, and decreased fats. These recommendations are broadly outlined in the 1985 Dietary Guidelines for Americans and specifically summarized in the 1977 Dietary Goals for the United States and the 1989 Diet and Health Statement from the National Research Council.

Tips for Modifying Recipes

Here are some ways to lower fat, sugar, and sodium and to increase fiber in the foods you fix. These tips reflect the Dietary Guidelines.

Modification	Effect
1. Remove fat from meats, skin from poultry before preparing.	Reduces fat
2. Broil, roast, or bake on a rack to allow fat to drip into a pan.	Reduces fat
3. Skim fat from stews and soups (refrigerate and let fat congeal on top, or place in freezer for 20 minutes).	Reduces fat
4. Instead of frying in oil, use no-stick pans or vegetable oil sprays, or stir-fry in water instead of oil. Limit batter-fried foods.	Reduces fat
5. Substitute plain low-fat yogurt for sour cream or mayonnaise in dips and dressings.	Reduces fat and cholesterol
6. Substitute skim milk for whole milk in baking and sauces.	Reduces fat and cholesterol
7. Substitute two egg whites for one whole egg in baking.	Reduces fat and cholesterol
8. Substitute skim milk-based white sauce for cream sauces or canned soups in casseroles.	Reduces fat and sodium
9. Use fresh, frozen, or no-salt-added canned vegetables to thicken casseroles and soups. Try grating, chopping, or puréeing them.	Reduces Calories and sodium
10. Reduce fat in recipes.*	Reduces fat
11. For seasoning, use herbs, spices, vinegar, fruit juices, flavoring extracts, fruit peel, or chopped vegetables rather than salt, seasoned salts, MSG, or soy sauce.	Reduces sodium
12. Cook cereal, vegetables, rice, or pasta in unsalted water. Try seasoning with spices and herbs instead.	Reduces sodium
13. Reduce salt in recipes to one-half or less.	Reduces sodium
14. Reduce sugar in recipes by up to one-third.*	Reduces added sugars
15. Substitute whole-wheat flour for part of the enriched white flour in recipes.** One cup whole-wheat flour = one cup enriched white flour.	Increases fiber and nutrients from whole grains

*Amounts and type of sugar, fat, and flour affect the structure, texture, and keeping quality of baked products. Cookies and quick breads such as pancakes and muffins are most readily modified. Experiment by reducing the proportions of fat and sugar gradually to maintain an acceptable product.

From *Better Eating for Better Health*, 1984, published by The American National Red Cross, Washington, D.C.

American Nutritional Concerns

The media has given much attention to these dietary reports from the U.S. government and professional organizations, especially during the 1980s. As a result, more and more Americans are considering their health as they select their foods from the supermarkets (36). Various surveys and studies show that a substantial number of consumers are at least concerned (if not always prompted into action) about several aspects of the diet.

In general, recent studies by the Food Marketing Institute and the **Food and Drug Administration** (FDA) demonstrate that concerns about Calories, sodium, fats, cholesterol, caffeine, and sugar have been increasingly noted, whereas concern about protein, vitamins, and minerals appears to have declined (37). In one recent national poll conducted by the Roper Organization, people were asked which of six items they were concerned about for health reasons. Seventy percent said they were "very" or "somewhat" concerned about salt, 65 percent about cholesterol, 63 percent about sugar, and 53 percent about caffeine.

The Food Marketing Institute (FMI), an organization of food retailers and wholesalers, including most big supermarkets and regional firms, conducts periodic surveys of food shoppers. In their 1986 survey, concerns about salt, sugar, and fat were greater than for additives and preservatives (37).

A 1986 Louis Harris and Associates Inc. survey on the health practices of Americans showed that 50 percent of adult Americans say

Some Recipes To Help You Put the Dietary Guidelines into Practice

Apple Crisp

4 servings, ½ cup each.
Calories per serving: about 230

Tart apples, pared, sliced	4 cups
Water	¼ cup
Lemon juice	1 tablespoon
Brown sugar, packed	¼ cup
Whole-wheat flour	¼ cup
Old-fashioned rolled oats	½ cup
Ground cinnamon	½ teaspoon
Ground nutmeg	¼ teaspoon
Margarine	3 tablespoons

1. Place apples in 8×8×2-inch baking pan.
2. Mix water and lemon juice, pour over apples.
3. Mix sugar, flour, oats, and spices.
4. Add margarine to dry mixture; mix until crumbly.
5. Sprinkle crumbly mixture evenly over apples.
6. Bake at 350° F (moderate oven) until apples are tender and topping is lightly browned, about 40 minutes.

Banana-Nut Bread

1 loaf, 18 slices.*
Calories per slice: about 135

Whole-wheat flour	1¾ cups
Sugar	½ cup
Baking powder	1 tablespoon
Salt	¼ teaspoon
Walnuts, chopped	½ cup
Oil	⅓ cup
Eggs	2
Bananas, mashed	2 medium (about 1 cup)

1. Preheat oven to 350° F (moderate).
2. Grease 9×5×3-inch loaf pan.
3. Mix flour, sugar, baking powder, salt, and nuts thoroughly.
4. Mix oil and eggs together. Mix in bananas.
5. Add dry ingredients to banana mixture. Stir until just smooth.
6. Pour into loaf pan.
7. Bake 45 minutes or until firmly set when lightly touched in center top.
8. Cool on rack. Remove from pan after 10 minutes.

From *Ideas for Better Eating, Menus and Recipes To Make Use of the Dietary Guidelines*, 1981. U.S. Department of Agriculture.

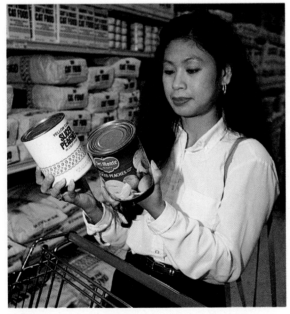
Surveys show that Americans are becoming increasingly concerned about the quality of their food.

they "try a lot" to watch eleven key aspects of nutrition. This ranged from 65 percent who reported they try a lot to eat vegetables in the cabbage family (for cancer prevention) to 31 percent who said they try a lot to eat fish twice a week (for heart disease prevention). Figure 2.17 summarizes the findings of this survey.

Overall, these surveys and polls tell us that the majority of Americans are concerned about health and nutrition and are doing something about their diets. These surveys are similar to the results of the 1980 USDA survey of 1,353 U.S. households, which revealed that three of five households had made a diet change in the preceding three years for health or nutrition reasons. In this survey, 21 percent of the households surveyed reported using less bacon and sausage, and four percent had stopped using these meats. Sixteen percent reported eating fewer hot dogs, less luncheon meats, and less beef and pork. Seventeen percent had increased their consumption of poultry.

FIGURE 2.17

Close to 50 percent of Americans say they "try a lot" to watch seven key aspects of nutrition.

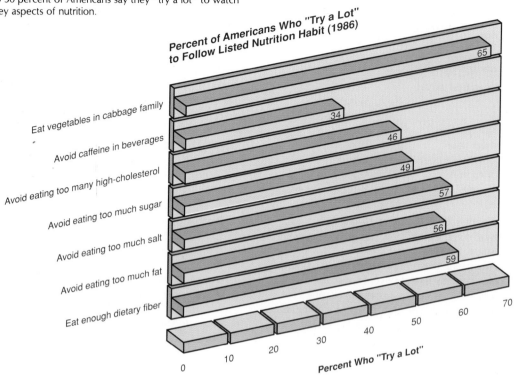

Percent of Americans Who "Try a Lot" to Follow Listed Nutrition Habit (1986)

- Eat vegetables in cabbage family — 34
- Avoid caffeine in beverages — 46
- Avoid eating too many high-cholesterol — 49
- Avoid eating too much sugar — 57
- Avoid eating too much salt — 56
- Avoid eating too much fat — 59
- Eat enough dietary fiber — 65

Percent Who "Try a Lot"

Healthy Trends in the American Diet

These increased concerns about various aspects of the diet have led to some improvements in the American diet (15). As shown in figures 2.1 through 2.10, there have been some healthy trends since 1970. These include the following.

Fresh fruits and vegetables have been one of the fastest-growing categories in U.S. supermarkets during the 1980s, accounting for $20 billion in sales in 1984. The biggest trend in fruits and vegetables is in the fresh produce department. The average number of items offered rose from 65 in 1972 to 173 in 1983. Consumers who are most concerned about nutrition, who exercise the most, and who are on special diets are most likely to eat fresh fruits and vegetables (36).

Although consumption of fresh fruits and vegetables has increased, use of potatoes is still very low when compared to 1910. Well over half of the potato consumption today is in the form of processed products, including potato chips and canned, frozen, shoestring, and dehydrated potatoes. A staggering 3.9 billion pounds of potatoes were made into frozen french fries in 1984, 3.4 billion pounds of them going to restaurants. Fresh potatoes may come back into popularity, however, thanks to the recent introduction of baked potatoes in fast-food outlets and to the increased use of microwave ovens in the home (one million units were sold in 1975; nine million in 1984).

Eggs and dairy products have traditionally been an important part of the American diet. Milk, butter, cheese, cream, and eggs accounted for almost one-fourth of the food the average American ate in 1985. Yet, over the last 30 years consumption of these foods has been falling. Not since the Great Depression of the 1930s have animal products such as milk, butter, lard, and eggs made up a smaller share of the U.S. diets than they do now.

Consumption of grain-based products is rising, including pasta and ready-to-eat breakfast cereals.

Americans are consuming less red meat but more poultry and fish than in previous years. People are eating poultry and fish at record rates. Beef consumption is down from its peak in 1975.

Diet soft drinks now represent 20 percent of the market, which should rise to 30–40 percent by 1990. Diet drinks are considered to be a healthier choice than regular soft drinks.

In 1984, 17.7 percent of all persons ten years and older were drinking decaffeinated coffee, up an amazing 342 percent from 1962. More than one out of five cups of coffee Americans drink is now decaffeinated.

Since 1950, consumption of fruit juices has tripled, from 2.1 to 7.1 gallons per person per year, with orange juice being number-one.

Factors behind These Healthy Dietary Trends

What is responsible for some of the changes taking place in the American diet? This is a complex question, but several factors include (38):

increased marketing (diet soft drinks, yogurt, for example);

technology (production efficiency in producing chickens, for example);

cost (prices for red meat and sucrose have risen, helping to decrease consumption);

health consciousness (more fruits and vegetables, less red meats, eggs, and dairy products, etc.);

changing life-styles (more leisure time, two-parent working families, more single-person households, more income, more education);

more eating out, especially in fast-food restaurants (increased use of cheese, frozen potatoes as french fries, for example);

desire to save time (convenience and time-saving factors have become very important, leading to increased use of fast foods, foods that can be microwaved, etc.).

In general, Americans are beginning to increase their consumption of poultry and fish, low-fat milk and yogurt, and fresh fruits and vegetables, while decreasing intake of eggs, coffee, whole milk, cream, and red meats. Even the National Restaurant Association has taken note of this trend (38). Americans are dining out more than

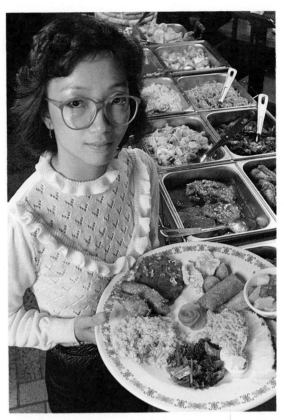

More and more restaurants are changing their menus to satisfy health-conscious clientele.

ever before, but growing numbers aren't leaving their desire for a healthy diet at home. In response, more and more restaurants are changing their menus to satisfy a calorie-counting and nutrition-conscious clientele. According to surveys by NRA, two of five Americans report that they have changed their eating habits while eating out. More restaurant patrons report eating more vegetables, less fat, less meat, fewer fried foods, less sugar and salt, and more fish and salads. Surveys show that the majority of restaurants now have healthful foods available and are willing to alter preparation methods when requested.

However impressive these figures are, much greater improvements must be realized by the majority of Americans before we can say that most Americans are healthy eaters. As noted in figures 2.11 and 2.12, the most popular foods in America are still items such as white bread, whole milk, doughnuts and cookies, sugar, soft drinks, cheeses, eggs, hot dogs, and hamburgers. Much work still remains in educating the majority of Americans to eat nutritiously and healthfully.

SUMMARY

1. Several important dietary trends have occurred during this century. Intake of carbohydrate has decreased, while intake of fat has increased. The decrease in carbohydrate is due to the decline in starch intake. Use of sugar, however, has increased sharply.

2. Major changes in individual food groups from 1910 to 1970 and 1985 were reviewed. Some highlights include the dramatic increase in use of poultry, plant oil, and sugar, and the decrease in intake of whole milk, potatoes, grain products, and eggs.

3. Despite the lower amounts of carbohydrate and higher amounts of fats being consumed by Americans, the levels of most vitamins and minerals in the food supply were higher in the 1980s than at the beginning of this century.

4. The average male in this country consumes 2,300–2,600 Calories per day, whereas the average female consumes 1,500–1,750 Calories per day. Calories from dietary fat range from 37–42 percent of total Calories for men and 37–41 percent for women.

5. The most frequently consumed food items in the U.S. are foods low in fiber and relatively high in salt, sugar, and fat. These include refined grain products, margarine, whole milk, fatty meats, and regular soft drinks. Meats contribute 41 percent of the total fat consumed by Americans.

6. Trends in food consumption have been accompanied by changes in eating patterns. Traditional family meals have been replaced in part by between-meal snacks and meals eaten away from home.

7. In response to American dietary trends from 1910 to the 1970s (see figures 2.1 through 2.10), several health agencies of the government and the public sectors published dietary guidelines for Americans, beginning in 1977. The first of several government reports was the *Dietary Goals for the United States*.

8. The majority of these reports have recommended that Americans reduce their intake of total fat, saturated fat, cholesterol, simple sugars, and salt, while moderating alcohol and Calories and increasing complex carbohydrate and dietary fiber.

9. In practice, Americans are urged to meet these dietary guidelines by increasing consumption of whole grains, fruits, and vegetables, and by decreasing use of fatty meats and high-fat dairy products.

10. The media has given much attention to these dietary reports from the U.S. government and professional organizations. As a result, more and more Americans are considering their health as they select their foods from the supermarkets. Various surveys and studies show that a substantial number of consumers are at least concerned (if not always prompted into action) about several aspects of the diet.

11. These increased concerns over various aspects of the diet have led to some improvements in American eating patterns. In general, Americans are beginning to increase their consumption of poultry and fish, low-fat milk and yogurt, and fresh fruits and vegetables, and to decrease intake of eggs, coffee, whole milk, cream, and red meats. Much work remains to be done, however, in improving the eating habits of Americans.

REFERENCES

1. Leveille, G. A. 1988. Current Attitude and Behavior Trends Regarding Consumption of Grains. *Food Technology.* (January):110–11.
2. Office of Disease Prevention and Health Promotion, U.S. Public Health Service, U.S. Department of Health and Human Services. 1988. *Disease Prevention/Health Promotion: The Facts.* Palo Alto: Bull Publishing.
3. Wolf I. D., and B. B. Peterkin. 1984. Dietary Guidelines: The USDA Perspective. *Food Technology.* (July):80–86.
4. U.S. Bureau of the Census. 1975. Historical Statistics of the United States, Colonial Times to 1970, Bicentennial Edition, Part 1. Washington, D.C.: U.S. Government Printing Office.
5. U.S. Bureau of the Census. 1987. Statistical Abstract of the United States. Washington, D.C.: U.S. Government Printing Office.
6. Lanza, E., et al. 1987. Dietary Fiber Intake in the U.S. Population. *American Journal of Clinical Nutrition* 46:790–97.
7. Morgan, K. J., V. J. Stults, and G. L. Stampley. 1985. Soft Drink Consumption Patterns of the U.S. Population. *Journal of the American Dietetic Association* 85:352–54.
8. Zamula, E. 1984. Basic to Our Food Chain Is Plain Old Field Corn. *FDA Consumer.* (November):24–27.
9. Welsh, S. O., and R. M. Martson. 1982. Review of Trends in Food Use in the U.S., 1909–1980. *Journal of the American Dietetic Association* 81:120.
10. Pennington, J. A. T. 1986. Dietary Patterns and Practices. *Clinical Nutrition* 5:17–26.
11. McDonald, J. T. 1986. Vitamin and Mineral Supplement Use in the United States. *Clinical Nutrition* 5:27–33.
12. Goor, R., et al. 1985. Nutrient Intakes Among Selected North American Populations in the Lipid Research Clinics Prevalence Study: Composition of Fat Intake. *American Journal of Clinical Nutrition* 41:299–311.
13. National Center for Health Statistics. 1963. Dietary Intake Source Data. United States 1976–80, Second National Health and Nutrition Examination Survey. Vital and Health Statistics. Series II—No. 231, by M. D. Carroll, S. Abraham, and C. M. Dresser. DHHS Pub. No. (PHS) 83-1681. Public Health Service. Washington, D.C.: U.S. Government Printing Office.
14. Consumer Nutrition Division, Human Nutrition Information Service, U.S. Department of Agriculture. 1984. Nutrient Intakes: Individuals in 48 States, Year 1977–78. Nationwide Food Consumption Survey 1977–78, Rept. No. I-2. Hyattsville, MD: U.S. Department of Agriculture.
15. U.S. Department of Agriculture, Human Nutrition Information Service. 1985. Nationwide Food Consumption Survey, Continuing Survey of Food Intakes by Individuals:

Women 19–50 Years and Their Children 1–5 Years, 1 Day, 1985. U.S. Department of Agriculture, Rept. No. 85-1. Men 19–50 Years, 1 Day, 1985. U.S. Department of Agriculture, Rept. No. 85-3.

16. Block, G., C. M. Dresser, A. M. Hartman, and M. D. Carroll. 1985. Nutrient Sources in the American Diet: Quantitative Data from the NHANES II Survey. *American Journal of Epidemiology* 122:27–40.

17. Crocetti, A. F., and H. A. Guthrie. 1986. Alternative Eating Patterns and the Role of Age, Sex, Selection, and Snacking in Nutritional Quality. *Clinical Nutrition* 5:34–42.

18. Morgan, K. J., and B. Goungetas. 1986. Snacking and Eating Away from Home. In *What is America Eating?* (Proceedings of a Symposium, Food and Nutrition Board, Commission on Life Sciences, National Research Council.) Washington, D.C.: National Academy Press.

19. Schoenborn, C. A., and B. H. Cohen. 1986. Trends in Smoking, Alcohol Consumption, and Other Health Practices Among U.S. Adults, 1977 and 1983. *Advancedata* (June 30): 118.

20. Dining Out with a Healthy Appetite. 1987. *FDA Consumer* (March): 19–23.

21. Ries, C. P., K. Kline, and S. O. Weaver. 1987. Impact of Commercial Eating on Nutrient Adequacy. *Journal of the American Dietetic Association* 87:463–68.

22. Liebman, B. 1985. What's New in Fast Food Nutrition. *Nutrition Action* (June): 4–7.

23. Dietary Goals for the United States. U.S. Government Printing Office, 1977, Washington, D.C., 20402. Stock No. 052-070-04376-8.

24. Behlen, P. M., and F. J. Cronin. 1985. Dietary Recommendations for Healthy Americans Summarized. *Family Economics Review* 3:17–24.

25. Miller, S. A., and M. G. Stephensen. 1985. Scientific and Public Health Rationale for the Dietary Guidelines for Americans. *American Journal of Clinical Nutrition* 42:739–45.

26. Truswell, A. S. 1987. Evolution of Dietary Recommendations, Goals, and Guidelines. *American Journal of Clinical Nutrition* 45:1060–72.

27. Palmer, S. 1983. Diet, Nutrition, and Cancer: The Future of Dietary Policy. *Cancer Research* 43(suppl):2509.

28. The Surgeon General's Report on Nutrition and Health. 1988. USDHHS (PHS) Publication no. 88-50211.

29. National Research Council. 1989. Diet and Health: Implications for Reducing Chronic Disease Risk. Washington, D.C.: National Academy Press.

30. U.S. Department of Agriculture/Department of Health and Human Services. 1985. Nutrition and Your Health: Dietary Guidelines for Americans, 1985. Pueblo, CO: Consumer Information Center, Dept. 622N.

31. Committee on Diet, Nutrition, and Cancer, Assembly of Life Sciences, National Research Council. 1982. *Diet, Nutrition, and Cancer.* Washington, D.C. National Academy Press.

32. American Cancer Society Special Report. 1984. *Nutrition and Cancer: Cause and Prevention.* (Ca-A Cancer J Clinicians) 34:1984.

33. National Institutes of Health. 1984. Consensus Development Conference Statement on Lowering Blood Cholesterol to Prevent Heart Disease. Bethesda, Maryland: National Heart, Lung, and Blood Institute, National Institutes of Health.

34. American Heart Association. 1988. Dietary Guidelines for Healthy American Adults: A Statement for Physicians and Health Professionals by the Nutrition Committee, American Heart Association. Circulation 77:721A–724A.

35. National Cholesterol Education Program. 1988. National Heart, Lung, and Blood Institute. National Institutes of Health. C-200. Bethesda, MD.

36. FDA Staff, Special Report. 1985. America's Changing Diet. *FDA Consumer* (October): 4–25.

37. Lecos, C. W. Shopping for the Second 50 Years. 1986. *FDA Consumer* (July–August):29–31.

38. Breidenstein, B. C. 1988. Changes in Consumer Attitudes toward Red Meat and Their Effect on Marketing Strategy. *Food Technology* (January):112–16.

*H*EALTH-PROMOTION ACTIVITY 2.1
How Do You Rate Your Diet?

Tables 2.6 through 2.9 in this health-promotion activity summarize the major source foods for various aspects of the diet. Study these tables, and then place a check mark in the blank by any of the "top five foods" in each table that apply to your regular diet. If you eat the particular food very seldom (less the three times per week), then do not place a check in the blank. If you consume the food *more than three times per week,* then check the blank by the food. Please note that some foods (whole milk, hamburgers, meat loaf, hot dogs, ham, lunch meats, beef steaks, roasts) are used more than once in the different lists. Make sure that you place a check by these foods for each category in which they are found.

Table 2.6
Sources of Fat in Our Diet

Food Category	Percentage of Dietary Fat
Meat	27.9
Dairy, eggs	18.3
Fats, oils	15.8
Desserts, snacks	12.6
Breads, grains, potatoes	11.2
Poultry, fish	4.9
Nuts, beans	3.1
Miscellaneous	6.2

Top Five Foods Supplying Fat to Americans

1. Hamburgers, meat loaf   _____

2. Hot dogs, ham, lunch meats   _____

3. Whole milk   _____

4. Doughnuts, cakes, cookies   _____

5. Beef steaks, roasts   _____

Note: Three of the five top fat-filled food groups in the average American's diet are meats. On a given day, almost 30 percent of the adult population eat a hot dog, ham, or lunch meat; 26 percent devour a hamburger, cheeseburger, or meat loaf; and 23 percent consume at least one serving of steak or roast beef. On a given day, 41 percent of the adult population drink two glasses of whole milk.

Table 2.7
Sources of Sodium in Our Diet

Food Category	Percentage of Dietary Sodium
Breads, cereals, pasta, potatoes	31.1
Meats	18.8
Dairy, eggs	14.2
Desserts, snacks	6.8
Soups	6.6
Fats, oils	5.4
Fish, poultry	3.5
Vegetables	2.9
Nuts, beans	1.8
Tomato condiments, ketchup	1.0
Miscellaneous	7.9

Top Five Foods Supplying Sodium to Americans

1. White bread, rolls, crackers _____
2. Hot dogs, ham, lunch meats _____
3. Soups _____
4. Cheeses _____
5. Potatoes (hash, fried, french fried) _____

Note: The figures above do not include the salt added in cooking or at the table. Refined bakery goods (white bread, crackers, rolls) are by far the greatest source of salt in the American diet. This is due to the large volume of such products that we consume. Close to 77 percent of all adults eat white breads two times every day. Processed meats (hot dogs, ham, and lunch meats) also supply a high amount of sodium. Soups, processed cheeses (American processed cheese slices), and processed potatoes round out the picture. Notice the key word here — *processed.* Manufacturers tend to add more salt than they should when they produce foods.

Table 2.8
Sources of Cholesterol in Our Diet

Top Five Foods	Percentage of Dietary Cholesterol	
Eggs	35.9	_____
Beef steaks, roasts	8.7	_____
Hamburgers, meat loaf	7.3	_____
Whole milk	5.4	_____
Hot dogs, ham, lunch meats	4.3	_____

Note: Every year 1,500,000 Americans have a heart attack. One reason is the high amounts of cholesterol that Americans consume (the other culprit is hard, saturated, animal fats.). Eggs are by far the largest source of cholesterol in the American diet. And meats and milk, foods that have also ranked high in the fat and sodium lists, supply most of the rest of the cholesterol Americans ingest.

Table 2.9
Sources of Sugar in Our Diet

Top Five Foods	Percentage of Dietary Sugar	
Soft drinks	21.0	_____
Sweets	18.4	_____
Bakery goods	13.3	_____
Milk products	9.6	_____
Bread, grain products	6.2	_____

Note: Soft drinks are the major source of sugar in the American diet. Sweets (syrups, jellies, jams, gelatin desserts, ices, and table sugar) run a close second. Bakery goods (cakes, cookies, pies, pastries, and sweet crackers), milk products (ice cream, milk shakes, flavored yogurt, chocolate milk), and bread and grain products (breads, pasta, rice, baby cereals, cooked cereals, crackers, and salty snacks) finish the top five. The reason bread and grain products, although relatively low in sugar content, rank somewhat high on the list is that Americans eat a large volume of such food.

Count the number of checks, and find your grade below.

Grade	Number of Checks (out of 20 possible)
A	0-2
B	3-4
C	5-6

More than six checks — keep studying your nutrition!

3

Nutritional Tools and Methods

INTRODUCTION

*H*ave you ever wondered what that sidebar label on your breakfast cereal box means when it says that your favorite cereal contains ``less than two percent of U.S. RDA of these nutrients?'' In this chapter, you will learn how to interpret this information and evaluate the quality of your diet.

Foods can be grouped into major and minor food groups. You may have heard of the Four Food Group plan from the United States Department of Agriculture (USDA). We'll discuss the pros and cons of this method of grouping.

Calculating the nutrient consumption in the American diet is a time-consuming and difficult process. This chapter will review the different techniques and survey methods used in nutritional assessment. The health-promotion activities of this chapter will guide you in evaluating your personal nutrient intake.

The Recommended Dietary Allowances—An Explanation

The **Recommended Dietary Allowances (RDA)**, established by the National Research Council of the National Academy of Sciences, have become the premier nutrient standard in both the U.S. and the world. More than 40 countries now have their own RDA, but many other countries use the U.S. RDA (1).

The RDA are a technical standard used for nutrition policies and decision making. Thus, the RDA are different from the Dietary Guidelines for Americans that we reviewed in the previous chapter. The Dietary Guidelines are used primarily for guiding people in making dietary decisions for the prevention of heart disease and cancer.

The RDA, however, are much more than a technical and scientific compilation of data. The RDA today are used for a wide variety of purposes, ranging from development of new food products to being the standard for federal nutrition assistance programs (2). The purposes of the RDA will be outlined after we review the definition in more detail.

Definition of RDA

The Recommended Dietary Allowances were first published in 1943 to "provide standards serving as a goal for good nutrition." The RDA have been revised about every five years since (3). RDA are the levels of intake of essential nutrients considered, in the judgment of the Committee on Dietary Allowances of the Food and Nutrition Board on the basis of available scientific knowledge, to be adequate to meet the known nutritional needs of practically all healthy persons. In other words, this group of nutrition experts has established mineral and vitamin intake criteria that Americans can use to judge the adequacy of their diet.

Several major principles behind the RDA can be outlined as follows.

1. RDA are the average daily amounts of nutrients that *population groups* should consume over a period of time. RDA are estimated to exceed the requirements of most *individuals* and thereby ensure that the needs of nearly *all* in the population are met. *Intakes below the RDA for a nutrient are thus not necessarily inadequate.* In other words, the RDA are "padded" to make sure that all Americans have adequate nutrient intakes. For this reason, not everyone needs to ingest 100 percent of RDA of all vitamins and minerals. Many researchers use 60 to 70 percent of RDA as the borderline between adequate and inadequate nutrient intake.

2. RDA are recommendations for *healthy* populations. Special needs for special groups (premature babies, individuals with infectious or chronic diseases) are not covered by the RDA. Registered dietitians who work in hospitals are trained to adapt the RDA for certain types of sick people.

3. RDA are intended to be met *by a diet of a wide variety of foods rather than by supplementation or by extensive fortification of single foods.* This is a very important point. The RDA only cover energy and 19 nutrients in the main tables, and 7 others in the additional table (see tables 3.1, 3.2, and 3.3). Some nutrients are left out because there is insufficient information to establish recommendations. Thus the RDA for vitamins and minerals are best met by eating food, not by taking pills.

4. The nutrient mix found in pills does not include all of the nutrients and substances found in fruits, vegetables, grains, nuts, dairy products, and meat products. This point will be discussed in much more detail in chapters 10 and 11.

Purposes of RDA

Table 3.4 outlines the major uses of the RDA. Many institutions, for example, schools, hospitals, and the military, use the RDA in planning and obtaining food supplies. National government dietary surveys like the Nationwide Food and Consumption Survey (NFCS) and the National Health and Nutrition Examination Survey (NHANES) use the RDA as their standard for comparison purposes. Government programs such as **Women, Infants, and Children (WIC)** or **Nutrition Education and Training (NET)** use the RDA as their standard for education.

TABLE 3.1
Median heights and weights and recommended energy intake

Category	Age (years) or Condition	Weight (kg)	Weight (lb)	Height (cm)	Height (in)	Average Energy Allowance (kcal)[b] REE[a] (kcal/day)	Average Energy Allowance (kcal)[b] Multiples of REE	Average Energy Allowance (kcal)[b] Per kg	Per day[c]
Infants	0.0–0.5	6	13	60	24	320		108	650
	0.5–1.0	9	20	71	28	500		98	850
Children	1–3	13	29	90	35	740		102	1,300
	4–6	20	44	112	44	950		90	1,800
	7–10	28	62	132	52	1,130		70	2,000
Males	11–14	45	99	157	62	1,440	1.70	55	2,500
	15–18	66	145	176	69	1,760	1.67	45	3,000
	19–24	72	160	177	70	1,780	1.67	40	2,900
	25–50	79	174	176	70	1,800	1.60	37	2,900
	51+	77	170	173	68	1,530	1.50	30	2,300
Females	11–14	46	101	157	62	1,310	1.67	47	2,200
	15–18	55	120	163	64	1,370	1.60	40	2,200
	19–24	58	128	164	65	1,350	1.60	38	2,200
	25–50	63	138	163	64	1,380	1.55	36	2,200
	51+	65	143	160	63	1,280	1.50	30	1,900
Pregnant	1st trimester								+0
	2nd trimester								+300
	3rd trimester								+300
Lactating	1st 6 months								+500
	2nd 6 months								+500

[a]Calculation based on FAO equations, then rounded.
[b]In the range of light to moderate activity, the coefficient of variation is ± 20%.
[c]Figure is rounded.

Reprinted with permission from: Food and Nutrition Board. Recommended Dietary Allowances. 10th rev. ed. 1989. Washington, DC: National Academy Press, 1989.

Food companies use the RDA to guide them in preparing food labels or in adding nutrients to food, which is called **food fortification.** Infant formulas, military combat rations, and even astronauts' rations are based on the RDA.

How RDA Are Estimated

When the Committee on Dietary Allowances meets to establish the RDA, it is faced with the very difficult task of establishing the RDA from a wide variety of scientific sources. Its report must then be approved by the governing board of the National Research Council, whose members are drawn from the councils of the National Academy of Sciences, the National Academy of Engineering, and the Institute of Medicine.

RDA estimation is not exact and has many limitations. Four steps are followed.

1. The average requirement of the population for a given vitamin or mineral is estimated. Unfortunately, the variability or range of individual needs for a given nutrient can be quite broad. Thus, the average is not always adequate for each person.

2. Because of this variability problem, the average requirement is next increased by an amount sufficient to meet the needs of nearly all members of the population.

3. For some nutrients, the RDA are increased even more to account for inefficient utilization by the body (poor absorption, for example) after the nutrient is consumed.

4. Finally, for some nutrients, common sense and judgment is used to interpret and extrapolate allowances when information on requirements is limited.

In chapters 10 and 11, a full description of the RDA for each nutrient will be given.

*T*ABLE 3.2

Food and Nutrition Board, National Academy of Sciences—National Research Council Recommended Dietary Allowances,[a] Revised 1989

Category	Age (years) or condition	Weight[b] (kg)	Weight[b] (lb)	Height[b] (cm)	Height[b] (in)	Protein (g)	Fat-Soluble Vitamins Vitamin A (μg RE)[c]	Vitamin D (μg)[d]	Vitamin E (mg α-TE)[e]	Vitamin K (μg)
Infants	0.0–0.5	6	13	60	24	13	375	7.5	3	5
	0.5–1.0	9	20	71	28	14	375	10	4	10
Children	1–3	13	29	90	35	16	400	10	6	15
	4–6	20	44	112	44	24	500	10	7	20
	7–10	28	62	132	52	28	700	10	7	30
Males	11–14	45	99	157	62	45	1,000	10	10	45
	15–18	66	145	176	69	59	1,000	10	10	65
	19–24	72	160	177	70	58	1,000	10	10	70
	25–50	79	174	176	70	63	1,000	5	10	80
	51+	77	170	173	68	63	1,000	5	10	80
Females	11–14	46	101	157	62	46	800	10	8	45
	15–18	55	120	163	64	44	800	10	8	55
	19–24	58	128	164	65	46	800	10	8	60
	25–50	63	138	163	64	50	800	5	8	65
	51+	65	143	160	63	50	800	5	8	65
Pregnant						60	800	10	10	65
Lactating	1st 6 months					65	1,300	10	12	65
	2nd 6 months					62	1,200	10	11	65

[a] The allowances, expressed as average daily intakes over time, are intended to provide for individual variations among most normal persons as they live in the United States under usual environmental stresses. Diets should be based on a variety of common foods in order to provide other nutrients for which human requirements have been less well defined.
[b] Weights and heights of Reference Adults are actual medians for the U.S. population of the designated age, as reported by NHANES II. The median weights and heights of those under 19 years of age were taken from Hamill et al. (1979) (see pages 16-17). The use of these figures does not imply that the height-to-weight ratios are ideal.

Reprinted with permission from: Food and Nutrition Board. Recommended Dietary Allowances. 10th rev. ed. 1989. Washington, DC: National Academy Press, 1989.

*T*ABLE 3.3

Estimated safe and adequate daily dietary intakes of selected vitamins and minerals[a]

Category	Age (years)	Vitamins Biotin (μg)	Pantothenic acid (mg)	Trace elements[b] Copper (mg)	Manganese (mg)	Fluoride (mg)	Chromium (mg)	Molybdenum (μg)
Infants	0–0.5	10	2	0.4–0.6	0.3–0.6	0.1–0.5	10–40	15–30
	0.5–1	15	3	0.6–0.7	0.6–1.0	0.2–1.0	20–60	20–40
Children	1–3	20	3	0.7–1.0	1.0–1.5	0.5–1.5	20–80	25–50
and	4–6	25	3–4	1.0–1.5	1.5–2.0	1.0–2.5	30–120	30–75
adolescents	7–10	30	4–5	1.0–2.0	2.0–3.0	1.5–2.5	50–200	50–150
	11+	30–100	4–7	1.5–2.5	2.0–5.0	1.5–2.5	50–200	75–250
Adults		30–100	4–7	1.5–3.0	2.0–5.0	1.5–4.0	50–200	75–250

[a] Because there is less information on which to base allowances, these figures are not given in the main table of RDA and are provided here in the form of ranges of recommended intakes.
[b] Since the toxic levels for many trace elements may be only several times usual intakes, the upper levels for the trace elements given in this table should not be habitually exceeded.

Reprinted with permission from: Food and Nutrition Board. Recommended Dietary Allowances. 10th rev. ed. 1989. Washington, DC: National Academy Press, 1989.

The RDA for energy (Calories) are treated differently from allowances for vitamins and minerals (3). *Average* energy needs for each age and sex group have been provided (see table 3.1). A surplus of energy from food is stored in the body as fat, which can lead to obesity and health problems (see chapters 8 and 9). The average energy needs of individuals vary widely based on physical activity, height and weight, and sex, for example. The energy RDA outlined in table 3.1 are provided with ranges to allow people to determine their unique requirements.

Water-Soluble Vitamins							Minerals						
Vitamin C (mg)	Thiamin (mg)	Riboflavin (mg)	Niacin (mg NE)[f]	Vita min B$_6$ (mg)	Folate (μg)	Vitamin B$_{12}$ (μg)	Cal- cium (mg)	Phos- phorus (mg)	Mag- nesium (mg)	Iron (mg)	Zinc (mg)	Iodine (μg)	Sele- nium (μg)
30	0.3	0.4	5	0.3	25	0.3	400	300	40	6	5	40	10
35	0.4	0.5	6	0.6	35	0.5	600	500	60	10	5	50	15
40	0.7	0.8	9	1.0	50	0.7	800	800	80	10	10	70	20
45	0.9	1.1	12	1.1	75	1.0	800	800	120	10	10	90	20
45	1.0	1.2	13	1.4	100	1.4	800	800	170	10	10	120	30
50	1.3	1.5	17	1.7	150	2.0	1,200	1,200	270	12	15	150	40
60	1.5	1.8	20	2.0	200	2.0	1,200	1,200	400	12	15	150	50
60	1.5	1.7	19	2.0	200	2.0	1,200	1,200	350	10	15	150	70
60	1.5	1.7	19	2.0	200	2.0	800	800	350	10	15	150	70
60	1.2	1.4	15	2.0	200	2.0	800	800	350	10	15	150	70
50	1.1	1.3	15	1.4	150	2.0	1,200	1,200	280	15	12	150	45
60	1.1	1.3	15	1.5	180	2.0	1,200	1,200	300	15	12	150	50
60	1.1	1.3	15	1.6	180	2.0	1,200	1,200	280	15	12	150	55
60	1.1	1.3	15	1.6	180	2.0	800	800	280	15	12	150	55
60	1.0	1.2	13	1.6	180	2.0	800	800	280	10	12	150	55
70	1.5	1.6	17	2.2	400	2.2	1,200	1,200	320	30	15	175	65
95	1.6	1.8	20	2.1	280	2.6	1,200	1,200	355	15	19	200	75
90	1.6	1.7	20	2.1	260	2.6	1,200	1,200	340	15	16	200	75

[c] Retinol equivalents. 1 retinol equivalent = 1 μg retinol or 6 μg β-carotene.
[d] As cholecalciferol. 10 μg cholecalciferol = 400 IU of vitamin D.
[e] α-Tocopherol equivalents. 1 mg d-α tocopherol = 1 α-TE.
[f] 1 NE (niacin equivalent) is equal to 1 mg of niacin or 60 mg of dietary tryptophan.

Should A New Basis for Determining RDA Be Utilized?

The RDA have traditionally represented the physiologic and metabolic requirements for vitamins and minerals (5,6). Recently, however, some have felt that the RDA should also reflect the relationship between diet and chronic disease prevention (heart disease and cancer, for example). During the early 1980s, scientific opinion on this question became so divisive that Dr. Frank Press of the National Research Council was forced to postpone publication of the tenth edition of the RDA, which was scheduled to be issued in 1985 (5). In 1989, the tenth edition was finally released. Six nutrients were at the center of the controversy: vitamins A, K, C, B$_{12}$, folate, and iron. For each of these nutrients, some experts recommended that the RDA be lowered to compare more closely with the Canadian and United Kingdom nutrient recommendations (see tables 3.5 and 3.6).

TABLE 3.4
Uses of the RDA

Category	Examples
Planning and obtaining food supplies for groups	Schools, hospitals, health care facilities; military and elderly
Sample diets for food programs	Thrifty Food Plan
Evaluation of dietary survey data and other scientific research	Reporting of NFCS, NHANES
Guide for food selection	Basic Four Food Groups
Food and nutrition information and education	WIC, NET
Food labeling	U.S. RDA
Food fortification	Standard fortification policies for white bread, milk
Developing new or modified food products	Military combat rations; space rations
Clinical dietetics	Therapeutic diets, when additional metabolic information is taken into account
Nutrient supplements and special dietary food	Infant formulas

TABLE 3.5
Summary examples of recommended nutrient intakes for Canadians, expressed as daily rates

Age	Sex	Weight (kg)	Energy (kcal)	Pro-tein (g)	Vit. A (RE[a])	Vit. D (µg)	Vit. E (mg)	Vit. C (mg)	Folate (µg)	Vit. B₁₂ (µg)	Cal-cium (mg)	Mag-nesium (mg)	Iron (mg)	Zinc (mg)	Thia-min (mg)	Ribo-flavin (mg)
Months																
0–4	Both	6.0	600	12[b]	400	10	3	20	25	0.3	250[c]	20	0.3[d]	2[d]	0.3	0.3
5–12	Both	9.0	900	12	400	10	3	20	40	0.4	400	32	7	3	0.4	0.5
Years																
1	Both	11	1100	13	400	10	3	20	40	0.5	500	40	6	4	0.5	0.6
2–3	Both	14	1300	16	400	5	4	20	50	0.6	550	50	6	4	0.6	0.7
4–6	Both	18	1800	19	500	5	5	25	70	0.8	600	65	8	5	0.7	0.9
7–9	M	25	2200	26	700	2.5	7	25	90	1.0	700	100	8	7	0.9	1.1
	F	25	1900	26	700	2.5	6	25	90	1.0	700	100	8	7	0.8	1.0
10–12	M	34	2500	34	800	2.5	8	25	120	1.0	900	130	8	9	1.0	1.3
	F	36	2200	36	800	2.5	7	25	130	1.0	1100	135	8	9	0.9	1.1
13–15	M	50	2800	49	900	2.5	9	30[e]	175	1.0	1100	185	10	12	1.1	1.4
	F	48	2200	46	800	2.5	7	30[e]	170	1.0	1000	180	13	9	0.9	1.1
16–18	M	62	3200	58	1000	2.5	10	40[e]	220	1.0	900	230	10	12	1.3	1.6
	F	53	2100	47	800	2.5	7	30[e]	190	1.0	700	200	12	9	0.8	1.1
19–24	M	71	3000	61	1000	2.5	10	40[e]	220	1.0	800	240	9	12	1.2	1.5
	F	58	2100	50	800	2.5	7	30[e]	180	1.0	700	200	13	9	0.8	1.1
25–49	M	74	2700	64	1000	2.5	9	40[e]	230	1.0	800	250	9	12	1.1	1.4
	F	59	1900	51	800	2.5	6	30[e]	185	1.0	700	200	13	9	0.8[f]	1.0[f]
50–74	M	73	2300	63	1000	5	7	40[e]	230	1.0	800	250	9	12	0.9	1.2
	F	63	1800	54	800	5	6	30[e]	195	1.0	800	210	8	9	0.8[f]	1.0[f]
75+	M	69	2000	59	1000	5	6	40[e]	215	1.0	800	230	9	12	0.8	1.0
	F[g]	64	1700	55	800	5	5	30[e]	200	1.0	800	210	8	9	0.8[f]	1.0[f]
Pregnancy (additional)																
1st Trimester			100	5	0	2.5	2	0	200	0.2	500	15	0	6	0.1	0.1
2nd Trimester			300	15	0	2.5	2	10	200	0.2	500	45	5	6	0.1	0.3
3rd Trimester			300	24	0	2.5	2	10	200	0.2	500	45	10	6	0.1	0.3
Lactation (additional)			450	20	400	2.5	3	25	100	0.2	500	65	0	6	0.2	0.4

[a] Retinol Equivalents
[b] Protein is assumed to be from breast milk and must be adjusted for infant formula.
[c] Infant formula with high phosphorus should contain 375 mg calcium.
[d] Breast milk is assumed to be the source of the mineral.
[e] Smokers should increase vitamin C by 50 percent.
[f] Level below which intake should not fall.
[g] Assumes moderate (more than average) physical activity.

Source: Health and Welfare Canada
Reproduced with permission of the Minister of Supply and Services Canada 1991.

TABLE 3.6
Recommended daily amounts of food energy and some nutrients for population groups in the United Kingdom

Age Range[a] (years)	Occupational Category	Energy[b] (MJ)	Energy[b] (Kcal)	Protein[c] (g)	Thiamin (mg)	Riboflavin (mg)	Nicotinic Acid Equivalents (mg)[d]	Ascorbic Acid (mg)	Vitamin A Retinol Equivalents (μg^e)	Vitamin D[f] Cholecalciferol (μg)	Calcium (mg)	Iron (mg)
1		5.0	1,200	30	0.5	0.6	7	20	300	10	600	7
2		5.75	1,400	35	0.6	0.7	8	20	300	10	600	7
3–4		6.5	1,560	39	0.6	0.8	9	20	300	10	600	8
5–6		7.25	1,740	43	0.7	0.9	10	20	300	f	600	10
7–8		8.25	1,980	49	0.8	1.0	11	20	400	f	600	10
9–11		9.5	2,280	57	0.9	1.2	14	25	575	f	700	12
12–14		11.0	2,640	66	1.1	1.4	16	25	725	f	700	12
15–17		12.0	2,880	72	1.2	1.7	19	30	750	f	600	12
1		4.5	1,100	27	0.4	0.6	7	20	300	10	600	7
2		5.5	1,300	32	0.5	0.7	8	20	300	10	600	7
3–4		6.25	1,500	37	0.6	0.8	9	20	300	10	600	8
5–6		7.0	1,680	42	0.7	0.9	10	20	300	f	600	10
7–8		8.0	1,900	47	0.8	1.0	11	20	400	f	600	10
9–11		8.5	2,050	51	0.8	1.2	14	25	575	f	700	12[h]
12–14		9.0	2,150	53	0.9	1.4	16	25	725	f	700	12[h]
15–17		9.0	2,150	53	0.9	1.7	19	30	750	f	600	12[h]
Men												
18–34	Sedentary	10.5	2,510	63	1.0	1.6	18	30	750	f	500	10
	Moderately active	12.0	2,900	72	1.2	1.6	18	30	750	f	500	10
	Very active	14.0	3,350	84	1.3	1.6	18	30	750	f	500	10
35–64	Sedentary	10.0	2,400	60	1.0	1.6	18	30	750	f	500	10
	Moderately active	11.5	2,750	69	1.1	1.6	18	30	750	f	500	10
	Very active	14.0	3,350	84	1.3	1.6	18	30	750	f	500	10
65–74	Assuming a	10.0	2,400	60	1.0	1.6	18	30	750	f	500	10
75+	sedentary life	9.0	2,150	54	0.9	1.6	18	30	750	f	500	10
Women												
18–54	Most occupations	9.0	2,150	54	0.9	1.3	15	30	750	f	500	12[h]
	Very active	10.5	2,500	62	1.0	1.3	15	30	750		500	12[h]
55–74	Assuming a	8.0	1,900	47	0.8	1.3	15	30	750	f	500	10
75+	sedentary life	7.0	1,680	42	0.7	1.3	15	30	750	f	500	10
Pregnancy		10.0	2,400	60	1.0	1.6	18	60	750	10	1,200[g]	13
Lactation		11.5	2,750	69	1.1	1.8	21	60	1,200	10	1,200	15

[a] Since the recommendations are average amounts, the figures for each age range represent the amounts recommended at the middle of the range. Within each age range, younger children will need less, and older children more, than the amount recommended.
[b] Megajoules (10^6 joules). Calculated from the relation 1 kilocalorie = 4.184 kilojoules, i.e., 1 megajoule = 240 kilocalories.
[c] Recommended amounts have been calculated as 10% of the recommendations for energy (paragraph 44 in original reference).
[d] 1 nicotinic acid equivalent = 1 mg available nicotinic acid or 60 mg tryptophan.
[e] 1 retinol equivalent = 1 µg retinol, 6 µg β-carotene, or 12 µg other biologically active carotenoids.
[f] No dietary sources may be necessary for children and adults who are sufficiently exposed to sunlight, but during the winter children and adolescents should receive 10 µg (400 i.u.) daily by supplementation. Adults with inadequate exposure to sunlight, for example those who are housebound, may also need a supplement of 10 µg daily.
[g] For the third trimester only.
[h] This intake may not be sufficient for 10% of girls and women with large menstrual losses.
Doubts have been expressed about the validity of the recommended daily amounts for folate and the figures have been withdrawn from this reprinted table. The Committee on Medical Aspects of Food Policy has decided that there is too little information at present upon which to base a practical recommendation for folate until further research has been done. A recommended daily amount for folate will be set as soon as sufficient information about folate requirements in the United Kingdom makes this possible.

From the *Report on Health and Social Subjects,* Department of Health and Social Security, Committee on Medical Aspects of Food Policy, 1979 (as per Third Impression, 1985). Reproduced with permission of the Controller of Her Britannic Majesty's Stationery Office, London.

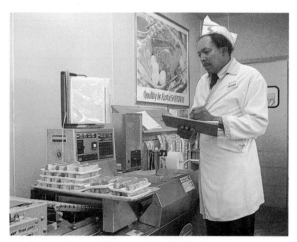
Food companies use RDA to guide them in the preparation of food to sell to consumers.

At the heart of the impasse were various nutrients that have been discovered to be important in cancer prevention. A specific example is vitamin A (6). Biochemical studies during the last fifteen years have given scientists a better basis for estimating the levels of dietary vitamin A required to maintain tissue at appropriate levels. This new information has led some experts to call for a *reduction* in the RDA for vitamin A. This comes at a time when an increase in the intake of vitamin A, or beta-carotene, for the possible prevention of certain types of cancer is being advocated by the American Cancer Society and the National Cancer Institute (see chapter 10, Health-Promotion Insight).

Should the RDA represent more than immediate needs for growth, development, prevention of deficiency diseases, and normal body function? Should the RDA also reflect the important association between diet and health? There are no easy answers. However, most nutrition experts feel that the RDA should reflect body needs for normal body function, whereas the Dietary Guidelines should promote the relationship between nutrient intake and high-level wellness, longevity, and chronic disease prevention (1). For example, study tables 3.2 and 3.3 carefully and notice that no RDA have been established for dietary fiber, fat, sugar, or cholesterol intake. However, these have been discussed thoroughly in the Dietary Goals and Dietary Guidelines (see chapter 2).

Estimated Safe and Adequate Intakes

Estimated safe and adequate intakes for two vitamins (pantothenic acid and biotin), and five trace elements (copper, chromium, fluoride, manganese, and molybdenum) are listed in table 3.3. Because of the increase in use of formulated foods, these nutrients have been given suggested intake ranges despite less-than-complete scientific data. Notice that table 3.7 gives the estimated minimum requirements for the three electrolytes—sodium, chloride, and potassium. Safe and adequate ranges are not provided for the three electrolytes because they are difficult to justify.

Conditions That May Require Adjustment in RDA

The RDA are intakes of nutrients that meet the needs of healthy people and do not take into account special needs that may require individual adaptation (3). Some of these conditions are:

1. *Physical activity.* Provided that foods are well selected, the increased need for various nutrients should be met by the larger quantities of food consumed (see chapter 12, Health-Promotion Insight).
2. *Climate.* Under most circumstances, adjustments in dietary allowances to compensate for temperature changes are not considered necessary (some consideration should be given for water, salt, and energy) (see chapter 12, Health-Promotion Insight).
3. *Aging.* As one ages, the lean body weight decreases as fat increases, lowering the basal energy metabolism (about two percent per decade after age 21) (see chapter 8). Since fewer Calories are expended, less food is needed. Unless food choices are made with great care, the amounts of essential nutrients consumed are likely to be less than desirable. In other words, each food choice should be rich in nutrients instead of high in fat and sugar Calories to ensure that enough vitamins and minerals are consumed despite the lowered Caloric intake. In addition, special dietary modifications may need to be made for people with various chronic diseases and for those who must take medication.

TABLE 3.7
Estimated sodium, chloride, and potassium minimum requirements of healthy persons[a]

Age	Weight (kg)[a]	Sodium (mg)[a,b]	Chloride (mg)[a,b]	Potassium (mg)[c]
Months				
0–5	4.5	120	180	500
6–11	8.9	200	300	700
Years				
1	11.0	225	350	1,000
2–5	16.0	300	500	1,400
6–9	25.0	400	600	1,600
10–18	50.0	500	750	2,000
>18[d]	70.0	500	750	2,000

[a]No allowance has been included for large, prolonged losses from the skin through sweat.

[b]There is no evidence that higher intakes confer any health benefit.

[c]Desirable intakes of potassium may considerably exceed these values (~3,500 mg for adults).

[d]No allowance included for growth. Values for those below 18 years assume a growth rate at the 50th percentile reported by the National Center for Health Statistics (Hamill et al., 1979) and averaged for males and females.

Reprinted with permission from: Food and Nutrition Board. Recommended Dietary Allowances. 10th rev. ed. 1989. Washington, DC: National Academy Press, 1989.

4. *Clinical problems.* The special nutritional needs of people with metabolic disorders, chronic diseases, injuries, and many other medical conditions, and the needs of premature infants, are not covered by RDA for healthy people. Infections, trauma, burns, and surgical procedures, for example, all increase the body's need for various nutrients.

Figure 3.1 shows the results from the National Health and Nutrition Examination Survey (NHANES II), a dietary survey that measures how the average American eats. From this figure you can see that the average American male obtains more than 100 percent of the RDA for each of the various nutrients, whereas the calcium and iron intakes of the average American female are marginal. These results will be discussed in greater detail in chapters 9 and 10.

The Concept of Nutrient Density

A **nutrient density** approach to evaluating the quality of diet has been developed at Utah State University (7,8). Nutrients are expressed on the basis of "per 1,000 Calories." Investigators in both Sweden and the U.S. have found that despite the sex or age of a person, nutrient requirements per 1,000 kcal are remarkably constant.

Table 3.8 outlines the single-value nutrient allowances per 1,000 Calories for all people one year of age and older. Expressing dietary allowances and the nutritional composition of foods or diets on this basis allows for a quick and accurate check of nutritional quality. Notice also that recommendations for fat, carbohydrate, added sugar, and cholesterol are given.

To see how to determine nutrient density of the diet, let us use Joe Brown as an example. Joe consumed 3,200 Calories of food on Sunday, primarily french fries, hamburgers, milkshakes, and snack chips. The total vitamin C and vitamin A intake for the day was 40 mg and 2,500 I.U., respectively. (I.U. = international units, see chapter 10.) To calculate the nutrient density for vitamin C, use the following formula:

$$\frac{40}{3,200} = \frac{X}{1,000} = \frac{40,000}{3,200} = 12.5 \text{ per 1,000 Calories}$$

Try to calculate the nutrient density for vitamin A on your own. (Your answer should be 781 I.U. per 1,000 Calories.) Notice that the recommended intakes in table 3.9 are much higher for both vitamin C (30 mg/1,000 Calories) and vitamin A (2,000 I.U./1,000 Calories). Joe's food choices were comparatively high in Calories but low in important nutrients.

The average American male and female consume more than
two-thirds the RDA for all major vitamins and minerals.

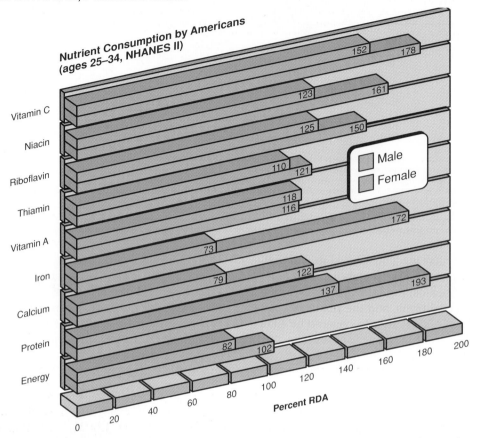

The United States Recommended Daily Allowances (U.S. RDA)

The **U.S. RDA** are a set of standards developed by the Food and Drug Administration (FDA) for use in regulating nutrition labeling. Although these standards were taken from the RDA, they are based on very few categories, and only 19 vitamins and minerals were chosen (see table 3.9). The values for adults and for children over the age of four were taken from the highest value given for each nutrient in the 1968 RDA tables for men and nonpregnant, nonlactating females. Separate U.S. RDA values were established for infants, children under four years of age, and pregnant or lactating women.

More and more foods now have nutrition labeling (see figure 3.2). Regulations adopted by the FDA in 1973 require manufacturers to provide nutrition information on their

TABLE 3.8

Single-value nutrient allowances per 1,000 kcal for heterogeneous populations 1 year of age and older

Nutrient	Allowance per 1,000 Kcal	
Protein	25	gm
Fat	39	gm
Carbohydrate	137.5	gm
Sugar, added	25	gm
Calcium	450	mg
Iron	8	mg
Magnesium	150	mg
Zinc	8	mg
Potassium	1,875	mg
Sodium	1,100	mg
Vitamin A	2,000	IU
Thiamin	0.5	mg
Riboflavin	0.6	mg
Vitamin B_6	1	mg
Vitamin B_{12}	1.5	μg
Vitamin C	30	mg
Folacin	200	μg
Cholesterol	175	mg

From R. G. Hansen et al. "Nutrient Density and Food Labeling." *Clinical Nutrition,*
4:164–170, 1985. Used with permission of Longman Group Ltd., Edinburgh.

TABLE 3.9
U.S. Recommended Daily Allowances (U.S. RDA)

Supplement	Adults and Children over 4 Years	Infants and Children under 4 Years	Pregnant or Lactating Women
Protein	65 g	25–28 g	65 g
Vitamin A	5,000 IU	2,500 IU	8,000 IU
Vitamin C	60 mg	40 mg	60 mg
Thiamin	1.5 mg	0.7 mg	1.7 mg
Riboflavin	1.7 mg	0.8 mg	2.0 mg
Niacin	20 mg	9.0 mg	20 mg
Calcium	1.0 g	0.8 g	1.3 g
Iron	18 mg	10 mg	18 mg
Vitamin D	400 IU	400 IU	400 IU
Vitamin E	30 IU	10 IU	30 IU
Vitamin B_6	2.0 mg	0.7 mg	2.5 mg
Folacin	0.4 mg	0.2 mg	0.8 mg
Vitamin B_{12}	6.0 μ	3 μ	8 μ
Phosphorus	1.0 g	0.8 g	1.3 g
Iodine	150 μ	70 μ	150 μ
Magnesium	400 mg	200 mg	450 mg
Zinc	15 mg	8 mg	15 mg
Copper	2.0 mg	1 mg	2 mg
Biotin	0.3 mg	0.15 mg	0.3 mg
Pantothenic acid	10 mg	5 mg	10 mg

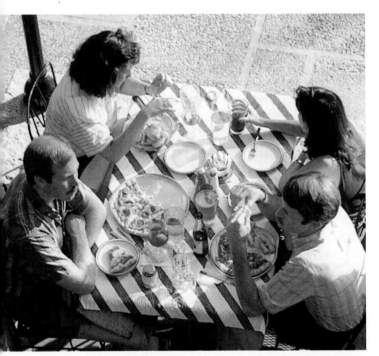

People's choice of food can be high in Calories but low in important nutrients.

product labels only if one or more nutrients are added to the food or if a nutritional claim is made about the product. Slightly more than half of all packaged foods today carry nutrition information, many of them voluntarily (9).

The nutrition information must include the number of Calories and the amount of protein, fat, carbohydrate, and sodium in a specified serving of a product. In addition, the label must show the protein content and the percentage of the U.S. RDA for seven essential vitamins and minerals in each serving. The FDA also requires that the ingredient present in the largest amount by weight is to be listed first, followed in order by other ingredients.

Nutrition labels and ingredient lists contain a wide array of technical and scientific terms. Surveys by the FDA show that while more than 80 percent of people have at least a functional understanding of such terms as cholesterol, calcium, and sodium, other such common terms as polyunsaturated fat, hydrogenated,

FIGURE 3.2

Food labels use percent U.S. RDA as their standard. Nutrition labels give nutrient information on a per serving basis.

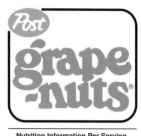

Nutrition Information Per Serving

Serving Size: 1 Oz.
(About 1/4 Cup) (28.35g)
Servings Per Package

	1 OZ. (28.35 g) Cereal	With 1/2 Cup (118 mL) Vitamin D Fortified Skim Milk
Calories	110	150
Protein	3 g	7 g
Carbohydrate	23 g	29 g
Fat	0	0 g
Sodium	190 mg	250 mg

Percentages of U.S. Recommended Daily Allowances (U.S. RDA)

Protein	4%	10%
Vitamin A	25%	30%
Vitamin C	**	**
Thiamine	25%	30%
Riboflavin	25%	35%
Niacin	25%	25%
Calcium	**	15%
Iron	15%	15%
Vitamin D	10%	25%
Vitamin B_6	25%	25%
Folic Acid	25%	25%
Vitamin B_{12}	25%	35%
Phosphorus	6%	15%
Magnesium	6%	10%
Zinc	8%	10%
Copper	6%	6%

**Contains less than 2% of the U.S. RDA of these nutrients.

Ingredients: Wheat, Malted Barley, Salt and Yeast.

Vitamins and Minerals: Vitamin A Palmitate, Niacinamide, Iron, Zinc Oxide (source of zinc), Vitamin B_6, Riboflavin (Vitamin B_2), Thiamine Mononitrate (Vitamin B_1), Vitamin B_{12}, Folic Acid and Vitamin D.

Carbohydrate Information

	1 OZ. Cereal	With 1/2 Cup Skim Milk
Complex Carbohydrates	18g	18g
Dietary Fiber	2g	2g
Maltose and Other Sugars*	3g	9g
Total Carbohydrate	23g	29g

*No sugar added. All sugars in GRAPE-NUTS® cereal occur naturally in the wheat and malted barley.

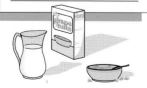

emulsifier, riboflavin, niacin, and potassium are understood by only a small minority. (In chapter 4 you will learn much more about food labels and food additives.) FDA surveys also show that Americans have great difficulty understanding the metric measurements used on food labels. For example, only six percent of Americans know that one gram is 1/28th of an ounce.

Study figure 3.2. Notice that the serving size of Grape Nuts is one ounce, or about one-fourth cup. A serving size is generally that amount of a particular food that an average adult male, engaged in light physical activity, would be expected to consume as a part of a meal.

The nutrition label must then list, on a per-serving basis, the amount of Calories, protein, carbohydrate, fat, and sodium. Notice that a serving of Grape Nuts has 110 Calories (without milk), three grams of protein, 23 grams of carbohydrate, and no fat. Sodium is 190 milligrams per serving.

Often nutritionists like to discuss the **percentage of total Calories** represented by protein, carbohydrate, and fat. This is useful to know and is calculated in the following manner:

$$1 \text{ gram carbohydrate} = 4 \text{ Calories}$$
$$1 \text{ gram protein} = 4 \text{ Calories}$$
$$1 \text{ gram fat} = 9 \text{ Calories}$$

In figure 3.2, Grape Nuts is represented as having 110 Calories per serving. To determine what percentage of the Calories is protein or carbohydrate or fat, the gram amount of each should be multiplied by the Calories/gram factor listed above, and then divided by the total energy (110 Calories). For example:

$$\text{Percent Calories as carbohydrate} = \frac{23 \text{ g} \times 4}{110 \text{ Calories}} = 83.6 \text{ percent}$$

$$\text{Percent Calories as protein} = \frac{3 \text{ g} \times 4}{110 \text{ Calories}} = 10.9 \text{ percent}$$

$$\text{Percent Calories as fat} = \frac{0 \text{ g} \times 9}{110 \text{ Calories}} = 0.0 \text{ percent}$$

Notice that the total percentage does not quite equal 100 percent. A common problem with food labels is that the gram amounts for the various nutrients are rounded off to the nearest whole number.

TABLE 3.10
Government agencies and congressional committees responsible for nutrition education and labeling activities and issues*

Education Area	House Committee	Senate Committee	Executive Branch
Nutrition Education and Training (NET)	Appropriations Education and Labor	Agriculture, Nutrition and Forestry Appropriations	Food and Nutrition Service, USDA
Dietary Guidance for the public (Dietary Guidelines)	Appropriations Agriculture Energy and Commerce	Agriculture, Nutrition and Forestry Appropriations Labor and Human Resources	Human Nutrition Information Service, USDA Office of Disease Prevention and Health Promotion, DHHS
Nutrition Education Resources	Appropriations Agriculture	Appropriations Agriculture, Nutrition and Forestry	Food and Nutrition Information Center, National Agriculture Library, USDA
Expanded Foods and Nutrition Education Program (EFNEP)	Agriculture Appropriations	Agriculture, Nutrition and Forestry Appropriations	Extensive Service, USDA
Sodium Reeducation Campaign	Energy and Commerce	Labor and Human Resources	Food and Drug Administration, DHHS
Cancer Communication Program	Appropriations Energy and Commerce	Appropriations Labor and Human Resources	National Cancer Institute, DHHS
National Cholesterol Education Project	Appropriations Energy and Commerce	Appropriations Labor and Human Resources	National Institute of Heart, Lung, and Blood, DHHS
Nutrition Labeling	Energy and Commerce	Labor and Human Resources	Food and Drug Administration, DHHS
Meat and Poultry Labeling	Agriculture	Agriculture, Nutrition and Forestry	Marketing and Inspection Service, USDA
Health Claims	Energy and Commerce	Labor and Human Resources Commerce, Science and Transportation	Food and Drug Administration, DHHS Federal Trade Commission

*This chart does not represent an exhaustive list of nutrition education activities conducted by the Federal government.

Notice that Grape Nuts has more than the required amount of vitamins and minerals listed and compared to the U.S. RDA. The listing of any other nutrient information is voluntary, and many manufacturers will list extra minerals and vitamins as well as carbohydrate information. The Post cereal company has listed dietary fiber, complex carbohydrates, and maltose and other sugars. (This information will be discussed in greater detail in chapter 5.)

What does it mean when the label says 15 percent U.S. RDA for iron? According to table 3.9, the U.S. RDA for iron is 18 milligrams.

Therefore, one serving of Grape Nuts has the following amount of iron:

$$15 \text{ percent} \times 18 \text{ mg} = 2.7 \text{ mg}$$

Calculate the amount of vitamin A in one serving of Grape Nuts. First take the U.S. RDA level from table 3.9 (5,000 I.U.), and then multiply it by 25 percent (percent U.S. RDA listed on the label for vitamin A). Your answer should be 1,250 I.U.

Various government agencies and congressional committees are responsible for nutrition education and food labeling activities and issues. These are outlined in table 3.10.

Major food groups, minor food groups, and examples of separate foods

Major Food Groups	Minor Food Groups	Sample Separate Foods	Major Food Groups	Minor Food Groups	Sample Separate Foods
Milk and milk products	Whole-milk products	Whole milk, chocolate milk, cheese (not cottage), cottage cheese (not low-fat)	Meat and meat alternates	Fish	Flounder, sole, anchovy, shrimp
	Low-fat milk products	Low-fat milk, skim milk, plain yogurt, fruit-flavored yogurt		Poultry	Chicken (except organ meat or luncheon meat), turkey (except organ meat or luncheon meat), poultry liver, poultry luncheon meat
Grain products	Whole-grain products	Shredded wheat, rye bread/rye rolls, brown rice, popcorn		Meat	Beef (except organ meat or luncheon meat), pork (except organ meat or luncheon meat), lamb, red meat liver
	Enriched products	White bread/white rolls, cornflakes, cookies, coffee cake		Eggs	All eggs
Fruits	Citrus, melon, and berries	Orange/orange juice, cantaloupe, strawberries, blueberries		Dried beans and peas	White beans, black beans, chickpeas, lentils
	Other fruits	Apples/ applesauce/apple juice, avocado, bananas, pears/ pear nectar		Nuts and seeds	Almonds, Brazil nuts, peanuts, sesame seeds
Vegetables	Dark green and deep yellow vegetables	Spinach, broccoli, carrots, squash	Fats, sweets, and alcohol	Fats	Bacon, salt pork, creams, oils
	Starchy vegetables	Potatoes, corn, plantain, potato chips		Sweets	Sugar, syrup, honey, popsicles
	Other vegetables	Cabbage, cauliflower, celery, cucumber		Alcohol	Beer, wine, liquor, liqueurs
			Miscellaneous foods		Plain gelatin, coffee, tea, bouillon

Daily Food Guides

Foods can be grouped into major and minor food groups. Table 3.11 outlines the types of divisions that are possible. In an attempt to translate nutritional information into easy-to-understand terms, the United States Department of Agriculture (USDA) has been publishing **Daily Food Guides** since 1917. The USDA has sought to define a "good diet" by recommending certain numbers of servings for the various food groups (see figure 3.3).

Most foods contain more than one nutrient, but no single food contains all the nutrients in the amounts needed. There is no such thing as a "perfect food." The Daily Food Guide suggests food combinations that together supply nutrients in the amounts needed. To use the Guide, one selects the main part of the diet from the four general food groups. To this, one adds other foods as desired to make meals appealing and satisfying. The additional foods should add enough Calories to meet energy needs, which will vary widely for different people. The

*F*IGURE 3.3

The USDA has sought to define a good diet by recommending certain numbers of servings for four food groups.

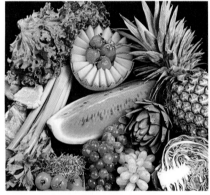

**Guide to Good Eating–
the Four Food Group Plan**

Bread-cereal group

Milk-cheese group

Vegetable-fruit group

Meat-poultry-fish-beans-nuts

Number in box = # of servings/day

Caution:

Fats, sweets, alcohol

*These foods provide Calories
but few nutrients*

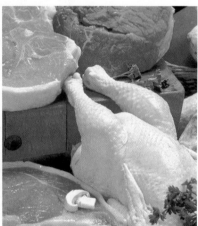

suggested number of servings in the food guide (4–4–2–2) will average about 1,200 Calories. One obtains additional Calories by increasing the number of servings in the various food groups.

The first food guide from the USDA was published in 1917 and contained five food groups: flesh foods, starch foods, fat foods, watery fruits and vegetables, and sweets (10). At that time, very little was known about vitamins, and emphasis was placed on energy from carbohydrate, fat, and protein.

During World War II, the Basic Seven Food Group Guide was formulated, which had three fruit and vegetable groups, along with groups represented by butter and margarine, grain products, dairy products, and meats. In 1958, the USDA published a daily food plan popularly called the Four Food Groups, which combined the three fruit and vegetable groups into a single group and eliminated the butter and margarine group. Finally, in 1979, the USDA published the Hassle-Free Guide to a Better Diet, which included a fifth food group—fats, sweets, and alcohol—for which no servings are recommended (11). Table 3.12 summarizes the Hassle-Free Guide from the USDA.

The Four Food Groups and the Hassle-Free Guide to a Better Diet have been criticized by many because it is possible to follow the basic

TABLE 3.12
Servings sizes used in the food group guides

Fruit and Vegetable Group (4 servings/day)

1 serving is:

½ cup

A small salad

A medium-sized potato

An orange

½ cantaloupe

½ grapefruit

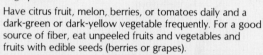

Have citrus fruit, melon, berries, or tomatoes daily and a dark-green or dark-yellow vegetable frequently. For a good source of fiber, eat unpeeled fruits and vegetables and fruits with edible seeds (berries or grapes).

Bread and Cereal Group (4 servings/day)

1 serving is:

1 slice of bread

½ to ¾ cup cooked cereal or pasta

1 ounce ready-to-eat cereal

Choose whole-grain products often.

Milk and Cheese Group (2 to 4 servings/day)

1 serving is:

1 cup milk or yogurt

1 ⅓ ounces cheddar or Swiss cheese

2 ounces processed cheese food

1 ½ cups ice cream or ice milk

2 cups cottage cheese

Skim, nonfat, and low-fat milk and milk products provide calcium and keep fat intake down.

Meat, Poultry, Fish, and Beans (2 servings/day)

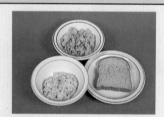

½ serving is:

1 to 1 ½ ounces lean, boneless, cooked meat, poultry, or fish

1 egg

½ to ¾ cup cooked dry beans, peas, lentils, or soybeans

2 tablespoons peanut butter

¼ to ½ cup nuts, sesame or sunflower seeds

Poultry and fish have less fat content than red meats.

Fats, Sweets, Alcohol (Caution)

These foods provide Calories but few nutrients.

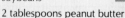

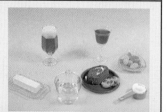

FIGURE 3.4
Australian nutrition foundation pyramid. This adopts the idea of the Swedish diet pyramid to combine Australian food groups and dietary guidelines.

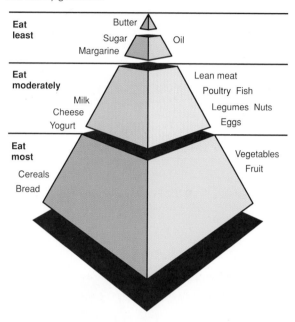

guide and still fail to eat a healthy diet. For example, a cheeseburger could give an adolescent a serving from each group (cheese for the milk and cheese group; a beef patty for the meat, poultry, fish, and beans group; a hamburger bun for the bread-cereal group; and onions and tomato for the vegetable-fruit group). However, intake of salt and fat would be high, and dietary fiber would be low.

Others have claimed that the Basic Four Food Groups plan is unnecessarily heavy in its emphasis on animal products (10). This emphasis became especially evident when the U.S. Dietary Goals and publications from the American Heart Association and American Cancer Society recommended that Americans decrease their intake of animal and high-fat dairy products and increase their intake of fruits, vegetables, and whole grains (see chapter 2).

Dr. Helen Guthrie conducted research on 212 young adults who were following the suggested number of servings from the Four Food Groups (13). Only one-third attained the RDA for vitamin E, vitamin B_6, iron, and zinc, and only two-thirds achieved the RDA for folacin and magnesium. If the goal of a food guide is to

TABLE 3.13
Combining the food guide with the dietary guidelines

Fruits and Vegetables: 4 servings/day	Milk and Cheese Group: adults, 2 servings; children, 2–4 servings
Serving = ½ cup, orange, small salad, medium-sized potato, ½ grapefruit, ½ cantaloupe. Major source of vitamins A and C, folic acid.	Serving = 1 cup milk or yogurt; 1 ⅓ ounces cheddar or Swiss cheese, 2 cups cottage cheese. Major source of calcium, riboflavin, protein, vitamin B_{12}, magnesium.
*Anytime (every day)	*Anytime (every day)
Most fruits and vegetables, raw, unseasoned frozen, or properly cooked (preferably steamed, low in fat and salt seasoning, with use of more herbs), especially: dark green and yellow vegetables (carrots, kale, yellow squash, collard greens, etc.), cruciferous vegetables (broccoli, cauliflower, brussels sprouts, cabbage), melons, and citrus fruits. Also dried fruits for those not needing to lose weight.	Skim milk (fresh or dry), nonfat or low-fat plain yogurt, low-fat cottage cheese, 1 percent low-fat milk.
*In Moderation (one to three times per week)	*In Moderation (one to three times per week)
Fruit juices and sauces (preferably unsweetened); unsalted vegetable juices; canned vegetables; seasoned frozen vegetables; cooked vegetables with light use of fat, salt, and spices; canned fruits in light syrup or own fruit juices; avocados; olives.	Low-fat cheeses such as part skim mozzarella, sapsago, farmer, part skim Swiss, buttermilk (made from skim milk), 2 percent low-fat milk, regular cottage cheese (4 percent milkfat), frozen low-fat yogurt, ice milk, low-fat yogurt (sweetened).
*Now and Then (once a week or less)	*Now and Then (once a week or less)
Vegetable and fruit products prepared with high fat, salt, sugar, and reduced fiber (potato chips, french fries, pickled vegetables, instant mashed potatoes, sweetened canned fruit, sweetened fruit juices).	Processed cheese and cheese foods, salty natural cheeses such as blue, camembert, cream, natural cheddar, and most other natural cheeses; sour cream; whole milk (fresh, evaporated, or dry); sweetened condensed milk; ice cream; fountain drinks made with ice cream; malted milk; cheese souffle; cheesecake; eggnog; puddings made with milk.

Bread and Cereal Group: 4 servings/day	Poultry, Fish, Meat, Eggs, Legumes, Nuts, and Seeds: 2 servings per day
Serving = 1 slice of bread, ½ to ¾ cup cooked cereal; 1 ounce ready-to-eat cereal. Major source of thiamin, niacin, iron, zinc.	Serving = 3 ounces meat, 1–1 ½ cups cooked dry beans, ½–1 cup nuts, sesame, or sunflower seeds. Major source of protein, iron, niacin, thiamin, vitamins B_6 and B_{12}, folic acid, magnesium, zinc.
*Anytime (every day)	*Anytime (every day)
Whole-grain products such as whole-wheat bread, brown rice, whole-grain hot and cold cereals low in sugar and salt (such as shredded wheat, Grape Nuts, and oatmeal), rye or pumpernickel bread, whole-wheat pasta.	Dried beans and peas, lentils, chick peas, soybeans, egg whites, fresh or frozen chicken or turkey (boiled or roasted, without skin), fresh or frozen fish prepared with little fat, tuna packed in water.
*In Moderation (one to three times a week)	*In Moderation (one to three times per week)
Low fiber grain products such as cornbread, flour tortilla, refined, unsweetened cereals, white bread and rolls, white rice, pasta, pizza, waffles or pancakes (unless whole wheat), crackers (unless whole grain and low in salt and fat).	Nuts, sunflower seeds, tofu, peanut butter, meat analogs, canned beans, various canned fish (drain well), shellfish, chicken or turkey with skin, eggs, lean cuts of meat (trim off all outside fat).
*Now and Then (once a week or less)	*Now and Then (once a week or less)
Grain products high in salt, fat, and/or sugar, and low in fiber (such as pretzels, salted crackers, pastries, doughnuts, presweetened breakfast cereals, croissants, cookies, and cake).	Fried chicken, frozen fish sticks, egg dishes (quiche, cheese omelet, souffle), bacon, organ meats, cold cuts, corned beef, ground beef, ham, frankfurters, spareribs, untrimmed red meats, sirloin steak, veal, sausage.

ensure an intake equal to the RDAs, a modification of the Four Food Groups guide is indicated to correct these shortcomings.

For these reasons, some nutritionists have developed food guides that combine the four food groups with the dietary guidelines. These types of food guides help people to make better choices within each category. Table 3.13 gives an adaptation of several of these. Figure 3.4 depicts the Australian nutrition foundation pyramid that adopts the idea of the Swedish diet pyramid to combine food group concepts with those from dietary guidelines.

Another problem associated with the Daily Food Guides is the confusion about serving sizes. Table 3.12 shows that servings within the milk group range from one cup of milk to two cups of cottage cheese. In the meat group, the USDA chooses to use the term "½ serving." Entire servings, therefore, would be one and one-half cups of dry beans, four tablespoons of

TABLE 3.14
Exchange lists

The reason for dividing food into six different groups is that foods vary in their carbohydrate, protein, fat, and Calorie content. Each exchange list contains foods that are alike; each choice contains about the same amount of carbohydrate, protein, fat, and Calories.

The following chart shows the amount of these nutrients in one serving from each exchange list.*

Exchange List	Carbohydrate (g)	Protein (g)	Fat (g)	Calories
Starch/bread	15	3	trace	80
Meat (lean)	—	7	3	55
(medium-fat)	—	7	5	75
(high-fat)	—	7	8	100
Vegetable	5	2	—	25
Fruit	15	—	—	60
Milk (skim)	12	8	trace	90
(low-fat)	12	8	5	120
(whole)	12	8	8	150
Fat	—	—	5	45

As you read the exchange lists (pages 61–67), you will notice that one choice often is a larger amount of food than another choice from the same list. Because foods are so different, each food is measured or weighed so the amount of carbohydrate, protein, fat, and Calories is the same in each choice.

*The exchange lists are based on material in the *Exchange Lists for Meal Planning* prepared by Committees of the American Diabetes Association, Inc. and the American Dietetic Association in cooperation with the National Institute of Arthritis, Metabolism, and Digestive Diseases and the National Heart and Lung Institutes of Health, Public Health Service, U.S. Department of Health and Human Services.

Reproduced with permission of the American Diabetes Association.

peanut butter, or one cup of nuts. The USDA decided to base serving size in the milk group on the amount of calcium contained in one cup of milk. Serving size in the meat group is based on the amount of protein in two to three ounces of meat. Thus, serving sizes of some foods in these two groups may be more than humans would typically consume.

Researchers have found that young adults often select servings of dry cereal, fruit juice, and breads that are larger than those given by the USDA. Servings for raw vegetables, meats, fish, and poultry tend to vary widely, and servings of milk usually are in the amounts recommended (13,14). In one national study, for a given 24-hour period only 63 percent of Americans were found to consume any type of fruit, and only 23 percent used whole-grain products (15). Only two and one-half servings of bread-cereal were consumed per day, versus the recommended four. Sweets and fats, however, were consumed by 82 percent and 97 percent of Americans, respectively. Ninety-six percent of Americans ate meat, but dried beans and peas were consumed by only eight percent.

In one other national study, the four food groups were used as the criteria for comparing three-day food intakes to the number of servings suggested from these groups. Only three percent of Americans were found to be averaging the number of servings recommended by the USDA. From these studies, it appears that U.S. diets do not measure up when the Daily Food Guide is used as the standard.

Food Exchange System

In one of the health-promotion activities at the end of this chapter, you will have an opportunity to calculate the nutrient composition of your diet. You may feel that using food composition tables to calculate your dietary quality is cumbersome, time consuming, and needlessly precise. You need not despair, however. Various professional groups have combined their expertise to produce what is known today as the **Food Exchange System.** The Exchange System was first developed in 1950, and then revised in 1976 and 1986 (16) (see table 3.14 and pages 61–67).

Starch/Bread List

Each item in this list contains about 15 g of carbohydrate, 3 g of protein, a trace of fat, and 80 Calories.

Whole-grain products average about 2 g of fiber per serving. Some foods are higher in fiber. Those foods that contain 3 or more g of fiber per serving are identified with the fiber symbol.†

You can choose your starch servings from any of the items on this list. If you want to eat a starch food that is not on this list, the general rule is that:

- ½ cup of cereal, grain, or pasta is one serving
- 1 ounce of bread product is one serving

Cereals/Grains/Pasta

Bran cereals†, flaked	½ cup
Bran cereals†, concentrated	⅓ cup
(such as Bran Buds, All Bran)	
Puffed cereal	1 ½ cup
Grapenuts	3 Tbsp
Shredded wheat	½ cup
Other ready-to-eat unsweetened cereals	¾ cup
Cooked cereals	½ cup
Bulgur (cooked)	½ cup
Grits (cooked)	½ cup
Pasta (cooked)	½ cup
Rice, white or brown (cooked)	⅓ cup
Cornmeal (dry)	2½ Tbsp
Wheat germ†	3 Tbsp

Dried Beans, Peas/Lentils

Beans† and peas† (cooked), e.g.,	⅓ cup
kidney, white, split, blackeye	
Lentils† (cooked)	⅓ cup
Baked beans†	¼ cup

Starchy Vegetables

Corn†	½ cup
Corn on cob†, 6″ long	1
Lima beans†	½ cup
Peas, green† (canned or frozen)	½ cup
Plantain†	½ cup
Potato, baked	1 small (3 oz)
Potato, mashed	½ cup
Squash, winter† (acorn, butternut)	¾ cup
Yam, sweet potato, plain	⅓ cup

Bread

Whole wheat	1 slice (1 oz)
Pita, 6″ across	½
Raisin, unfrosted	1 slice (1 oz)
Rye†, pumpernickel†	1 slice (1 oz)

Bread (continued)

White (including French, Italian)	1 slice (1 oz)
Bagel	½ (1 oz)
Bread sticks, crisp, 4″ long × ½″	2 (⅔ oz)
Croutons, low-fat	1 cup
English muffin	½
Plain roll, small	1 (1 oz)
Frankfurter or hamburger bun	½ (1 oz)
Tortilla, 6″ across	1

Crackers/Snacks

Animal crackers	8
Graham crackers, 2½″ square	3
Matzoth	¾ oz
Melba toast	5 slices
Oyster crackers	24
Popcorn (popped, no fat added)	3 cups
Pretzels	¾ oz
Rye crisp, 2″ × 3½″	4
Saltine-type crackers	6
Whole-wheat crackers, no fat added	2–4 slices
(crispbreads, such as Finn,	(¾ oz)
Kavli, Wasa)	

Starch Foods Prepared With Fat (Count as 1 starch/bread serving plus 1 fat serving)

Biscuit, 2½″ across	1
Chow mein noodles	½ cup
Corn bread, 2″ cube	1 (2 oz)
Cracker, round butter type	6
French fried potatoes, 2″ to 3½″ long	10 (1½ oz)
Muffin, plain, small	1
Pancake, 4″ across	2
Waffle, 4½″ square	1
Stuffing, bread (prepared)	¼ cup
Taco shell, 6″ across	2
Whole-wheat crackers, fat added	4–6 (1 oz)
(such as Triscuits)	

†3 g or more of fiber per serving.

Meat List

Each serving of meat and substitutes on this list contains varying amounts of fat and Calories. The list is divided into three parts based on the amount of fat and Calories: lean meat, medium-fat meat, and high-fat meat. One ounce (one meat exchange) of each of these includes:

	Carbohydrate (g)	Protein (g)	Fat (g)	Calories
Lean	0	7	3	55
Medium-fat	0	7	5	75
High-fat	0	7	8	100

You are encouraged to use more lean and medium-fat meat, poultry, and fish in your meal plan. This will help decrease your fat intake, which may help decrease your risk for heart disease. The items from the high-fat group are high in saturated fat, cholesterol, and Calories. You should limit your choices from the high-fat group to three (3) times per week. Meat and substitutes do not contribute any fiber to your meal plan. Meat and meat substitutes that have 400 mg or more of sodium are identified with a § symbol.

Tips:

1. Bake, roast, broil, grill, or boil these foods rather than frying them with added fat.
2. Use a nonstick pan spray or a nonstick pan to brown or fry these foods.
3. Trim off visible fat before and after cooking.
4. Do not add flour, bread crumbs, coating mixes, or fat to these foods when preparing them.
5. Weigh meat after removing bones and fat, and after cooking. Three ounces of cooked meat is about equal to 4 ounces of raw meat. Some examples of meat portions are:

   2 oz meat (2 meat exchanges) = 1 small chicken leg or thigh
   ½ cup cottage cheese or tuna

   3 oz meat (3 meat exchanges) = 1 medium pork chop
   1 small hamburger
   ½ chicken breast (1 side)
   1 unbreaded fish fillet
   cooked meat, about the size of a deck of cards

6. Restaurants usually serve prime cuts of meat, which are high in fat and Calories.

Lean Meat and Substitutes

(One exchange is equal to any one of the following items)

Beef:	USDA Good or Choice grades of lean beef, such as round, sirloin, and flank steak, tenderloin, and chipped beef§	1 oz
Pork:	Lean pork, such as fresh ham; canned, cured, or boiled ham; Canadian bacon§, tenderloin	1 oz
Veal:	All cuts are lean except for veal cutlets (ground or cubed). Examples of lean veal are chops and roasts.	1 oz
Poultry:	Chicken, turkey, Cornish hen (without skin)	1 oz
Fish:	All fresh and frozen fish	1 oz
	Crab, lobster, scallops, shrimp, clams (fresh, or canned in water§)	2 oz
	Oysters	6 medium
	Tuna§ (canned in water)	¼ cup
	Herring (uncreamed or smoked)	1 oz
	Sardines (canned)	2 medium
Wild Game:	Venison, rabbit, squirrel	1 oz
	Pheasant, duck, goose (without skin)	1 oz
Cheese:	Any cottage cheese	¼ cup
	Grated Parmesan	2 Tbsp
	Diet cheese§ with less than 55 Calories per oz	1 oz
Other:	95% fat-free luncheon meat§	1 oz
	Egg whites	3 whites
	Egg substitutes with less than 55 Calories per ¼ cup	¼ cup

Medium-Fat Meat and Substitutes

(One exchange is equal to any one of the following items)

Beef:	Most beef products fall into this category. Examples are all ground beef, roast (rib, chuck, rump), steak (cubed, Porterhouse, T-bone), and meatloaf	1 oz
Pork:	Most pork products fall into this category. Examples are chops, loin roast, Boston butt, cutlets	1 oz
Lamb:	Most lamb products fall into this category. Examples are chops, leg, and roast	1 oz
Veal:	Cutlet (ground or cubed, unbreaded)	1 oz
Poultry:	Chicken (with skin), domestic duck or goose (well-drained of fat), ground turkey	1 oz
Fish:	Tuna§ (canned in oil and drained), salmon§ (canned)	¼ cup
Cheese:	Skim or part-skim milk cheeses, such as	
	ricotta	¼ cup
	Mozzarella	1 oz
	Diet cheeses§ with 56–80 Calories per oz	1 oz
Other:	86% fat-free luncheon meat§	1 oz
	Egg (high in cholesterol, limit to 3 per week)	1
	Egg substitutes with 56–80 Calories per ¼ cup	¼ cup
	Tofu (2½″ × 2¾″ × 1″)	4 oz
	Liver, heart, kidney, sweetbreads (high in cholesterol)	1 oz

Meat List *(continued)*

High-Fat Meat and Substitutes

Remember, these items are high in saturated fat, cholesterol, and Calories, and should be used only three (3) times per week. (One exchange is equal to any one of the following items)

Beef:	Most USDA Prime cuts of beef, such as ribs, corned beef§	1 oz
Pork:	Spareribs, ground pork, pork sausage§ (patty or link)	1 oz
Lamb:	Patties (ground lamb)	1 oz
Fish:	Any fried fish product	1 oz
Cheese:	All regular cheese,§ such as American, blue, cheddar, Monterey, Swiss	1 oz
Other:	Luncheon meat,§ such as bologna, salami, pimento loaf	1 oz
	Sausage,§ such as Polish, Italian, knockwurst, smoked	1 oz
	bratwurst§	1 oz
	Frankfurters§ (turkey or chicken)††	1 frank (10/lb).
	Peanut butter (contains unsaturated fat)	1 Tbsp

§400 mg or more of sodium per exchange.
††Frankfurter (beef, pork or combination). Count as one high-fat meat plus one fat exchange: 1 frank (10/lb).

Fruit List

Each item on this list contains about 15 g of carbohydrate and 60 Calories. Fresh, frozen, and dry fruits have about 2 g of fiber per serving. Fruits that have 3 g or more of fiber per serving have a † symbol. Fruit juices contain very little dietary fiber.

The carbohydrate and Calorie content for a fruit serving are based on the usual serving of the most commonly eaten fruits. Use fresh fruits, or fruits frozen or canned without sugar added. Whole fruit is more filling than fruit juice, and may be a better choice for those who are trying to lose weight. Unless otherwise noted, the serving size for fruit is:

- ½ cup of fresh fruit or fruit juice
- ¼ cup of dried fruit

Fresh, Frozen, and Unsweetened Canned Fruit

Apple (raw, 2″ across)	1 apple	Persimmon (medium, native)	2 persimmons
Applesauce (unsweetened)	½ cup	Pineapple (raw)	¾ cup
Apricots (medium, raw)	4 apricots	Pineapple (canned)	⅓ cup
Apricots (canned)	½ cup, or 4 halves	Plum (raw, 2″ across)	2 plums
Banana (9″ long)	½ banana	†Pomegranate	½ pomegranate
†Blackberries (raw)	¾ cup	†Raspberries (raw)	1 cup
†Blueberries (raw)	¾ cup	†Strawberries (raw, whole)	1-¼ cup
Cantaloupe (5″ across)	⅓ melon	†Tangerine (2-½″ across)	2 tangerines
(cubes)	1 cup	Watermelon (cubes)	1-¼ cup
Cherries (large, sweet, raw)	12 cherries	*Dried Fruit*	
Cherries (canned)	½ cup		
Figs (raw, 2″ across)	2 figs	†Apples	4 rings
Fruit cocktail (canned)	½ cup	†Apricots	7 halves
Grapefruit (medium)	½ grapefruit	Dates	2-½ medium
Grapefruit (segments)	¾ cup	†Figs	1-½
Grapes (small)	15 grapes	†Prunes	3 medium
Honeydew melon (medium)	⅛ melon	Raisins	2 Tbsp
(cubes)	1 cup	*Fruit Juices*	
Kiwi (large)	1 kiwi		
Mandarin oranges	¾ cup	Apple juice/cider	½ cup
Mango (small)	½ mango	Cranberry juice cocktail	⅓ cup
†Nectarine (1-½″ across)	1 nectarine	Grapefruit juice	½ cup
Orange (2-½″ across)	1 orange	Grape juice	⅓ cup
Papaya	1 cup	Orange juice	½ cup
Peach (2-¾″ across)	1 peach, or ¾ cup	Pineapple juice	½ cup
Peaches (canned)	½ cup, or 2 halves	Prune juice	⅓ cup
Pear	½ large, 1 small		
Pears (canned)	½ cup, or 2 halves		

Vegetable List

Each vegetable serving on this list contains about 5 g of carbohydrate, 2 g of protein, and 25 Calories. Vegetables contain 2–3 g of dietary fiber. Vegetables that contain 400 mg or more of sodium per serving are identified with a § symbol.

Vegetables are a good source of vitamins and minerals. Fresh and frozen vegetables have more vitamins and less added salt. Rinsing canned vegetables will remove much of the salt.

Unless otherwise noted, the serving size for vegetables is:

- ½ cup of cooked vegetables or vegetable juice
- 1 cup of raw vegetables

Artichoke (½ medium)	Eggplant	Rutabaga
Asparagus	Greens (collard, mustard, turnip)	Sauerkraut§
Beans (green, wax, Italian)	Kohlrabi	Spinach, cooked
Bean sprouts	Leeks	Summer squash (crookneck)
Beets	Mushrooms, cooked	Tomato (one large)
Broccoli	Okra	Tomato/vegetable juice§
Brussels sprouts	Onions	Turnips
Cabbage, cooked	Pea pods	Water chestnuts
Carrots	Peppers (green)	Zucchini, cooked
Cauliflower		

Starchy vegetables such as corn, peas, and potatoes are found on the Starch/Bread list.

For free vegetables, see Free Food list.

Milk List

Each serving of milk or milk products on this list contains about 12 g of carbohydrate and 8 g of protein. The amount of fat in milk is measured in percent (%) of butterfat. The Calories vary, depending on what kind of milk you choose. The list is divided into three parts based on the amount of fat and Calories: skim/very low-fat milk, low-fat milk, and whole milk. One serving (one milk exchange) of each of these includes:

	Carbohydrate (g)	Protein (g)	Fat (g)	Calories
Skim/Very low-fat	12	8	trace	90
Low-fat	12	8	5	120
Whole	12	8	8	150

Milk is the body's main source of calcium, the mineral needed for growth and repair of bones. Yogurt is also a good source of calcium. Yogurt and many dry or powdered milk products have different amounts of fat. If you have questions about a particular item, read the label to find out the fat and Calorie content.

Milk is good to drink, but it can also be added to cereal and to other foods. Many tasty dishes such as sugar-free pudding are made with milk (see the Combination Foods list). Plain yogurt is delicious with one of your fruit servings mixed with it.

Skim and Very Low-Fat Milk

- 1 cup skim milk
- 1 cup ½% milk
- 1 cup 1% milk
- 1 cup low-fat buttermilk
- ½ cup evaporated skim milk
- ⅓ cup dry nonfat milk
- 8-oz carton plain nonfat yogurt

Low-Fat Milk

- 1 cup fluid 2% milk
- 8-oz carton plain low-fat yogurt
(with added nonfat milk solids)

Whole Milk

The whole-milk group has much more fat per serving than the skim and low-fat groups. Whole milk has more that 3¼% butterfat. Try to limit your choices from the whole-milk group as much as possible.

- 1 cup whole milk
- ½ cup evaporated whole milk
- 8-oz carton whole plain yogurt

Fat List

Each serving on the fat list contains about 5 g of fat and 45 Calories.

The foods on the fat list contain mostly fat, although some items may also contain a small amount of protein. All fats are high in calories and should be carefully measured. Everyone should modify their fat intake by eating unsaturated fats instead of saturated fats. The sodium content of these foods varies widely. Check the label for sodium information.

Unsaturated Foods		Saturated Fats	
Avocado	⅛ medium	Butter	1 tsp
Margarine	1 tsp	Bacon#	1 slice
Margarine, diet#	1 Tbsp	Chitterlings	½ oz
Mayonnaise	1 tsp	Coconut, shredded	2 Tbsp

Fat List *(continued)*

Unsaturated Foods		Saturated Fats	
Mayonnaise, reduced-Calorie#	1 Tbsp	Coffee whitener, liquid	2 Tbsp
Nuts and seeds:		Coffee whitener, powder	4 tsp
Almonds, dry roasted	6 whole	Cream (light, coffee, table)	2 Tbsp
Cashews, dry roasted	1 Tbsp	Cream, sour	2 Tbsp
Pecans	2 whole	Cream (heavy, whipping)	1 Tbsp
Peanuts	20 small, 10 large	Cream cheese	1 Tbsp
Walnuts	2 whole	Salt pork#	¼ oz
Other nuts	1 Tbsp		
Seeds, pine nuts, sunflower (without shells)	1 Tbsp		
Pumpkin seeds	2 tsp		
Oil (corn, cottonseed, safflower, soybean, sunflower, olive, peanut)	1 tsp		
Olives#	10 small, 5 large		
Salad dressing, mayonnaise-type	2 tsp		
Salad dressing, mayonnaise-type, reduced-Calorie	1 Tbsp		
Salad dressing (all varieties)#	1 Tbsp		
Salad dressing, reduced-Calorie (two tablespoons of low-Calorie is a free food)§	2 Tbsp		

#If more than one or two servings are eaten, foods have 400 mg or more of sodium.

Free Foods

A free food is any food or drink that contains 20 Calories or less per serving. You can eat as much as you want of those items that have no serving size specified. You may eat two or three servings per day of those items that have a specific serving size. Be sure to spread them out through the day.

Drinks

Bouillon§ or broth without fat†
Bouillon, low-sodium
Carbonated drinks, sugar-free
Carbonated water
Club soda
Cocoa powder, unsweetened (1 Tbsp)
Coffee/Tea
Drink mixes, sugar-free
Mineral water
Tonic water, sugar-free

Nonstick pan spray

Fruit

Cranberries, unsweetened (½ cup)
Rhubarb, unsweetened (½ cup)

Vegetables (raw, 1 cup)

Cabbage
Celery
Chinese cabbage†
Cucumber
Green onion
Hot peppers
Mushrooms
Radishes
Zucchini†
Salad greens:
Endive
Escarole
Lettuce
Romaine
Spinach

Sweet Substitutes

Candy, hard, sugar-free
Gelatin, sugar-free
Gum, sugar-free
Jam/jelly, sugar-free (2 tsp)
Pancake syrup, sugar-free (¼ cup)
Sugar substitutes (saccharin, Equal)
Whipped topping, low-Calorie

Condiments

Catsup (1 Tbsp)
Horseradish
Mustard
Pickles§, dill, unsweetened
Salad dressing, low-Calorie (2 Tbsp)
Taco sauce (1 Tbsp)
Vinegar

Seasonings can be very helpful in making food taste better. Be careful of how much sodium you use. Read the label and choose those seasonings that do not contain sodium or salt.

Basil (fresh)
Celery seeds
Cinnamon
Chili powder
Chives
Curry
Dill
Flavoring extracts (e.g., vanilla, lemon, almond, walnut, peppermint, butter)

Garlic
Garlic powder
Herbs
Hot pepper sauce
Lemon
Lemon juice
Lemon pepper
Lime
Lime juice
Mint

Onion powder
Oregano
Paprika
Pepper
Pimento
Spices
Soy sauce§
Soy sauce, low-sodium
Wine, used in cooking (¼ cup)
Worcestershire sauce

Combination Foods

Much of the food we eat is mixed together in various combinations. These combination foods do not fit into only one exchange list. It can be difficult to tell what is in a certain casserole dish or baked food item. This is a list of average values for some typical combination foods. This list will help you fit these foods into your meal plan. Ask your dietitian for information about any other foods you'd like to eat. The *American Diabetes Association/American Dietetic Association Family Cookbooks* and the *American Diabetes Association Holiday Cookbook* have many recipes and further information about many foods, including combination foods. Check your library or local bookstore.

Food	Amount	Exchanges
Casseroles, homemade	1 cup (8 oz)	2 starch, 2 medium-fat meat, 1 fat
Cheese pizza§ thin crust	¼ of 15 oz or ¼ or 10″	2 starch, 1 medium-fat meat, 1 fat
Chili with beans†§ (commercial)	1 cup (8 oz)	2 starch, 2 medium-fat meat, 2 fat
Chow mein† (without noodles or rice)	2 cups (16 oz)	1 starch, 2 vegetable, 2 lean meat
Macaroni and cheese§	1 cup (8 oz)	2 starch, 1 medium-fat meat, 2 fat
Soup		
Bean†	1 cup (8 oz)	1 starch, 1 vegetable, 1 lean meat
Chunky, all varieties	10-¾ oz can	1 starch, 1 vegetable, 1 medium-fat meat
Cream§ (made with water)	1 cup (8 oz)	1 starch, 1 fat
Vegetable§ or broth§	1 cup (8 oz)	1 starch
Spaghetti and meatballs§ (canned)	1 cup (8 oz)	2 starch, 1 medium-fat meat, 1 fat
Sugar-free pudding (made with skim milk)	½ cup	1 starch
If beans are used as a meat substitute:		
Dried beans,† peas,† lentils†	1 cup (cooked)	2 starch, 1 lean meat

Foods for Occasional Use

Moderate amounts of some foods can be used in your meal plan, in spite of their sugar or fat content, as long as you can maintain blood glucose control. The following list includes average exchange values for some of these foods. Because they are concentrated sources of carbohydrate, you will notice that the portion sizes are very small. Check with your dietitian for advice on how often and when you can eat them.

Food	Amount	Exchanges
Angel food cake	1/12 cake	2 starch
Cake, no icing	1/12 cake, or a 3″ square	2 starch, 2 fat
Cookies	2 small (1-¾″ across)	1 starch, 1 fat
Frozen fruit yogurt	⅓ cup	1 starch
Gingersnaps	3	1 starch
Granola	¼ cup	1 starch, 1 fat
Granola bars	1 small	1 starch, 1 fat
Ice cream, any flavor	½ cup	1 starch, 2 fat
Ice milk, any flavor	½ cup	1 starch, 1 fat
Sherbet, any flavor	¼ cup	1 starch
Snack chips,§ all varieties	1 oz	1 starch, 2 fat
Vanilla wafers	6 small	1 starch, 1 fat

§If more than one serving is eaten, these foods have 400 mg or more of sodium.

Management Tips

Some food you buy uncooked will weigh less after you cook it. This is true of most meats. Starches often swell in cooking, so a small amount of uncooked starch will become a much larger amount of cooked food. The following table shows some of the changes:

Food (starch group)	Uncooked	Cooked
Oatmeal	3 level Tbsp	½ cup
Cream of wheat	2 level Tbsp	½ cup
Grits	3 level Tbsp	½ cup
Rice	2 level Tbsp	⅓ cup
Spaghetti	¼ cup	½ cup
Noodles	⅓ cup	½ cup
Macaroni	¼ cup	½ cup
Dried beans	3 Tbsp	⅓ cup
Dried peas	3 Tbsp	⅓ cup
Lentils	2 Tbsp	⅓ cup

Food (meat group)		
Hamburger	4 oz	3 oz
Chicken	1 small drumstick	1 oz
	½ breast (1 side)	3 oz

- Read food labels. Remember — *dietetic* does not mean *diabetic!* When you see the word "dietetic" on a food label, it means that something has been changed or replaced. It may have less salt, less fat, or less sugar. It does not mean that the food is sugar-free or Calorie-free. Some dietetic foods may be useful. Those that contain 20 Calories or less per serving may be eaten up to three times a day as free foods.
- Know your sweeteners. Two types of sweeteners are on the market: those with Calories and those without Calories. Sweeteners with Calories, such as fructose, sorbitol, and mannitol, when used in large amounts, may cause cramping and diarrhea. Remember, these sweeteners do have Calories that add up. Sweeteners without Calories include saccharin and aspartame (Equal, Nutrasweet) and may be used in moderation.

The food groups in the Exchange System are similar to, yet slightly different from, the groups in the Hassle-Free Guide to a Better Diet. Vegetable and fruit exchanges are separate. Table 3.14 gives the average protein, fat, carbohydrate, and energy values for each exchange. These values are averages of the nutrient values of the foods in a group, with more weight given to foods that are used more often. Average values for minerals and vitamins have not been calculated for the Exchange System because of the wide variations within each exchange.

The Exchange System makes planning a diet much easier. As you can see in table 3.15, by following the recommended number of exchanges for each food group, one can follow the energy and recommendations for percent Calories as carbohydrate, protein, and fat. When specific Calorie-controlled diets are given to patients, dietitians will use the Exchange System to recommend a set number of servings per food group. Many weight-management programs and diabetic diet plans are based on the Exchange System because it simplifies the task of counting Calories. The Exchange System allows more personal freedom by providing a list of foods from which to choose within each category, rather than specifying a food choice.

Methods to Measure How the Diet Compares with the RDA Standard

The Food Exchange System gives an idea of the number of Calories and grams of carbohydrate, fat, and protein in a diet. However, if the mineral and vitamin quality of the diet is to be calculated, other methods must be used.

Calculating the nutrient consumption of the diet is time consuming and difficult (17). Even when the exact amount of food a person eats is known, many other factors can affect the accuracy of the final mineral and vitamin levels in the body. For example, the nutrient content of food can be affected by heat, light, storage time, and cooking preparation (see chapter 10). Therefore, using an average value from a reference book could be inaccurate. Also, the analytical techniques for many nutrients are inadequate. Finally, the percentage of nutrients absorbed from the food that is inside the small intestine varies from person to person. All of these factors together mean that measurement of nutrient consumption can be imprecise.

Study of the human diet has taken on two forms: use of **food disappearance studies** and **household consumption studies.** These are discussed in the following sections.

Food Disappearance

This is the measurement of food that "disappears" into the civilian food supply. Sometimes it is referred to as the U.S. per capita food supply. The data are collected annually by the Economic Research Service of the USDA. The nutritive value of these amounts of foods is estimated by the Agricultural Research Service of the USDA. Since 1909, the Consumer Nutrition Center of the USDA has published annual estimates of the nutrient content of the national food supply (see chapter 2). The quantities are measures of approximately 350 foods that "disappear" into the food distribution system. Although these figures are good for year-to-year comparisons, they tend to overestimate the actual food eaten by people. For example, although data suggest that about 3,500 Calories are

TABLE 3.15

Sample diet plans using the exchange lists for meal planning

Food Group	Serving #	Carbohydrate (grams)	Protein (grams)	Fat (grams)
1,500 Kilocalorie Diet				
Starch/bread	7	105	21	0
Meat/cheese (2 lean/ 2 med)	4	0	28	16
Vegetable	4	20	8	0
Fruit	4	60	0	0
Milk (Low-fat)	2	24	16	10
Fat	3	0	0	15
Total grams		209	73	41
Percent total kcal		56%	19%	25%
2,000 Kilocalorie Diet				
Starch/bread	10	150	30	0
Meat/cheese (2 lean/ 3 med)	5	0	35	21
Vegetable	4	20	8	0
Fruit	6	90	0	0
Milk (low-fat)	2	24	16	10
Fat	5	0	0	25
Total grams		284	89	56
Percent total kcal		57%	18%	25%
2,500 Kilocalorie Diet				
Starch/bread	15	225	45	0
Meat/cheese (2 lean/ 3 med)	5	0	35	21
Vegetable	6	30	12	0
Fruit	6	90	0	0
Milk (low-fat)	2	24	16	10
Fat	7	0	0	35
Total grams		369	108	66
Percent total kcal		59%	17%	24%

Note: Don't forget to follow the serving sizes closely, and remember that one exchange of meat is only one ounce.

available in the U.S. food supply for each person each day, the average American male actually ingests only 2,750 Calories per day, and the average female consumes 1,630 Calories per day. Many of these Calories are lost in the marketplace and in the home. Most studies show that three to seven percent of available Calories coming into the home are wasted, averaging $150 per household per year (18).

Household Consumption Studies

Some researchers go to the homes of Americans and measure what they actually consume. Table 3.16 outlines all the various dietary studies being conducted by the government under what is called the National Nutrition Monitoring System.

Two large-scale national surveys of the food consumption of individuals are the Nationwide Food Consumption Survey (NFCS), conducted by the USDA, and the National Health

TABLE 3.16
The national nutrition monitoring system

Activity	Principal Agency	Frequency
1. Food production surveillance	USDA	Annual
2. Food composition analyses	FDA	Annual
Total diet study	USDA	Continuous
National nutrient data bank		
3. Food consumption surveys		
Nationwide Food Consumption Survey (NCFS)	USDA	Continuous
National Health and Nutrition Examination Survey (NHANES)	NCHS	Each decade
4. Retail marketplace surveillance	FDA	Every 2 years
5. Clinical nutrition status		
NHANES	NCHS	Each decade
State surveillance program	CDC	Continuous
6. Public interests and practices	FDA	Annual
7. Nutrition information and education systems	USDA/DHHS	Continuous
8. Adverse effects surveillance	FDA	Continuous
9. Special studies		
Vitamin and mineral supplement-use surveys	FDA/NCHS	Periodically
Infant feeding practices survey	FDA	Ad hoc
10. Methods development	NIH/FDA/USDA/CDC	Continuous

and Nutrition Examination Survey (NHANES), conducted by the U.S. Department of Health and Human Services (HHS) (19,20).

The NFCS gathers information on food consumption in households and on individuals within those households. The recent 1977–78 sample was a study of about 15,000 households and 34,000 individuals surveyed in 48 states. Food-use data for households was obtained for a seven-day period. Individuals gave a 24-hour dietary recall, and most of them kept food-intake records for the following two days. The NFCS is conducted every ten years, and data from the recent survey is still being analyzed.

NHANES is also conducted every ten years on an average sample of Americans. People are asked to recall their food intake from the previous day. In addition, clinical and body-composition measurements of the people are taken, and blood samples are collected.

Data from these two studies represent the best information the U.S. has on the eating habits of Americans and the quality of their diets. Figure 3.1 of this chapter used information from NHANES. Results from the NFCS and NHANES will be reviewed in detail in chapters 10 and 11.

How to Measure the Diet

Several methods are being used to measure the diets of Americans. These include **dietary recall, dietary records,** and **dietary history** and are discussed in the following sections.

Dietary Recall

In this method the subject recalls, in as much detail as possible, food consumption for a specified period of time. The recall period may vary from one day to several weeks, and the 24-hour period is most commonly used. One limitation of the 24-hour recall, however, is that the interview covers food consumption for the previous day only, which might not represent long-term normal intake. Also, intakes vary from day to day and according to the day of the week, and they tend to be greater on weekends than on weekdays. In spite of these limitations, the 24-hour recall method is believed to give fairly reliable data on the current food consumption of a large group, although it can be inaccurate for individuals.

Dietary Records

The individual using this method must record all foods and beverages consumed in a three- to seven-day period. Often a person carries the diet record throughout the day to record every mouthful consumed. The problem with this method is that when people are asked to record their food intake, they tend to eat differently than normal. People are frequently concerned that they will be judged poor eaters and may try to eat better than normal. Another problem is that it is difficult for people to accurately record the exact portion sizes of the food they eat.

Dietary History

The major benefit of this method is that it reveals long-range dietary intake. The individual, with the help of a trained dietician, fills out a form concerning the usual intake of different types of foods for a given period of time (usually the previous three months or year). Using food models, the dietician records frequency of intake (per day, week, or month) and usual size portions, in addition to the kinds of food. Respondents sometimes find it difficult to recall usual frequency of food intake, however. "Averaging" is necessary, and some people find this mental arithmetic difficult. (One of the health-promotion activities at the end of this chapter will ask you to fill out a dietary history form.)

Food Composition Tables as a Tool for Assessing Dietary Practices

Food composition tables give the average energy, protein, fat, carbohydrate, mineral, and vitamin content of a defined amount of food. In general, the figures given in food composition tables are only representative values and apply to food as it is usually produced and marketed for year-round and countrywide use by the consumer. The actual amount of a nutrient in any food an individual may eat may vary substantially from the average. (For example, the vitamin C content in tomato juice can vary from 3.2 to 21.7 mg/dL between different samples.) Factors such as genetic variation, maturity, part of the plant consumed, seasonal or geographical differences, length and type of storage, food processing, and new varieties of foods all affect food composition, and so the tables must be seen as giving only approximate values.

　　Following is a discussion of commonly used food composition tables, including **USDA Handbook No.8, USDA Handbook No. 456, USDA Bulletin No. 72,** and **Food Values of Portions Commonly Used.**

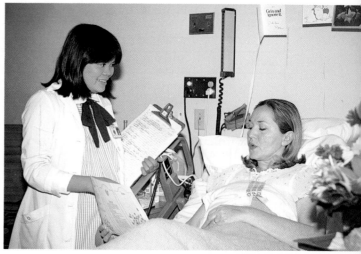
A dietician can assist people in determining their food intake.

USDA Handbook No. 8

Since its original publication in 1950, USDA Handbook No. 8 has been the most widely used food composition table. It was revised in 1963. The latest revision is being published in separate books, each of which contains a table of nutrient data for a major food group. To facilitate continual and rapid updating, the handbook is prepared in looseleaf form, and each page contains the nutrient profile for a single food item. Values are listed for energy, water, protein, fat, carbohydrate, nine minerals (calcium, iron, magnesium, phosphorus, potassium, sodium, zinc, copper, and manganese), nine vitamins (ascorbic acid, thiamin, riboflavin, niacin, pantothenic acid, vitamin B_6, folacin, vitamin B_{12} and vitamin A), individual fatty acids (total saturated, monounsaturated, and polyunsaturated fatty acids), cholesterol, and eighteen amino acids.

USDA Handbook No. 456

The figures in USDA Handbook No. 456 are calculated from the 1963 edition of Handbook No. 8, with a limited amount of updating for some nutrients. No. 456 is unique because it uses volume measurements of food, with weight of food in grams given for the various measurements.

USDA Bulletin No. 72

This consumer bulletin contains food values for over 730 foods, based on average servings or common household units. The figures are derived from Handbook No. 8, 1963 edition.

Food Values of Portions Commonly Used

This food composition table, now in its 13th edition, is commonly referred to as Bowes and Church because Anna dePlanter Bowes, a nutritionist, and Dr. C. F. Church were the authors of the first edition, published in 1937. The latest edition is authored by Dr. Pennington and Dr. Church. The nutrient values given in this table have been derived from a variety of sources, including Handbook No. 8. This publication differs from Handbook No. 8 in that the food items are listed by groups, for example, breads, cereals, and cereal products. In addition, the household measure as well as the gram weights are given, and brand names are used for some items.

Summary

1. The RDA are a technical standard used for nutrition policies and decision making. Thus the RDA are different from the Dietary Guidelines for Americans, which are primarily used for guiding people in making dietary decisions for prevention of disease and promotion of health.
2. RDA are the levels of intake of essential nutrients considered, in the judgment of the Committee on Dietary Allowances of the Food and Nutrition Board on the basis of available scientific knowledge, to be adequate to meet the known nutritional needs of practically all healthy persons.
3. RDA are used by many organizations and institutions to plan and obtain food supplies. Government programs use the RDA as their standard for education, and food companies used the RDA to guide them in preparing food labels.
4. The U.S. RDA are a set of standards developed by the FDA for use in regulating nutrition labeling. Regulations adopted by the FDA in 1973 require manufacturers to provide nutrition information on their product labels only if one or more nutrients are added to the food or if a nutritional claim is made about the product.
5. The USDA has published food guides since 1917. Their latest version is the Hassle-Free Daily Food Guide, which gives recommended numbers of servings from five different food groups. Some nutritionists recommend food guides that combine the four food groups with the dietary guidelines to assist people in making better food choices within each food group.
6. The Food Exchange System makes planning a diet relatively simple. Foods are divided into six different groups. Each exchange list within a food group contains foods that are alike, with each choice containing about the same amount of carbohydrate, protein, fat, and Calories.
7. Study of the human diet has taken on two forms: use of food disappearance data and household food consumption data. Several methods were reviewed, including dietary recall, dietary record, and dietary history.
8. Food composition tables give the average energy, protein, fat, carbohydrate, mineral, and vitamin content of a defined amount of food. The USDA has published several types of food composition tables.

References

1. Truswell, A. S. 1987. Evolution of Dietary Recommendations, Goals, and Guidelines. *American Journal of Clinical Nutrition* 45:1060-72.
2. Smith, J., and J. S. Turner. 1986. A Perspective on the History and Use of the Recommended Dietary Allowances. *Currents* 2(1):4-11.
3. Food and Nutrition Board. Recommended Dietary Allowances. 10th rev. ed. 1989. Washington, D.C.: National Academy Press, 1989.
4. AMA Council on Scientific Affairs. 1987. Vitamin Preparations as Dietary Supplements and as Therapeutic Agents. *Journal of the American Medical Association* 257:1929-36.
5. Press, F. 1985. Postponement of the Tenth Edition of the RDAs. *Journal of the American Dietetic Association* 85:1644-45.
6. Shils, M. E., and V. R. Young. 1988. *Modern Nutrition in Health and Disease,* 7th ed. Philadelphia: Lea & Febiger.
7. Hansen, R. G., C. T. Windham, and B. W. Wyse. 1985. Nutrient Density and Food Labeling. *Clinical Nutrition* 4:164-70.
8. Wyse, B. W., C. T. Windham, and R. G. Hansen. 1985. Nutrition Intervention: Panacea or Pandora's Box? *Journal of the American Dietetic Association.* 85:1084-90.
9. Lecos, C. W. 1988. Food Labels: Test Your Food Label Knowledge. *FDA Consumer* (March): 16-21.
10. Haughton, B., J. D. Gussow, and J. M. Dodds. 1987. An Historical Study of the Underlying Assumptions for United States Food Guides from 1917 through the Basic Four Food Group Guide. *Journal of Nutrition Education* 19(4):169-75.
11. U.S. Department of Agriculture. Science and Education Administration. 1979. Food, by C. A. Davis, et al. Home and Garden Bulletin No. 232. Washington, D.C.: Government Printing Office.
12. Guthrie, H. A., and J. C. Scheer. 1981. Nutritional Adequacy of Self-Selected Diets That Satisfy the Four Food Groups Guide. *Journal of Nutrition Education* 13(2):46-49.
13. Guthrie, H. A. 1984. Selection and Quantification of Typical Food Proportions by Young Adults. *Journal of the American Dietetic Association* 84:1440-44.
14. Krebs-Smith, S. M., and H. Smiciklas-Wright. 1985. Typical Serving Sizes: Implications for Food Guidance. *Journal of the American Dietetic Association* 85:1139-41.
15. Brewer, E. R., et al. 1987. Food Group System of Analysis with Special Attention to Type and Amount of Fat Methodology. *Journal of the American Dietetic Association* 87:584-92.

16. Committees of the American Diabetes Association, Inc., and the American Dietetic Association, in cooperation with the National Institute of Arthritis, Metabolism, and Digestive Diseases and the National Heart and Lung Institute of Health, Public Health Service, U.S. Department of Health and Human Services. 1986. Exchange Lists for Meal Planning. American Diabetes Association.

17. Swan, P. B. 1983. Food Consumption by Individuals in the United States. *Annual Review of Nutrition* 3:413–32.

18. Van Garde, S. J., and M. J. Woodburn. 1987. Food Discard Practices of Householders. *Journal of the American Dietetic Association* 87:322–29.

19. Wotecki, C. E., R. R. Briefel, and R. Kuczmarski. 1988. Contributions of the National Center for Health Statistics. *American Journal of Clinical Nutrition* 47:320–28.

20. Sims, L. S. 1988. Contributions of the United States Department of Agriculture. *American Journal of Clinical Nutrition* 47:329–32.

HEALTH-PROMOTION ACTIVITY 3.1
How Does Your Diet Rate for Variety?

The following quiz, based on material prepared by the U.S. Department of Agriculture's Human Nutrition Information Service, will help you determine how well-balanced your diet is. For a free copy of "Dietary Guidelines for Americans: Eat a Variety of Foods," from which this quiz was adapted, request Home and Garden Bulletin No. 232-1 from USDA, HNIS, Room 360, 6506 Belcrest Rd., Hyattsville, Md. 20782.

Check the box that best describes your eating habits.

How often do you eat:	Seldom or never	1 or 2 times a week	3 to 4 times a week	Almost daily
1. at least six servings of bread, cereals, rice, crackers, pasta or other foods made from grains (a serving is one slice of bread or a half cup cereal, rice, etc.) per day?	☐	☐	☐	☐
2. foods made from whole grains?	☐	☐	☐	☐
3. three different kinds of vegetables per day?	☐	☐	☐	☐
4. cooked dry beans or peas?	☐	☐	☐	☐
5. a dark-green vegetable, such as spinach or broccoli?	☐	☐	☐	☐
6. two kinds of fruit or fruit juice per day?	☐	☐	☐	☐
7. two servings (three if teenager, pregnant, or breast-feeding) of milk, cheese, or yogurt per day?	☐	☐	☐	☐
8. two servings of lean meat, poultry, fish, or alternates, such as eggs, dry beans or nuts per day?	☐	☐	☐	☐

Answer Box

Compare your answers to the best answer, listed below.

1. **Almost daily.** Many people believe that eating breads and cereals will make you fat. That's not true for most of us. Extra Calories often come from the fat and/or sugar you MAY eat with them. Both whole-grain and enriched breads and cereals provide starch and essential nutrients.

2. **Almost daily.** Whole-grain breads and cereals contain vitamins, minerals and dietary fiber that are low in the diets of many Americans. Select whole-grain cereals and bakery products — those with a whole grain listed first on the ingredient label. Or make your own and use whole-wheat flour.

3. **Almost daily.** Vegetables vary in the amounts of vitamins and minerals they contain. So, it's important to include several kinds every day.

4. **3 to 4 times a week.** Dry beans and peas fit into two food groups because of the nutrients they provide. They can be used as an alternate to meat, poultry, and fish. And they are also an excellent vegetable choice.

5. **3 to 4 times a week.** Popeye gulped down spinach to build his superior strength. Although this effect of spinach was exaggerated, spinach and other dark-green leafy vegetables are excellent sources of some nutrients that are low in many diets.

6. **Almost daily.** Fruits are nature's sweets. They taste good and are good for you. Choose several different kinds each day.

7. **Almost daily.** Adults as well as children need the calcium and other nutrients found in milk, cheese and yogurt.

8. **Almost daily.** Most Americans include some meat, poultry or fish in their diets regularly. Dry beans and peas, peanuts (including peanut butter), nuts and seeds, and eggs can be used as alternates.

---

*H*EALTH-PROMOTION ACTIVITY 3.2
Measurement of Your Diet Using the Dietary History Approach

For this activity you will fill out the dietary history questionnaire on the following pages, and then enter your data into a computer for analysis. Your teacher will need to arrange the purchase of computer software from:

Wellsource
P.O. Box 569
15431 SE 82 Dr, Ste E
Clackamas, OR 97015
(503) 656-7446

As you fill out the questionnaire, it is very important that you follow the instructions carefully. Try to average your usual intake over the past three months. Pay close attention to the listed portion sizes.

Review the computer printout results with your instructor.

Instructions

Read each question carefully and write in your answer in the space provided. Check to be sure no questions are skipped. The accuracy of your report depends on the correctness of your answers.

Biographical Data

Name (Print) _____

Mail Address _____

City _____ State _____ Zip _____

Date today _____ - _____ - _____

_____ Group ID No. (Skip if unknown)

_____ Age

_____ Sex (M = 1, F = 2)

_____ Height (inches, note: 5 ft. = 60 in.)

_____ Weight (lbs.)

Frame size:
_____ Small = 1, Med. = 2, Large = 3

Eating Habits Survey

Instructions: Mark the answer that best describes your *usual* eating behavior.

1. How often do you eat a good breakfast (something more than coffee and a sweet roll)?
   1 [ ] Always
   2 [ ] Usually
   3 [ ] Sporadically
   4 [ ] Seldom

2. How often do you eat snack foods between meals?
   1 [ ] Regularly, more than once per day
   2 [ ] Once per day
   3 [ ] Occasionally
   4 [ ] Seldom or never eat between meals

3. What is your *usual* dinner eating pattern?
   1 [ ] Large evening meal, major source of Calories for the day
   2 [ ] Average size evening meal
   3 [ ] Light evening meal
   4 [ ] Seldom eat an evening meal

4. Indicate the kind of meals you *generally* eat.
   1 [ ] Regular mixed diet including meat
   2 [ ] Regular mixed diet with fish or fowl but no red meat
   3 [ ] Vegetarian diet with eggs and/or milk but no meat, fish, or fowl
   4 [ ] Total vegetarian diet, no animal foods

5. What kind of bread do you *usually* eat?
   1 [ ] Typical white bread and rolls
   2 [ ] Whole-wheat breads
   3 [ ] Use both about the same
   4 [ ] Seldom ever eat bread

6. What kind of breakfast cereals do you *usually* eat?
   1 [ ] Typical sweetened dry cereals
   2 [ ] Whole-grain cereals (cooked or dry)
   3 [ ] Use both about the same
   4 [ ] Seldom ever eat cereals

7. What kind of milk do you *usually* drink?
   1 [ ] Whole milk
   2 [ ] Low-fat or skim milk
   3 [ ] Soy milk
   4 [ ] Never drink milk

8. Primary kind of spread you *usually* use?
   1 [ ] Butter
   2 [ ] Hard stick margarine
   3 [ ] Soft tub margarine
   4 [ ] Don't use any typical spreads

9. Primary kind of fats you *usually* use?
   1 [ ] Shortening
   2 [ ] Vegetable oil
   3 [ ] Use both about the same
   4 [ ] Don't use any fats

10. How do you *usually* salt your food?
   1 [ ] Freely
   2 [ ] Moderately
   3 [ ] Sparingly
   4 [ ] Don't add salt

11. Kind of red meat you *usually* eat?
   1 [ ] Marbled cuts of red meat
   2 [ ] Regular cuts of red meat
   3 [ ] Only lean cuts
   4 [ ] Don't eat red meat

12. How much water do you *usually* drink per day?
   1 [ ] Seldom ever drink water
   2 [ ] 1-2 cups/day
   3 [ ] 3-5 cups/day
   4 [ ] 6+ cups/day

13. Kind of soft drinks you *usually* have?
   1 [ ] Cola drinks
   2 [ ] Caffeine-free
   3 [ ] Drink both
   4 [ ] Never drink soft drinks

14. Kind of coffee you *usually* drink?
   1 [ ] Brewed coffee
   2 [ ] Instant coffee
   3 [ ] Decaffeinated coffee
   4 [ ] Never drink coffee

Physical Activity Status

Indicate how many hours per day you typically spend in each of the following categories. If your activity level fluctuates, use average values. *Total must equal 24 hours.* Decimals can be used (eg. 30 min. = 0.5 hrs.)

15. _____ Sleeping or lying still; relaxed, napping, lying down watching TV

16. _____ Sitting or standing still; eating, watching TV, writing, reading, sewing, typing, desk work

17. _____ Very light activity; driving a car, slow walking on level ground, most office work, laboratory work, playing musical instruments

18. _____ Light activity; normal walking (2.5 to 3 mph), most housework, electrical trades, carpentry, golf, sailing, table tennis, volleyball, active gardening (raking, weeding)

19. _____ Moderate activity; Brisk walking (3.5 to 4 mph), heavy construction, hard gardening (hoeing, digging), loading and stacking bales, cycling, skiing, tennis, active dance

20. _____ Heavy activity; tree felling, work with pick and shovel, basketball, x-c skiing, running, hill climbing with a pack, fast swimming

   _____ TOTAL; must equal 24 hours

21. During your free time, how often do you get vigorous, sustained, aerobic exercise of 20 plus minutes per session?
   1 [ ] Don't have a regular exercise program
   2 [ ] 1-2 times/week
   3 [ ] 3-4 times/week
   4 [ ] 5 plus times/week

22. Concerning your present weight, do you consider yourself . . .
   1 [ ] Definitely overweight
   2 [ ] Somewhat overweight
   3 [ ] About right
   4 [ ] Somewhat underweight

23. Indicate your present condition:
   1 [ ] Male
   2 [ ] Pregnant
   3 [ ] Currently nursing a child
   4 [ ] Female other than above

24. How often do you eat cruciferous type vegetables? These include broccoli, Brussel sprouts, cabbage, kohlrabi, and cauliflower.
   1 [ ] Never
   2 [ ] 1 to 2 times each week
   3 [ ] 3 to 5 times each week
   4 [ ] Nearly every day

25. How often do you eat cured or smoked foods? These include conventionally smoked foods such as hams, some varieties of sausages, and fish; salt-cured or pickled foods and nitrite-cured foods.
   1 [ ] Seldom or never
   2 [ ] About once a week
   3 [ ] 2-5 times each week
   4 [ ] Nearly every day

26. Mark any program that you are interested in and would like to recieve more information.
   1 [ ] Nutrition education class
   2 [ ] Weight control program
   3 [ ] Exercise class
   4 [ ] Low calorie cooking
   5 [ ] Low cholesterol cooking
   6 [ ] Coronary risk reduction program
   7 [ ] Comprehensive nutritional evaluation
   8 [ ] Nutrition counselling
   9 [ ] Other, list below:

Food Intake History

Instructions: Indicate the usual *number of servings* you eat from each food group listed below. Foods eaten less than daily should be marked under the weekly or monthly column, but mark only *one column* per food group. Notice the serving size and adjust your number of servings reported accordingly. Use decimals to indicate partial servings, e.g., .5 for ½ or 1.5 for 1-½. Be sure to include *all* foods, snacks, salad dressings, etc.

Example

If you regularly eat an orange and a half a tomato daily and cooked vegetables 4 times per week, then mark as shown below.

Number of servings per

	Day	Week	Month		
1.	[1.5]	[ ]	[ ]	Foods rich in vitamin C	1 orange, ½ grapefruit, 2 tangerines, 1 lemon, green pepper, 1 C fresh strawberries, 1 tomato
8.	[ ]	[4]	[ ]	Cooked vegetables	½ C green beans, cabbage, beets, asparagus, summer squash, cauliflower, Chinese vegetables

Number of servings per

	Day	Week	Month	**Fruits**	**Serving Sizes of Selected Foods**
1.	[ ]	[ ]	[ ]	Foods rich in vitamin C	1 orange, ½ grapefruit, 2 tangerines, 1 lemon, green pepper, 1 C fresh strawberries, 1 tomato, slice honeydew or watermelon
2.	[ ]	[ ]	[ ]	Drinks rich in vitamin C	¾ C orange, grapefruit or lemon drink, 1 C tomato or vegetable cocktail juice
3.	[ ]	[ ]	[ ]	Unsweetened fruits	1 medium apple, banana or pear, 2 plums, 1 C cherries or grapes, 3 T raisins, 2–3 dates, 2–3 pieces of dried fruit
4.	[ ]	[ ]	[ ]	Sweetened fruits	½ C applesauce, peaches, pears, plums, berries, pineapple, cherries, fruit cocktail
5.	[ ]	[ ]	[ ]	Other fruit juices	¾ C apple, grape, cranapple, apricot nectar
				Vegetables	
6.	[ ]	[ ]	[ ]	Foods rich in vitamin A	½ C cooked or 1 C fresh dark, leafy green and dark yellow foods; greens, squash, carrots, apricots, broccoli, sweet potatoes
7.	[ ]	[ ]	[ ]	Salads/raw vegetables	Medium salad bowl (no dressing) lettuce and other raw vegetables, celery, radishes, onions, sprouts, cabbage, endive

Number of servings per

	Day	Week	Month	Vegetables	Examples and Serving Sizes
8.	[ ]	[ ]	[ ]	Cooked vegetables	½ C green beans, cabbage, beets, asparagus, summer squash, cauliflower, Chinese vegetables
9.	[ ]	[ ]	[ ]	Starchy vegetables	1 medium potato (baked or boiled), 1 medium ear corn, ⅔ C corn, green peas, yams
10.	[ ]	[ ]	[ ]	Dry peas/beans	⅔ C beans, lentils, garbanzos, split peas
				Bread and Grains	
11.	[ ]	[ ]	[ ]	Bread, whole grain	1 slice, roll, muffin, whole-grain crackers, etc.
12.	[ ]	[ ]	[ ]	Breads, other	1 slice, roll, biscuit, French bread, English muffin, etc.
13.	[ ]	[ ]	[ ]	Quick breads	1 slice or piece cornbread, roll, biscuit, pancake, 2 tortillas, crackers (4–5), ½ waffle
14.	[ ]	[ ]	[ ]	Cooked cereals	¾ C cooked oatmeal, rice, Cream of Wheat, or other cooked cereal
15.	[ ]	[ ]	[ ]	Dry cereals (sweetened)	1 C Frosted Flakes, Kix, Fruit Loops, Sugar Puffs, etc.
16.	[ ]	[ ]	[ ]	Dry cereals (low sugar)	1 C Wheat Chex, Shredded Wheat, Nutrigrain, Cheerios, ⅓ C Grape Nuts or granola, 2 C unbuttered popcorn
17.	[ ]	[ ]	[ ]	Pasta	½ C cooked spaghetti, macaroni, noodles, other pasta (report sauce or toppings in appropriate group)
				Dairy Products	
18.	[ ]	[ ]	[ ]	Milk products	1 C whole milk, yogurt, ⅔ C cottage cheese
19.	[ ]	[ ]	[ ]	Skim milk	1 C skim milk, low-fat yogurt, buttermilk
20.	[ ]	[ ]	[ ]	Cream	1 T heavy cream, 2 T light cream, 2 T sour cream, 1 T cream cheese
21.	[ ]	[ ]	[ ]	Ice cream	1 C ice cream, 1 medium cone or ice cream bar
22.	[ ]	[ ]	[ ]	Butter (real)	1 T (include butter used in cooking, too)
23.	[ ]	[ ]	[ ]	Hard cheese	1 oz. or 1 slice sandwich size
24.	[ ]	[ ]	[ ]	Eggs	1 egg fried, scrambled, or boiled
				Protein Rich Foods	
25.	[ ]	[ ]	[ ]	Red meats	3–4 oz. beef, lamb, pork, steak, roast, 1 hamburger patty
26.	[ ]	[ ]	[ ]	Lunch meats/franks	1 frankfurter, slice luncheon meat, 2 slices bacon, slice salami
27.	[ ]	[ ]	[ ]	Fowl	3–4 oz. chicken, turkey
28.	[ ]	[ ]	[ ]	Fish/shellfish	3–4 oz. tuna, halibut, salmon, oysters, shrimp, caviar, lobster, crab, abalone
29.	[ ]	[ ]	[ ]	Organ meats	3–4 oz. liver or other
30.	[ ]	[ ]	[ ]	Meat substitutes	3–4 oz. glutenburger, soy product, weiners, steak, chicken-like slices

Number of servings per

	Day	Week	Month	Protein Rich Foods	Examples and Serving Sizes
31.	[ ]	[ ]	[ ]	Vegetarian entrees	(No milk/eggs) ¾ C roast or patties
32.	[ ]	[ ]	[ ]	Vegetarian entrees	With milk/eggs/cheese, ¾ C roast/patties
				Fat Rich Foods	
33.	[ ]	[ ]	[ ]	Nuts	½ oz. or 2 T peanuts, almonds, sunflower seeds, 1 T peanut butter, Tahini, coconut
34.	[ ]	[ ]	[ ]	Fats	1 T shortening, vegetable oil, 2–3 T gravy
35.	[ ]	[ ]	[ ]	Spreads/dressings	1 T margarine, 1-½ T salad dressing, mayonnaise, (include all fats added to bread, vegetables, salads, etc.)
36.	[ ]	[ ]	[ ]	Avocado/olives	¼ avocado; 6–7 olives
				Miscellaneous Foods	
37.	[ ]	[ ]	[ ]	Soups	1 C vegetable, chicken, mushroom, or tomato soup
38.	[ ]	[ ]	[ ]	Soft drinks	12 oz. 7-Up, Coca Cola, Pepsi, Kool Aid (omit nonnutritive or artificially sweetened drinks)
39.	[ ]	[ ]	[ ]	Coffee/tea	1 C (mark sugar and cream separately)
40.	[ ]	[ ]	[ ]	Alcoholic beverages	12 oz. beer, 4 oz. wine, 1.5 oz. whiskey, gin
41.	[ ]	[ ]	[ ]	Candy/sweets	1 oz., e.g., candy, mints, caramels, chocolates
42.	[ ]	[ ]	[ ]	Sugar/sweeteners	1 T sugar, honey, jam, jelly, syrups
43.	[ ]	[ ]	[ ]	Baked goodies	2 cookies, brownie, doughnut, small pastry
44.	[ ]	[ ]	[ ]	Desserts	1/6 pie, 1 C custard dessert, 1 piece cake
45.	[ ]	[ ]	[ ]	Snacks	1 oz. potato chips, Fritos, Cheezettes, deep-fried onions, 1 C buttered popcorn, small order fries
46.	[ ]	[ ]	[ ]	Fast foods	1 regular serving pizza, hamburger, hot dog, taco, burrito

Nutrition Profile

Description

Nutrition Profile carefully assesses the patient's eating habits to determine nutritional status. It then recommends areas for improvement based on the individual's age, sex, and special needs.

Uses

Nutrition awareness programs. Develops a receptive attitude that in turn promotes individual responsibility for one's well-being.

Weight control classes
Employee wellness programs
Nutrition counseling

Benefits

Provides an easy way to assess a patient's general nutritional state. Only five to ten minutes to complete the questionnaire, and then immediate results. Oriented toward nutrition as a source of health promotion and disease prevention.

Generates business revenue and interest in nutrition education programs.

Permits provider to offer a new health service.

Simple to operate.

Helps people become aware of nutritional needs, and makes recommendations tailored for their personal requirements.

Furnishes the means for monitoring change, either personal or corporate. Documents the effects of a nutritional promotion program.

Input Information

The profile is prepared from information obtained in a two-part questionnaire. The "Eating Habits Survey" covers eating patterns, quality of food choices, use of salt, and refined food choices, along with physical activity level.

A "Food Intake History" estimates the number of servings eaten per day of various food groups with common nutritional content. This program does not require food coding.

Features

Recommended range shown for each nutritional factor. Create your own nutritional data base and norms for comparison with your group.

HEALTH-PROMOTION ACTIVITY 3.3
Measurement of Your Diet Using the Food Record Approach

Using the worksheet below, record all foods you consume for one day, being very careful to accurately assess portion sizes. It might help you to use a cup and tablespoon to more accurately visualize and measure your intake.

After recording your food intake for one day, use the nutrient information from appendix B and fill in the nutrient quantities for each food listed, and then calculate the total intake. Finally, compare your one-day results with the RDA (see tables 3.2 and 3.3).

Worksheet to Calculate Nutrient Intake for One Day

Food Description	Portion Size	Food Energy (kcal)	Protein (gm)	Fat (gm)	Carbohydrate (gm)	Calcium (mg)	Iron (mg)	Vit. A (I.U.)	Thiamine (mg)	Vit. C (mg)
Totals										
RDA Comparison										

4

Food Safety and Labeling

OUTLINE

INTRODUCTION

When it comes to deciding what is safe to eat, most consumers prefer to rely on themselves. This was the consensus of 48 percent of those interviewed in 1986 by the Food Marketing Institute of Washington, D.C. (see figure 4.1). Twenty-nine percent of those respondents relied on the federal government as their second choice in assuring food safety (1).

Self-reliant consumers need to be familiar with safe food purchases, food-handling practices, storage techniques, processing concerns, and possible food contaminants. Although our food supply is safer than it has ever been, consumers today must be skeptical about "scientific claims" and counterclaims concerning various products. Informed consumers can ask questions about food safety and advertising claims and can be prepared to report concerns to the appropriate government agencies.

This chapter provides information about food safety and consumer copying strategies to reduce the health risks associated with food.

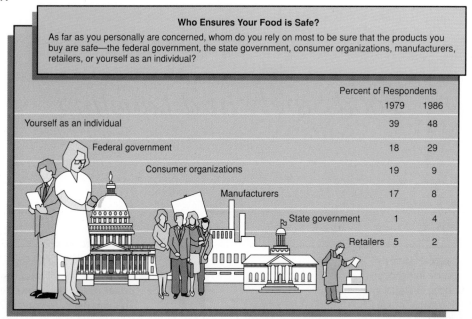

Who Ensures Your Food is Safe?

As far as you personally are concerned, whom do you rely on most to be sure that the products you buy are safe—the federal government, the state government, consumer organizations, manufacturers, retailers, or yourself as an individual?

	Percent of Respondents	
	1979	1986
Yourself as an individual	39	48
Federal government	18	29
Consumer organizations	19	9
Manufacturers	17	8
State government	1	4
Retailers	5	2

Microbiological Hazards

Data from the Food and Drug Administration (FDA) and Centers for Disease Control (CDC) show that the number of cases of foodborne disease is rising. Of the 20,000 cases reported to CDC annually, nearly one-half are due to microorganisms (2). Because doctors are not legally required to report cases of food poisoning and because victims do not always seek medical treatment, the actual number of cases is probably in the millions. It is estimated that this year, one in every ten Americans will have a bout with diarrhea that is related to food that is eaten (3). Since problems persist in this area, a discussion of the offending organisms and their sources is justified (see figure 4.2). Several bacteria are responsible, and they cause problems in two different ways.

Foodborne Infections

Foodborne infections are caused by foods that are contaminated by large numbers of living organisms, the most common of which are *Salmonella* bacteria. These bacteria can be found in the feces of humans or animals, including pets and livestock. The largest outbreak in 1986 resulted from raw milk ingestion (2). Certified raw milk is often a culprit because it is not pasteurized (sterilized). Raw or undercooked meats can also be contaminated with *Salmonella* bacteria.

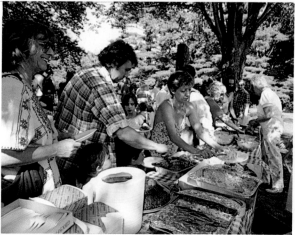

Picnics can be a food-poisoner's feast.

Another source is raw eggs (which are often mixed in milkshakes or breakfast shakes). Infected feces can enter through any crack in the shell during or after laying of the egg.

Salmonellosis, the type of food poisoning that is caused by *Salmonella* bacteria, is estimated to affect two million people annually in the United States. Symptoms include diarrhea, abdominal pain, vomiting, dehydration, fever, and chills. The onset occurs within 12 to 36 hours after a person eats contaminated food. Symptoms may last for several days and vary in severity, but fatalities are rare.

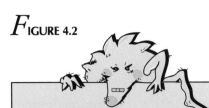

*F*IGURE 4.2

Understanding the Food Poisoners

What is food poisoning? Food poisoning, caused by harmful bacteria, normally produces intestinal flu-like symptoms lasting a few hours to several days. But in cases of botulism, or when food poisoning strikes infants, the ill or the elderly, the situation can be serious.

Where do these bacteria come from, and how can they be stopped? Food poisoning bacteria, microscopic in size, surround us - in the air, soil , and water, and in our own digestive tracts and in those of many animals. The only way they can effectively be stopped is by careful attention to food handling rules like those outlined in this booklet.

Bacteria	How it attacks	Symptoms	Prevention
Staphylococcus aureus (Staph)	Staph spreads from someone handling food. It is found on the skin and in boils, pimples and throat infections. At warm temperatures, staph produces a poison.	2-8 hours after eating, you could have vomiting and diarrhea lasting a day or two.	Cooking won't destroy the staph poison, so: -- Wash hands, utensils before preparing food. -- Don't leave food out over 2 hours. --Susceptible foods are meat, poultry, meat and poultry salads, cheese, egg products, starchy salads (potato, macaroni, pasta and tuna), custards, cream-filled desserts.
Salmonella	You can get salmonella when infected food - meat, poultry, eggs, fish - is eaten raw or undercooked. Other cases? When cooked food comes in contact with infected raw food, or when an infected person contaminates food.	In 12-36 hours you could have diarrhea, fever and vomiting lasting 2-7 days.	Keep raw food away from cooked food, and: -- Thoroughly cook meat, poultry, fish. -- Be especially careful with poultry, pork, roast beef, hamburger. -- Don't drink unpasteurized milk.
Clostridium perfringens	This "buffet germ" grows rapidly in large portions of food that are cooling slowly. It can also grow in chafing dishes which may not keep food sufficiently hot, and even in the refrigerator if food is stored in large portions which do not cool quickly.	In 8-24 hours you could have diarrhea and gas pains, ending usually in less than a day. But older people and ulcer patients can be badly affected.	Keep food hot (over 140° F) or cold (under 40° F),and: -- Divide bulk cooked foods into smaller portions for serving and cooling. -- Be careful with poultry, gravy, stews, casseroles.
Campylobacter jejuni	You drink untreated water on an outing.Your pet becomes infected and spreads it to the whole family, or you eat raw or undercooked meat, poultry or shellfish.	In 2-5 days you could have severe (possibly bloody) diarrhea, cramping, fever and headache lasting 2-7 days.	Don't drink untreated water or unpasteurized milk,and: -- Thoroughly clean hands, utensils and surfaces that touch raw meats. -- Thoroughly cook meat, poultry and fish.
Clostridium botulism	Often occurs in home-canned or any canned goods showing warning signs-clear liquids turned milky, cracked jars, loose lids, swollen or dented cans or lids. Beware of any jar or can that spurts liquid or has an off-odor when opened.	In 12-48 hours your nervous system could be affected. Symptoms? Double vision, droopy eyelids, trouble speaking and swallowing, difficult breathing. Untreated, botulism can be fatal.	Carefully examine home-canned goods before use, and: -- Don't use any canned goods showing danger signs. -- If you or a family member has botulism symptoms, get medical help immediately.

Note: While the chart highlights the preventive measures most important in avoiding each type of bacteria, you should understand that all the rules of prevention should be followed with all foods.

Foodborne Bacterial Intoxications

Bacteria may also cause illness by producing toxins in foods. *Staphylococcus aureus, Clostridium perfringens,* and *Clostridium botulinum* are three bacteria that produce such toxins.

   Staphylococcus aureus is commonly found in pimples, boils, wound infections (cuts and scrapes), hangnails, sputum, and sneeze droplets. Humans, therefore, are a major reservoir of these organisms. They flourish in foods containing protein, such as cooked meats; sauces; gravies; chicken, ham, and egg salads; cream pies; and pastries. *Staphylococcus* bacteria grow in these foods and produce an **enterotoxin,** which is a poison of the intestinal tract. Although cooking or heating foods may kill the bacteria, it does not damage the toxin. Because the toxin is what causes the illness, not the multiplication of organisms, the onset of symptoms is rapid. Vomiting and diarrhea may occur within 30 minutes, although two to eight hours is more common. Illness is brief, lasting for a day or two. Severity differs, depending on the susceptibility of the individual.

Clostridium perfringens toxin can be found in cooked meat and poultry that has been left unrefrigerated for several hours. The toxin must be ingested in large amounts to produce illness. The onset of symptoms is usually between 8 to 24 hours, with severe discomfort lasting only a day.

The most serious of all bacterial food-borne illnesses is botulism, produced by the spore-forming soil bacterium *Clostridium botulinum*. A neurotoxin is produced by the bacteria under **anaerobic** (without oxygen) conditions. Outbreaks of botulism are most frequently associated with home-canned, low-acid foods such as green beans, beets, corn, spinach, mushrooms, and peas. The affected food does not necessarily smell or look unusual, making it impossible to detect the bacteria. Since spores of *Clostridium botulinum* are heat resistant, a long processing time is needed to kill them. If the spores are not killed, they will grow in the oxygen-free medium and produce the deadly toxin. The botulism toxin can be destroyed if the food that contains it is boiled for 20 minutes; however, many of these items are only briefly warmed before eating. Cans that are dented, bulging, or buckled should be discarded, because this may indicate that gas has formed within the can from *C. botulinum*.

Botulism is first evidenced by unusual gastrointestinal distress within 12 to 48 hours. Neurological symptoms follow and include double vision; difficulty in swallowing, speaking, and breathing. Respiratory paralysis leading to death can occur. Recent advances in respiratory therapy, and prompt administration of the antitoxin, have significantly increased a victim's chance for survival (4).

Infants under the age of one are susceptible to botulism in a peculiar way. Unlike adults, their gastrointestinal tracts provide the right environmental conditions that allow the bacteria to produce toxin. The symptoms that result are similar to those in an adult and can result in death. Honey and corn syrup are two products in which *C. botulinum* spores have been found, and therefore are not recommended for children under the age of one (5).

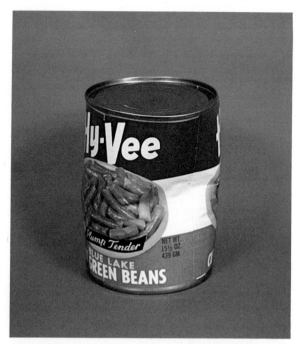

What food poison do you suspect from the dented can?

Food Handling for Health Promotion

Centers for Disease Control report that five practices contribute to the majority of foodborne illness (6). In order of frequency they are

1. improper holding temperature,
2. food from an unsafe source,
3. inadequate cooking,
4. poor personal hygiene on the part of food handlers, and
5. contaminated equipment.

Therefore, strategies to avoid foodborne illnesses must include particular attention to the selection, preparation, and storage of foods.

Food Selections

When selecting food from the supermarket, carefully examine each item. Fruits and vegetables should be clean, without dirt or manure still clinging. Examine eggs to assure that they are free from cracks. Milk and cheeses should be pasteurized and sealed in leakproof containers. Breaks in the seals indicate potential sites where bacteria can enter. Cans and plastic containers should be sealed, with no leaks or dents. Expansion of a container could mean that bacteria are multiplying inside. Expiration dates on products should be heeded. Meats should have a bright color and no foul odor. Refrigerated

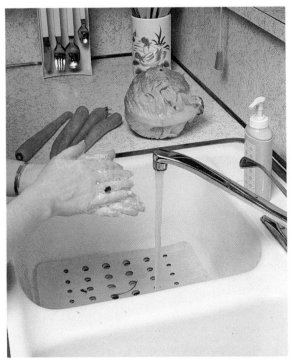
Handwashing can stop the spread of microorganisms.

products should be located where adequate cool air will circulate around the items. Selecting wholesome foods is the first step in avoiding foodborne illness.

Food Preparation
In the preparation of food, cleanliness is essential; food handlers can be a source of contamination. Washing the hands with soapy water is necessary after using the bathroom, sneezing or coughing, and nose blowing. In addition, people who have colds or other contagious illnesses should not prepare food.

Utensils also need thorough cleaning when switching from raw to cooked foods and from meats to other foods. For example, the same plate that carried raw meat should not be used for cooked meat. Hot, soapy water can be used to clean preparation areas and utensils. However, simply washing a wooden cutting board with this water will not kill all the bacteria because they can remain in the crevices of the wood and be difficult to remove. Therefore, plastic cutting boards should be used for meats. A cleansing solution of one part bleach to eight parts of water will help kill many bacteria and can be followed by a clear water rinse. Sponges and dishcloths should also be soaked in this solution for short periods because they harbor many microorganisms.

To safely defrost frozen foods or meats, place them in the refrigerator or the microwave, depending on the amount of time available before preparation. Eating raw or rare meat compounds the chance of getting food poisoning. Once the meat is cooked, it should be served immediately. Even foods that have just been cooked contain bacterial spores that will begin germinating as soon as the food cools down to the "danger zone" temperatures of 125–60 degrees F (see figure 4.3).

Boiling suspicious foods is certainly better than warming them briefly, but it needs to be done for 20 minutes to destroy toxins. However, it would be better not to eat foods that you suspect are contaminated with microbes, because the toxins of staphylococcus or perfringens are not destroyed by heat.

Food Storage
Improper storage of food results in considerable bacterial growth and is the most common contributing factor in restaurant food poisonings (6). Cooked food can last only two hours maximum at room temperature before the safety limits are reached. The practice of preparing macaroni, ham, chicken, potato, and other salads or custard pies for picnics and allowing them to sit out for hours is unsafe. It is also risky to allow sandwiches (chicken, turkey, tuna, ham, egg), or fried chicken to remain unrefrigerated for hours.

Precautions should be taken to keep foods at temperatures either above 140 degrees F or below 40 degrees F. Of course this is not always practical, especially at buffets or picnics or for brown-bag lunches. Under these circumstances, foods should be considered safe for only two to three hours at the danger zone temperatures. After this time has elapsed, it is better not to eat the food.

A simple check of the refrigerator-freezer can help improve its ability to prevent food poisoning. The refrigerator should be kept clean so it will not become a breeding ground for microorganisms. Refrigeration and freezing do not kill microorganisms but simply slow down their growth. Weekly "search-and-seizures" of spoiled foods in the refrigerator can help to reduce microbial growth (see figure 4.4). The refrigerator temperature should remain below 40 degrees F, and the freezer must be below 32 degrees F. If storing foods in the freezer for more than a few weeks, the temperature should be 0 degrees F or below, not varying more than 10 degrees above this.

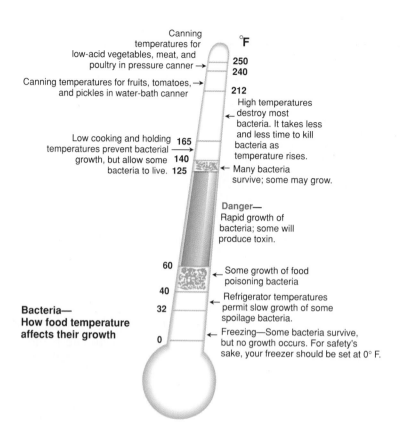

Canning temperatures for low-acid vegetables, meat, and poultry in pressure canner → 250 / 240

Canning temperatures for fruits, tomatoes, and pickles in water-bath canner → 212

High temperatures destroy most bacteria. It takes less and less time to kill bacteria as temperature rises.

Low cooking and holding temperatures prevent bacterial growth, but allow some bacteria to live. 165 / 140 / 125

Many bacteria survive; some may grow.

Danger— Rapid growth of bacteria; some will produce toxin.

60

Some growth of food poisoning bacteria

40

Refrigerator temperatures permit slow growth of some spoilage bacteria.

Bacteria— How food temperature affects their growth

32

Freezing—Some bacteria survive, but no growth occurs. For safety's sake, your freezer should be set at 0° F.

0

Food Canning

Most botulism cases reported today are a result of improper canning techniques. Reviewing current canning methods provided by the United States Department of Agriculture is critical. These change periodically, and it is extremely important to follow the procedures exactly. Reputable cookbooks on canning, as well as your state agricultural extension office, can provide current information.

Natural Toxins in Food

The widely held belief that "natural" foods are safe and nutritious is not always true. Because plants are unable to escape from their animal predators, their mechanism of defense is often to concentrate poisons in their leaves, roots, or stems. This has a wide variety of effects when the plant is eaten, including burning or inflaming the

mouth, irritating the digestive tract, inactivating enzymes, interfering with hormonal activity, and a quick death. There is a long roster of commonly eaten plants, both wild and cultivated, that contain poisons.

The mushroom is a gourmet's delight, provided that it is not of the poisonous variety. Although folklore provides helpful hints on telling the difference, there is no good rule of thumb for distinguishing between poisonous and nonpoisonous varieties. Of the thousands of species available in North America, only 100 are poisonous, and they often look like their nonpoisonous counterparts. Both poisonous and nonpoisonous varieties can even grow in the same places. Antidotes are available for many poisonous species, but a few have no cure. Symptoms may vary from intestinal upset to liver and kidney damage. If symptoms appear in less than three hours, the mushroom was one of the less toxic varieties. Symptoms that occur more than five hours to three weeks later could mean major trouble (7).

FIGURE 4.4

Food Storing Chart

Product	Storage period (to maintain its quality)	
	Refrigerator 35° to 40° F. Days	Freezer 0 ° F. Months
Fresh meats		
Roasts (Beef and Lamb)....	3 to 5	8 to 12
Roasts (Pork and Veal)......	3 to 5	4 to 8
Steaks (Beef)....................	3 to 5	8 to 12
Chops (Lamb and Pork).....	3 to 5	3 to 4
Ground and Stew Meats....	1 to 2	2 to 3
Variety Meats....................	1 to 2	3 to 4
Sausage (Pork).................	1 to 2	1 to 2
Processed meats		
Bacon.................................	7	1
Frankfurters.......................	7	1/2
Ham (Whole)......................	7	1 to 2
Ham (Half).........................	3 to 5	1 to 2
Ham (Slices)......................	3	1 to 2
Luncheon Meats................	3 to 5	
Sausage (Smoked)............	7	Freezing not recom-mended
Sausage (Dry and Semi - Dry).....	14 to 21	
Cooked meats		
Cooked Meats and Meat Dishes...........................	1 to 2	2 to 3
Gravy and Meat Broth........	1 to 2	2 to 3
Fresh poultry		
Chicken and Turkey............	1 to 2	12
Duck and Goose.................	1 to 2	6
Giblets................................	1 to 2	3
Cooked poultry		
Pieces (Covered with Broth)	1 to 2	6
Pieces (Not Covered)..........	1 to 2	1
Cooked Poultry Dishes........	1 to 2	6
Fried Chicken......................	1 to 2	4

In case of emergency

If power fails or the freezer stops operating normally, try to determine how long before the freezer will be back in operation.

A fully loaded freezer usually will stay cold enough to keep foods frozen for 2 days if the cabinet is not opened. In a cabinet with less than half a load, food may not stay frozen more than 1 day.

If normal operation cannot be resumed before the food will start to thaw, use dry ice. If dry ice is placed in the freezer soon after the power is off, 25 pounds should keep the temperature below freezing for 2 to 3 days in a 10-cubic-foot cabinet with half a load, 3 to 4 days in a loaded cabinet.

Place the dry ice on cardboard or small boards on top of packages, and do not open freezer again except to put in more dry ice or to remove it when normal operation is resumed.

Or move food to a locker plant, using insulated boxes or thick layers of paper to prevent thawing.

Another naturally occurring poison is aflatoxin, which is produced by a fungus that grows on peanuts, pistachios, corn, rice, and certain other grains and nuts. This toxin-producing mold is one of the most powerful carcinogens known. In parts of Africa and Southeast Asia this fungus, *Aspergillus flavus,* is thought to be responsible for high rates of liver cancer.

Several different types of food poisoning are associated with eating certain marine fish and shellfish. Ciguatoxin, which has been responsible for many food poisonings in Florida and Hawaii, results from the consumption of bottom-dwelling fish such as barracuda, grouper, sea bass, eel, and red snapper. Cooking does not destroy the poison, and symptoms include cramps, vomiting, diarrhea, numbness, and other signs of nervous disorders, appearing one to six hours after ingestion. Paralytic shellfish poisoning (PSP) results from eating shellfish that come from sewage-contaminated waters. PSP is characterized by numbness, gastric distress, and possibly difficulty in speaking and walking. Symptoms occur within 30 minutes to three hours. Proper inspection and sanitation is needed to prevent these poisonings.

Refer to Sidebar 4.1 for instructions on what to do if poisoning occurs.

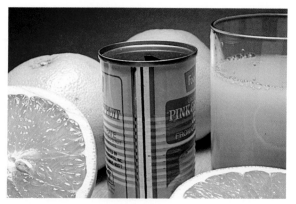

Acidic foods should not be stored in cans because the lead solder might leach out into the food.

Environmental Contaminants

Along with the poisons that occur naturally in our food supply, a considerable number of chemicals contaminate our foods accidentally. The sources of these chemicals include cookware, food containers, agricultural residues, and industrial wastes. This important topic could be discussed at considerable length; however, only lead and pesticide residues are presented here but will illustrate the complexity of the problem.

Lead

Today lead is used in a wide range of industries, most importantly for making storage batteries and as an antiknock additive in gasoline. It is found throughout the environment, in soil, water, air, and food.

Several sources of lead in the food supply should be noted. Canned foods are a potential source of lead for humans. Lead solder is used to seal cans along the seams. Acidic foods such as tomato products, fruits, fruit juices, and pickles leach out the lead from the solder into the food. Exposure to oxygen accelerates the process, so storing acidic foods in the can after

opening is dangerous. The Food and Drug Administration (FDA) recommends that a child consume no more than 100 micrograms of lead per day. An open can of orange juice in the refrigerator may contain 34 to 420 micrograms of lead per ounce, depending on how long it has been in the refrigerator (8). A half-cup serving ranging from 136 to 1,680 micrograms would be far above the FDA maximum recommendation for children. Immediately transferring canned foods to glass containers after opening would reduce the risk of lead exposure.

Another potential hazard to our food supply is using earthenware containers to store or serve acidic foods. If the glaze on these containers has not been fired sufficiently, lead can leach from the glaze and poison the food. Earthenware produced commercially in this country is not a concern, but caution should be taken with items bought in other countries or made at home. Only lead-free glazes should be used on food containers that you make. If foreign purchases are questionable, do not use them for acidic foods.

Lead affects health in a number of adverse ways; it can cause sterility, miscarriage, birth defects, and anemia. The most serious manifestation is damage to the central nervous system, resulting in mental retardation, convulsions, coma, and death. Most cases have resulted from the consumption of lead-based paint chips from old (before 1940) interior paints. However, new evidence reveals that chronic exposure to levels of lead previously considered safe can result in lower scores on tests of intelligence, verbal skills, attention span, language development, as well as more unruly classroom behavior (9).

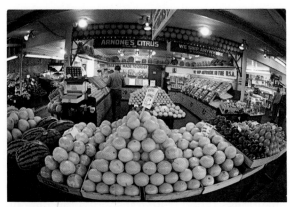
Fruits and vegetables are inspected for pesticide residues before public consumption.

Pesticide Residues

Pesticides have been widely used in the United States since the 1950s to protect food crops from insects, weeds, and destructive diseases. There are 300 chemical compounds that are active ingredients in pesticides. As the use of pesticides became more widespread, evidence mounted that some of these chemicals not only destroyed pests but also were harmful to humans and to the environment.

The use of pesticides is regulated by two agencies. The Environmental Protection Agency (EPA) is responsible for the environment, and the FDA monitors pesticide residues in foods. A Roper poll in 1984 shows that 59 percent of the public sees a need for even more regulation than is currently practiced by these agencies (10). The public lists residues of pesticides as one of its major concerns. Of those surveyed by the Food Marketing Institute, 77 percent said that chemical residues such as pesticides and herbicides are a serious hazard, and 18 percent described them as something of a hazard (11).

The process of assuring safety involves balancing the risks and the benefits. The EPA sets "tolerances" for pesticide levels in food, based on research data and on the residue that will be left on food when it reaches the consumer. Tolerances are maximum levels of residue allowed that will still ensure the public safety. The EPA must weigh the risk of residues against the benefit of pesticide use. The U.S. Department of Agriculture estimates that without pesticides, crop production would drop at least 25 percent, and food prices would rise 50 percent (12).

The FDA enforces the residue tolerances by frequent sampling of fruits, vegetables, fish, milk and dairy products, grains, and animal feeds. Special sampling is conducted when problems are suspected or information on a food commodity or pesticide is needed. The FDA inspects and samples food in the field, on route to market, at the marketplace, and at the supermarket. The purpose of inspecting food at the supermarket is to evaluate the pesticide consumption of a total diet. Surveillance of domestic and imported foods shows that almost all samples comply with the residue limits (10). Periodic problems do occur, though, and crops may be turned away, for example, at the border of Mexico during import, or seized at our own markets and destroyed.

Food Additives

The FDA: Safeguarding Our Food Supply

A novel by Upton Sinclair (*The Jungle*) illustrated that the conditions in Chicago's meatpacking industry at the turn of the century were repulsive. Moldy, spoiled meat was doused with borax and glycerine to cover up the smell and create a fresh look. Public outrage at these and other practices of the food industry stimulated the passage in 1906 of this nation's first Food and Drug Act. This act stated that only additives that were proved to be safe and effective could be used in foods. While an important start, the act was difficult to enforce due to limited testing of foods for residues of additives and pesticides. Government inspection of processing plants was allowed only if prior agreement was made with the management.

The authority of the FDA was extended in 1938 with the passage of the Federal Food, Drug, and Cosmetic Act. The act provided for **standards of identity** for 200 foods. These define what ingredients must be used in particular foods, such as mayonnaise, ketchup, peanut butter, and ice cream. Ingredients of foods that have standards of identity do not need to be listed on the label. Some consumers disapprove of the standards of identity because the ingredient list is not easily available to them. Also under this act, additives could be used by the food industry unless they were proven unsafe by the FDA, a laborious and expensive task that did not give priority to the nation's health.

In 1958, the Food Additives Amendment was added to the 1938 Food, Drug, and Cosmetics Act. The 1958 law enforced manufacturers, rather than the FDA, to provide evidence of safety for each additive.

The GRAS List

More than 600 additives that were in common use before the Food Additives Amendment of 1958 were exempt from the requirement to prove they were harmless. This group of chemicals was titled "generally recognized as safe" **(the GRAS list).** Although it appeared reasonable to allow salt, sugar, and spices to be added to foods, a number of additives with questionable or untested safety appeared on the list.

If the FDA questions the safety of a chemical on the GRAS list, it must provide evidence that it is unsafe before it can be removed. For example, cyclamate, an artificial sweetener, was shown to cause bladder cancer in mice and rats, and it was removed from the list in 1969. About thirteen certified food colors have also been removed. Additives that remain on the GRAS list have for the most part stood the test of time. Controversy exists concerning the potential for dangerous chemicals to be hidden behind this list while an unsuspecting public consumes them.

The Delaney Clause

The Delaney Clause was another amendment to the Pure Food, Drug, and Cosmetics Act. It was passed by Congress in 1958 to protect the public from additives found to be **carcinogenic.** The amendment states that a substance that causes cancer in either a human or an animal at any dosage, no matter how small, must not be added to food. If additives on the GRAS list, previously tested additives, or new additives are found to cause cancer, they must be banned. The FDA has no discretionary power on this point. Outside pressures from the food industry therefore cannot influence the decision of the FDA.

Support is growing to amend the Delaney Clause or to apply the concept of *de minimis non curat lex* ("the law takes no account of trifles"). Frank E. Young, commissioner of the FDA in 1988, concluded that the FDA has the discretion to apply the *de minimis* concept under the Color Additive Amendments of 1960 (13). Based on the threshold principle of carcinogenesis, such interpretation would allow the addition of substances at a level so low that it would not have significant (if any) health risk. Additives might then be divided into high-, moderate-, and low-risk categories, leaving different options for regulation. The high-risk additives would be banned, but the low-risk additives may only carry a warning label. Like other additives, carcinogens would then be weighted on a risk-benefit ratio scale. Financial benefits are still difficult to measure against health risks.

The Function of Food Additives

The role of food additives has become more prominent in recent years due to the changes that have occurred in the American life-style. As Americans moved from farms to cities, large-scale production of food was necessary. Great quantities of food were transported throughout the country and stored for long periods. Women began to pursue careers outside the home, which created a demand for prepared, processed, and convenience foods. Technology became more sophisticated, and seasonal products were available year-round. Greater buying power, along with sophisticated marketing techniques, has expanded the demand for new products. Thus our supermarkets are bursting with a wider variety of food selections, but the price is more food additives.

Food additives are any substances that become part of a food product or that otherwise affect the characteristics of any food, directly or indirectly through producing, processing, treating, packaging, transporting or storing. Some 2,800 substances are intentionally added to foods, whereas 10,000 other compounds find their way into our foods during processing, packaging, or storage (14).

Our ancestors used salt to preserve meat and fish, and large amounts of sugar helped preserve fruit. Today sugar and salt are still the most widely used additives. These two, along with corn syrup and dextrose, account for over 90 percent by weight of the food additives used in our country (15) (see table 4.1).

Intentional uses of food additives are designated for the following four purposes:

to maintain or improve nutritional value,
to maintain product quality,
to make food more appealing, and
to help in processing or preparation.

Additives to Improve Nutritional Value

Over the past 50 years, diseases such as goiter, pellagra, beriberi, and rickets have nearly disappeared in the United States. Most of us have not seen nor experienced them, due in part to the addition of vitamins and minerals to flour, milk, cereals, and breads.

TABLE 4.1
Annual per capita consumption of the most common food additives in the United States

Additive	Amount (in lbs)
Sugar	100.0
Salt	15.0
Corn syrup	8.0
Dextrose	4.0
Flavor enhancers	
MSG	1.5
Mustard	0.8
Black pepper	0.4
Hydrolyzed vegetable protein, etc.	0.2
Stabilizers/thickeners	
Sodium caseinate	0.4
Modified starch	0.8
Leavening agents	
Sodium/calcium carbonate	0.3
Dicalcium/disodium phosphate	0.1
Acidity control	
Sodium bicarbonate	0.3
Hydrogen chloride	0.3
Citric acid	0.2
Emulsifiers	
Lecithin	0.2
Mono- or diglycerides	0.9
Miscellaneous	
Sulfur dioxide (preservative)	0.5
Carbon dioxide (effervescent)	0.2
Calcium sulfate (processing acid)	0.2
Caramel	0.3

Adapted from B. Caballero, "Food Additives in the Pediatric Diet." *Clinical Nutrition*, 4:200–206, 1985. Used with permission of Longman Group L., Edinburgh.

Several terms are used when discussing the enhancement of the nutrient value of foods. **Restoration** is the addition of nutrients to food to compensate for losses during processing. **Fortification** is the addition of nutrients at levels higher than those found in the original food and includes adding nutrients that were not present in the original food. For example, vitamin D is added to milk, and vitamin A is added to margarine. **Enrichment** is the addition of nutrients to levels specified in the standards of identity. When white flour is milled, some of the nutrients are removed and several of them (thiamine, niacin, riboflavin, and iron) are then replaced to meet the standard of identity. Enrichment, then, is incomplete restoration of foods.

Nutrient fortification of foods probably started in 1833, when a French chemist advocated the addition of iodine to salt to prevent **goiter,** an enlargement of the thyroid gland due to lack of iodine in the diet. Goiter was prevalent in the Great Lakes area of the United States because the soil, water, and crops were devoid of iodine. In 1924, iodine began being added to salt in the United States.

During World War I, vitamin A deficiency became apparent in Denmark, and shortly thereafter margarine was fortified with vitamin A. Vitamin D fortification of whole milk began in 1931 to help prevent rickets, a childhood deficiency disease in which the bones fail to grow properly.

In the 1940s evidence of widespread deficiency diseases in the United States was developing. The National Research Council established what is now known as the Food and Nutrition Board. This committee soon endorsed a program to enrich grains with iron and the B-complex vitamins thiamine, riboflavin, and niacin. This was a public health measure to prevent such diseases as iron-deficiency anemia, **beriberi** (a thiamine deficiency that results in partial paralysis of the extremities), and **pellagra** (a niacin deficiency resulting in skin eruptions, digestive and nervous system disturbances, and mental deterioration). Staple foods are often fortified or enriched to ensure affecting the greatest number of consumers. Currently, calcium is being added to a variety of products, including flour, milk, and some soft drinks, in hopes that it will help prevent **osteoporosis** (a disease in which the density of bones decreases with age and they become brittle). Fiber is another recent additive to breads and breakfast cereals.

The Food and Nutrition Board continues to endorse nutrient fortification and enrichment under the following conditions.

1. The intake of the nutrient is below the desirable level in a significant number of people.
2. The fortified food will be consumed in quantities that will make a considerable input on the diet of the target population.
3. The addition of the nutrient will not cause an imbalance in other essential nutrients.
4. The nutrient added is stable during storage of the food.
5. The nutrient is physiologically available from the food.
6. There is little risk of toxicity due to excessive intake (16).

Controversy about fortification does exist in regard to the cost and the health benefits. Although fortification is useful for selected groups of individuals, not everyone needs fortified foods. In some instances toxicity could result from fortification of products in combination with a diet that is already sufficient. The fortification of cereals at 100 percent of the U.S. RDA is one case in which the benefits may be less than the cost.

Consumers can tell which food products are enriched or fortified because they must be labeled. The FDA requires the labeling of additives for nutritional value. Packages for "enriched flour" or "fortified milk" must list the specific nutrients included and the amounts of each.

Additives That Maintain Product Quality

The group of additives that prevent food spoilage is known as **preservatives.** Although this group is more often maligned than most of the others, the majority of preservatives are quite harmless; in fact they are beneficial.

There are basically two ways in which food spoils. One type of spoilage is caused by mold, bacteria, fungi, and yeast and leads to possible food poisoning. The other type occurs when foods are exposed to oxygen, which leads to changes in color and/or flavor. For instance, oxidation causes sliced peaches to become brown and butter to taste rancid when left on the counter for too long. Two categories of preservatives are designed to prevent spoilage.

Antimicrobial agents inhibit the growth of microorganisms in food. These have helped to dramatically reduce the cases of food poisoning in our country. Some of these agents have been used since history was recorded. Salt, for instance, was used to preserve meats, fish, and vegetables. Sugar has also long been used to preserve fruits. Other preservatives in this category are calcium or sodium propionate, sodium benzoate, sodium nitrate, potassium sorbate, and sodium bisulfite (17). Table 4.2 describes the function and sources of these additives.

Antioxidants are the group of additives that retard rancidity in foods. They scavenge oxygen on the surface of foods so that it is not available for attacking food ingredients. This helps to extend the shelf life of a product. Many manufacturers use safe additives like vitamin E and vitamin C. At home you may use lemon juice or vinegar to keep sliced apples from browning. Commercially, three of the most widely used antioxidants, butylated hydroxyanisole (BHA), butylated hydroxytoluene (BHT), and propylgallate are of questionable safety (18) (see table 4.2).

Additives That Make Food More Appealing

Colors and flavors are often added to foods to make them more appealing. Both strongly influence food selection, judgment of food quality, and decisions about whether to eat the food again.

Colors Almost all processed foods contain color additives. They must be listed as ingredients (except when present in butter, cheese, or ice cream), and cannot be used in excessive amounts or to cover up unwholesome products.

There are two classes of color additives (19). Uncertified colors are derived from natural sources such as vegetables, animals, and minerals, or synthetic duplications of these colors. Certified colors are synthetic chemicals produced in laboratories and undergo a more stringent approval process. By far these are the most widely used of the two. The synthetic colors are stronger and therefore can be used in smaller amounts, and thus at a lower cost.

Red No. 40 and Yellow No. 5 are two of the most frequently used food colors. Controversy exists over their use because both pose health risks for humans. Red No. 40 is suspected of causing cancer of the lymph tissue. Yellow No. 5 causes allergic reactions (rashes and sniffles) in 50,000 to 90,000 Americans (14) (see table 4.2).

Flavors Flavor additives have been criticized less than color additives, probably because they have a more direct link to the acceptability of food (see table 4.2). Synthetic flavors are cheaper and more abundant than their natural counterparts. Also, people who have adverse reactions to synthetic flavors are likely to react to the natural ones too, because of similar chemical composition.

Products containing any artificial flavorings must note it on the label, for example, "artificial flavors or spices." "Artificially flavored peach yogurt" means that it contains artificial flavors, whereas "peach yogurt" contains only natural flavorings and peaches. "Peach-flavored yogurt" means a product contains only the natural flavor of the peaches but no actual fruit (20).

TABLE 4.2
Food additives

Purpose: To Improve or Maintain Nutritional Value
Class: Nutrients

Some Additives	Where You Might Find Them	Their Functions
B vitamins: thiamine, thiamine hydrochloride, thiamine mononitrate; riboflavin; niacin, niacinamide	Flour, breads, cereals, rice, macaroni products	*Enrich:* Replace vitamins and minerals lost in processing.
Beta carotene (source of vitamin A)	Margarine	or
Iodine, potassium iodide	Salt	
Iron	Grain products	*Fortify:* Add nutrients that may be lacking in the diet.
Alpha tocopherols (vitamin E)	Cereals, grain products	
Vitamin A	Milk, margarine, cereals	
Vitamin D, D_2, D_3	Milk, cereals	
Vitamin C (ascorbic acid)	Beverages, beverage mixes, processed fruit	

Purpose: To Maintain Product Quality
Class: Preservatives (Antimicrobials)

Some Additives	Where You Might Find Them	Their Functions
Ascorbic acid (vitamin C)	Fruit products, acidic foods	Prevent food spoilage from bacteria, molds, fungi, and yeast; extend shelf life; or protect natural color/flavor.
Benzoic acid, sodium benzoate	Fruit products, acidic foods, margarine	
Citric Acid	Acidic foods	
Lactic acid, calcium lactate	Olives, cheese, frozen desserts, some beverages	
Parabens: butylparaben, heptylparaben, methylparaben, propylparaben	Beverages, cake-type pastries, salad dressings, relishes	
Propionic acid: calcium propionate, potassium propionate, sodium propionate	Breads and other baked goods	
Sodium diacetate	Baked goods	
Sodium erythorbate	Cured meats	
Sodium nitrate, sodium nitrite	Cured meats, fish, poultry	
Sorbic acid: calcium sorbate, potassium sorbate, sodium sorbate	Cheeses, syrups, cakes, beverages, mayonnaise, fruit products, margarine, processed meats	

Purpose: To Maintain Product Quality
Class: Preservatives (Antioxidants)

Some Additives	Where You Might Find Them	Their Functions
Ascorbic acid (vitamin C)	Processed fruits, baked goods	Delay or prevent undesirable changes in color, flavor, or texture — enzymatic browning or discoloration due to oxidation; delay or prevent rancidity in foods with unstable oils.
BHA (butylated hydroxyanisole) BHT (butylated hydroxytoluene)	Bakery products, cereals, snack foods, fats and oils	
Citric acid	Fruits, snack foods, cereals, instant potatoes	
EDTA (ethylenediaminetetraacetic acid)	Dressings, sauces, margarine	
Propyl gallate	Cereals, snack foods, pastries	
TBHQ (tertiary butylhydroquinone)	Snack foods, fats and oils	
Tocopherols (including vitamin E)	Oils and shortening	

Source: U.S. Department of Health and Human Services, Public Health Service, Food and Drug Administration, 1979. More Than You Ever Thought You Would Know about Food Additives. *FDA Consumer.* (May and June). HHS Publication No. (FDA) 79-2118 (May, Part II) and 79-2119 (June, Part III). Washington, D.C.: U.S. Government Printing Office.

TABLE 4.2
continued

Purpose: To Aid in Processing or Preparation
Class: Emulsifiers

Some Additives	Where You Might Find Them	Their Functions
Carrageenan	Chocolate milk, canned milk drinks, whipped toppings	Help to evenly distribute tiny particles of one liquid into another, e.g., oil and water; modify surface tension of liquid to establish a uniform dispersion or emulsion; improve homogeneity, consistency, stability, texture.
Lecithin	Margarine, dressings, chocolate, frozen desserts, baked goods	
Mono/diglycerides	Baked goods, peanut butter, cereals	
Polysorbate 60, 65, 80	Gelatin/pudding desserts, dressings, baked goods, nondairy creams, ice cream	
Sorbitan monostearate	Cakes, toppings, chocolate	
Dioctyl sodium sulfosuccinate	Cocoa	

Purpose: To Aid in Processing or Preparation
Class: Stabilizers, Thickeners, Texturizers

Some Additives	Where You Might Find Them	Their Functions
Ammonium alginate Calcium alginate Potassium alginate Sodium alginate	Dessert-type dairy products, confections	Impart body, improve consistency, texture; stabilize emulsions; affect appearance/mouth feel of the food; many are natural carbohydrate which absorb water in the food.
Carrageenan	Frozen desserts, puddings, syrups, jellies	
Cellulose derivates	Breads, ice cream, confections, diet foods	
Flour	Sauces, gravies, canned foods	
Furcelleran	Frozen desserts, puddings, syrups	
Modified food starch	Sauces, soups, pie fillings, canned meals, snack foods	
Pectin	Jams/jellies, fruit products, frozen desserts	
Propylene glycol	Baked goods, frozen desserts, dairy spreads	
Vegetable gums: guar gum, gum arabic, gum ghatti, karaya gum, locust (carob) bean gum, tragacanth gum, larch gum (arabinogalactan)	Chewing gum, sauces, desserts, dressings, syrups, beverages, fabricated foods, cheese, baked goods	

Purpose: To Aid in Processing or Preparation
Class: Leavening Agents

Some Additives	Where You Might Find Them	Their Functions
Yeast	Breads, baked goods	Affect cooking results; texture and increased volume; also some flavor effects.
Baking powder, double-acting (sodium bicarbonate, sodium aluminum sulfate, calcium phosphate)	Quick breads, cake-type baked goods	
Baking soda (sodium bicarbonate)	Quick breads, cake-type baked goods	

Purpose: To Aid in Processing or Preparation
Class: pH Control Agents

Some Additives	Where You Might Find Them	Their Functions
Acetic acid/sodium acetate	Candies, sauces, dressings, relishes	Control (change/maintain) acidity or alkalinity; can affect texture, taste, wholesomeness.
Adipic acid	Beverage/gelatin bases, bottled drinks	
Citric acid/sodium citrate	Fruit products, candies, beverages, frozen desserts	
Fumaric acid	Dry dessert bases, confections, powdered soft drinks	
Lactic acid	Cheeses, beverages, frozen desserts	
Calcium lactate	Fruits/vegetables, dry/condensed milk	
Phosphoric acid/phosphates	Fruit products, beverages, ices/sherbets, soft drinks, oils, baked goods	
Tartaric acid/tartrates	Confections, some dairy desserts, baked goods, beverages	

Purpose: To Aid in Processing or Preparation
Class: Humectants

Some Additives	Where You Might Find Them	Their Functions
Glycerine	Flaked coconut	Retain moisture.
Glycerol monostearate	Marshmallow	
Propylene glycol	Confections, pet foods	
Sorbitol	Soft candies, gum	

Purpose: To Aid in Processing or Preparation
Class: Maturing and Bleaching Agents, Dough Conditioners

Some Additives	Where You Might Find Them	Their Functions
Azodicarbonamide	Cereal flour, breads	Accelerate the aging process (oxidation) to develop the gluten characteristics of flour; improve baking qualities.
Acetone peroxide	Flour, breads & rolls	
Benzoyl peroxide		
Hydrogen peroxide		
Calcium/potassium bromate	Breads	
Sodium stearyl fumarate	Yeast-leavened breads, instant potatoes, processed cereals	

Purpose: To Aid in Processing or Preparation
Class: Anticaking Agents

Some Additives	Where You Might Find Them	Their Functions
Calcium silicate	Table salt, baking powder, other powdered foods	Help keep salts and powders free-flowing; prevent caking, lumping, or clustering of a finely powdered or crystalline substance.
Iron ammonium citrate	Salt	
Silicon dioxide	Table salt, baking powder, other powdered foods	
Yellow prussiate of soda	Salt	

Purpose: To Affect Appeal Characteristics
Class: Flavor Enhancers

Some Additives	Where You Might Find Them	Their Functions
Disodium guanylate	Canned vegetables	Substances which supplement, magnify, or modify the original taste and/or aroma of a food — *without* imparting a characteristic taste or aroma of its own.
Disodium inosinate	Canned vegetables	
Hydrolyzed vegetable protein	Processed meats, gravy/sauce mixes, fabricated foods	
MSG (monosodium glutamate)	Oriental foods, soups, foods with animal protein	
Yeast-malt sprout extract	Gravies, sauces	

Purpose: To Affect Appeal Characteristics
Class: Flavors

Some Additives	Where You Might Find Them	Their Functions
Vanilla (natural)	Baked goods	Make foods taste better; improve natural flavor; restore flavors lost in processing.
Vanillin (synthetic)	Baked goods	
Spices and other natural seasonings and flavorings, e.g., clove, cinnamon, ginger, paprika, turmeric, anise, sage, thyme, basil	No restrictions on usage in foods — found in many products	

Purpose: To Affect Appeal Characteristics
Class: Sweeteners

Some Additives	Where You Might Find Them	Their Functions
Nutritive Sweeteners: Mannitol — sugar alcohol Sorbitol — sugar alcohol	Candies, gum, confections, baked goods	Make the aroma or taste of a food more agreeable or pleasurable.
Dextrose Fructose Glucose Sucrose (table sugar)	Cereals, baked goods, candies, processed foods, processed meats.	
Corn syrup/corn syrup solids Invert sugar	Cereals, baked goods, candies, processed foods, processed meats.	
Non-nutritive sweeteners: Saccharin	Special dietary foods, beverages	

Flavor Enhancers Substances that modify the way food tastes without contributing a flavor of their own are called **food enhancers.** Monosodium glutamate (MSG) is one of the best-known food enhancers. It is heavily used in Chinese restaurants and can cause a burning sensation in the neck and forearms, tightness in the chest, and a headache in some people. Several years ago MSG was removed from baby foods because studies showed that large amounts destroy brain cells in mice.

Sweeteners Sweeteners are divided into two categories—non-nutritive (Calorie-free) and nutritive (providing Calories).

Cyclamate and saccharin top the list of non-nutritive sweeteners. Cyclamate was banned by the FDA in 1969 after studies showed it causes cancer in animals. Saccharin was removed from the GRAS list in the early 1970s due to evidence that it was a health hazard. A ban was proposed by the FDA in 1977 after a Canadian government study showed it produced bladder cancer in rats. Saccharin is used in dietetic foods and diet soft drinks, but the proposed removal from the latter

TABLE 4.2
continued

Purpose: To Affect Appeal Characteristics
Class: Natural/Synthetic (N/S) Colors

Some Additives	Where You Might Find Them	Their Functions
N Annatto extract (yellow-red)	No restrictions	Increase consumer appeal and product acceptance by giving a desired, appetizing, or characteristic color. Any material which imparts color when added to a food. Generally *not* restricted to certain foods or food classes. May *not* be used to cover up an unwholesome food, *or* used in excessive amounts.
N Dehydrated beets/beet powder	No restrictions	
S Ultramarine Blue	Animal feed only .5% by wt.	
N/S Canthaxanthin (orange-red)	Limit = 30 mg/lb of food	
N Caramel (brown)	No restrictions	
N/S Beta-apo-8' carotenal (yellow-red)	Limit = 15 mg/lb of food	
N/S Beta carotene (yellow)	No restrictions	*Must* be used in accordance with FDA Good Manufacturing Practice Regulations.
N Cochineal extract/carmine (red)	No restrictions	
N Toasted partially defatted cooked cottonseed flour (brown shades)	No restrictions	
S Ferrous gluconate (turns black)	Ripe olives	
N Grape skin extract (purple-red)	Beverages only	
S Iron oxide (red-brown)	Pet foods only .25% or less by wt.	
N Fruit juice/vegetable juice	No restrictions	
N Dried algae meal (yellow)	Chicken feed only	
N Tagetes (Aztec Marigold)	Chicken feed only	
N Carrot oil (orange)	No restrictions	
N Corn endosperm (red-brown)	Chicken feed only	
N Paprika/paprika oleoresin (red-orange)	No restrictions	
N/S Riboflavin (yellow)	No restrictions	
N Saffron (orange)	No restrictions	
S Titanium dioxide (white)	Limit = 1% by wt.	
N Turmeric/Turmeric oleoresins (yellow)	No restrictions	
S FD&C Blue No. 1	No restrictions	Synthetic color additives subject to certification; inspected and tested for impurities.
S Citrus Red No. 2	Orange skins of mature, green, eating-oranges. Limit = 2 ppm.	
S FD&C Red No. 3	No restrictions	
S FD&C Red No. 40	No restrictions	
S FD&C Yellow No. 5	No restrictions	

caused a public outcry. Congress passed a moratorium on the ban, and as of today it is still sold in bulk and added to foods and beverages. Acesulfame potassium received approval in July 1988 as a new Calorie-free sweetener and will compete in the artificial-sweetener market.

The nutritive sweeteners include sucrose, fructose, glucose, and sugar alcohols such as mannitol, xylitol, and sorbitol. Natural sugars not only flavor foods but may help them to brown or give them a certain texture.

Sugar alcohols are variants of sugar commonly found in diabetic or low- or no-sugar products. Although they taste sweet, their absorption and metabolism differs from sugar. Sorbitol is the most widely distributed and can be found in chewing gums, candies, and dietetic ice cream.

In the early 1980s, aspartame, a nutritive sweetener, gained approval from the FDA, and its sales have now surpassed those of saccharin's. Marketed under the name of Nutra-Sweet, it is two hundred times sweeter than table sugar. Its amazing popularity may be attributed to a taste similar to that of sugar, without the bitter aftertaste of saccharin. What are the health consequences of this product? Although many symptoms have been reported by consumers, research has not shown any significant problems in healthy or diabetic adults.

Aspartame is composed of two amino acids, phenylalanine and aspartic acid, that are broken down in the digestive tract and then absorbed. The fact that these two amino acids can accumulate in the blood may be cause for concern, although no health or behavioral effects have yet been consistently shown. People with the genetic disease phenylketonuria (PKU), however, should not ingest aspartame. These individuals are unable to metabolize the amino acid phenylalanine, and it can build up to toxic levels in their bloodstream. (PKU is further discussed later in this chapter.)

FDA approval of aspartame was based on the assumption that adults would not consume more than 34 milligrams per kilogram of body weight per day. A 130-pound female could then use 60 packs of this sweetener each day. Although that sounds like a tremendous amount, one 12-ounce soft drink contains the equivalent of five to six packs. (Some people do drink up to ten cans of soft drink per day. This high intake should be reduced and soft drinks replaced with water, for example.) The FDA assumes that infants and children would not consume large amounts of such products.

Additives That Help in Processing or Preparation

The final category of food additives includes those that aid in processing and/or preparation of foods. They are responsible for some of the characteristics that we commonly associate with foods. The rising of baked goods, the thickening of jams, the lack of crystals in ice cream, and the lack of separation between the dry and oily portions of some peanut butters are all qualities achieved with the use of additives. Alginate, brominated vegetable oil, carrageenan, gelatin, gums, lecithin, mono- and diglycerides, polysorbate 60, sodium carboxymethylcellulose, and starch are just such texture-improving agents. Table 4.2 provides information on their uses.

Food Labels

Although we might be fearful of what is in a particular food, the label is a reliable source of this information. A product label may state the nutritional makeup, an ingredient list, how long the product has been on the supermarket shelf, and the expiration date. In some cases the FDA requires that certain information be listed, but other information often is included voluntarily by the manufacturer.

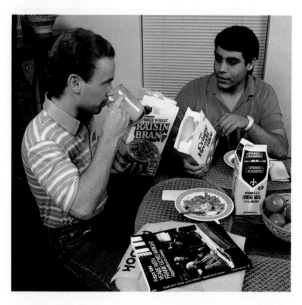

*F*IGURE 4.5
Comparing ingredients.

List of Ingredients

Most foods must contain a list of ingredients by common names. The ingredient present in the largest amount must be listed first, followed in descending order by the others (see figure 4.5). Additives also must be listed; however, general language can be used, such as, "artificial colors" and "artificial flavors." The exception is Yellow No. 5 (tartrazine), which must be identified specifically because it causes allergic reactions in some people. Those foods that have standards of identity need not list their ingredients. A standard of identity describes the ingredients a food must contain. Mayonnaise, ice cream, peanut butter, and ketchup, for example, have standards of identity. Only the mandatory contents are included in the standard of identity; any extra ingredients that are not part of the standard must be listed on the product label.

Nutrition Information

Nutrition information is required for all products that add protein, vitamins, or minerals, or if a nutritional claim is made on the label (for example, "contains no cholesterol"). The amount of protein, carbohydrate, and fat in a specified serving is listed on many products. Beginning in 1986, the sodium content was also required to be listed on all labels. See table 4.3 for a summary of mandatory and optional items found on product labels.

TABLE 4.3
Summary of nutrition labeling requirements

Description	Reporting Requirement
Mandatory Items	
Serving size	Varies
Servings per container	Varies
Calorie content	0–20 Kcal to the nearest 2 Kcal; 21–50 Kcal to the nearest 5 Kcal; 51+ Kcal to the nearest 10 Kcal
Protein content	For 1 gram or more, grams per serving to the nearest gram
Carbohydrate	For 1 gram or more, grams per serving to the nearest gram
Fat	For 1 gram or more, grams per serving to the nearest gram
Sodium	Milligrams per serving
Percentage of U.S. RDA for protein, vitamin A, vitamin C, thiamine, riboflavin, niacin, calcium, iron	In 2% increments to 10% level; 5% increments to 50% level; 10% increments above 50%; less than 2% indicated by 0 or other appropriate notation
Optional Nutrients	
Percentage of U.S. RDA for vitamins D, E, and B$_6$, folic acid, vitamin B$_{12}$, phosphorous, iodine, magnesium, zinc, copper, biotin, pantothenic acid	
Information on potassium, cholesterol, and fatty acids may also be presented, the latter two with the data on fat.	

Note: Nutrition information must be presented in this order.

Data from Code of Federal Regulations. Title 21. Part 101.9 (1985).

The label must state the amount per serving of each nutrient. The serving size should be stated in cups, teaspoons, or other common measures, and the number of servings per container must be shown. Protein, fat, and carbohydrate content are expressed in grams, whereas sodium is listed in milligrams.

Look closely at the label on a product from your own cupboard. Notice the percentages of the U.S. RDA for protein, five vitamins (vitamins A, C, thiamine, riboflavin, and niacin), and two minerals (iron and calcium). Optional listing of 12 other nutrients, if they contribute at least two percent of the U.S. RDA, is possible. If any of these 19 nutrients is added or the package makes a claim about them, they must be included on the label.

Use labels to your advantage. Suppose the cereal you eat contains 25 percent of the U.S. RDA for iron. (The U.S. RDA of iron is 18 milligrams.) If you ate one serving of the cereal, you consumed 4.5 milligrams of iron. Check all the cereals in your cupboard; do some provide more iron than others?

FIGURE 4.6
Always check for the expiration date before using perishable products.

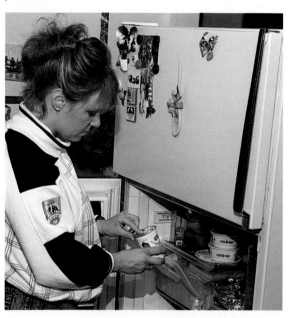

Addition of Nutrients to Food

The FDA supports the addition of nutrients to food for fortification, enrichment, or restoration. These include vitamin A fortification of margarine, vitamin D fortification of milk, and enrichment of grains with B vitamins and iron. The FDA considers it inappropriate to add nutrients to fresh produce or meats, sugars, snack foods, candy, and carbonated beverages.

Product Dating

When buying products, especially perishables, check the product date for safety. Four types of dating are commonly used. The **pack date** is the day the product was manufactured. The **pull or sell date** is more informative to the supermarket, since it indicates the last date the product should be sold. This provides some time for home storage before it is safely eaten. The **expiration date** is important to check in the home because it is the last date the food can safely be consumed (see figure 4.6). Last, the **freshness date** is used for baked goods, which may safely be eaten for a short time after the date but may not taste the same.

Label Usage

More Americans claim to use the information provided on nutrition labels—80 percent more than in the early 1970s (21). Unfortunately, they do not always use it to make better food choices. Some of the reasons for this include:

label comprehension is low,
brand loyalty and price complicate nutritious food selections,
clever advertising often detracts from nutritious choices, and
descriptive terms on product labels ("naturally sweet" for example) are equally influential with labeling (21).

Learning how to interpret the information on product labels can help you distinguish between healthy products and those that rely on marketing gimmicks. Table 4.4 explains terms found on labels, and figure 4.7 explains how to use nutrition information.

Food Allergies

About 17 percent of Americans suffer from some type of allergy. The most common is hay fever (7 percent), followed by asthma (4 percent). Food allergies are most prevalent in infants, with an incidence ranging from 0.3 percent to 20 percent (22). Fortunately, most children outgrow food allergies.

Immunological Reactions to Food

Protein and other large molecules are usually broken down in the digestive tract before being absorbed. Occasionally, these large molecules are absorbed without being broken down, causing an **allergic reaction.** This means that the immune system has initiated a defensive attack on the substance (an antigen), by producing antibodies, histamine, or other defensive agents. Allergic reactions can cause various symptoms: 70 percent of people report gastrointestinal disturbances (swelling of the throat, nausea, cramping pain, abdominal distention, vomiting, and diarrhea); 24 percent report skin reactions (hives and eczema); and 4 percent report respiratory problems (hay fever and asthma) (23). **Anaphylactic shock,** the most dangerous allergic reaction, can occur within

TABLE 4.4
Terms used on food labels

Diet	The product contains no more than 40 Calories per serving or has at least one-third fewer Calories than a product it replaces or resembles.
Low-Calorie	Products can have no more than 40 Calories per serving or 0.4 Calories per gram of food.
Reduced Calorie	Must contain at least one-third fewer Calories than the product it replaces or resembles. The label must show a comparison with the standard product.
Light or Lite	No legal definition. Possibly less Calories, fat, or salt; may simply be lighter in color.
Natural	Meat and poultry that contain no artificial flavors, colors, or preservatives. Processed products that have "natural" on their labels may contain artificial ingredients or additives because there is no legal definition in processed foods.
Organic	No legal definition exists.
Naturally Sweetened	There is no regulation on this term, so a product bearing this on the label may contain sugar or other refined sweeteners.
Sugar Free	This product does not contain sucrose but may contain honey, fructose, or other sweeteners.
No Cholesterol	This product contains no cholesterol but may contain large amounts of saturated fats (coconut or palm oil).
Sodium Free	The product has less than 5 milligrams per serving of sodium.
Very Low Sodium	35 milligrams or less per serving.
Reduced Sodium	The usual level of sodium was reduced by 75% in this product.
Unsalted or No Salt Added	No salt is added during processing, but the product may still contain salt because of the use of sodium-containing ingredients.
Extra Lean	No more than 5% fat by weight in meat and poultry products.
Lean	No more than 10% fat by weight in meat and poultry products. Lean may be used as part of a brand name with no restriction.
Leaner	25% less fat than the standard product for meat and poultry.

FIGURE 4.7

How You Can Use Nutrition Information

■ The day's diet should provide the many nutrients the body needs. You can be sure of an adequate intake of key nutrients if the total amount of each nutrient from *all* foods eaten during the day is 100% of the U.S. Recommended Daily Allowance. This amount provides the quantity of nutrients needed by healthy people every day, plus an excess to allow for individual variations.

■ Labels show the amount of Calories, protein, carbohydrate, and fat, plus at least seven of the vitamins and minerals considered to be essential in the day's diet.

■ The amount of each listed nutrient supplied by a single serving of this food is shown as a percentage of the total amount recommended for each day (U.S. Recommended Daily Allowance—U.S. RDA).

■ Since cereals are eaten with milk, nutrition information is shown for the cereal alone and for a serving of the cereal with milk.

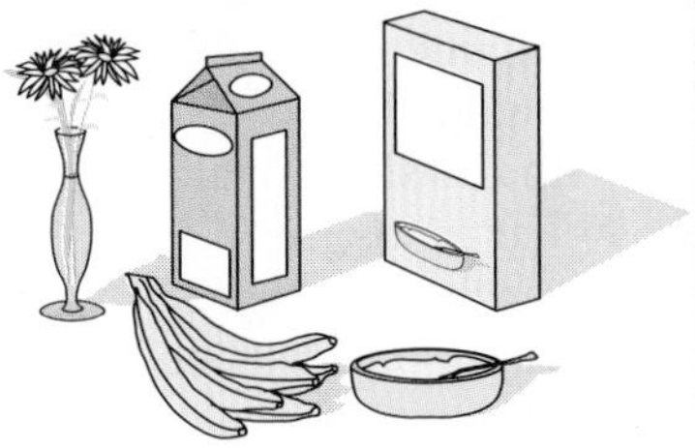

Example of Nutrition Information on Cereal Package

NUTRITION INFORMATION PER SERVING

SERVING SIZE: One ounce (1 1/2 cup) Corn flakes alone and in combination with 1/2 cup vitamin D fortified whole milk.
SERVINGS PER CONTAINER: 12

CORN FLAKES	1 oz.	with 1/2 cup whole milk
CALORIES	110	190
PROTEIN	2 gm	6 gm
CARBOHYDRATE	24 gm	30 gm
FAT	0 gm	4 gm

PERCENTAGE OF U.S. RECOMMENDED DAILY ALLOWANCE (U.S. RDA)

CORN FLAKES	1 oz.	with 1/2 cup whole milk
PROTEIN	2	10
VITAMIN A	25	25
VITAMIN C	25	25
THIAMINE	25	25
RIBOFLAVIN	25	35
NIACIN	25	25
CALCIUM	*	16
IRON	10	10
VITAMIN D	10	25
VITAMIN B_6	25	25
FOLIC ACID	25	25
PHOSPHORUS	*	10
MAGNESIUM	*	4

*Contains less than 2 percent of the U.S. RDA of these nutrients.

---

minutes to hours after eating a food. Symptoms include abdominal pain, nausea, a drop in blood pressure, chest pain, diarrhea, and shock, and death can occur.

Considering the number of different foods available to us, those that are reported to cause allergic reactions are surprisingly few. Adults frequently suffer from allergies to shellfish, peanuts, nuts, and grains. The foods that most commonly cause allergies among infants and children are cow's milk, chicken eggs, legumes (peanuts and soybeans), wheat, tree nuts (filberts and cashews) and fish (22). Infants are introduced to single-ingredient foods slowly so that symptoms of potential allergies can be observed. The gut of the infant is not yet mature, and proteins are more capable of being absorbed into the body undigested, creating an immune response. About 40 percent of food allergies that occur before the age of three will be "outgrown." Tolerances of milk, egg, and soy,

for example, usually develop with time. Food allergies that begin after the age of three are more persistent (24). Individuals who suspect that they have food allergies should consult a physician.

Diagnosing true food allergies can be very difficult. Table 4.5 lists the assessment procedures used. Of the several immunological tests used, the most reliable are the skin-prick test, the radioallergosorbent test (RAST), and the enzyme-linked immunosorbent assay (ELISA). The cytotoxic test, which is popular today for diagnosis of food allergies and other maladies, is unreliable and is not an accepted clinical procedure (25).

These tests should always be followed by an elimination diet and a food-challenge test. An **elimination diet** excludes from the diet the foods that are suspected of causing the food allergy. If no satisfactory results occur, more extensive elimination of foods is necessary.

TABLE 4.5
Food allergy assessment

History

Provides detailed description of symptoms, time from ingestion of food to onset of symptoms, most recent reaction, quantity of food necessary to produce a reaction, and suspected foods. Includes family history.

Physical Examination

Food and Symptom Diary For 2 Weeks

Immunological Testing

Trial Elimination Diet For 2 to 4 Weeks or Until Symptoms Clear

Nutritionally sound.
Begins with only suspected foods being eliminated.

Food Challenge

Returns suspect foods to diet, one at a time, after symptoms have cleared for 2 to 4 weeks. Neither the patient nor physician know which food is being given (to prevent placebo effects).

Adapted from S. N. Butkus and L. K. Mahan, "Food Allergies: Immunological Reactions to Food." *Journal of the American Dietetic Association,* 86:604, 1986.

A careful record of food intake and symptoms accompanies this diet. After symptoms have cleared for two to four weeks, the suspected foods are returned to the diet, one at a time, to check for reactions. This is known as a **food challenge.**

Nonimmunological Reactions to Food

Adverse reactions to food may be caused by gastrointestinal disorders, enzyme deficiencies, psychosomatic reactions, bacterial or chemical contamination, or noxious elements in the food. (Some books refer to these as food intolerances.) Typical symptoms are abdominal pain, vomiting, diarrhea, asthma, and headaches.

The belief that food additives are responsible for many adverse reactions to foods is not substantiated in the literature. The relationship of food additives to hyperactivity in children was suggested by Dr. Benjamin Feingold in 1973. Five to ten percent of young, school-aged children manifest **hyperactivity,** a cluster of symptoms that include attention deficit, impulsiveness, excitability, and general behavior problems in the absence of mental illness. When food additives were tested in controlled, double-blind studies with hyperactive children, no changes in behavior could be attributed to the additives in foods. Other therapies therefore should be followed (see chapter 14).

Sulfites are also food additives that have recently concerned the public. **Sulfites** are a group of sulfur-based substances that have widespread use in the food industry. Sodium sulfite, potassium sulfite, sulfur dioxide, sodium bisulfite, potassium bisulfite, and sodium or potassium metabisulfite are all examples. They are used as preservatives and antioxidants to prevent the spoilage and discoloration of food. For example, lettuce will wilt and turn brown if left in a salad bar, but sulfites help it stay crisper and greener for a longer period of time.

In 1986, the FDA took two measures to restrict the usage of sulfitic agents. These preservatives can no longer be used on fruits and vegetables, and many processed foods that contain them will have to include them on the label. As of early 1987, any food containing ten parts per million of sulfites must disclose it on the label. This value was chosen because it is the lowest level at which sulfitic agents can readily be detected (26). The ban on their use on fruits and vegetables is targeted at restaurant salad bars and supermarkets. Other foods that you may find at the salad bar may still contain sulfites, such as potato and shrimp salads, canned vegetables, and pickled foods.

Sulfitic agents are a possible health hazard for one million Americans, most of them asthmatics. Their allergic-type reactions to this food additive range from mild to severe and have resulted in death for a few. Table 4.6 lists foods commonly containing sulfites.

Another example of a nonimmunological reaction to food is phenylketonuria (PKU). The essential amino acid phenylalanine is necessary for proper growth. However, people with the genetic disorder PKU (phenylketonuria) are unable to tolerate high levels of phenylalanine in their bloodstream. Their diet must be carefully monitored, therefore, to limit intake of foods with a high phenylalanine content.

Untreated PKU can cause severe mental retardation and damage to the central nervous system in children. Newborns are routinely given a blood test for the disease, however, and if PKU is diagnosed, a special diet is required until the baby's brain and nervous system are fully developed. Also, an adult female who has PKU must be careful during pregnancy, because phenylalanine buildup in her bloodstream can cause brain damage to the fetus.

TABLE 4.6
Common foods with sulfites

Food Category	Examples	Food Category	Examples
Alcoholic beverages	Wine, beer, cocktail mixes, wine cooler	Processed vegetables	Vegetable juices; canned, pickled, or dried vegetables; instant mashed potatoes; frozen potatoes; potato salad
Baked goods	Cookies, crackers, mixes with dried fruits or vegetables, pie crust, pizza crust, quiche crust, flour tortillas	Gelatins, pudding, fillings	Fruit fillings, all gelatin, pectin, jelling agents
Beverage bases	Dried citrus fruit beverage mixes	Grain products and pasta	Cornstarch, modified food starch, spinach pasta, gravies, hominy, breadings, batters, noodle/rice mixes
Condiments and relishes	Horseradish, onion and pickle relishes, pickles, olives, salad-dressing mixes, wine vinegar		
Confections and frostings	Any sugar derived from sugar beets, brown, raw, powdered, or white	Jams and jellies	Jams and jellies
		Nuts and nut products	Shredded coconut
Fish and shellfish	Canned clams; fresh, frozen, canned, or dried shrimp; frozen lobster; scallops; dried cod	Plant protein products	Soy protein products
		Snack foods	Dried fruit snacks, filled crackers
Fresh fruit and vegetables	Banned by FDA regulation (7/9/86), but fresh precut potatoes excluded from ban	Soups and soup mixes	Canned soups, dried soup mixes
Processed fruits	Canned, bottled, or frozen fruit juices; dried fruit; canned, bottled, or frozen dietetic fruit or fruit juices; maraschino cherries; glazed fruit	Sweet sauces, toppings	Corn syrup, maple syrup, fruit toppings, pancake syrup, molasses
		Tea	Instant and liquid tea concentrates

Note: Not all manufacturers of these foods use sulfites.

From C. W. Lecos, "Sulfites: FDA Limits Uses, Broadens Labeling." *FDA Consumer,* October 1986, pp. 11–13.

HEALTH-PROMOTION INSIGHT
Food Faddism and Quackery

Since ancient times, people have desired a quick, simple solution to better health. This year Americans will spend 25 billion dollars on products that don't do anything, don't do what we expect, or perhaps even do harm to us (27). This insight is designed to help you take a look at why food faddism persists, the harm it does, some current practices, and strategies for combating quackery.

Definitions

Just what is food faddism? It is an exaggerated belief in the effects of nutrition on maintaining health. On the other hand, food quackery applies to people or advertisers who are sincere but misguided in their beliefs about a product. They believe in and spread the news of food faddism.

Why Food Faddism Persists

One reason food faddism persists is that it targets the Achilles heel of many Americans: loss of performance or youth. Advertisements often claim that a product will enhance beauty or sexual prowess. For example, vitamin E captured 17 percent of the vitamin market, a leading seller, because of its mythical association with sexual rejuvenation (28). Some products claim to retard the aging process (wrinkles, loss of hair, loss of energy), and others to cure or bring relief from disease.

Another popular market for food faddism is athletes. People in this group are vulnerable because of their great desire to gain a decisive edge over their competitors. Nine percent of athletes take protein powder with the belief that supplementation will produce an increase in muscle mass (29).

Food faddism also persists because erroneous beliefs exist about the inadequacy of our food supply. According to an FDA study, most people believe the fallacies upon which faddism is established (30) (see table 4.7).

Table 4.7

Percentage agreeing with statements about food supply healthfulness

Statement	Percentage Agreeing
1. The chemicals added to our manufactured food take away much of its value for health. (False)	48
2. Manmade vitamins are just as good as natural vitamins. (True)	35
3. Much of our food has been so processed and refined that it has lost its value for health. (False)	60
4. Chemical sprays that farmers use make our food a danger to health, even if they are used carefully. (False)	57
5. There is no difference in food value between food grown in poor, worn-out soil and food grown in rich soil. (True)	15
6. Many foods lose a lot of their value for health because they are shipped so far and stored so long. (False)	73
7. Food grown with chemical fertilizers is just as healthful as food grown with natural fertilizers. (True)	44

Food and Drug Administration, 1972. *A Study of Health Practices and Opinions.* Philadelphia: National Analysts, Inc. Part II, p. 65.

The High Price of Food Faddism

High Cost

The food faddism industry is profitable. Foods that are labeled ''natural,'' ''organic,'' or ''health foods'' carry a high price tag because of smaller demand and higher distribution costs. Although these terms imply that a product is safer and more nutritious than one that is grown conventionally, there is little agreement on the definitions of these terms. In fact the one thing that foods labeled ''natural,'' ''organic,'' or ''health food'' do have in common is a higher price, as much as 70 percent more than their conventional counterparts (28).

Harm to Our Health

Food faddism not only robs us of our money but also can steal our health. Deaths have resulted from strict diet regimes such as the Zen Macrobiotic diet. Fatal poisonings have occurred from laetrile, a drug derived from apricot pits. Laetrile, purported to be a cancer cure, has also been responsible for neglect of conventional cancer treatments. Several deaths have resulted. Many herbal preparations promoted by the health-food industry, such as ginseng, licorice root, mate tea, senna tea, tansy ragwort tea, and bee pollen are also potentially harmful and sometimes lethal. Another danger to our health is the promotion of megadoses of vitamins and minerals. Food faddism encourages us to focus on nonscientific-based cures or preventions; as a result, the facts are ignored, and our health is harmed.

Current Practices

With billions of dollars at stake, it is not surprising that efforts to exploit the consumer are well organized. Professionals, reputable companies, marketing campaigns, and the media at times work to create false beliefs. Some organized efforts to undermine the consumer should be noted.

Professionals

Some clinical professionals such as physicians, dentists, psychologists, and physical therapists support unorthodox nutritional therapies. These include chelation therapy, cytotoxic food allergy testing, hair analysis, colonic irrigation, and vitamin megadoses. Many such professionals have little or no background in nutrition, and their ''expertise'' in this area is questionable.

Pseudo-Nutrition Experts

The term ''nutritionist'' is still unregulated in many states. This means that anyone can call him- or herself a nutritionist even though he or she may not have a diploma from an accredited college or university. Several diploma mills offer credentials (bachelor of science, master of science, or doctor of philosophy) for a fee. These schools are not approved or accredited by recognized accrediting agencies, but they often state that they are ''authorized'' to issue such credentials. The credentials have no validity. One report states that in 1982 these diploma mills granted more PH.D.'s in nutrition than all the legitimate schools combined (28). Between 1982 and 1985, the National Council Against Health Fraud carried out a study of yellow-pages advertising and found that 87 percent of self-advertised ''nutritionists'' were not qualified (31).

Pharmaceutical Companies

Pharmaceutical companies try to increase their sale of food supplements in several ways. Many people consider drugstores to be an authority about all medications and supplements, and they are thus the number-one sellers of vitamin and mineral supplements. Health-food stores rank second in sales, and supermarkets are third. Pharmaceutical companies also rely on direct advertising, creating the belief that people are not quite healthy or not quite getting every nutrient they may need. They often purport that there is nothing a supplement can't cure. The pharmaceutical companies also advertise in professional journals and send sales representatives to visit selected professionals personally. Free samples and other incentives are available to practitioners who participate in promotions.

Pyramid Sales Promotions
Many people, with hopes of financial success, have been drawn into pyramid sales promotions. These involve companies that use marketing and distributing methods to maximize sales. Many levels of sales personnel are involved in a pyramid organizational structure. These schemes have been devised to sell food supplements, herbs, weight-loss products, and other fraudulent items. These products sound too good to be true, and usually are.

Health Literature
Magazine articles and health books sometimes participate in ''hidden advertising'' for food faddist products. Articles will encourage the use of supplements or weight-loss regimes when good nutritional eating may be more appropriate.

Many people believe that advertising is screened for truthfulness by some government agency, but this is not the case. Enforcement agencies can take action against fraudulent claims only after they appear. Furthermore, not all claims are harmful enough to warrant action by enforcement agencies. As a result, there are products on the market that may not harm your health, only your pocketbook.

Products that claim a ''money-back guarantee'' are not necessarily more reputable. For example, refund demands are ignored by many quacks. Or, by the time a request arrives in the mail, the address of the scam operation has changed.

Consumer Protection

Government Agencies
Three major government agencies help protect the consumer from health fraud: the Food and Drug Administration (FDA), the Federal Trade Commission (FTC), and the United States Postal Service (USPS).

The FDA is responsible for consumer protection in the areas of safety and effectiveness of all drugs and food additives. It protects the consumer against misrepresented or worthless medical devices or drugs. Food contaminants are also regulated by the FDA. Complaints can be addressed to: Director, Consumer Communications, FDA, 5600 Fishers Lane, Rockville, Md. 20857.

The FTC safeguards the consumer against deceptive claims in advertising. Most violations involve misrepresentation or mislabeling of a product. Claims are commonly filed against over-the-counter drugs, cosmetics, medical devices, hearing aids, contact lenses, hair restorers, bust developers, and weight-loss products. Although the process is tedious, collecting good evidence is the key to filing a claim. Complaints may be filed in writing to: Office of the Secretary, Federal Trade Commission, Washington, D.C. 20580.

If products are misrepresented, harmful, or worthless and are sold through the mail, the USPS will investigate for mail fraud. Again, collecting appropriate evidence is a must. Initiate the complaint by contacting: Consumer Advocate, U.S. Postal Service, Washington, D.C. 20260.

Private Agencies
The Better Business Bureau is a nonprofit corporation supported by private business. This organization can assist consumers in several ways. The Better Business Bureau will mediate between consumers and businesses, investigate advertising misinformation and questionable activity, and serve as a resource for factual information on businesses throughout the country.

Professional associations such as the American Dietetic Association, the American Medical Association, and the American Dental Association are instrumental in preventing health fraud. Your city's health department may also be able to provide information on local resources. Another valuable private organization is the National Council Against Health Fraud, Inc., P.O. Box 1276, Loma Linda, CA 92354. This organization publishes a bimonthly newsletter and has several state affiliates.

Protecting Yourself
When deciding whether to purchase and use a product, consumers need to be healthy skeptics. Remember the standard second opinion from the FDA: If it sounds too good to be true, it's probably

the medical equivalent of buying the Brooklyn Bridge (32). The next time you are trying to judge a particular product, ask yourself the following questions:

- Does the product appeal to basic human needs, such as fear and love, or is it presented objectively?
- Is the cure quick and painless?
- Is the formula "secret," "ancient," or "foreign" and only available through one supplier?
- Does the advertiser use case histories or testimonials as the main proof that the product works?
- Is the product a cure-all for a wide variety of ailments?

- Has a new "scientific breakthrough" created this product?
- Is the medical community accused of not releasing information or of overlooking the proof of this product?
- Is unclear information used, such as "hospital tests showed . . .", "doctors recommend . . ." or "a major study revealed" without these sources being identified? Claims should be supported by scientific evidence, and the research should be consistent with other investigators.

A "yes" answer to any of the above questions should make the consumer skeptical. Insist on hard evidence before buying.

S I D E B A R 4.2

Examine a popular magazine to find nutrition advertisements. Evaluate the advertisements, keeping in mind the questions listed under "Protecting Yourself." What did you discover? Is there any distortion in the claims for the product? Locate one advertisement that seems accurate and free of unsupported claims.

Summary

1. This chapter reviewed the microbiological and chemical safety of foods. An insight on food quackery was also presented.
2. The most common type of foodborne infection is caused by *Salmonella* bacteria. Raw or undercooked meat, and poultry, eggs, or fish are potential sources of this bacteria.
3. *Staphylococcus* are bacteria that produce a toxin in foods containing protein, such as meat, poultry, cheese, egg products, pasta or potato salads, custards, and cream-filled desserts. This toxin causes vomiting and diarrhea if present in sufficient quantity.
4. Botulism is caused by another bacteria, *Clostridium botulinum,* that produces a toxin under anaerobic conditions. Dented, bulging, or buckling cans could harbor the deadly toxin and should be discarded.
5. To prevent foodborne illness, care should be taken when selecting foods. Examine the food and check expiration dates. Any break in the skin or packaging of a food could lead to contamination with bacteria.

6. Cleanliness of the food preparer's hands, all utensils, and cutting boards is essential in food preparation. Frozen meats should be given sufficient time to defrost in the refrigerator.
7. When storing cooked foods, place them in the refrigerator immediately, before cooling. Cooked foods are safe for two hours maximum at room temperature and should then be discarded. Refrigerators should remain below 40 degrees F and freezers at 0 degrees F.
8. Natural toxins do exist in food and can be found in some types of mushrooms, fish, nuts, and grains, as well as in many herbs.
9. Environmental contaminants can be quite harmful in our food supply and may enter accidentally from agricultural residues, food containers, cookware, and industrial wastes.
10. The Food and Drug Administration safeguards our food supply by approving additives that can be used in foods. More than 600 additives, however, are exempt from having to prove their safety because they were in common use prior to a 1958 act that demanded such proof from all future additives. This group of commonly used additives is known as the GRAS list (Generally Recognized as Safe).
11. If any additive, including those on the GRAS list, is found to cause cancer in an animal or human, it may not be added to food. This amendment to the Pure Food and Drug Act of 1938 is known as the Delaney Clause.
12. Food additives are approved for four purposes: to maintain or improve nutritional value, to maintain product quality, to make food more appealing, and to help in processing or preparation.
13. Food labels provide a valuable source of nutrition information. They may include a list of ingredients, nutrient information, and product dating.

14. Food allergies are more prevalent in the pediatric population than in adults. Symptoms include 70 percent gastrointestinal disturbances (nausea, cramping pain, abdominal distention, vomiting, diarrhea), 24 percent skin reactions (hives, eczema) and 4 percent respiratory problems (hay fever, asthma).

15. An accumulation of evidence is needed to diagnose a food allergy. Assessment should include a history, physical examination, a food and symptom diary, and a diagnostic test. These should be followed up by an elimination diet and food-challenge test.

16. Sulfites can cause severe reactions for some individuals and were banned for use on the fresh fruits and vegetables at salad bars. However, they may still be found in a variety of foods, including dried fruits, potatoes, canned vegetables, and pickled foods.

17. Food faddism and quackery persist for many reasons. In particular, they target our fear of loss of performance or youth. Products and schemes not only rob people of their money, but also of their health.

18. Government agencies (The Food and Drug Administration, The Federal Trade Commission, and the United States Postal Service), private agencies (Better Business Bureau, American Dietetic Association, National Council Against Health Fraud) and the individual consumer can stop quackery.

*R*EFERENCES

1. Lecos, C. W. 1986. Shopping for the Second 50 Years. *FDA Consumer* (July–August).
2. MacDonald, K. L., and P. M. Griffin. 1986. Foodborne Disease Outbreaks. *Journal of Food Protection* 49:933.
3. Nightingale, S. L. 1987. Foodborne Disease: An Increasing Problem. *American Family Physician* 35:353.
4. U.S. Department of Health, Education, and Welfare, Public Health Service, Centers for Disease Control. 1979. Botulism in the United States, 1899–1977, R. A. Gunn, ed.
5. Arnon, S. S., et al. 1979. Honey and Other Environmental Risk Factors for Infant Botulism. *Journal of Pediatrics* 94:331.
6. U. S. Department of Health, Education, and Welfare, Public Health Service, Centers for Disease Control. 1983. Foodborne Disease Outbreaks. Washington, D.C.: U.S. Government Printing Office.
7. The Wild Mushroom: An Endangering Species. 1980. *Emergency Medicine.* (September 15): p. 73.
8. Johnson, E. Children Shoulder the Burden of Lead. 1982. *Nutrition Action* (March): p. 3.
9. Needleman, H. L., et al. 1979. Deficits in Psychological and Classroom Performance of Children with Elevated Dentine Lead Levels. *New England Journal of Medicine* 300:689–95.
10. Thompson, R. C. 1984. The Search for Pesticide Residues. *FDA Consumer* (July–August).
11. Lecos, C. W. 1984. Pesticides and Food: Public Worry No. 1. *FDA Consumer* (July–August).
12. Nadakavukaren, A. 1986. *Man and Environment.* Prospect Heights, Ill.: Waveland Press.
13. Middekauff, R. D., 1985. Delaney Meets de minimis. *Food Technology* 39:62.
14. Lehman, P. 1982. More Than You Thought You Would Ever Know About Food Additives. *FDA Consumer* (February).
15. Caballero, B. 1985. Food Additives in the Pediatric Diet. *Clinical Nutrition* 4:200–206.
16. Leveille, G. A. 1984. Food Fortification — Opportunities and Pitfalls. *Food Technology* (January): p. 59.
17. Dziezak, J. D. 1986. Preservatives: Antimicrobial Agents. *Food Technology* (September): p. 104–11.
18. Jacobson, M. F., 1986. Antioxidants. *Nutrition Action* (January): p. 6–7.
19. Meggos, H. N. 1984. Colors — Key Food Ingredients. *Food Technology* (January): p. 70–74.
20. Lindsay, R. C. 1984. Flavor Ingredient Technology. *Food Technology* (January): p. 76–81.
21. Ellefson, W. 1986. The Impact of Nutrition Labeling. *Nutrition Forum* 3:41–45.
22. Butkus, S. N., and L. K. Mahan. 1986. Food Allergies: Immunological Reactions to Food. *Journal of the American Dietetic Association* 86:601–608.
23. Minford, A. M. B., A. MacDonald, and J. M. Littlewood. 1982. Food Intolerance and Food Allergy in Children: A Review of 68 Cases. *Archives of Disease in Childhood* 57:742.
24. Bock, S. A. 1982. The Natural History of Food Sensitivity. *Journal of Allergy and Clinical Immunology* 69:173.
25. Thompson, R. C. 1984. The Flaw in Cytotoxic Testing: There's No Proof It Works. *FDA Consumer* (October).
26. Lecos, C. W. 1988. An Order of Fries — Hold the Sulfites. *FDA Consumer* (March): p. 9–11.
27. Cowart, V. S. 1988. Health Fraud's Toll: Lost Hopes, Misspent Billions. *Journal of the American Medical Association* 259:3229.
28. Jarvis, W. T. 1983. Food Faddism, Cultism, and Quackery. *Annual Review of Nutrition* 3:35–52.
29. Parr, R. B., M. A. Porter, and S. C. Hodgson. 1984. Nutrition Knowledge and Practice of Coaches, Trainers, and Athletes. *Physician and Sportsmedicine* 12:3:127–38.
30. FDA. 1972. A Study of Health Practices and Opinions. Part II, p. 65. Philadelphia: National Analysts, Inc.
31. National Council Against Health Fraud Newsletter. 1986. 9:1:2.
32. Grigg, W. 1988. Quackery: It Costs More Than Money. *FDA Consumer* (July–August).

*H*EALTH-PROMOTION ACTIVITY 4.1
Food Safety in Your Kitchen

Developing safe food-storage habits is essential to assure product safety and quality. Using this list, check for any "violations" in your kitchen.

Cabinets and Counters

___ Is food stored underneath the kitchen sink, or in cabinets where water or heat pipes enter or leave the house? Foods here are a possible feast for rodents and insects.

___ Is food stored near containers of household chemicals such as cleaning solution, oven cleaner, or medications? This can be a serious mistake.

___ Is any food thawing or warming on the counter? Place the milk back as soon as you use it.

The Food Cupboard

___ Look for expiration dates on products in the cupboard and toss out old goods.

___ Keep cans dusted so a can opener won't push the dirt to the inside.

___ If cans stick to the shelf, they may be leaking. Cans that leak, bulge, or are otherwise odd should be returned to the store and reported to the FDA.

___ Do you taste foods that don't seem quite right? This could be a deadly practice.

___ If products in your cupboard should have been refrigerated, discard them.

The Refrigerator and Freezer

___ Do a "search-and-seizure" of any food that has been stored for more than a week in the refrigerator. Start placing a date on all foods stored in the refrigerator or freezer.

___ Thoroughly clean the refrigerator compartment with hot, soapy water to prevent bacteria from breeding.

___ Check the temperatures in the refrigerator (less than 45 degrees F) and the freezer (0 degrees F).

___ All foods should be covered, except produce, and circulation of cool air must be maintained. Packing foods carelessly can lead to spillage and little air movement.

HEALTH-PROMOTION ACTIVITY 4.2
What You Can Learn from Labels

Are you bothered by the fact that many foods contain additives, preservatives, and other chemicals? Do you often buy foods that are claimed to have "no preservatives" because you believe they contain no additives? One way to determine whether the foods that you commonly consume are a reason for concern is to look at the label.

Select three processed foods or drinks that you consume frequently, and collect the following information from the labels.

General Information

Brand, size of container, type of container, price, net weight

Unit Price

Cost per standard unit of net measure (per pound, per quart)

Nutrition

Serving size; number of servings; Calories; grams of protein, carbohydrate, and fat per serving; presence or absence of fatty acids, cholesterol, and sodium; percent of U.S. RDA for protein, vitamins A and C, thiamin, riboflavin, niacin, calcium, and iron.

Ingredients

In order of decreasing quantity, including sugar and sugar substitutes

In table 4.2, find the additives that are listed on your label. Why are they being used?

What else have you learned about these products?

If you are still concerned about what you are eating, list several healthy substitutions that you will try.

HEALTH-PROMOTION ACTIVITY 4.3
Just Too Sweet

Manufacturers are enjoying an expanding market for sugar substitutes as Americans become even more weight and sugar conscious. However, a product is not necessarily safe just because it doesn't contain sugar. How many products that you eat regularly contain either saccharin or aspartame (NutraSweet)?

Product	Quantity (per day)
Soft drinks	_____
Cocoa or shakes	_____
Other presweetened beverages	_____
Packages or pills	_____
Gelatin desserts	_____
Puddings	_____
Candy	_____
Cookies or cakes	_____

Drinking seven cans of diet soft drink per day, or the equivalent in any combination of products, would be an excessive intake of sugar substitutes. What else could you substitute?

Energy in Nutrition

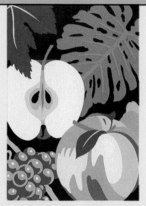

Carbohydrate, fat, and protein are the nutrients that supply our bodies with fuel for energy. The amount of energy that these three nutrients provide is usually expressed in Calories. Energy balance in the body is dependent on the amount of Calories consumed versus the Calories expended.

These nutrients not only supply energy but also serve other essential roles in the body. Carbohydrate provides bulk and helps in the making of various structures and compounds in the body. Fats, along with other lipids, are needed by the body for insulation, protection, transport of fat-soluble vitamins, and structural components of the body. Protein also provides structure and regulates body functions.

Our diets are a complex mixture of carbohydrate, fat, and protein. The contribution that each of these nutrients makes in our diets does affect our health. Therefore, each chapter in this section will examine both the quality and quantity of each nutrient needed to promote the health of Americans.

5

Carbohydrate

OUTLINE

INTRODUCTION

Carbohydrate-rich foods are perhaps the most misunderstood. Many people believe that potatoes are fattening or that rice and beans are "too starchy." On the contrary, high-carbohydrate foods are not the high-Calorie culprits, but the company they often keep usually is. Butter, gravy, sour cream, and other high-fat extras all too often smother the low-Calorie carbohydrate foods, causing the food item to double or even triple in Calories.

Even though many Americans try to limit their carbohydrate intake, people still consume 46 percent of their Calories in the form of carbohydrate. Take a moment to remember what you've eaten so far today. Were there any fruits, vegetables, cereals, breads, or pasta? All of these contribute greatly to our carbohydrate intake during the day — or at least should.

Both the quantity and quality of the carbohydrate we eat plays an important role in health promotion. For example, a diet high in sugar is related to higher rates of tooth decay in children. On the other hand, diets high in fiber-rich foods have been associated with a lower risk of colon cancer.

Carbohydrate can serve us well in promoting our health. This chapter will examine just how carbohydrate can perform such a task.

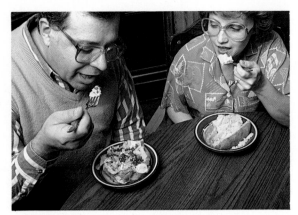

A simple baked potato triples in kilocalories after being smothered in high-fat extras.

Carbohydrate Structure and Function

Carbohydrate is a group of molecules that primarily contain the atoms carbon, hydrogen, and oxygen. The latter two are always found in the same proportion as in water; that is, two hydrogen and one oxygen. Carbohydrates differ mainly in their size and will be discussed from the smallest carbohydrate (the monosaccharides) to the largest (the polysaccharides).

The Monosaccharides

Monosaccharides are the simplest carbohydrate, containing only one subunit of sugar (mono-one; saccharide-sugar). Three monosaccharides are important in our discussion of nutrition: glucose, fructose, and galactose (see figure 5.1). Each of these contains 6 carbons, 12 hydrogen, and 6 oxygen; however, the arrangement of these atoms is different in the three sugars.

Glucose is found in honey and several fruits. It is also the most common way that carbohydrate is transported in the bloodstream. Because it is a very simple molecule, the body can easily break it down to make energy.

Fructose can also be found in honey and fruit. It is sweeter than glucose and is purported to be a Calorie saver. However, although this property holds true in cold, slightly acidic drinks, the sweetness of fructose becomes equal to glucose in hot beverages or in baked goods. For this reason, and because of the difficulty in processing fructose, its potential popularity in the marketplace has decreased.

Three monosaccharides. Boxed areas demonstrate how glucose differs from the other monosaccharides.

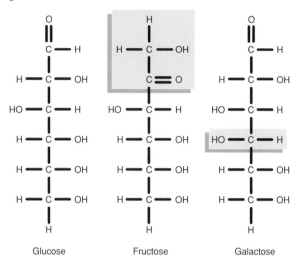

Glucose   Fructose   Galactose

FIGURE 5.2
Two monosaccharides combine to form each disaccharide: maltose, sucrose, and lactose.

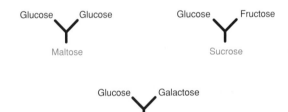

Galactose does not exist free in nature but is commonly found together with glucose as lactose, the sugar found in milk.

The Disaccharides

When two of the monosaccharides combine, they form a **disaccharide** (two sugars) (see figure 5.2). Only three biologically important disaccharides are typically found in food: sucrose, lactose, and maltose.

Sucrose is a combination of glucose and fructose. This is the most common disaccharide obtained from the refining of sugarcane or sugar beets. Sucrose is the familiar table sugar. Americans use 86 pounds per capita, per year of this sugar, more than all others combined (1). Sucrose also occurs in many fruits and vegetables, for example, carrots and pineapple.

Table 5.1

Relative sweetness of selected sugars compared to sucrose*

Sweetener	Relative Sweetness
Saccharin	200–600
Aspartame	180–220
Cyclamate	30
Fructose	1.5
Glucose	0.75
Sorbital	0.54
Lactose	0.5

*Sucrose is given a rating of 1.0

From G. E. Inglett, "Sweeteners: A Review." *Food Technology* 35:(3)37–41, March 1981. Used with permission.

Lactose, a disaccharide of glucose and galactose, is also known as the sugar of milk. The combination of two glucose molecules produces yet another disaccharide, maltose, which can be found in sprouting grains or partially digested grains like corn syrup. The flavor of maple syrup, beer, and malted milk can be attributed in part to maltose.

Both the monosaccharides and the disaccharides are considered simple sugars, or simple carbohydrate. They will dissolve readily in water, crystallize, and have a sweet taste. Table 5.1 compares the relative sweetness of the various sugars. The significance of such a comparison is that if a sweeter tasting sugar is added to foods, less may be used, thus saving some Calories. Even though sucrose is twice as sweet as maltose, equal weights will contain the same number of Calories. Therefore, half as much sucrose would be needed to give the same desired sweetness as maltose, yet provide only half the Calories. Problems with manufacture, availability, and cost may limit the choices of what sweetener can be used in food products.

The Polysaccharides

The **polysaccharides** are known as "complex carbohydrate" because they are made up of many monosaccharides (see figure 5.3). These long chains of sugars can contain thousands of monosaccharide subunits. Their properties are quite the opposite of simple sugars, however; they do not dissolve in cold water, crystallize, or taste particularly sweet. The polysaccharides include starch, glycogen, and fiber. Although most polysaccharides are composed of glucose molecules alone, they differ from one another in length and in arrangement of the molecules.

Figure 5.3

A complex carbohydrate is made up of many monosaccharides. (Each sphere represents the monosaccharide glucose.)

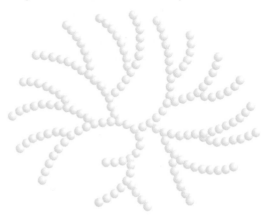

Starch

Plants store energy in the form of starch. Starch can be found in seeds, where it provides nourishment for the developing embryo plant, and in the roots of some plants such as potatoes and turnips, where it provides energy through long winters. Three sources of starch are the "staff of life" for most people in the world. The cereal grains wheat, rice, oats, and corn are valued as staple crops. Potatoes and legumes (dried peas and beans) are also important sources of Calories for people in many countries.

The starch in plants is made of long, sometimes branched chains of glucose. Although not soluble in cold water, starches will become thick, gelatinous, and more digestible when they are cooked. Cornstarch is a familiar form of pure starch that demonstrates this property well, and it is frequently used to thicken gravies or other sauces.

Glycogen

Animals can also store carbohydrate energy in the form of glycogen. Glycogen is made up of highly branched glucose molecules and is stored in either the liver or the muscles. The amount that can be stored in these two sites varies quite a bit, but the energy supply for one-half day (about 1,200 Calories) is usually available to meet energy needs (2).

Fiber

The third type of polysaccharide is **dietary fiber,** which comes from plant sources. Fiber cannot be digested by the enzymes in the human

TABLE 5.2
The dietary fibers

Soluble Fibers	Insoluble Fibers
Gums	Cellulose
Mucilages	Lignin
Pectin	Some hemicelluloses
Some hemicelluloses	
Algal polysaccharides	

digestive tract, although some can be broken down by intestinal bacteria. It is for this reason that dietary fiber is essential for the body to function properly, as we will see later.

Of the seven main types of dietary fiber (see table 5.2), six are actually carbohydrate. Lignin is a noncarbohydrate dietary fiber and comes from the extremely woody portions of plants. It can also be found as part of fruit and vegetable skins or whole grains.

Cellulose is the most abundant fiber, forming the cell walls of many plants. Although it is formed from long chains of glucose, the type of chemical bond that holds the glucose molecules together in cellulose cannot be broken by human digestive enzymes. Therefore, cellulose cannot be digested or provide Calories to the body. Cellulose, along with lignin, is referred to as **water-insoluble fiber.**

Interestingly, some microorganisms can break the bonds in the cellulose chain. Animals like cattle and sheep, which house these microorganisms in their digestive tract, are able to digest grasses and other leaves that contain large amounts of cellulose.

The other five types of fiber are not fibrous or woody but gelatinous or gummy, and they are known as **water-soluble fibers.** They include hemicellulose, pectin, gums, mucilages, and algal polysaccharides. The ability of pectin to gel is a good example of the characteristics of these five fibers. Pectin that is extracted from fruit is used to assist in the making of jellies and jams.

Due to the difficulty and expense of measuring all seven types of fiber in food, complete tables that give food fiber composition data are not available (3). For many years, crude fiber, which consists of cellulose and lignin, was reported on product labels and in tables. Unfortunately, the chemical tests used to measure fiber content of food were inaccurate, only measuring a part of the cellulose and lignin in a food, and not the other fibers (4). Better analytical techniques, however, have provided reports of dietary fiber content that includes all seven fibers. Preferably, all product labels would include information about dietary fiber or the content of individual fiber. Until that time, using crude fiber measurements to evaluate fiber content of products is not reliable.

Carbohydrate Functions

Energy

Of the three major functions of carbohydrate, the most important is to provide fuel to the body. Each gram of digestible carbohydrate contains four Calories. About half of our energy each day is supplied by carbohydrate.

Protein and fat can also provide fuel, but the body uses carbohydrate much more efficiently. In fact, carbohydrate is said to spare protein, meaning that as long as adequate fuel is available in the form of carbohydrate, the body will not use its precious protein for fuel. Protein is better used to build and maintain tissue.

Even when fat is the primary fuel source, such as during long-term aerobic exercises (marathon running, bicycling, swimming), carbohydrate is needed to spark the complete burning of fat as fuel. Low carbohydrate stores can cause incomplete fat combustion (5). A toxic by-product of this incomplete combustion is called ketone bodies. When ketone bodies are allowed to accumulate in the bloodstream, a condition known as ketosis can result. Symptoms of this metabolic disorder are nausea, headache, appetite loss, and dehydration. Indeed, this is a potentially life-threatening condition. Caution should be taken to avoid the popular low-carbohydrate diets for just such a reason.

Bulk

Water-insoluble fibers provide bulk to the diet, which helps the large intestine to move its contents along faster and with less effort. Also, some water-soluble fibers favorably influence the speed of absorption of nutrients by slowing it down in the small intestine (6). The importance of these functions will be discussed later in the chapter.

Special Functions

The carbon structure of carbohydrate can also be used in the making of nonessential amino acids, fats, components of hereditary material, DNA and RNA, and other structures and compounds in the body.

Digestion, Absorption, and Transport of Carbohydrate

Glucose is the basic carbohydrate unit that helps fuel all of the cells of the body. During digestion the body must be equipped to convert any monosaccharide, disaccharide, or polysaccharide into the usable form of glucose. Let's take a look at how this occurs (see table 5.3).

The Mouth and Stomach

Digestion begins in the mouth, where chewing action mechanically breaks food down into smaller particles, allowing more surface area of the food to be exposed to salivary juices containing an enzyme called **amylase.** Amylase is responsible for breaking the long chains of glucose molecules in starches into smaller units. The resulting products of this glucose-splitting activity are maltose and smaller starch chains known as dextrins.

Food does not remain in the mouth for long before it is swallowed and moves into the stomach. The high acidity of the stomach deactivates amylase, so no further digestion of carbohydrate takes place until the food moves into the small intestine.

The Small Intestine

As carbohydrate enters the small intestine, enzymes that are produced in the pancreas and in the wall of the small intestine complete the digestive process. These enzymes, known as amylase and disaccharidases, break down both disaccharides and polysaccharides into monosaccharides for absorption.

One of these enzymes, **lactase,** splits lactose into glucose and galactose before absorption. Absence of this enzyme in individuals is common throughout the world. Without lactase, lactose remains in the digestive tract and is fermented by microbes in the lower intestine. This produces gas, causing abdominal bloating, flatulence, and cramps.

TABLE 5.3
Carbohydrate digestion

Location	Enzyme	Substrate	End Product
Mouth	Amylase	Polysaccharides	Monosaccharides
Small intestine	Amylase	Polysaccharides	Monosaccharides
	Disaccharidases	Polysaccharides	Monosaccharides

Some individuals with lactose intolerance can still consume some milk and milk products (7). For those who cannot tolerate milk at all, several alternatives are available. For example, an enzyme can be purchased to mix with milk that will convert the lactose into glucose and galactose. Also, yogurt, kefir, and buttermilk have little lactose available because they contain microbes that break down the lactose. Cheeses are another good dairy product for individuals who are lactose intolerant because they are made from the portion of milk that contains little or no lactose. On the other hand, sweet acidophilus milk is not tolerated well by lactose-intolerant individuals, despite some suggestions to the contrary.

Absorption and Transport

Absorption of carbohydrate takes place as monosaccharides move across the intestinal lining and into the bloodstream. Absorption can be slowed by the presence of water-soluble fibers, which makes it difficult for enzymes to act quickly in breaking down polysaccharides (6). This property of water-soluble fibers is beneficial and will be discussed later in this chapter. Once in the bloodstream, fructose and galactose will be converted to glucose by the liver.

Blood Glucose

Both monosaccharides and disaccharides are absorbed from the small intestine into the bloodstream within minutes. But even starches that take longer to be broken down by enzymes show up in the bloodstream within just 30 to 60 minutes. Blood glucose is often measured by taking a sample of blood from an individual and analyzing the sample for the amount of glucose per 100 milliliters. High blood-glucose values could mean different things. For example, a person may have consumed a carbohydrate meal or snack in the previous hour, and the blood glucose may be elevated due to the absorption of this meal or snack. On the other hand, in a fasting individual, elevated blood-glucose levels could indicate diabetes. **Diabetes mellitus** is a metabolic abnormality in which there are high levels of glucose in the bloodstream even when an individual is in a fasting state. (See the Health-Promotion Insight at the end of this chapter.)

Glucose is the primary means by which carbohydrate is transported in the body. The brain in particular requires glucose exclusively for energy, utilizing up to 25 percent of the body's supply of glucose. (Muscles and other cells need glucose as a ready supply of energy, but they can use other sources.) It is no wonder, then, that carbohydrate makes up the largest proportion of the Calories in our diets.

Regulation of Blood Glucose

Insulin

Although all cells use glucose as an energy source, the hormone **insulin** regulates its passage from the blood to the body cells. After a carbohydrate-rich meal, blood glucose rises rapidly, which triggers insulin to be released from the pancreas. Insulin influences the body cells to allow glucose to enter, thereby decreasing the blood glucose. If the blood glucose is not needed immediately for energy, the surplus that the cells do not take up is stored in the liver, which converts glucose to either glycogen or fat, and in muscle, which converts it to glycogen. Then, when the blood glucose level is too low, the stored glucose can be used.

Glucagon, Epinephrine, and Growth Hormone

If blood glucose were to continue to fall due to the effect of insulin, the body would suffer from the maldistribution of fuel. In order to maintain a relatively stable level of functioning (homeostasis), other hormones cooperate to cause blood glucose to rise. **Glucagon, epinephrine,** and **growth hormone** are the three hormones that elevate blood-glucose levels in the body. They are able to do this by increasing the utilization of fat inside cells, thus freeing glucose for transport. These hormones also increase the breakdown of glycogen into glucose in the liver, where it is stored. Hormones intricately balance one another to stabilize fluctuations in blood glucose while still allowing glucose to be absorbed into the bloodstream and transported to organs of the body where it is needed (see figure 5.4).

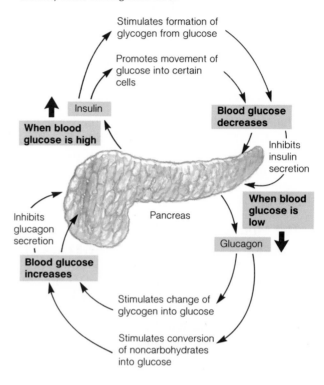

*F*IGURE 5.4
Insulin and glucagon function together to help maintain a relatively stable blood glucose level.

The Hypothalamus

Although your appetite is affected by internal and external factors, hunger has a more physiological basis. The hypothalamus is a gland at the base of the brain that has the ability to measure the blood-glucose level. If a person has not eaten for several hours, the blood-glucose level begins to drop. When the level hits a critical low, the hypothalamus signals the brain that it's time to eat. It is not surprising that the brain has a sensor for blood glucose—the brain is dependent on glucose as a source of fuel and cannot use fats.

Other Factors

Other factors can also influence blood glucose. Some of the most common include stress, tobacco, and caffeine. These act to stimulate the hormones that will convert liver glycogen into blood glucose. Stress, for example, triggers epinephrine levels to increase so that the body can prepare to respond to a stressor. Epinephrine, as was mentioned in the previous section, stimulates the liver to break down glycogen stores to glucose. This glucose enters the bloodstream, providing fuel for the response to a stressor.

FIGURE 5.5

Aerobic metabolism of carbohydrate utilizes oxygen to yield much more energy (36 ATP) than anaerobic metabolism (2 ATP).

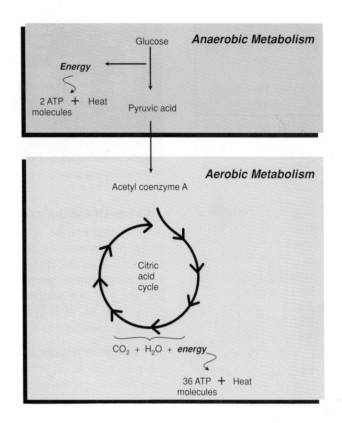

Tobacco and caffeine also have a similar effect on liver glycogen, which helps explain why having a cigarette and a cup of coffee in the morning can make a person feel as if he or she has obtained enough nourishment without having eaten a good breakfast. Unfortunately, the higher blood-glucose level soon returns to its low state, and no carbohydrate was eaten to furnish the depleted stores from the evening fast.

Metabolism and Storage

Glucose Metabolism

A chain of metabolic reactions in the cell quickly changes glucose into energy. In the **cytoplasm,** a cell's vital fluid interior, glucose molecules are broken in half, and some of the energy is released. Because no oxygen is required for this reaction, it is called anaerobic metabolism (energy derived without oxygen). At this point these molecular halves can be reassembled to form glucose again (but this will take energy), or be further broken down. In the latter process, the two halves of the glucose molecule move

into the **mitochondria.** These are the energy-producing "furnaces" within the cytoplasm of the cell. The molecular halves are further burned to produce more energy, with the resulting end products of carbon dioxide (CO_2) and water (H_2O). This latter process utilizes oxygen to yield much more energy than anaerobic metabolism, and it is therefore referred to as aerobic metabolism (energy derived using oxygen) (see figure 5.5).

Glucose Storage

When more than enough glucose is available, the excess will be put into storage. As the first alternative, glucose units will be assembled into longer chains for short-term storage as glycogen in either the liver or muscles. When these storage facilities are full, the liver will convert glucose to fat for long-term storage in body tissue.

Since there are only about 80 Calories of blood glucose available, these storage sites for energy are extremely important. As blood glucose falls, glycogen provides an immediate source of new glucose molecules to resupply the

TABLE 5.4

Estimated carbohydrate stores of energy in the body of a 154-pound male

Carbohydrate	Grams Present	Calories Available
Glucose in the blood	20	80
Glycogen		
Liver	85	340
Muscle	350	1,400
Total carbohydrate stores	455	1,820

From D. C. Nieman, *The Sports Medicine Fitness Course.* © 1986. Bull Publishing Co., Palo Alto, CA. Reprinted by permission.

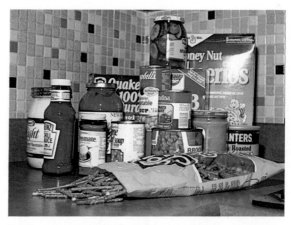

Simple sugars may be hidden in many products.

blood. Liver and muscle glycogen can be broken down into glucose units with just one enzymatic reaction when the need arises. Fat, on the other hand, cannot be broken down into glucose units, and the glucose that is stored in this fashion will not be available to refurnish blood glucose.

Just how much energy is stored in the form of glycogen varies considerably among individuals. For the typical 154-pound male, approximately 85 grams (or 340 Calories) of glycogen are stored in the liver, and 350 grams (or 1,400 Calories) are stored in the muscles. This storage may then last for about three-fourths of a day (2) (see table 5.4).

The Large Intestine

Not all carbohydrate is absorbed into the body. Fiber, which is indigestible, proceeds through the digestive tract into the large intestine, or colon. Some of this fiber is broken down by bacteria and absorbed. Cellulose, lignins, and some hemicelluloses have properties of holding onto water and swelling, resulting in a stool that feels large and stimulates peristalsis, the wavelike muscular action of the digestive tract which is responsible for moving the contents along in the large intestine. The water-insoluble fibers, therefore, help to move the stool through faster. This is advantageous in several respects and will be discussed later in this chapter.

Dietary Guidelines for Carbohydrate Consumption

Now that we have discussed the function of carbohydrate in the body, this section will focus on how to obtain carbohydrate and on making the best choices to achieve the dietary guidelines.

Sources of Carbohydrate

A great abundance of food contains carbohydrate; it is present in all four food groups. Carbohydrate can also be found in the group known as "limited extras," in which various sweeteners are placed. The sources are divided into two groups for discussion: simple carbohydrate and complex carbohydrate.

Simple Carbohydrate

Derived from sugar beets and sugarcane, affordable table sugar has been available for about one hundred years. As the technique for refining sugar improved, table sugar was produced in large quantities. The refining process shreds, strains, boils, centrifuges, dissolves, clarifies, filters, crystallizes, and dries sugarcane and sugar beets into a concentrated end product known as raw sugar. Raw sugar is not commonly used due to contaminants in the product, and it must be sanitized.

In the United States, consumption of sugar averages 18 percent of an American's Calories, or about 125 pounds per person each year (8). Most people don't believe that they eat that shocking amount; however, the simple sugars have a number of different names and are hidden in many products that don't necessarily taste sweet. When you are in the supermarket someday, check labels for the following terms, which equate with simple sugars: honey, brown sugar, dextrose, sucrose, maltose, molasses, fructose, levulose, corn syrup, and high fructose corn syrup. The latter of these, which is produced from corn, has gained popularity in the food industry and is used extensively in processed foods. In 1985 the annual per capita consumption of high fructose corn syrup was 38 pounds, compared to five pounds in 1975 (8).

TABLE 5.5
Some hidden sources of sugar

Food	Size Portion	No. Teaspoons Granulated Sugar	Food	Size Portion	No. Teaspoons Granulated Sugar
Cola drinks	1 (6 oz. bottle or glass)	3½	Ginger snaps	1	3
Cordials	1 (¾ oz. glass)	1½	Macaroons	1	6
Ginger ale	6 oz.	5	Nut cookies	1	1½
Orange-ade	1 (8 oz. glass)	5	Oatmeal cookies	1	2
Root beer	1 (10 oz. bottle)	4½	Sugar cookies	1	1½
Seven-up	1 (6 oz. bottle)	3¾	Chocolate eclair	1	7
Soda pop	1 (8 oz. bottle)	5	Cream puff	1	2
Sweet cider	1 cup	6	Donut (plain)	2	3
CAKES AND COOKIES			Donut (glazed)	1	6
Angel food	1 (4 oz. piece)	7	Snail	1 (4 oz. piece)	4½
Applesauce cake	1 (4 oz. piece)	5½	CANDIES		
Banana cake	1 (2 oz. piece)	2	Av. chocolate milk bar (ex. Hershey)	1 (1½ oz.)	2½
Cheesecake	1 (4 oz. piece)	2	Chewing gum	1 stick	½
Chocolate cake (plain)	1 (4 oz. piece)	6	Chocolate cream	1 piece	2
Chocolate cake (iced)	1 (4 oz. piece)	10	Butterscotch chew	1 piece	1
Coffee cake	1 (4 oz. piece)	4½	Chocolate mints	1 piece	2
Cupcake (iced)	1	6	Fudge	1 oz. square	4½
Fruit cake	1 (4 oz. piece)	5	Gum drop	1	2
Jelly-roll	1 (2 oz. piece)	2½	Hard candy	4 oz.	20
Orange cake	1 (4 oz. piece	4	Lifesavers	1	½
Pound cake	1 (4 oz. piece)	5	Peanut brittle	1	3½
Sponge cake	1 (1 oz. piece)	2	CANNED FRUITS & JUICES		
Strawberry shortcake	1 serving	4	Canned apricots	4 halv. & 1 T syr.	3½
Brownies unfrosted	1 (¾ oz.)	3	Canned fruit juices sweetened	½ cup	2
Chocolate cookies	1	1½	Canned peaches	2 halv. & 1 T syr.	3½
Fig newtons	1	5	Fruit salad	½ cup	3½
			Fruit syrup	2 T	2½
			Stewed fruits	½ cup	2

From American Foundation for Medical-Dental Science, Los Angeles.

Additionally, some products that are obviously sweet contain more sugar than one might expect. For example, table 5.5 shows the number of teaspoons of sugar that can be found in some commonly eaten foods. A 12-ounce can of soft drink contains about nine teaspoons, and a banana-split ice-cream sundae has a whopping 25 teaspoons. The average per capita consumption of sugar is about 20 teaspoons per day (8). Children eat even more sugar, with much of their intake originating from soft drinks, juices, and sugared cereals.

Soft drinks are now the number-one beverage used in the United States. The annual per capita consumption in 1982 was 39.5 gallons—double the consumption in 1962. Children 5–12 years of age average 5.6–7.7 ounces per day of regular soda; adolescents 13–18 years of age consume 8.6–12.6 ounces per day, and adults 19–44 years of age average 8.1–13.0 ounces per day (9). It is alarming to note that soft drinks, pastries, and sugar contribute almost 20 percent of the total carbohydrate intake in America (10). Health-Promotion Activity 5.1 will help you discover how much sugar you are currently consuming and where it is coming from.

TABLE 5.5
continued

Food	Size Portion	No. Teaspoons Granulated Sugar	Food	Size Portion	No. Teaspoons Granulated Sugar
DAIRY PRODUCTS			Prune pie	1 slice	6
Ice cream	⅓ pt. (3½ oz.)	3½	Pumpkin pie	1 slice	5
Ice cream bar	1	1-7 accord. to size	Rhubarb pie	1 slice	4
Ice cream cone	1	3½	Banana pudding	½ cup	2
Ice cream soda	1	5	Bread pudding	½ cup	1½
Ice cream sundae	1	7	Chocolate pudding	½ cup	4
Malted milk shake	1 (10 oz. glass)	5	Cornstarch pudding	½ cup	2½
JELLIES & JAMS			Date pudding	½ cup	7
Apple butter	1 T	1	Fig pudding	½ cup	7
Jelly	1 T	4-6	Grapenut pudding	½ cup	2
Orange marmalade	1 T	4-6	Plum pudding	½ cup	4
Peach butter	1 T	1	Rice pudding	½ cup	5
Strawberry jam	1 T	4	Tapioca pudding	½ cup	3
DESSERTS MISC.			Berry tart	1	10
Apple cobbler	½ cup	3	Blanc mange	½ cup	5
Blueberry cobbler	½ cup	3	Brown Betty	½ cup	3
Custard	½ cup	2	Sherbet	½ cup	9
French pastry	1 (4 oz. piece)	5	SYRUPS & ICINGS & SUGAR		
Jello	½ cup	4½	Brown sugar	1 T	3
Apple pie	1 slice, average	7	Chocolate icing	1 oz.	5
Apricot pie	1 slice	7	Chocolate sauce	1 T	3½
Berry pie	1 slice	10	Corn syrup	1 T	3
Butterscotch pie	1 slice	4	Granulated sugar	1 T	3
Cherry pie	1 slice	10	Honey	1 T	3
Cream pie	1 slice	4	Karo syrup	1 T	3
Lemon pie	1 slice	7	Maple syrup	1 T	5
Mincemeat pie	1 slice	4	Molasses	1 T	3½
Peach pie	1 slice	7	White icing	1 oz.	3

Complex Carbohydrate

Complex carbohydrate is rich in starch, fiber, or both. Starch and fiber are usually found together in unprocessed foods, and the food is referred to as "whole." Whole starches have not been concentrated or separated from the parent plant. **Legumes** (dried beans and peas), potatoes, fruits, vegetables, and whole grains can be found in this category.

Refinement is a process that extracts the starch or endosperm of grains, discarding the other cereal parts. A cereal grain has three main parts: the germ, the endosperm, and the bran. The germ contains the embryo plant and is rich in B-vitamins, vitamin E, and protein. The endosperm contains mostly starch and protein. The grain is surrounded by a protective bran layer, which is a good source of fiber, B-vitamins, and minerals. Paradoxically, it is the endosperm that is used to make flour, cereal, and other products, while the bran and germ are often used for animal feed.

Refinement does change the characteristics of a particular food. For example, refining the wheat grain creates the familiar white flour that produces a light, fluffy texture in baked products. The wheat grain is a good source of fiber and nutrients, but after refinement it is mainly a source of Calories.

When refinement of wheat flour began in the United States, white bread was expensive and a luxury item. Gradually, as white flour became cheaper to produce, it was used in great quantity. Because bread is a staple in this

TABLE 5.6

Nutrient differences between one slice (one ounce) of enriched and whole-grain bread

Nutrients	Whole Wheat	White Enriched
Iron (mg)	0.86	0.68
Riboflavin (mg)	0.05	0.07
Niacin (mg)	1.0	0.9
Thiamine (mg)	0.09	0.11
B_6 (mg)	0.05	0.01
Folacin (mcg)	14.0	8.0
Pantothenic acid (mg)	0.18	0.10
Copper (mg)	0.4	0.03
Zinc (mg)	0.56	0.15
Fiber (g)	0.4	Trace

From J. A. T. Pennington and H. N. Church. *Food Values of Portions Commonly Used.* © 1985. J. B. Lippincott Co., Philadelphia.

country, deficiency diseases such as anemia became evident because of the removal of iron during the refinement process.

Today, all refined grains have four different nutrients added back to the final refined product: thiamine, riboflavin, niacin, and iron. The process of adding nutrients to a product that were originally in the grain but removed during processing is known as **enrichment.** This term can be found on bread, pasta, and cereal product labels.

Other nutrients are removed during milling that are not replaced (see table 5.6). Fiber is one such nutrient that is not added back in the enrichment process. The consumption of highly refined diets, then, has led to a decrease in the amount of fiber that Americans eat. In response to this problem, many manufacturers add fiber (usually wheat bran), to some grain products. Breakfast cereals are probably the main source of added fiber on the market. This is not really enrichment, but fortification. **Fortification** means that something is added to a food that was not originally present or not present in such large quantities.

Grains are not the only carbohydrate-rich food that succumb to the removal of fiber and other nutrients. Potatoes, fruits, and vegetables are also processed in this fashion. The removal of skins from these sources of carbohydrate reduces both their fiber and nutrient concentration. The comparison of fiber in apple slices and apple juice in figure 5.6 demonstrates the dramatic reduction in fiber with processing.

FIGURE 5.6

There is a dramatic reduction in fiber when a product is processed.

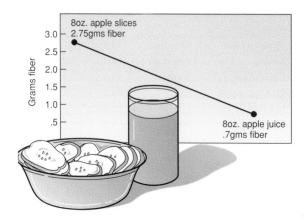

FIGURE 5.7

Percent of Calories from carbohydrate.

One cup of apple slices has 2.75 grams of fiber in comparison to .7 grams in one cup of apple juice. This is nearly a four-fold difference. Of course, such processing is not only done by manufacturers but also by the home food preparer. For example, people often leave the skin from a baked potato on their plate or peel an apple or carrot before eating it.

Recommended Carbohydrate Intake

In the national food supply, carbohydrate currently contributes 46 percent of the Calories (see figure 5.7). Chapter 2 discussed how this has decreased since the early 1900s. At the same time, the contribution of simple carbohydrate as a portion of the 46 percent has increased. Fiber and starches have actually decreased in this percentage. Of the seven U.S. Dietary Goals, two are directed at correcting the balance of starch, fiber, and sugar in the American diet. The first requires an increase in complex carbohydrate from the current 28 percent to about 48 percent of an

TABLE 5.7
Foods and the amount of dietary fiber they contain

Food	Amount	Grams of Dietary Fiber	Calories	Food	Amount	Grams of Dietary Fiber	Calories
Fruits				Kidney beans, cooked	½ cup	7.3	110
Apple (w/skin)	1 medium	3.5	81	Lima beans, cooked	½ cup	4.5	64
Banana	1 medium	2.4	105	Lentils, cooked	½ cup	3.7	97
Cantaloupe	¼ melon	1.0	30	Navy beans, cooked	½ cup	6.0	112
Cherries, sweet	10	1.2	49	*Breads, pastas, and flours*			
Peach (w/skin)	1	1.9	37				
Pear (w/skin)	½ large	3.1	61	Bagels	1 bagel	0.6	145
Prunes	3	3.0	60	Bran muffins	1 muffin	2.5	104
Raisins	¼ cup	3.1	108	French bread	1 slice	0.7	102
Raspberries	½ cup	3.1	35	Oatmeal bread	1 slice	0.5	63
Strawberries	1 cup	3.0	45	Pumpernickel bread	1 slice	1.0	66
Orange	1 medium	2.6	62	Whole-wheat bread	1 slice	1.4	61
Vegetables, cooked							
Asparagus, cut	½ cup	1.0	15	Rice, brown, cooked	½ cup	1.0	97
Beans, string, green	½ cup	1.6	16	Spaghetti, cooked	½ cup	1.1	155
Broccoli	½ cup	2.2	20	*Nuts and seeds*			
Brussels sprouts	½ cup	2.3	28	Almonds	10 nuts	1.1	79
Parsnips	½ cup	2.7	51	Peanuts	10 nuts	1.4	105
Potato (w/skin)	1 medium	2.5	106	Filberts	10 nuts	0.8	54
Spinach	½ cup	2.1	21	Popcorn, popped	1 cup	1.0	54
Sweet potato	½ medium	1.7	80	*Breakfast cereals*			
Turnip	½ cup	1.6	17	All-Bran	⅓ cup	8.5	71
Zucchini	½ cup	1.8	11	Bran Buds	⅓ cup	7.9	73
Vegetables, raw				Bran Chex	⅔ cup	4.6	91
Celery, diced	½ cup	1.1	10	Corn Bran	⅔ cup	5.4	98
Cucumber	½ cup	0.4	8	40% Bran-type	¾ cup	4.0	93
Lettuce, sliced	1 cup	0.9	7	Raisin Bran-type	¾ cup	4.0	115
Mushrooms, sliced	½ cup	0.9	10	Shredded wheat	⅔ cup	2.6	102
Tomato	1 medium	1.5	20	Oatmeal, regular, quick and instant, cooked	¾ cup	1.6	108
Spinach	1 cup	1.2	8				
Legumes							
Baked beans	½ cup	8.8	155	Cornflakes	1¼ cup	0.3	110
Dried peas, cooked	½ cup	4.7	115				

Source: E. Lanza and R. R. Butrum. "A Critical Review of Food Fiber Analysis and Data." *Journal of the American Dietetic Association*, 86: 737, 1986.

individual's energy intake. The second asks Americans to reduce their consumption of sugars from a very high 18 percent to about 10 percent of the energy intake (11). This would increase overall carbohydrate consumption to 58 percent of the Calories.

These changes would also increase fiber consumption. The average American today consumes about 10 to 20 grams of dietary fiber per day. The goal of the National Cancer Institute is for Americans to consume 25 to 35 grams of fiber per day by the year 2000 (12).

The American Dietetic Association also recommends a diet that is high in complex carbohydrate, low in fat, and that contains 20 to 35 grams of dietary fiber from a wide variety of sources (see table 5.7). Fiber supplements are not recommended because they are devoid of other nutrients and may not be related to the beneficial effects of dietary fiber in natural food sources. Large consumption of fiber (50 or more grams per day), may in fact have some adverse effects, according to the American Dietetic Association. These include decreased availability of vitamins and minerals such as copper, zinc, and iron (3).

The Athlete's Diet

The demand for carbohydrate during exercise is tremendous. The harder and longer the exercise (such as long-distance bicycling), the greater the need for carbohydrate by the working muscles. Exercise draws on muscle glycogen, and these stores are the limiting factor in the ability to perform hard exercise.

Do athletes then need a higher percentage of carbohydrate as energy in their diet than average healthy adults? Many researchers have confirmed that during heavy training a diet of 70 percent carbohydrate would help the glycogen stores to remain at a high level. Certainly, the athlete who consumes the average 46 percent would suffer from chronic depletion of the muscle glycogen stores and would perform poorly.

Another consideration for the endurance athlete is that exercising for longer than 75 minutes will substantially decrease glycogen stores to affect performance. Glycogen stores can be increased by a modified carbohydrate-loading regime. This involves eating a mixed 50 percent carbohydrate diet for three days, while gradually tapering down on exercise training. The last three days before an athletic event are spent resting and consuming a 70 percent carbohydrate diet to replenish and increase glycogen stores.

For those individuals who are regular exercisers, but not high-performance athletes, the recommended 58 percent of energy consumption would be adequate to fuel the body's need for more energy. The Health-Promotion Insight in chapter 12 is on sports nutrition and will further discuss the athlete's diet.

Achieving the Dietary Guidelines

The dietary guidelines for carbohydrate suggest the following changes in food selection and preparation (see table 5.8).

TABLE 5.8

Recommended servings from high-fiber, complex-carbohydrate food groups

Food Group	Number of Servings
Whole-grain products	4–6 per day
Fresh fruits	2+ per day
Vegetables	2+ per day
Legumes	3+ per week

Source: J. W. Anderson, N. J. Gustafson, and J. Tietyen-Clark. "Dietary Fiber and Diabetes: A Comprehensive Review and Practical Application." *Journal of the American Dietetic Association* 87:1189–97, 1987.

1. Increase the consumption of whole fruits and vegetables and whole grains. Decrease consumption of juices, which usually have the fiber removed.
2. Don't remove edible peels from fruits or vegetables unless absolutely necessary. Wash the fruits and vegetables well.
3. When choosing breads, cereals, pasta, crackers, and other grain products, look for the term *whole* before the listing of the grain. This indicates that the bran layer and germ are still present in the food product. "Rolled" is often used to mean the whole oat grain. The term "enriched" before a grain indicates that the product is refined and probably contains little fiber.
4. Read ingredient labels and screen for sugars and refined carbohydrate. Remember that the ingredients are listed by amount on the label, with the larger amounts in the product listed first. Avoid foods that are high in sugars and refined carbohydrate (see table 5.5 for hints on which foods are high-sugar sources).
5. Drink more water. Soft drinks are high in sugar, so substitute juices and beverages in which you can control the amount of sugar that is added (e.g., lemonade).
6. Choose cereals, drinks, fruits, and desserts that allow the individual to add sugar. Add sugar sparingly.
7. Include legumes in your diet.

Carbohydrate for Health Promotion

For Americans, there are dire consequences of not achieving the recommended dietary guidelines for carbohydrate. Let's examine some of the most common of these problems and their causes.

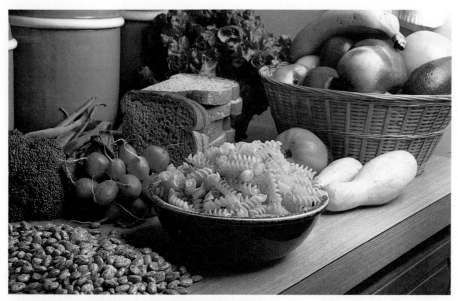

Include a variety of complex carbohydrate in your daily diet.

Too Much Sugar

Many of the major degenerative diseases in the United States have in part been blamed on our rising sugar consumption. Although this is not true, the high sugar consumption of Americans is highly undesirable. Sugar contains pure carbohydrate. Even though it provides Calories, it does not contain any of the other important nutrients, such as vitamins and minerals. This forces the body to depend on 83 percent of its Calories to supply 100 percent of its vitamin and mineral needs. In addition, the sugar consumption itself is linked to two important health problems.

Dental Caries

The health problem most widely accepted as being associated with consuming too much sugar is dental caries, or tooth decay (12). The American Dental Association estimates that 98 percent of American children have some tooth decay and that by age 55, about 50 percent of Americans have no natural teeth (13). Tooth decay begins with dental plaque, the sticky film that continuously forms in the mouth. Bacteria that are present in plaque are responsible for the breakdown of food, particularly sugars, into organic acids. These acids attack the enamel of the teeth and cause tooth decay.

Three factors determine the extent to which this acid will cause tooth decay: the hardness of the tooth enamel; the strength of the acids; and the length of time that acid is on the teeth. Acids work on the enamel for about 15 to 20 minutes after food is eaten. Just three meals a day provide one hour of "acid attack" per day. This does not account for any snacking, which may increase daily exposure to acid.

Cavities, fortunately, do not occur overnight. Changing your diet and dental-health habits can help prevent decay. Good dental health guidelines include:

1. Reduce consumption of sugars and foods high in sugar.
2. Avoid snacking when possible. Choose fresh fruits and raw vegetables, rather than sticky or sweet foods, if you do snack.
3. Brush and floss teeth or rinse your mouth after meals and snacks, especially after eating sweet or sticky snack foods.
4. Children should use a fluoride toothpaste because it increases the strength of the enamel and prevents calcium from leaving the tooth.

Reactive Hypoglycemia

Reactive hypoglycemia is a condition in which abnormally low blood sugar results from an overproduction of insulin after consuming an ordinary carbohydrate meal. The result of the increased insulin is a below-normal drop in blood glucose (hypoglycemia) between two to four hours after a meal (see figure 5.8). Since the brain in particular is dependent on glucose for fuel, some definite symptoms result. These include sweating, hunger, weakness, anxiety, lack of concentration, and palpitations.

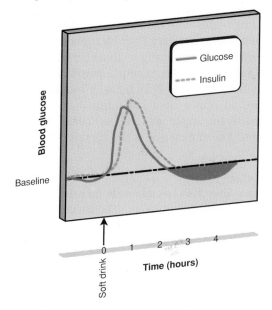

*F*IGURE 5.8

In reactive hypoglycemia, an overproduction of insulin, due to a rapid rise in blood glucose, causes a below-normal rebound in blood glucose (shaded area) in two to three hours.

A physician should be consulted if these symptoms consistently occur after carbohydrate meals. Since the condition seems to be worse if simple carbohydrate is eaten, it should be avoided or eaten with other foods. Symptoms may also be lessened by eating smaller and more frequent meals.

Too Little Fiber

Americans eat far too little fiber. This is mainly a result of an increase in consumption of sugar and refined-carbohydrate and a decrease in consumption of unrefined carbohydrate. Dietary-fiber intake is related to the prevention of several diseases.

Constipation and Hemorrhoids

Fiber initially became considered as an important dietary constituent because of its link to several diseases of the large intestine. Large epidemiological studies indicated that people in countries that consumed large amounts of dietary fiber, such as Africa, have lower incidence of constipation, hemorrhoids, and colon cancer than did people in developed countries. Metabolic studies have provided some explanations of this observation.

Water-insoluble fibers in the large intestine will absorb water and swell (8). The larger, softer stool will stimulate peristalsis to occur.

This will cause the stool to move faster through the tract, with less pressure. The latter is a result of less pressure needed to expel a softer stool. **Transit time** (the time it takes for food to move from the mouth and exit as waste through the anus) is usually 24 to 72 hours with adequate intakes of fiber, but can be longer if a low-fiber diet is consumed. Individuals who eat larger quantities of plant foods have been found to suffer less from both constipation and hemorrhoids (14).

Diverticular Disease

Another disease that is associated with low water-insoluble fiber intakes is diverticular disease. Approximately one-third of the U.S. population over the age of 60 suffer from this disease. Outpouchings, or **diverticuli,** occur in the wall of the large intestine. These are thought to be caused by the increased pressure needed to move a small, hard stool along the intestinal tract. Food sometimes gets caught in these diverticuli and becomes a source of irritation. This eventually will become inflamed and is called diverticulitis.

High-fiber diets tend to reduce the pressure needed to move the stool along the intestinal tract because the stool is softer and larger. A larger stool stimulates peristalsis. Certainly, high-fiber diets can relieve some of the symptoms of this disease, but many researchers believe that high-fiber diets can also prevent diverticular disease. Apart from diet, an increase in fluid consumption and exercise may also improve fecal elimination.

Colon Cancer

Colon cancer is one of the top two leading causes of cancer deaths in the United States. Numerous epidemiological studies now suggest that high dietary-fiber intake is associated with the prevention of colon cancer. Again the association is linked to the ability of fiber to decrease the transit time through the digestive tract. One theory suggests that the faster the feces goes through the digestive tract, the less time there will be for the exposure of the lining to any fecal carcinogens (15).

Dietary fiber is not the only dietary factor that has been linked to colon cancer. High fat and high Calories have also been associated. Despite some uncertainty, the National Cancer Institute recommends that Americans eat a variety of fiber to help prevent colon cancer.

Cardiovascular Diseases

The water-soluble fibers are associated with a lowered cardiovascular disease rate. This is primarily the result of the effect of water-soluble fiber on two of the primary risk factors for cardiovascular disease—high blood pressure and high serum cholesterol levels (3). Numerous research studies have related reductions in total serum cholesterol levels and in blood pressure after following diets high in water-soluble fibers for several months (16,17).

Exactly how water-soluble fibers affect these risk factors is not fully understood. In the case of cholesterol, water-soluble fibers bind the cholesterol released into the digestive tract in the form of **bile.** Bile helps to absorb fat into the body and is usually reabsorbed itself in the large intestine. If water-soluble fibers bind this cholesterol, it will be taken out of the body in the feces. The removal of cholesterol in the feces is a major excretion pathway. Thus water-soluble fiber can contribute to the reduction of serum cholesterol by increasing its excretion.

The relationship between the consumption of water-soluble fibers and the reduction in blood pressure is not as easily explained. Some researchers suggest that as bacteria act on the fiber in the digestive tract, they produce metabolites. These metabolites are then absorbed into the body and have an effect on the hormonelike substances that play a role in controlling blood pressure.

Obesity

Diets that are high in dietary fiber are usually lower in Calories and are less likely to contribute to obesity. Obesity is a critical factor in the development of many chronic diseases, including cardiovascular disease, diabetes, and hypertension. Dietary fiber increases satiety and delays gastric emptying so that one will feel full and eat less (3). An example may help to illustrate this concept: Which takes longer to consume, an apple or a half cup of apple juice? Probably the apple, which also "sticks with you" longer. The difference is the dietary fiber in the apple.

Diabetes

Dietary fiber also has a beneficial role in the regulation of blood glucose. For instance, carbohydrate that contains water-soluble fibers will form a gummy or gel-like substance in the small intestine. Enzymes have a difficult time penetrating the water-soluble fibers and breaking apart the polysaccharides for absorption, so it takes longer. The end result is a slower and less sharp rise in blood glucose, with a corresponding slower and less sharp rise in insulin. Water-soluble fibers are beneficial in reducing the extreme variations in blood glucose and insulin that individuals with diabetes often experience. This aids them in better control of their diabetic condition. The Health-Promotion Insight about diabetes, which follows, will provide more detail on this disease.

---

*H*EALTH-PROMOTION INSIGHT
Diabetes

Diabetes mellitus is the sixth leading cause of death in the United States, and 500,000 new cases are diagnosed each year. The medical costs attributed to this disease alone are estimated at $20.4 billion annually, and they continue to skyrocket (18). Although the statistics sound bleak, diabetes has potential as a manageable and, in many cases, preventable disease.

Definitions and Classifications
Diabetes is a disorder in which not enough insulin is present in the bloodstream to move glucose into the cell and use it for energy. As a result of the ineffective levels of insulin, blood glucose rises. The symptoms and complications of diabetes are caused by this high blood glucose.

There are two major types of diabetes mellitus: insulin-dependent diabetes and non-insulin-dependent diabetes.

Insulin-Dependent Diabetes Mellitus
The pancreas of individuals with **insulin-dependent diabetes mellitus** (IDDM) does not make insulin. Without insulin, the body cannot burn glucose for energy and must try to use fat alone. The combustion of fat results in acid wastes called **ketones.** As these ketones build up in the blood supply, a serious metabolic condition known as **ketoacidosis** can occur. If untreated, this condition will result in death. This type of diabetes usually occurs in young children or adolescents and is also known as Type I or juvenile-onset diabetes. Only

about ten percent of all diabetes diagnosed is IDDM. Individuals with this type of diabetes require an external source of insulin to sustain life.

Non-Insulin-Dependent Diabetes Mellitus

The pancreas of individuals with **non-insulin-dependent diabetes mellitus** (NIDDM) make some insulin, but it is either insufficient or not effective. While these individuals are not prone to the life-threatening ketoacidosis, they may still require insulin from an external source for correction of high blood glucose if this cannot be achieved by diet and exercise. Of all the cases of diabetes, 85 percent are NIDDM. NIDDM usually occurs after the age of 40, and 85 percent of those diagnosed are obese. The obesity is thought to reduce the effectiveness of insulin in the body, with each cell being less sensitive to insulin.

Symptoms and Diagnosis

The risk of developing diabetes increases with age and is 60 times more likely in people older than 65 years than in those under 17 years. Diabetes is also 50 percent more common in women than in men. The symptoms of diabetes include frequent urination and thirst, extreme hunger, rapid weight loss, blurred vision or a sudden change in visual acuity, easy tiring, drowsiness, or general weakness. These symptoms may recur or persist.

A simple fasting (12 hours) blood test can be used to diagnose diabetes. An elevated fasting glucose concentration of more than 140 mg/dL on more than one occasion indicates diabetes. A normal fasting blood glucose is less than 115 mg/dL. If there is any question about the blood test, a physician may order a more sophisticated test for more conclusive results.

Complications

An estimated 11 million individuals in the U.S. have diabetes, 45 percent of which remain unaware of their illness. While high blood glucose is a serious problem in itself, the long-term complications of this disease are deadly.

Diabetic women who are pregnant have a higher risk of infant mortality, birth defects, respiratory problems, prematurity, and other health disorders. Individuals with diabetes suffer from coronary artery disease, running two to three times the risk of suffering a heart attack or stroke than those without the disease (19). Fifteen years after diagnosis, 80 percent of diabetic individuals have some degree of **retinopathy,** a hemorrhage in the

capillaries of the retina of the eye. Due to this disease, diabetes is the number-one cause of blindness in the U.S. Diabetes contributes to 17 times more kidney disease, with half of all diabetic children dying of kidney failure within 25 years of diagnosis. Diabetes is also responsible for nerve damage. Furthermore, diabetes gives rise to peripheral vascular disease, in which the extremities of the body do not get enough blood, leading to tissue death. The resulting gangrene is five times more likely to occur in diabetic individuals than nondiabetic individuals and often requires amputation (20).

Management of Diabetes

The management of diabetes should focus on blood-glucose regulation and on the prevention of cardiovascular disease, since diabetes accelerates the atherosclerotic process. Therefore, management is directed to four areas: nutrition, exercise, medication (if needed), and other heart disease risk factors (see figure 5.9).

Nutrition

There are four nutritional goals of diabetes management.

1. Maintain appropriate blood glucose levels.
2. Achieve and maintain healthy blood lipid levels.
3. Achieve and maintain reasonable weight.
4. Practice good nutritional habits.

Interestingly, the principles of a health-promoting diet that are beneficial for all adults will also serve to meet the nutritional goals of diabetes management. The American Diabetic Association urges that the diabetic diet be varied, nutritious, adapted to individual needs, integrated with medication regimens, reduced in saturated fats and cholesterol, high in fiber, reduced in sodium, and low in alcohol (21). The following specific guidelines apply.

Eat less fat. Eat fish, skinless poultry, and other lean meats, being cautious to limit your portion sizes to two to three ounces. Eat fewer high-fat items like cold cuts, bacon, nuts, gravy, salad dressing, mayonnaise, margarine, and solid shortening. Use low-fat dairy products. A low saturated fat diet reduces the blood cholesterol and triglyceride values.

Eat more complex carbohydrate. Include whole-grain breads and cereals, and whole fresh fruits and vegetables in your daily diet. Eat more legumes (lentils, dried peas, and beans). Dietary fiber that can be found in these foods has been found to reduce insulin requirements, improve blood-glucose control, lower fasting blood cholesterol and triglyceride values, and promote weight loss (19).

FIGURE 5.9
Diabetes management involves four parts: nutrition, exercise, medication (if needed), and other heart disease risk factors.

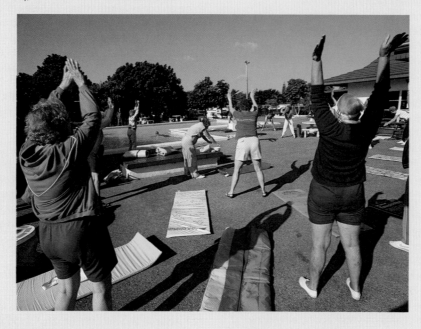

Eat less sugar. All people should eat less sugar. Although sugar does not cause diabetes and there has been considerable debate on the effect of various sources of sugar on blood glucose, there are several problems with the current consumption patterns of Americans. Sugar has many Calories and no vitamins, minerals, or fiber. Overconsumption of sugar certainly makes it more difficult to attain a reasonable weight, too. Foods high in sugar include desserts, sugared breakfast cereals, soft drinks, and added sugars such as table sugar, honey, and syrups. Unfortunately, only 25 percent of the sugar eaten is added at home; 75 percent is already contained in a purchased product (1). A decision not to purchase sugary foods is then a major point of control.

Use less salt. Most of us eat too much salt. High blood pressure, a major risk factor for heart disease and stroke, may worsen as salt causes the body to retain water. Try using less salt in cooking or at the table. Foods that are high in sodium are processed meats, condiments, cheeses, chips, fast foods, convenience meals, crackers, and nuts.

Use alcohol in moderation. Alcohol is another source of Calories that is devoid of nutrients. It is best to avoid alcoholic beverages if possible.

The Diabetic Meal Plan

A dietitian can assist the diabetic individual in creating a plan for daily eating that will incorporate good nutrition. A meal plan shows how many food choices or exchanges a person can eat for each meal or snack. The plan should be based on 50 to 60 percent of the daily Calories as carbohydrate, 15 percent as protein, and the remainder as fat (22).

The exchange lists help a meal plan work because they provide a wide variety of food to select from in fulfilling an exchange. The portion sizes of each exchange are listed in the exchange lists in chapter 3, along with instructions on their use.

In making a meal plan, consistency in daily routine is essential for the individual with IDDM. This means that meals should be eaten at the same times each day. The amount and types of food should also be the same. This will help to balance insulin injections.

On the other hand, the individual with NIDDM must strive to achieve and maintain reasonable weight. Many NIDDM individuals will cease to demonstrate high blood glucose episodes if they reach a reasonable weight.

Exercise

A regular aerobic exercise program has four important benefits in diabetes management.

Improved diabetic control. A regular aerobic exercise program will decrease the need for insulin by 30–50 percent in well-controlled IDDM individuals and by 100 percent in NIDDM individuals. Each cell seems to increase its sensitivity to the insulin that is present (23).

Correction or prevention of obesity. Aerobic exercise is related to a decrease in body fat and an increase in resting metabolic rate.

Effect of blood lipids. Exercise decreases total cholesterol, improves the ratio of low-density lipoprotein to high-density lipoprotein cholesterol (see chapter 6), and reduces blood triglycerides, all of which reduce the risk of heart disease (24).

Reduced risk of coronary heart disease. A reduced risk of coronary heart disease has been consistently associated with physical activity. Physical activity may reduce blood lipids, blood pressure, smoking habits, stress levels, and body weight, which would in turn decrease the risk of coronary heart disease.

Medication

Effective treatment of diabetes centers around the control of blood-glucose levels within the narrow limits that a healthy pancreas would maintain. About one-fourth of known diabetic individuals in the U.S. are being treated with insulin, about half are receiving an oral agent that stimulates the pancreas to secrete insulin, and about one-fourth are not receiving any antidiabetic medication. Yet it is estimated that with optimum long-term diet and exercise therapy, only about 25 percent of diabetics would need any medication (25). The American Dietetic Association and The American Diabetic Association consider diet, exercise, and medication when needed to be an integral triad in the effective management of diabetes.

Other Heart Disease Risk Factors

There are two other risk factors that are included in the prevention of heart disease that should be mentioned. Individuals with diabetes should strive to reduce their smoking and stress (19).

SUMMARY

1. Carbohydrate differs mainly in size. The smallest units are called monosaccharides. The disaccharides are made up of two monosaccharides. The polysaccharides are made of many monosaccharides, even thousands, and are therefore called complex carbohydrate.

2. Most polysaccharides are made up of glucose molecules alone, but differ in their arrangement and bonding. Polysaccharides include starch, a plant's storage form of carbohydrate; glycogen, an animal's storage form of carbohydrate; and fiber, complex plant material that cannot be digested.

3. Carbohydrate has three major functions: providing energy and bulk, and helping to make other structures and compounds in the body.

4. Although carbohydrate digestion begins in the mouth, enzymes in the small intestine are largely responsible for the breakdown of carbohydrate into monosaccharides for digestion.

5. Glucose is absorbed from the small intestine and is the major transport form of carbohydrate in the bloodstream. Insulin is the hormone that regulates blood glucose levels by allowing glucose into cells and by promoting glycogen production and fat storage from surplus glucose. Glucagon, epinephrine, and growth hormone balance the effects of insulin by causing an increase in blood glucose when needed.

6. The hypothalamus is a gland at the base of the brain that stimulates hunger when blood glucose is low.

7. When newly absorbed glucose enters the bloodstream, it has three alternatives. The glucose may be used to replenish blood glucose first. Next the glucose will be assembled into glycogen for short-term storage in the liver or muscles. Finally, when these storage facilities are full, glucose will be converted to fat for long-term storage.

8. Fiber is indigestible and proceeds into the large intestine, where some will be degraded by bacteria and absorbed. The insoluble fibers will absorb water and swell, creating a soft, large stool. The pressure of the larger stool on the walls of the intestine will trigger peristalsis, which helps to move the stool through the intestine faster.

9. Americans consume 125 pounds of sugar per person per year. Alarmingly, soft drinks, desserts, and sugar contribute 20 percent of the total carbohydrate intake in the U.S. Product labels may

indicate hidden sugars with the following ingredients: sucrose, fructose, maltose, molasses, dextrose, levulose, corn syrup, brown sugar, and honey.

10. Whole grains, whole fruits and vegetables, and legumes are excellent sources of complex carbohydrate that still contain the original fiber. When grains are refined, the bran and the germ are discarded, and the endosperm or starch remains. Unfortunately, only some of the B-vitamins and iron are added back in the enrichment process, but not the fiber or other nutrients.

11. Americans should strive to increase their current carbohydrate consumption from 46 percent to 58 percent of their total Calories, with no more than 10 percent of the Calories as simple sugars. This diet should also include 20 to 35 grams of dietary fiber from a wide variety of sources.

12. A high sugar intake is related to dental caries. Sugar is devoid of vitamins, minerals, and fiber.

13. A low dietary fiber intake is related to several diseases including constipation and hemorrhoids, diverticular disease, colon cancer, cardiovascular diseases, obesity, and diabetes.

14. Diabetes is the sixth leading cause of death in the U.S. It results when not enough insulin is manufactured by the body to properly metabolize and transport glucose. Retinopathy, blindness, nerve damage, gangrene, kidney disease, and cardiovascular disease are serious complications of diabetes.

15. The management of diabetes involves nutrition, exercise, medication (if needed), and other heart disease risk factors.

16. The nutritional goals for diabetes are similar to the health-promoting goals for all adults. The four are to maintain appropriate blood-glucose levels, to achieve and maintain healthy blood-lipid levels, to achieve and maintain reasonable weight, and to practice good nutritional habits.

REFERENCES

1. Anderson, T. A. 1982. Recent Trends in Carbohydrate Consumption. *Annual Review of Nutrition* 2:113-32.
2. Williams, M. H. 1983. *Nutrition for Fitness and Sport*. Wm. C. Brown Publishers, Dubuque, Iowa. pp. 25-26.
3. Gorman, M. A., and C. Bowman. 1988. Position of The American Dietetic Association: Health Implications of Dietary Fiber. *Journal of the American Dietetic Association* 88 (2):216-21.
4. Olson, A., G. M. Gray, and M. Chiu. 1987. Chemistry and Analysis of Dietary Fiber. *Food Technology* (February): 71-80.
5. MacDonald, I. 1987. Metabolic Requirements for Dietary Carbohydrate. *American Journal of Clinical Nutrition* 45:1193-96.
6. Schneeman, B. O. 1987. Soluble vs. Insoluble Fiber — Different Physiological Responses. *Food Technology* (February): 71-80.
7. McDonough, F. E., et al. 1987. Modification of Sweet Acidophilus Milk to Improve Utilization by Lactose-Intolerant Persons. *American Journal of Clinical Nutrition* 45:570-74.
8. Glinsman, W. H., H. Irausquin, and Y. K. Park. 1986. Executive Summary: Evaluation of Health Aspects of Sugars Contained in Carbohydrate Sweeteners. Report of Sugars Task Force, 1986. *Journal of Nutrition* 116: (11 suppl) :S1-S216.
9. Morgan, K. J., V. J. Stults, and G. L. Stampley. 1985. Soft Drink Consumption Patterns of the U.S. Population. *Journal of the American Dietetic Association* 85:(3):352-54.
10. Block, G., et al. 1985. Nutrient Sources in the American Diet: Quantitative Data from the NHANES II Survey. *American Journal of Epidemiology* 122:27-40.
11. Wolf, I. D., and B. B. Peterkin. 1984. Dietary Guidelines: The USDA Perspective. *Food Technology* (July): 80-86.
12. Slavin, J. L., 1987. Dietary Fiber: Classification, Chemical Analysis, and Food Sources. *Journal of the American Dietetic Association* 87:1164-1171.
13. Mayer, J. 1976. The Bitter Truth about Sugar. *New York Times Magazine* (June 20): 26.
14. Klurfeld, D. M. 1987. The Role of Dietary Fiber in Gastrointestinal Disease. *Journal of the American Dietetic Association* 87:1172-1177.
15. Greenswald, P., E. Lanza, and G. A. Eddy. 1987. Dietary Fiber in the Reduction of Colon Cancer Risk. *Journal of the American Dietetic Association* 87:1178-1188.
16. Ullrick, I. H. 1987. Evaluation of High-Fiber Diet in Hyperlipidemia: A Review. *Journal of the American College of Nutrition* 6:19-25.
17. Behall, K. M., et al. 1987. Mineral Balance in Adult Men: Effect of Four Refined Fibers. *American Journal of Clinical Nutrition* 46:307-14.
18. American Diabetes Association. 1988. Diabetes Facts and Figures. Alexandria, VA: Diabetes Information Service Center.
19. Anderson, J. W., N. J. Gustafson, and J. Tietyen-Clark. Dietary Fiber and Diabetes: A Comprehensive Review and Practical Application. *Journal of the American Dietetic Association* 87 (9)1189-1197.
20. National Diabetes Advisory Board. 1980. The Treatment and Control of Diabetes: A National Plan to Reduce Mortality and Morbidity. NIH Publication No. 81-2284.
21. American Diabetes Association and American Dietetic Association. 1986. Exchange Lists for Meal Planning. Alexandria, VA: Diabetes Information Service Center.
22. Nuttall, F. Q. 1979. Principles of Nutrition and Dietary Recommendations for Individuals with Diabetes Mellitus. *Diabetes* 28:1028-1029.
23. Rauramaa, R. 1984. Relationship of Physical Activity, Glucose Tolerance, and Weight Management. *Preventive Medicine* 13:37-46.
24. Wheeler, M. L., L. Delahanty, and J. Wylie-Rosett. 1987. Diet and Exercise in Noninsulin Dependent Diabetes Mellitus: Implications for Dietitians from the NIH Consensus Development Conference. *Journal of the American Dietetic Association* 87:480-85.
25. West, M. W. 1983. Diabetes Mellitus. In *Nutritional Support of Medical Practice*. H. A. Schneider, et al., eds. Philadelphia: Harper and Row, Publishers.

HEALTH-PROMOTION ACTIVITY 5.1
The Sweet Truth

1. Record what you've eaten on one weekday and one weekend day.
2. For each food listed on your diet history, look up the teaspoons of sugar in the food in table 5.5. (Even if you do not suspect that a food contains sugar, check to be sure. List any sugar source below.)

Food	Sugar (in teaspoons)
_____	_____
_____	_____
_____	_____
_____	_____
_____	_____
_____	_____
_____	_____
_____	_____
_____	_____

3. Add up the teaspoons of sugar you ate in one day.
   _____ teaspoons
   If you consumed less than ten teaspoons for each of the two days, congratulations. However, if you consumed more than ten teaspoons of sugar in a day, what would you be willing to change to reduce your sugar consumption?

4. List two alternative foods to those that you ate that are high in sugar (greater than three teaspoons).

HEALTH-PROMOTION ACTIVITY 5.2
Putting More Fiber into Your Day

The following is an example of a 15-gram fiber diet. Use table 5.7 and appendix B to select foods that will increase the fiber content of this diet to 25 to 30 grams.

Breakfast	Amount	Fiber (g)	Breakfast	Amount	Fiber (g)
Egg, fried	1	—	_____		
Special K	1 cup	0.1	_____		
Milk, low-fat	1 cup	—	_____		
White bread	1 slice	0.8	_____		
Margarine	2 tsp	—	_____		
Orange juice	4 oz	0.6	_____		

Lunch	Amount	Fiber (g)	Lunch	Amount	Fiber (g)
Turkey	2 oz	—			
Mayonnaise	1 tbsp	—			
Lettuce	1 leaf	0.2			
Salad					
Lettuce	3/4 cup	0.8			
Tomato	1/4 cup	0.5			
Cucumber	1/3 cup	0.2			
Italian dressing	1 tbsp	—			
Apple juice	6 oz	0.3			
Peach	1	1.1			

Dinner	Amount	Fiber (g)	Dinner	Amount	Fiber (g)
Steak	4 oz	—			
Baked potato					
with skin	1 med	5.2			
Margarine	1 tbsp	—			
Green beans	1/2 cup	1.4			
White roll	1 oz	0.8			
Sherbet	1/2 cup	—			
Grapes	10	0.4			

Snack	Amount	Fiber (g)	Snack	Amount	Fiber (g)
Graham crackers	2	1.3			
Soft drink	12 oz	—			

List two ways to add more fiber into your daily diet.

The labels of two popular cold cereals are provided. Compare the ingredient list and the carbohydrate information and answer the following questions.

1. Which cereal is a better choice for getting dietary fiber? How many grams of dietary fiber does each cereal provide? What term on the cereal ingredient lists tells you that the cereal may be a good source of fiber?

2. Compare the ingredients on the list and tell which cereal is lowest in sugar.

3. Now look at the carbohydrate information. How many grams of sucrose are in each cereal per serving? Divide the grams of sucrose and other sugars by the grams of total carbohydrate.

   __ g sugars/ __ g total carbohydrate = __
   Multiply this number by 100 percent to see which cereal has the greatest percentage of its carbohydrate as sugar.

4. A label can reveal quite a lot of information on carbohydrate. While both cereals in this activity are high in dietary fiber, #2 is much lower in sugar. Ideally, your morning would be high in dietary fiber and low in sugar. Look at the label on one of your favorite cereals and compare the nutritional label to the two cereals provided in this activity. Do you need to make any adjustments to your choice of cereal? Are some in your cupboard better than others?

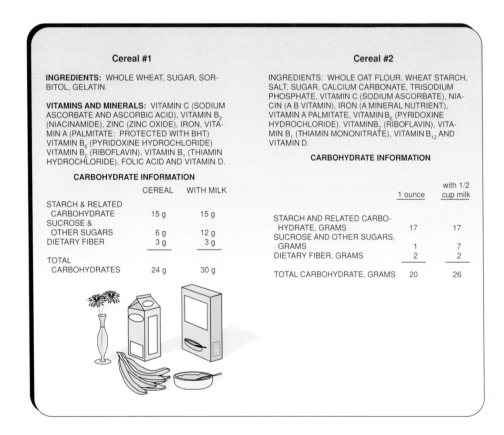

Cereal #1

INGREDIENTS: WHOLE WHEAT, SUGAR, SORBITOL, GELATIN.

VITAMINS AND MINERALS: VITAMIN C (SODIUM ASCORBATE AND ASCORBIC ACID), VITAMIN B_2 (NIACINAMIDE), ZINC (ZINC OXIDE), IRON, VITAMIN A (PALMITATE: PROTECTED WITH BHT) VITAMIN B_6 (PYRIDOXINE HYDROCHLORIDE) VITAMIN B_2 (RIBOFLAVIN), VITAMIN B_1 (THIAMIN HYDROCHLORIDE), FOLIC ACID AND VITAMIN D.

CARBOHYDRATE INFORMATION

	CEREAL	WITH MILK
STARCH & RELATED CARBOHYDRATE	15 g	15 g
SUCROSE & OTHER SUGARS	6 g	12 g
DIETARY FIBER	3 g	3 g
TOTAL CARBOHYDRATES	24 g	30 g

Cereal #2

INGREDIENTS: WHOLE OAT FLOUR, WHEAT STARCH, SALT, SUGAR, CALCIUM CARBONATE, TRISODIUM PHOSPHATE, VITAMIN C (SODIUM ASCORBATE), NIACIN (A B VITAMIN), IRON (A MINERAL NUTRIENT), VITAMIN A PALMITATE, VITAMIN B_6 (PYRIDOXINE HYDROCHLORIDE), VITAMINB_2 (RIBOFLAVIN), VITAMIN B_1 (THIAMIN MONONITRATE), VITAMIN B_{12} AND VITAMIN D.

CARBOHYDRATE INFORMATION

	1 ounce	with 1/2 cup milk
STARCH AND RELATED CARBOHYDRATE, GRAMS	17	17
SUCROSE AND OTHER SUGARS, GRAMS	1	7
DIETARY FIBER, GRAMS	2	2
TOTAL CARBOHYDRATE, GRAMS	20	26

6

Lipids

INTRODUCTION

*H*ave you ever thought about eating a tuna-fish sandwich without the mayonnaise, mashed potatoes without the gravy, or perhaps a salad with just vinegar and herbs? The usual toppings on these foods consist of a large proportion of lipid. Lipids are an integral part of our diet, adding flavor and nutrients to the foods we eat. However, they have recently received a bad reputation for being related to several chronic diseases, as well as for providing hidden Calories to our foods. Nonetheless, lipids are essential in our diet and keep us satisfied for a longer period of time after a meal.

This chapter will discuss the types and functions of lipids in the body. It will also reveal the sources of and the dietary recommendations for lipids in a healthy diet.

*F*IGURE 6.1

Structure of a triglyceride. Three molecules of fatty acids bond to one molecule of glycerol to form a triglyceride.

```
Glycerol —Fatty acid
        —Fatty acid
        —Fatty acid
```

Lipid Structure and Function

Lipid is a general term used for several different compounds that include both solid fats and liquid oils. The three major classes of lipids are triglycerides, phospholipids, and sterols.

Triglycerides

Ninety-five percent of the lipids found in foods are **triglycerides.** These are composed of a three-carbon glycerol molecule, to which is attached three fatty acids (see figure 6.1). Occasionally only one or two fatty acids are attached, and these are called monoglycerides or diglycerides, respectively. The fatty-acid portion of the molecule is responsible for its characteristics. The fatty acids differ from one another in chain length and degree of saturation.

Chain length refers to the number of carbon atoms linked together in the fatty-acid skeleton. Fatty acids may have between 4 and 22 carbon atoms.

The degree of saturation refers to the bonding between the carbon atoms. Four bonds surround every carbon atom in the chain. Figure 6.2 illustrates that a fatty acid with only single bonds around each carbon atom is called a **saturated fatty acid** (SFA). If one of the carbons is connected to another carbon by a double bond, the fatty acid is considered unsaturated. If the double bonds were to be broken, there would be room for more hydrogen atoms on the chain. A fatty acid with one double bond is referred to as a **monounsaturated fatty acid** (MUFA), whereas a fatty acid containing two or more double bonds is considered a **polyunsaturated fatty acid** (PUFA).

Triglycerides that contain mostly saturated fatty acids are usually solid at room temperature (like the fat around a beef steak), whereas those containing mostly polyunsaturated fatty acids are liquid (like corn or soybean

*F*IGURE 6.2

Unsaturated fatty acids differ from saturated fatty acids in that they contain one or more double bonds between carbon atoms. Sources of each fatty acid are listed.

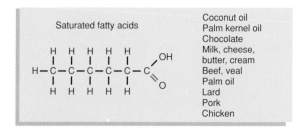

Saturated fatty acids — Coconut oil, Palm kernel oil, Chocolate, Milk, cheese, butter, cream, Beef, veal, Palm oil, Lard, Pork, Chicken

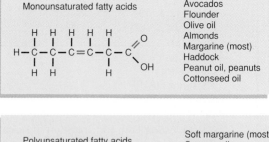

Monounsaturated fatty acids — Avocados, Flounder, Olive oil, Almonds, Margarine (most), Haddock, Peanut oil, peanuts, Cottonseed oil

Polyunsaturated fatty acids — Soft margarine (most), Sesame oil, Mayonnaise, Soybean oil, Corn oil, Sunflower oil, Safflower oil

oil). There are several exceptions to the rule. Coconut and palm oils are mostly saturated fatty acids, and fish fat contains a large proportion of polyunsaturated fatty acids.

Phospholipids

Phospholipids are found in all cells of the body. They are similar to triglycerides but contain only two fatty acids and one phosphorus-containing substance. **Lecithin** is a common phospholipid in the body that may act as an **emulsifier.** Emulsifiers have the property of mixing well with both fats and water and are used in many aspects of the food industry. For example, emulsifiers are used to keep salad dressings from separating.

Sterols

Sterols are unlike other lipids in their structure but qualify because of their physical properties. One of the most familiar sterols is cholesterol. Others include vitamin D, estrogen, testosterone, and other hormones.

Figure 6.3

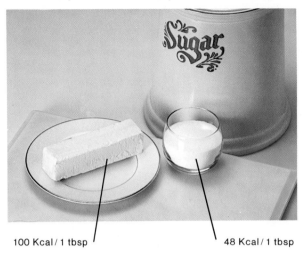

Fat is a concentrated source of energy, providing more than twice as many kilocalories as carbohydrate.

100 Kcal / 1 tbsp   48 Kcal / 1 tbsp

Lipid Functions

Lipids function in the body in six important ways.

Energy

Fat is a concentrated source of energy, providing nine Calories per gram. This is more than twice the amount that either protein or carbohydrate (four Calories per gram each) offer. Therefore, it is an excellent storage form of energy in the body (see figure 6.3).

Essential Fatty Acids

Lipids also include several **essential fatty acids:** linoleic acid and linolenic acid. Arachidonic acid is also considered essential by some authors. According to the National Research Council, these must be supplied by the diet because the body cannot synthesize them in significant amounts. Fortunately, the essential fatty acids are widespread in food sources, and it is unlikely for adults to become deficient. Infants should not be fed skim milk as their main source of food, or they may experience deficiency symptoms.

Transport of Fat-Soluble Vitamins

Lipids aid in the absorption of the fat-soluble vitamins A, D, E, and K.

Structural Components of the Body

Besides being stored for energy in **adipose tissue** (fat), lipids are also structural components of cell membranes, digestive secretions, hormones, and nerve coverings. Actually lipids help to maintain the integrity of our skin and hair to keep us looking healthy.

Insulation

To help maintain the inner temperature of the body, about half of the adipose tissue acts as insulation. It is stored directly under the skin in what is called the subcutaneous fat layer. It is advantageous in controlling temperature and in creating a pleasant appearance. However, too much subcutaneous fat may not be appealing or healthy.

Protection

Adipose tissue also acts to cushion and protect vital body organs from bruises or damage.

Digestion, Absorption, and Transport of Lipids

There are a wide variety of lipids to be transported into the body, but this section will focus on just two. Triglycerides will be discussed because they are the most common lipid in foods, and dietary cholesterol because of the current concern about heart disease.

The Small Intestine

When triglycerides are consumed, the first digestive enzymes they encounter are in the stomach. However, the majority of digestion takes place in the small intestine. Two substances found there help in the digestive and absorptive processes.

    Bile is the first of these substances. It is made in the liver, stored in the gallbladder, and released into the small intestine upon the entrance of triglycerides. Bile is composed of cholesterol, lecithin, and bile salts (sterols). Large droplets of triglycerides are emulsified, or broken down into smaller droplets, by bile. This increases the surface area that can be exposed to digestive enzymes.

    Lipases are digestive enzymes produced in the pancreas and small intestine. They break down the triglycerides into glycerol, fatty acids, and monoglycerides. These products are then incorporated with bile salts in a package called a **micelle.** Micelles deliver their contents of the intestinal cell membrane for transport into the body.

    Dietary cholesterol is usually attached to a fatty acid in foods. This is first removed in the small intestine by lipases; then cholesterol can also be incorporated into the micelles. Again the micelles deliver the cholesterol to the intestinal cell for transport into the body.

The absorption of triglycerides is dependent on the availability of bile salts. If sufficient quantities are present, 97 percent of all fat will be absorbed. In contrast, only 50 percent of cholesterol is commonly absorbed. Its absorption is dependent on the presence of micelles to move it into the intestinal cells.

Transport from the Intestine

There are two mechanisms for the transport of the products of lipid digestion into the bloodstream, based on the solubility of these products in water. The blood is a water medium and can therefore transport only water-soluble forms of lipid material.

Glycerol and fatty acids with short- and medium-length chains are water soluble. They may be transported from the cells of the small intestine directly to the liver, moving through the bloodstream via the portal vein.

Long-chain fatty acids, cholesterol, and phospholipids are insoluble in water. If they were to enter the bloodstream, they could potentially clump together and clog blood vessels. A water-soluble packaging must therefore be constructed for transport. The long-chain fatty acids are reformed into triglycerides and packaged along with cholesterol, phospholipids, and protein. This results in a soluble aggregate known as a **lipoprotein.** This particular type of lipoprotein is approximately 85 percent triglyceride and is called a **chylomicron.** Chylomicrons are the principal lipoproteins made in the intestinal wall. They are released into the lymphatic system and soon link with the bloodstream. The fate of the triglycerides in the chylomicrons is that they will be used for energy production or for storage as fat in muscle, adipose, or liver tissue (see figure 6.4).

Transport between Body Tissues

The level of lipids in the bloodstream is not only determined by those absorbed by the intestine but also by those released from the liver. The liver can take fatty acids directly from the bloodstream or synthesize them from other nutrients, such as glucose, amino acids, or alcohol. These fatty acids are combined with glycerol to form

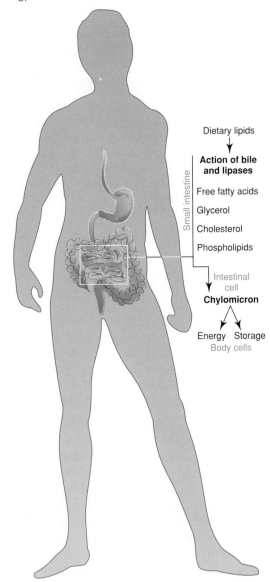

FIGURE 6.4
Dietary lipids enter the body and are eventually used for energy or stored as fat.

triglycerides. The triglycerides are packaged with cholesterol, phospholipids, and protein before being released to the bloodstream. These protein packets are known as lipoproteins and are necessary to allow lipids to move through the water medium of the blood.

There are three major lipoproteins in addition to the chylomicrons mentioned in the last section (see figure 6.5):

Composition of the four major lipoproteins.

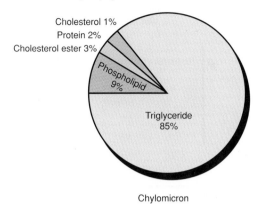

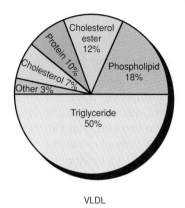

Chylomicron

VLDL

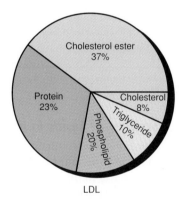

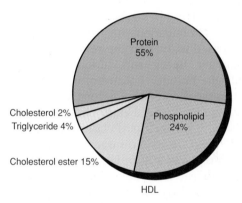

LDL

HDL

Very Low Density Lipoproteins (VLDL) consist mainly of triglycerides that are being transported to provide fatty acids and glycerol to tissues.

Low Density Lipoproteins (LDL) contain a high proportion of cholesterol. LDL transport cholesterol from the liver to other body cells. LDL are often referred to as "bad" cholesterol because they may be taken up by muscle cells in arteries and have been implicated in the development of **atherosclerosis,** a hardening of the arteries that leads to coronary heart disease, stroke, and other diseases (1,2).

High Density Lipoproteins (HDL) are dense because they are made up of a large proportion of protein. They also contain a high proportion of cholesterol; however, HDL transport cholesterol in the opposite

direction from LDL. HDL remove cholesterol from peripheral tissues and return it to the liver for possible degradation. This function is beneficial to the prevention of atherosclerosis and coronary heart disease, so HDL are often referred to as "good" cholesterol (3).

Dietary Guidelines for Lipid Consumption

Americans consume about 40 percent of their Calories from lipid sources, an increase of nine percent since the early 1900s. The fact is that many of the foods that Americans love are high in fat, but many favorite recipes can be modified to comply with the dietary guidelines for lipid consumption without much change in taste. This section will consider the current recommendations for lipid consumption as well as foods to add to your diet and foods to avoid.

Recommended Lipid Intake

The lipid-consumption pattern of Americans is unhealthy and has been related to heart disease, some cancers, diabetes, and obesity. Not only do Americans eat too much fat (40 percent of their Calories), but they also eat the wrong types of fat (4). Currently 15 to 20 percent of their total Calories are from saturated fats, whereas many healthy populations in other countries consume less than seven percent of their Calories from these fats. Monounsaturated fats contribute 15 to 20 percent of the Calories in the American diet, and polyunsaturated fats contribute five to seven percent of the total. Along with high fat intake is an average dietary cholesterol consumption of 600 mg per day.

Recommendations for healthy lipid intakes are based mainly on the relationship between dietary lipids and blood-cholesterol levels. Elevated blood cholesterol is one of the three primary risk factors for coronary heart disease. Saturated fats and dietary cholesterol are associated with higher blood-cholesterol levels. Polyunsaturated fats, monounsaturated fats, and **omega-3-fatty acids** (found in fish oils) are associated with lower blood-cholesterol levels. Note that excess consumption of the latter three is not recommended because PUFA consumption may be related to some cancers, and evidence of safety for the others is not conclusive.

The Nutrition Committee of the American Heart Association has set forth the following dietary guidelines for the consumption of lipids (4) (see figure 6.6).

1. Total fat intake should be less than 30 percent of the total Calories.
2. Saturated fat intake should be less than ten percent of the total Calories.
3. Polyunsaturated fat intake should be no more than ten percent of the total Calories.
4. Dietary cholesterol intake should be less than 100 mg/1,000 Calories, not to exceed 300 mg/day.

FIGURE 6.6

Percent of kilocalories from fat in the U.S. diet.

TABLE 6.1

Major sources of fat in the U.S. diet

Top Five Foods That Provide Fat	Percentage of Calories as Fat
Burgers, meatloaf	63
Hot dogs, ham, lunch meats	58
Whole milk, whole-milk beverages	54
Doughnuts, cakes, cookies	54
Beef steaks, roasts	50

Data from U.S. Department of Agriculture, Human Nutrition Information Service, 1985.

Sources of Lipids in the Diet

The first step in improving lipid consumption is to know which foods are high or low in triglycerides, the main source of lipid. Table 6.1 shows the top five foods eaten in the United States that contribute the most fat to an average adult's diet. Three out of the five are meats. On a typical day, almost 30 percent of adults eat a hot dog, ham, or lunch meat; 26 percent consume meatloaf or a burger of some kind; and 23 percent have at least one serving of steak or roast beef (5).

Table 6.2 reveals the percentage of Calories from fat in various food choices. (See Health-Promotion Activity 6.1.) In general, whole fruits and vegetables have little or no fat, with avocados and olives being notable exceptions (containing about 80 percent of their Calories as fat). Red meats, whole-milk dairy products, and eggs contain considerable amounts of fat. Other sources of dietary fat are more obvious, for example, gravies, butter or margarine, salad dressings, mayonnaise, sour cream, creamed soups, and sauces.

TABLE 6.2
Dietary cholesterol and saturated fat in foods

Food	Amount	Percent Calories from Total Fat	Percent Calories from Saturated Fat	Cholesterol (milligrams)
Fruits		Low	Low	0
Vegetables		Low	Low	0
Grains		Low	Low	0
Nuts		High	Moderate	0
Avocado		88	17	0
Coconut, dried		88	76	0
Milk, nonfat	1 cup	—	—	5
Milk, low-fat	1 cup	30	17	22
Cottage cheese, 4% fat	½ cup	35	20	24
Cheese – pasteurized type	1 oz	73	40	25
Cream (half & half)	¼ cup	79	58	26
Ice cream, regular	½ cup	49	27	27
Cheese, cheddar	1 oz	72	40	28
Milk, whole	1 cup	48	27	34
Butter	1 tbsp	100	55	35
Margarine	1 tbsp	100	18	0
Tuna, canned	3 oz	38	10	55
Chicken, cooked	3 oz	19	6	74
Pork, cooked	3 oz	73	26	76
Beef, cooked	3 oz	77	37	80
Lamb, cooked	3 oz	61	34	83
Egg yolk	One	71	43	250
Liver, fried	2 oz	43	13	250

Source: U.S. Department of Agriculture, *Nutritive Value of Foods*, Handbook No. 456.

Saturated Fat
The American Heart Association recommends a 30 to 50 percent reduction in the amount of saturated-fat Calories that Americans currently eat. This will take considerable effort. A person who now eats 2,200 Calories per day would have to consume no more than 220 Calories, or 25 grams, as saturated fat. Table 6.3 shows the number of grams of saturated fat in some commonly eaten foods.

Most foods that contain fat have a combination of saturated and unsaturated fats. Some general rules apply for pinpointing foods that are made up of more saturated than unsaturated fats. Saturated fats are usually solid at room temperature. For example, think about the fat surrounding a piece of steak; it doesn't melt at room temperature. Some saturated fats are surrounded by watery mediums, and this particular property is not obvious; whole milk, for instance.

Saturated fats tend to raise blood-cholesterol levels. Foods high in saturated fats include beef, pork, lamb, whole-milk products and butter, many solid and hydrogenated (saturated) vegetable shortenings, coconut, and coconut and palm oils (often used in commercial baked goods).

Polyunsaturated Fat
Although polyunsaturated fats are associated with lower blood-cholesterol levels, the American Heart Association guidelines recommend a maximum consumption of ten percent of the total Calories. This caution is necessary because overconsumption of polyunsaturates may be related to other diseases, like cancers (6).

Polyunsaturated fats are usually liquid at room temperature like most of the plant oils. Both coconut and palm oils are highly saturated and are exceptions to the rule. They are often used in food processing because of their flavor and low cost. (Figure 6.2 lists sources of polyunsaturated fats.)

TABLE 6.3
Amounts of total fat, saturated fat, and dietary cholesterol in foods

Dairy Products	Total Fat (grams)	Saturated Fat (grams)	Cholesterol (milligrams)	Dairy Products	Total Fat (grams)	Saturated Fat (grams)	Cholesterol (milligrams)
Milk, Yogurt, and Cheese				*Cream and Coffee Creamers*			
Milk, whole, 1 cup	8.1	5.1	33	Sour cream, 1 tbsp	2.5	1.6	5
Milk, 2% fat, with nonfat milk solids, 1 cup	4.7	2.9	18	Cream, half-and-half, 1 tbsp	1.⁻	1.1	6
Milk, 1% fat, with nonfat milk solids, 1 cup	2.4	1.5	10	Coffee creamer with coconut or palm oil, dry powder, 1 tsp	—	.6	0
Skim milk with nonfat milk solids, 1 cup	.6	.4	5	*Desserts*			
				Vanilla ice cream, ½ cup	⁻.2	4.4	30
Cottage cheese, creamed, ½ cup	5.2	3.3	17	Vanilla ice milk, ½ cup	2.8	1.8	9
Natural cheddar cheese, 1 oz	9.4	6.0	30	Frozen yogurt, ½ cup	1.5	1.0	6
Mozzarella cheese, part skim milk, 1 oz	4.5	2.9	16	Orange sherbet, ½ cup	1.9	1.2	7

Meat, Poultry, Fish, Beans, and Eggs	Total Fat (grams)	Saturated Fat (grams)	Cholesterol (milligrams)	Meat, Poultry, Fish, Beans, and Eggs	Total Fat (grams)	Saturated Fat (grams)	Cholesterol (milligrams)
Beef rib roast, choice grade, roasted, 2 oz				*Light meat without skin*	2.6	.7	48
Lean and fat	18.4	7.8	48	*Dark meat with skin*	9.0	2.5	52
Lean only	8.1	3.5	46	*Dark meat without skin*	5.6	1.5	53
Beef rump, choice grade, roasted, 2 oz				Turkey, roasted, without skin, 2 oz			
Lean and fat	8.9	3.5	47	*Light meat*	1.8	.6	39
Lean only	4.4	1.6	46	*Dark meat*	4.1	1.4	48
Ground-beef patty, cooked, 2 oz				Halibut fillets, broiled, 2 oz	.8	.1	35
Regular	11.7	4.6	51	Tuna, canned, oil pack, drained, 2 oz	4.6	1.2	37
Lean	10.5	4.1	49				
Extra lean	9.3	3.6	48	Great northern or navy beans, cooked, ½ cup	.4	.1	0
Pork loin, lean, roasted, 2 oz							
Lean and fat	13.8	5.0	51	Canned beans without pork, ½ cup	.6	.2	0
Lean only	7.9	2.7	51				
Liver, beef, cooked with fat added, 2 oz	4.5	1.6	273	Egg, large, 1			
				Whole	5.6	1.7	274
Chicken, roasted, 2 oz				*Yolk*	5.6	1.7	274
Light meat with skin	6.2	1.7	48	*White*	Trace	0	0

Fats and Oils	Total Fat (grams)	Saturated Fat (grams)	Cholesterol (milligrams)	Fats and Oils	Total Fat (grams)	Saturated Fat (grams)	Cholesterol (milligrams)
Animal Fats, 1 tbsp				Margarine			
Butter	11.5	7.2	31	Hard (stick)	11.4	2.1	0
Vegetable Oils, 1 tbsp				Soft (tub)	11.4	1.8	0
Corn	13.6	1.7	0	Vegetable shortening, hydrogenated	12.8	3.9	0
Peanut	13.5	2.3	0	Salad Dressings, 1 tbsp			
Safflower	13.6	1.2	0	Mayonnaise	11.0	1.6	8
Soybean	13.6	2.0	0	Italian	7.1	1.0	0
Olive	13.5	1.8	0	Blue cheese	8.0	1.5	3
Coconut	13.6	11.8	0	French	6.4	1.5	0
Palm	13.6	6.7	0	Thousand Island	5.6	.9	4

Selected Snacks	Total Fat (grams)	Saturated Fat (grams)	Cholesterol (milligrams)	Selected Snacks	Total Fat (grams)	Saturated Fat (grams)	Cholesterol (milligrams)
Cracker and Chip Types				Peanuts, dry-roasted, salted, ¼ cup	17.6	3.1	0
Potato chips, 10	8.0	2.0	0	Peanut butter, 2 tbsp	15.3	2.8	0
French fries, salted, 10 long strips	10.3	2.6	0	Sunflower seeds, roasted, salted, ¼ cup	16.8	3.2	0
Corn chips, ½ cup	6.1	1.3	0	Dessert Type			
Popcorn, plain, 1 cup	.3	Trace	0	Chocolate chip cookies, 2	4.4	1.3	8
Popcorn, salted and buttered, 1 cup	2.0	.9	4	Frosted brownie, 1	6.6	2.2	12
Butter crackers, 4	2.3	.8	0	Gingersnaps, 2	1.2	.3	5
Saltine crackers, 4	1.4	.3	0	Sandwich-type cookies, chocolate or vanilla, 2	4.5	1.2	8
Whole-wheat crackers, 4	2.2	.5	0	Chocolate-frosted cupcake, 1	4.5	1.8	17
Pretzels, salted, 10 thin sticks	.1	Trace	0	Doughnut, raised, 1	11.2	2.8	10
Nuts and Seeds							
Peanuts, roasted, salted, ¼ cup	17.9	3.9	0				

One ounce = approximately 28 grams.

From *Food 3*, published by the American Dietetic Association based on material developed by the U.S. Department of Agriculture, 1982.

One group of polyunsaturated fats is experiencing considerable publicity recently. The omega-3-fatty acids, which are commonly found in fish oils, are apparently beneficial in reducing blood pressure and blood cholesterol (7). The omega-3-fatty acids promote the production of one type of **prostaglandin,** a hormonelike substance that seems to play a regulatory role for blood pressure and blood-cholesterol levels in the body. Fatty fish (herring, mackerel, salmon, lake trout, tuna, and whitefish) are the best natural sources of the omega-3-fatty acids.

Consumers should not purchase supplements containing fish oils or omega-3-fatty acids. Such extracts are expensive, have not been proven effective, and have not been tested for safety. Incorporating fish meals into weekly menus would be a better strategy for increasing omega-3-fatty acids in the diet.

TABLE 6.4
Polyunsaturated/saturated fat ratios of foods

Food	P/S Ratio	
Walnuts	10.3	Excellent
Sunflower seeds	6.3	
Margarine (safflower, soft)	5.3	
Vegetable oil (corn)	4.6	
Wheat germ	3.5	
Pumpkin seeds	2.4	Good
Peanut butter	1.8	
Hard stick margarine	1.6	
Brazil nuts	1.5	
Vegetable shortening	1.0	
Turkey	.9	Fair
Cashews	.9	
Olive oil	.6	
Ham	.5	Poor
Pork	.4	
Lard	.3	
Beef gravy	.08	
Cream	.06	
Whole milk	.06	
Cheddar cheese	.04	
Parmesan cheese	.03	

From *Fatty Acids in Food Fats.* Home Economics Research Report No. 7. U.S. Department of Agriculture.

Polyunsaturated/Saturated-Fat Ratio

The polyunsaturated to saturated fat ratio (p/s) can be used to determine what type of fat a particular product contains. Favorable ratios are greater than or equal to one (see table 6.4). Many food product labels today list the breakdown of fats, and p/s ratios can therefore be calculated. For example, meat, margarine, salad dressing, and mayonnaise may contain such a listing. (Appendix B also provides this information for some products.)

Another way to find out about the type of fat in a product is to read the ingredient list. For instance, on a margarine label, the first fat listed should be a liquid oil.

Hydrogenated Fat

Polyunsaturated liquid oil is often changed into a saturated fat by a process known as **hydrogenation.** The double bonds that characterize a polyunsaturated fat are broken by adding hydrogen atoms, thus creating a saturated fat. The body is not able to tell the difference between a hydrogenated fat and a saturated fat. Hydrogenated fats have the same detrimental effects on blood cholesterol as do saturated fats. Margarine, vegetable shortening, and processed foods are the major sources of hydrogenated fats in our diet.

One reason the food industry changes an unsaturated fat to a saturated fat is, for example, to make margarine spreadable (it would otherwise be liquid). The hydrogenated fat allows margarine to be more solid at room temperature. This property may at times be beneficial for the texture of baked or cooked products.

Why use margarine instead of butter if the hydrogenated fat in the margarine is really saturated? Margarine is made up of both hydrogenated and polyunsaturated fat. To make the best choice in margarine, the one lowest in saturated and hydrogenated fats, determine whether the p/s is greater than one. (Hydrogenated fats are included with the saturated fat grams in a product.) Also, check the ingredient list on the product for the terms hydrogenated or partially hydrogenated corn, soybean, or another oil (see figure 6.7). If the liquid oil is listed before the hydrogenated oil, the food probably has a p/s that is greater than one.

Monounsaturated Fat

The American Heart Association recommendations do not limit the percentage of Calories that are derived from monounsaturated fatty acids (MUFA) above the 30 percent total fat limitation. This is based on recent research that has shown that MUFA lower total and LDL cholesterol but not HDL. This research is consistent with evidence that MUFA are safe and effective in lowering heart disease risk in Mediterranean countries (8). (Figure 6.2 lists sources of monounsaturated fats in foods.)

Cholesterol

A major function of cholesterol in the body is to become part of bile. Because the role of bile is to help absorb fats from the intestine, it is found only in animals. (Plants do not eat fat or need to absorb it.) Animal products such as meat, milk, cheese, eggs, and anything that is made from these sources contain cholesterol.

A food can contain mostly saturated fat but no cholesterol. For instance, coconut oil and hydrogenated vegetable oil (two saturated fats) are from plant sources and therefore contain no cholesterol. It is important to know that a "cholesterol-free" food may contain saturated fats that contribute to higher blood-cholesterol levels.

FIGURE 6.7

Although this margarine contains hydrogenated soybean oil, which is equivalent to saturated fat, it would be a good choice. Note that the first ingredient is liquid soybean oil and the polyunsaturated to saturated fat ratio is 3/2, or 1.5.

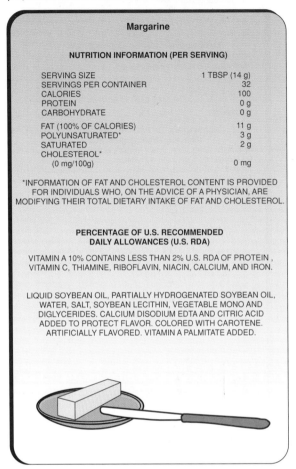

Margarine

NUTRITION INFORMATION (PER SERVING)

SERVING SIZE	1 TBSP (14 g)
SERVINGS PER CONTAINER	32
CALORIES	100
PROTEIN	0 g
CARBOHYDRATE	0 g
FAT (100% OF CALORIES)	11 g
POLYUNSATURATED*	3 g
SATURATED	2 g
CHOLESTEROL*	
(0 mg/100g)	0 mg

*INFORMATION OF FAT AND CHOLESTEROL CONTENT IS PROVIDED FOR INDIVIDUALS WHO, ON THE ADVICE OF A PHYSICIAN, ARE MODIFYING THEIR TOTAL DIETARY INTAKE OF FAT AND CHOLESTEROL.

PERCENTAGE OF U.S. RECOMMENDED
DAILY ALLOWANCES (U.S. RDA)

VITAMIN A 10% CONTAINS LESS THAN 2% U.S. RDA OF PROTEIN , VITAMIN C, THIAMINE, RIBOFLAVIN, NIACIN, CALCIUM, AND IRON.

LIQUID SOYBEAN OIL, PARTIALLY HYDROGENATED SOYBEAN OIL, WATER, SALT, SOYBEAN LECITHIN, VEGETABLE MONO AND DIGLYCERIDES. CALCIUM DISODIUM EDTA AND CITRIC ACID ADDED TO PROTECT FLAVOR. COLORED WITH CAROTENE. ARTIFICIALLY FLAVORED. VITAMIN A PALMITATE ADDED.

Refer to table 6.2. Note that most meats have the same amount of dietary cholesterol per three-ounce portion even though they differ in fat content. Eggs, liver, organ meats, and shellfish are high in dietary cholesterol. Fruits, nuts, and vegetables have no dietary cholesterol.

Achieving the Dietary Guidelines

Each person must devise his or her own plan for achieving the dietary guidelines. Foods that contain visible fats, or the ones that you can see, are often the easiest to change first. These include gravies, sour cream, sauces, salad dressings, margarine, and the fat around meat. Surprisingly though, as much as 60 percent of the fat that Americans eat is invisible fat and can go unnoticed. The fat inside of meat (known as marbling), ice cream, cheese, baked goods, and

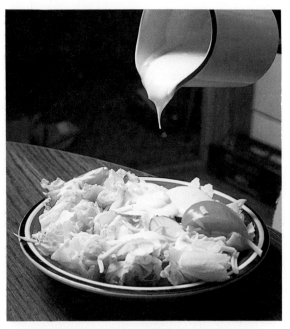

Visible fats like salad dressing are obvious targets for change in achieving lower fat and cholesterol recommendations.

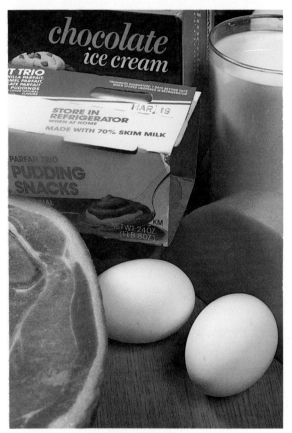

Many foods contain a large proportion of invisible fat kilocalories.

casseroles are in this category. Both visible and invisible sources of fat need to be examined when developing a plan to reduce fat intake.

The following are practical suggestions for cutting down on visible and invisible fats and dietary cholesterol.

Foods to Eat More Often

1. *Fish and Poultry (without the skin).* They're low in saturated fat, so try substituting them more often for beef, lamb, or pork.
2. *Lean Cuts of Meat.* When you do eat red meat, choose lean cuts and trim visible fat.
3. *Fruits, Nuts, and Raw Vegetables (except coconut and avocado).* Try them as refreshing and convenient snacks.
4. *Skim Milk or Low-Fat Dairy Products.* Skim milk or low-fat milk and low-fat cheese offer a triple treat—less saturated fats, dietary cholesterol, and Calories.
5. *Grains and Starchy Foods.* These will help stretch your meat budget and give you important vitamins, minerals, and fiber.
6. *Liquid Vegetable Oils and Margarines High in Polyunsaturated or Monounsaturated Fats.* Go easy on all fats, but when you do use them, substitute these fats because they help to lower blood cholesterol.

Foods to Eat Less Often

7. *Fatty Luncheon and Variety Meats and Organ Meats.* Sausage, bacon, salami, bologna, liver, and kidney are high in fat and dietary cholesterol.
8. *Egg Yolks.* People who are concerned about cholesterol should eat fewer egg yolks, which are particularly high in dietary cholesterol.
9. *Butter.* When you do have to use fat, try a margarine that is high in polyunsaturated and/or monounsaturated fat instead.

Foods to Beware Of

10. *Processed and Convenience Foods.* Read the labels on foods, and don't assume that "cholesterol free" means "good for you." Many products with no dietary cholesterol are filled with saturated fat. Remember that coconut and palm oils are saturated fats that are used in many processed foods. The terms "light," "lean," or "lower fat" may also be misleading. Interpret the label for fat content (see figure 6.8).

*F*IGURE 6.8

Interpreting labels for fat content. Cream cheese offers a high percentage of its kilocalories as fat. Calculate the fat percentage of another product from your own kitchen.

Cream cheese

NUTRITION INFORMATION PER PORTION

PORTION SIZE...2 TBSP. (28 g)
PORTIONS PER CONTAINER...8
CALORIES...100
PROTEIN...2 GRAMS
CARBOHYDRATE...2 GRAMS
FAT...10 GRAMS
SODIUM...100 mg

PERCENTAGE OF U.S. RECOMMENDED DAILY ALLOWANCES (U.S. RDA)

PROTEIN	4	RIBOFLAVIN	2
VITAMIN A	4	NIACIN	*
VITAMIN C	*	CALCIUM	2
THIAMINE	*	IRON	*

CONTAINS LESS THAN 2% OF THE U.S. RDA OF THESE NUTRIENTS.

INGREDIENTS: MILK, CREAM, CHEESE CULTURE, SALT AND VEGETABLE GUM.

KEEP REFRIGERATED

Grams of fat = 10 grams/2 TBSP of cream cheese

Percent of Kilocalories as fat

$$= \frac{10 \text{ grams of fat} \times 9 \text{ Kcal/gm of fat}}{2 \text{ TBSP cream cheese}}$$

100 Kcal per 2 TBSP of cream cheese

$$= \frac{90 \text{ Kcal of fat/2 TBSP of cream cheese}}{100 \text{ Kcal per 2 TBSP of cream cheese}}$$

= 90% of the Kilocalories are from fat

11. *Fast Foods.* Avoid deep-fried foods. Appendix B lists fast-food selections and the amount of fat in each.

Ways to Prepare Food

12. *Broiling, Boiling, Roasting, and Stewing.* These cooking methods help remove fat from food.

Incorporating these suggestions into your diet may be difficult at first. Table 6.5 provides some helpful tips. (See Health-Promotion Activity 6.2.)

1. Make changes gradually. You may try changing the way you eat one meal at a time. For instance, just work on making breakfast a low-fat meal. Or you might try changing one type of food at a time, such as substituting low-fat milk for whole milk. The goal is to make permanent changes that you can live with throughout life.
2. Yes, you do have choices. Having only one ounce of cheese rather than four may satisfy your craving but still keep you within a reasonable saturated-fat level for the day. Having cereal with low-fat milk and a banana for breakfast may allow you to save some saturated-fat Calories for the evening meal.
3. Plan to succeed. Evaluate your weekly activities and budget your Calorie expenditures throughout each day and week. If you plan to attend a birthday party on Friday night, for example, have light desserts and no red meats on Thursday.
4. Eat a balanced diet each day. It is not necessary (or desirable) to eliminate any food groups when planning a healthy diet. Include wise choices from each of the four food groups each day; then extras can be planned for if desired.
5. If you need help, a dietitian or nutritionist can analyze your diet and help you to work out a personal plan. Agencies like the American Heart Association have cookbooks, pamphlets, and other free materials to help you.
6. Be honest. You may fool yourself (``Just this once won't hurt''), but you can't fool your blood-cholesterol level. Establish a goal of having a blood-cholesterol level of less than 200 mg/dL, and achieve it. New eating patterns are for life.

Artificial Fats

The development of two new artificial fats may help some individuals reduce their total fat consumption. **Olestra** is a Calorie-free fat replacement that was formerly known as sucrose polyester. Although Olestra is a synthetic combination of sucrose and fatty acids, it is not digestible. Olestra passes through the digestive tract unabsorbed but will interfere with the absorption of dietary cholesterol and cholesterol that is being recycled from bile. This results in a reduction in blood cholesterol.

Olestra looks, feels, and tastes like dietary fat and has some similar cooking properties. It can be used in oils, margarine, snacks, and desserts. Current research suggests that Olestra is safe, with only one undesirable effect—it interferes with the absorption of vitamin E. Vitamin E may be fortified in products that contain Olestra. The FDA is currently reviewing this product.

The second fat substitute that the FDA is reviewing is **Simplesse.** This product is manufactured from the protein of egg white or milk. In a manufacturing process the protein is altered into tiny round particles that feel creamy on the tongue. Simplesse provides one and one-third Calories per gram, a substantial reduction from the nine Calories per gram offered by fat. If approved, Simplesse will be available only to manufacturers and used in products such as ice cream, yogurt, sour cream, and oil-based products. Since Simplesse gels when heated, it is unsuitable for products that are heated or baked.

Food researchers are attempting to meet the demand for low-Calorie, good-tasting foods that will not elevate disease risk factors. Perhaps fat substitutes will someday be as commonplace as artificial sweeteners.

Lipids for Health Promotion

Although a few people may still suffer the consequences of having too little lipid in their diets, the majority of Americans must work to reduce their lipid consumption.

Insufficient Lipid Consumption

Insufficient lipid consumption (less than three percent of the total Caloric intake) most often occurs in infants who are fed low-fat or nonfat milk or formulas made from these. Overzealous parents may also try to restrict the lipid consumption of an infant or toddler under the age of two for health benefits. Parents need to be cautioned that limitations in lipids are not meant for individuals under the age of two years. As was discussed in the section on function of lipids, essential fatty acids are needed in the diet. This is particularly important for growth stages. If a child does not get enough of the essential fatty acids, his or her growth will be impaired. Older children and adults may only experience rough and scaly skin.

Excess Lipid Consumption

Four major threats to the health of Americans are associated with excess lipid consumption.

Obesity

There is good reason to believe that much of the obesity today is in part due to Calorie-rich foods that are high in fat. Both animal and human research studies provide evidence to support this theory.

The most commonly used means of inducing obesity in laboratory rats is feeding them a high-fat diet (9). Lean human subjects had difficulty gaining weight on a mixed diet but gained weight easily on a high-fat diet. Research also shows that it costs the body less energy to store dietary fat as body fat (three percent of ingested Calories) than to store carbohydrate as body fat (23 percent of ingested Calories) (10).

Calories from any source can create obesity, but many researchers suggest that a high-carbohydrate, low-fat diet will help individuals remain lean or lose excess fat (11,12). See chapter 9 for a discussion on obesity and how to achieve and maintain reasonable weight.

Cardiovascular Disease

Cardiovascular disease is a group of heart and blood-vessel diseases that include heart attack, stroke, high blood pressure, and atherosclerosis. They are responsible for one of every two deaths in the United States. A major risk factor for all four of these dieases is high blood-cholesterol levels (13). The consumption of total fat, saturated fat, and dietary cholesterol are associated with elevations in blood cholesterol. Most of the guidelines on lipid consumption are influenced by this strong association. The Health-Promotion Insight at the end of the chapter will provide more detail on these diseases and on reducing blood-cholesterol levels.

Diabetes

Individuals with diabetes have twice the risk of developing cardiovascular disease that those without the disease have. Therefore, a diet low in total fat, saturated fat, and cholesterol that is consistent with the American Heart Association guidelines discussed in this chapter is recommended for individuals with diabetes. In addition, by restricting fatty foods, individuals are better able to decrease their body weight. When many individuals with diabetes lose weight, their metabolic disorder returns to normal (14). The Health-Promotion Insight on diabetes at the end of chapter 5 provides more detail on this disease.

Cancer

Dietary fat is also associated with the second leading cause of death in the U.S.—cancer. A diet high in total fat may be a factor in the development of breast, colon, rectal, uterine, and prostate cancer (6). Chapter 10 provides more information on preventing cancer through diet.

HEALTH-PROMOTION INSIGHT
Cardiovascular Disease

According to the American Heart Association statistics, more than 63 million people (nearly one in four Americans) have one or more forms of heart or blood-vessel disease, including heart disease, high blood pressure, and stroke (13). These diseases are not only debilitating but deadly. Almost half of Americans die of cardiovascular disease. This creates a severe economic burden, estimated at $85.2 billion. Although there has been a drop in deaths from cardiovascular disease since 1968, each of us still has a 50 percent chance of developing some form of cardiovascular disease in our lifetime. Premature heart disease, before the age of 65, has remarkable potential for prevention.

Atherosclerosis

The single biggest cause of heart and blood-vessel disease is atherosclerosis, or "hardening of the arteries." Atherosclerosis is characterized by **plaque** formation on the inner walls of arteries (see figure 6.9). One commonly accepted theory of plaque formation suggests that there is a minor injury to the lining of a blood vessel. Lipid material is deposited at the injured spot and covered by **platelets,** the clotting mechanism of the blood. The blood vessel in turn produces more cells to cover over this area. As the process continues, hardening or calcification occurs. This newly formed material is called plaque.

Figure 6.9

Progressive atherosclerosis buildup on artery walls.

Normal artery

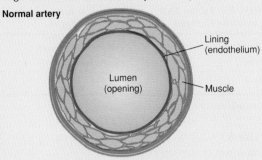

Lining (endothelium)

Lumen (opening)

Muscle

Early injury

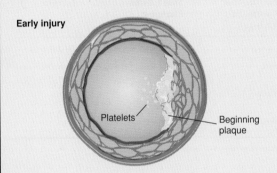

Platelets

Beginning plaque

Atherosclerosis

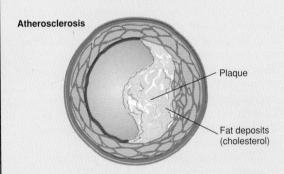

Plaque

Fat deposits (cholesterol)

Arteries undergoing plaque formation soon lose their ability to expand and contract, and their diameter also narrows, making blood flow more difficult.

There are three possible consequences to the continued plaque formation. The first is a narrowing of the artery to the point that a total blockage occurs. Any tissue beyond that point would lose its oxygen and nutrient supply. The tissue would quickly die, and if it were a large organ or one important enough to the functioning of the body, the person may die. Otherwise, varying degrees of functioning may be impaired.

Another consequence is that a blood clot could form on top of the plaque. This itself may occlude or block an artery and is known as a **thrombus.** A thrombus may break loose into the bloodstream, then referred to as an **embolus,** and can lodge in a smaller artery. This results in a sudden loss of blood to the area the artery previously supplied.

Any area of the body could be effected by atherosclerosis, but two of particular concern are the heart and brain. Interruption of blood flow to the brain results in a **cerebrovascular accident,** or stroke. In the heart, **myocardial infarction,** or a heart attack, occurs if blood flow through the coronary arteries that supply the heart muscle is blocked (see figure 6.10).

The Roots of Atherosclerosis

Many people mistakenly believe that heart disease develops in old age. Autopsy data from the Korean and Vietnam wars have indicated that even men under the age of 20 have varying degrees of plaque in their arteries (15). Atherosclerosis actually begins at puberty and continues throughout life. Heredity and life-style contribute to the rate at which atherosclerosis develops.

The optimal time for intervention in the atherosclerotic process appears to be shortly after birth, with most prevention strategies acceptable by age two. Life-style factors that increase the accumulation of plaque should be avoided or be modified early to slow the disease process.

Risk Factors

Risk factors are characteristics associated with the greater likelihood of developing a specific health problem. They are usually discovered through animal or epidemiological (population) research studies. They are not necessarily causative.

Extensive clinical and statistical studies have identified several risk factors for cardiovascular disease. Table 6.6 lists the risk factors for stroke, and table 6.7 lists those for heart disease. Some of the risk factors cannot be changed, such as heredity, sex, race, or age. The three primary risk factors for heart disease are changeable: cigarette smoking, high blood pressure, and high blood-cholesterol levels.

*F*IGURE 6.10

Atherosclerosis in the coronary arteries, which supply blood to the heart, can lead to total blockage. A heart attack or myocardial infarction may result.

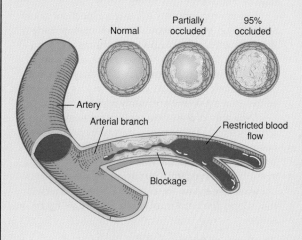

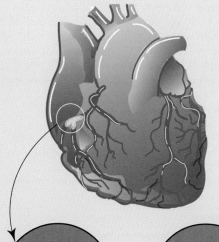

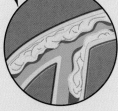

Narrowed
coronary artery

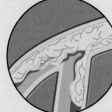

Blocked
coronary artery

Table 6.6
Risk factors of stroke

Major Risk Factors That Cannot Be Changed	Major Risk Factors That Can Be Changed
Heredity	High blood pressure
Sex	Heart disease
Race	Diabetes mellitus

From *Heart Facts*, 1987. American Heart Association.

Table 6.7
Risk factors of coronary heart disease

Major Risk Factors That Cannot Be Changed	Major Risk Factors That Can Be Changed	Contributing Factors
Heredity	Cigarette smoking	Obesity
Sex	High blood pressure	Lack of exercise
Race	High blood cholesterol	Stress
Age	Diabetes	

From *Heart Facts*, 1987. American Heart Association.

Cigarette Smoking

The recent Surgeon General's report on the cardiovascular disease consequences of smoking has stated: "Cigarette smoking should be considered the most important of the known modifiable risk factors for coronary heart disease in the United States" (16). This report estimates that smokers (average one pack per day) have a 70 percent greater coronary heart disease (CHD) death rate than nonsmokers. Heavy smokers who consume more than two packs per day experience death rates from CHD more than 200 times that of nonsmokers.

The lighted cigarette generates about two thousand compounds; of these, carbon monoxide, tar, and nicotine are judged as most likely to contribute to the health hazards of smoking. Carbon monoxide, tar, and nicotine might produce irregular rhythms to occur in the heart rate, increase the clumping of platelets, and decrease blood-vessel-wall oxygen supply, thus increasing the coronary arteries' permeability to cholesterol (17). Cigarette smoking also decreases the important HDL cholesterol (18).

A person who stops smoking reduces his or her CHD death risk to that of nonsmokers within approximately fifteen years.

High Blood Pressure

In most Western societies, average blood pressure increases with age. In a few tribal communities there is little change in blood pressure with age (19). From these studies and migration studies showing that life-style and environment are important determinants of blood pressure, various strategies for preventing hypertension have been developed.

Weight reduction provides a powerful means of reducing high blood pressure (20). This occurs even if ideal weight is not achieved. The mechanisms involved in the development of hypertension in overweight persons are not yet fully clarified.

Salt restriction is another method of decreasing high blood pressure. The average American consumes 7.5 to 10 grams of salt per day, which is about double the recommended intake (21). Controlled intervention studies with hypertensives have provided better evidence that changing salt consumption usually results in a decrease in blood pressure (22,23). As a result of these studies and others, the Joint National Committee on Detection, Evaluation, and Treatment of High Blood Pressure has recommended that even moderate dietary salt restriction of 5 grams per day may reduce elevated blood pressure.

A major study recently demonstrated that a combination of weight loss and salt restriction allowed 39 percent of hypertensive individuals to be reclassified as normotensive (22).

Several other life-style factors have been associated with a decrease in high blood pressure, including high calcium and magnesium intake, a high polyunsaturated/saturated-fat ratio, high potassium, high dietary fiber, and aerobic exercise (24). (See the Health-Promotion Insight in chapter 11.)

High Blood-Cholesterol Levels

The third primary risk factor for coronary heart disease is high blood-cholesterol level. Although many studies have suggested that lowering blood cholesterol in individuals would produce a reduction in cardiovascular disease, they have not been conclusive (25,26). Recently, a $150 million, 12-year study by the National Heart, Lung, and Blood Institute provided the first truly solid evidence that the reduction of blood cholesterol leads to a decrease in heart disease (27). This research concluded that a 49 percent drop in coronary heart disease incidence can be predicted for individuals who reduce their blood-cholesterol levels by 25 percent.

Blood Cholesterol Measurement. Blood-cholesterol level is determined by analyzing a small sample of blood. A typical blood test will usually include a measurement of blood cholesterol. The average blood-cholesterol level for middle-aged adults is 215 mg/dL (29). This means that there are 215 mg of cholesterol in every one-tenth liter of blood. An optimal level of total blood cholesterol is 160 mg/dL, with 190 mg/dL being an attainable level for most Americans, according to the Heart, Lung, and Blood Institute (30).

If your physician tells you that your total blood cholesterol is "normal," make sure that he or she does not mean "average." In America, it does not pay to be average when it comes to blood cholesterol — one in every five Americans has a high blood-cholesterol level (see figure 6.11).

A more sophisticated report will include measurements of LDL and HDL cholesterol. The ratio of LDL cholesterol to HDL cholesterol (LDL-C/HDL-C) has been found to be highly predictive of heart disease risk, more so than total blood cholesterol alone (3). When LDL is not available, the total blood cholesterol to HDL cholesterol ratio can be used. Individuals with a LDL-C/HDL-C of 1.0 or a total blood cholesterol/HDL-C of 3.4 have about one-half the heart-disease risk of the average American (see figure 6.12).

If you do not currently know your blood-cholesterol level but have had a blood test recently, call your doctor to find out. Other alternatives are to request a blood test at your next visit or to take advantage of a local health fair that may be doing blood tests (see Health-Promotion Activity 6.2). Any questions that arise should be directed to a local health professional.

Lowering Total Blood Cholesterol/LDL Cholesterol. Factors that help to lower LDL cholesterol include (31,32,33):

1. Decrease dietary cholesterol
2. Decrease saturated fats
3. Increase P/S ratio
4. Increase MUFA
5. Decrease Calories from fat
6. Increase water-soluble fibers in the diet (mainly found in fruits, vegetables, grains, and legumes)
7. Weight reduction
8. Aerobic exercise

Figure 6.11

Understanding your blood cholesterol readings.

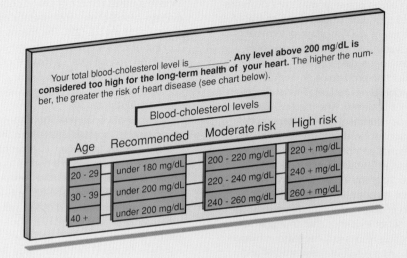

Your total blood-cholesterol level is_____. **Any level above 200 mg/dL is considered too high for the long-term health of your heart.** The higher the number, the greater the risk of heart disease (see chart below).

Blood-cholesterol levels

Age	Recommended	Moderate risk	High risk
20 - 29	under 180 mg/dL	200 - 220 mg/dL	220 + mg/dL
30 - 39	under 200 mg/dL	220 - 240 mg/dL	240 + mg/dL
40 +	under 200 mg/dL	240 - 260 mg/dL	260 + mg/dL

Figure 6.12

The risk of death from coronary heart disease increases as the ratio of total or LDL cholesterol to HDL cholesterol increases.

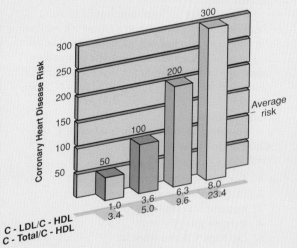

Raising HDL Cholesterol. High amounts of HDL cholesterol in the bloodstream are strongly associated with lower heart-disease risk (34). Several intervenable factors have been shown to increase HDL cholesterol (31,32,35):

1. Aerobic exercise
2. Cessation of smoking
3. Weight reduction

Tracking

Tracking of both blood pressure and cholesterol in individuals has shown interesting results. Those individuals who have high blood pressure and blood-cholesterol levels at a younger age are also most likely to rank high when they are older, even though everyone's blood pressure and blood cholesterol tends to increase with age (see figure 6.13).

Both high blood pressure and blood cholesterol are controllable and do not have to increase with age, because early detection and intervention are possible (36).

Multiple Risk Factors

Although each of the primary risk factors can independently increase the risk of CHD, many investigators believe that slightly high values in several of the risk factors better explains the incidence (new cases) of CHD. Table 6.8 illustrates that the dangers of heart attack increase with the number of risk factors present.

FIGURE 6.13

Although everyone's blood cholesterol level will increase with age, those who rank highest in blood cholesterol levels at younger ages will usually continue to rank highest as they age.

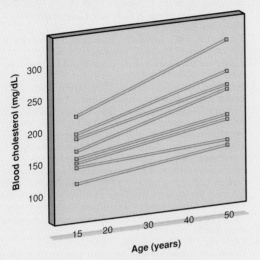

A person who has a total blood cholesterol of 235 mg/dL and a systolic blood pressure of 150 and who smokes half a pack of cigarettes per day may have as high a risk of CHD as someone who has only one risk factor — a person who smokes two and one-half packs of cigarettes per day.

Prevention

One of the first steps in decreasing the risk of CHD for our population is to assess the risk factors. Health-Promotion Activity 6.3 is a simplified scale that allows one to see if he or she is or will be at risk for

Table 6.8

The danger of a heart attack increases with the number of the three primary risk factors present.

Primary Risk Factors	Risk
None	77
Cigarette smoker	120
Cigarette smoker, high cholesterol level	236
Cigarette smoker, high cholesterol level, and high blood pressure	384

Note: The average American has a risk of 100. The person who is a cigarette smoker and has high cholesterol and high blood pressure has a risk of 384. This means that he or she is 3.84 times as likely to have a heart attack as the average American.

From The Framingham, Massachusetts, Heart Study.

a heart attack or stroke. Take the test to see if your life-style needs modification. Assess your smoking habits, and find out what your blood pressure and blood-cholesterol level are. Keep track of these as you age. Any changes in life-style, whether positive or negative, will also affect these values.

Once the risk factors have been assessed, take responsibility for the life-style factors that can change these values. Always consult your physician about a plan of action. A medical professional can recommend appropriate resources to help with specific risk factors and can help you monitor your progress.

Refer to the appropriate chapters in this text for help and suggestions on modifying the dietary habits that have been mentioned in this section.

SUMMARY

1. In this chapter the types and functions of lipids were discussed. Dietary recommendations for lipids were also presented, along with the methods to achieve such recommendations.
2. The three major classes of lipids are triglycerides, phospholipids, and sterols. Triglycerides make up 95 percent of the lipids found in foods.
3. Triglycerides are composed of a glycerol molecule with three fatty acids attached. Fatty acids can differ in the degree of saturation in their carbon chain. A saturated fatty acid has no double bonds between carbon atoms, whereas unsaturated fatty acids have one or more.
4. Lipids have six important functions in the body: energy, essential fatty acids, transport fat-soluble vitamins, structure, insulation, and protection.
5. Lipases break down triglycerides in the small intestine into glycerol and fatty acids for absorption. Bile helps in this process by emulsifying large droplets of fat into smaller droplets, increasing the surface area that lipases can act on.
6. The products of lipid digestion are incorporated into a micelle, a water-soluble package that delivers the contents into the body.
7. Chylomicrons are formed in the intestinal cells from the products of digestion, fatty acids, glycerol, cholesterol, and phospholipids. The chylomicron is responsible for the delivery of these lipids from the intestinal cell to body tissues.

8. Three major protein packets other than chylomicrons transport lipids in the body: very low density lipoproteins, low density lipoproteins, and high density lipoproteins. Low density lipoproteins are associated with increased atherosclerosis, while high density lipoproteins serve to decrease atherosclerosis.

9. The lipid consumption pattern of Americans is unhealthy and is related to heart disease, some cancers, diabetes, and obesity. We not only eat too much fat but also the wrong kinds of fat.

10. The American Heart Association has set forth four guidelines specifically directed at the consumption of lipids. They are: reduce total fat to less than 30 percent of total Calories; reduce saturated fat to less than 10 percent of total Calories; consume no more than 10 percent of polyunsaturated fat; and consume no more than 300 mg/day of dietary cholesterol.

11. Foods high in saturated fat include beef, pork, lamb, whole-milk products and butter, many solid and hydrogenated vegetable shortenings, and coconut and palm oils. Saturated fats are associated with elevated blood-cholesterol levels.

12. Foods high in polyunsaturated fats include most oils except coconut and palm, vegetables, legumes, nuts, and most margarines.

13. Hydrogenated fats are made when an unsaturated fat is processed into a saturated fat. The body can not distinguish hydrogenated fats from saturated fats. Vegetable shortenings and margarines contain different amounts of these fats.

14. Monounsaturated fats may be beneficial in lowering heart disease risk. Sources include olive oil, peanut oil, almonds, avocado, and haddock.

15. Dietary cholesterol can be found in all animal food sources, such as eggs, milk, cheese, meat, chicken, shellfish, and foods made from them.

16. Invisible fats contribute significantly more Calories to the American diet than do visible foods. Invisible fats are hidden in marbled meats, whole-milk products, baked goods, and casseroles.

17. In order to reduce lipid consumption, Americans must be aware of food selection and food preparation techniques.

18. Nearly one in every four Americans has one or more forms of cardiovascular disease that is not only debilitating but also deadly.

19. The single largest cause of cadiovascular disease is atherosclerosis, or "hardening of the arteries." Atherosclerosis is cumulative throughout life, *beginning at puberty.* Optimal time for prevention is two years of age, before life-style factors are ingrained. However, it is never too late.

20. The three primary risk factors for coronary heart disease include cigarette smoking, high blood pressure, and high blood cholesterol.

21. All Americans should know their blood cholesterol. Blood cholesterol levels can be changed. There are several intervenable factors to raise HDL cholesterol and to lower LDL cholesterol.

References

1. Simons, L. A., and J. C. Gibson. 1980. Plasma Lipids and Lipoproteins. In *Lipids: A Clinicians' Guide.* Baltimore: University Park Press.

2. Patsch, J. R. 1982. Metabolic Aspects of Subfractions of Lipoproteins. In *Metabolic Risk Factors in Ischemic Cardiovascular Disease.* L. A. Carlson and B. Panow, eds. New York: Raven Press.

3. American Health Foundation. 1980. *Plasma Lipids: Optimal Levels for Health.* New York: Academic Press.

4. American Heart Association. 1986. Dietary Guidelines for Healthy American Adults: A Statement for Physicians and Health Professionals by the Nutrition Committee, American Heart Association. Dallas: American Heart Association.

5. U.S. Department of Agriculture, Human Nutrition Information Service. 1985. Nationwide Food Consumption Survey, Continuing Survey of Food Intakes by Individuals: Women 19–50 Years and Their Children 1–5 Years, 1 Day, 1985. U.S. Department of Agriculture, Rept. 85–1. Men 19–50 Years, 1 Day, 1985. U.S. Department of Agriculture, Rept. 85–3.

6. Greenwald, P., and E. Sondik. 1986. Diet and Chemoprevention in NCI's Research Strategy to Achieve National Cancer Control Objectives. *Annual Review of Public Health* 7:267–91.

7. Hartog, J. M., et al. 1987. Comparison of Mackerel-Oil and Lard-Fat Enriched Diets on Plasma Lipids, Cardiac Membrane Phospholipids, Cardiovascular Performance, and Morphology in Young Pigs. *American Journal of Clinical Nutrition* 46:258–66.

8. Grundy, S. M. 1987. Monounsaturated Fatty Acids, Plasma Cholesterol, and Coronary Heart Disease. *American Journal of Clinical Nutrition* 45:1168–1175.

9. Sclafani, 1980. In *Obesity,* A. J. Stunkard, ed. Philadelphia: W. B. Saunders.

10. Danforth, E. 1985. Diet and Obesity. *American Journal of Clinical Nutrition* 41:1132–1145.

11. Bray, G. A. 1983. The Energetics of Obesity. *Medicine and Science in Sports and Exercise* 15:32–40.

12. Duncan, K. H., J. A. Bacon, and R. L. Weinsier. 1983. The Effects of High and Low Energy Density Diets on Satiety, Energy Intake, and Eating Time of Obese and Nonobese Subjects. *American Journal of Clinical Nutrition* 37:763–67.

13. American Heart Association. 1987 Heart Facts. Dallas: American Heart Association.

14. Consensus Development Conference on Diet and Exercise in Non-Insulin Dependent Diabetes Mellitus. 1987. *Dietetic Currents* 14 (4):17–20.

15. Enos, W. F., R. H. Holmes, and J. Beyer. 1953. Coronary Disease Among United States Soldiers Killed in Action in Korea. *Journal of the American Medical Association* 152:1090–1093.

16. U.S. Department of Health and Human Services. Office on Smoking and Health, Public Health Service. 1983. The Health Consequences of Smoking: Cardiovascular Disease. A Report of the Surgeon General. Washington, D.C.: U.S. Government Printing Office.

17. Murphy, G. P., and R. Sciandra. 1983. Helping Patients Withdraw from Smoking. *New York State Journal of Medicine* 83:1353–1360.

18. Benbassat, J., and P. Froom. 1986. Blood Pressure Response to Exercise as a Predictor of Hypertension. *Archives of Internal Medicine* 146:2053-2055.
19. World Health Organization Scientific Group. 1983. Primary Prevention of Essential Hypertension. Geneva: World Health Organization.
20. Wilber, J. A. 1982. The Role of Diet in the Treatment of High Blood Pressure. *American Dietetic Association Journal* 80:25-29.
21. Holbrook, J. T., et al. 1984. Sodium and Potassium Intake and Balance in Adults Consuming Self-Selected Diets. *American Journal of Clinical Nutrition* 40:786.
22. Stamler, R., et al. 1987. Nutritional Therapy for High Blood Pressure: Final Report of a Four-Year Randomized Controlled Trial — The Hypertension Control Program. *Journal of the American Medical Association* 257:1484-1491.
23. Miller, J. Z., et al. 1987. Heterogeneity of Blood Pressure Response to Dietary Sodium Restriction in Normotensive Adults. *Journal of Chronic Diseases* 40:245-50.
24. Kaplan, N. M. 1986. Dietary Aspects of the Treatment of Hypertension. *Annual Review of Public Health* 7:503-19.
25. Reports of Inter-Society Commission for Heart Disease Resources. 1984. Circulation 70:155A-205A.
26. Borhani, N. O. 1985. Prevention of Coronary Heart Disease in Practice: Implications of the Results of Recent Clinical Trials. *Journal of the American Medical Association* 254:257-62.
27. Lipid Research Clinics Program: The Lipid Research Clinics Coronary Primary Prevention Trial Results, I and II. 1984. 251:351-74.
28. Glatter, T. R. 1984. Hyperlipidemia. *Postgraduate Medicine* 76:49-59.
29. National Center for Health Statistics — National Heart, Lung, and Blood Institute Collaborative Lipid Group. 1987. Trends in Serum Cholesterol Levels Among U.S. Adults Ages 20-74 Years. *Journal of the American Medical Association* 257:937-42.
30. Consensus Conference. 1985. Lowering Blood Cholesterol to Prevent Heart Disease. *Journal of the American Medical Association* 253:2080-2086.
31. Reports of Inter-Society Commission for Heart Disease Resources. 1984. Circulation 70:155A-205A.
32. Nicoll, A., N. E. Miller, and B. Lewis. 1980. High-Density Lipoprotein Metabolism. *Advances in Lipid Research* 17:53-96.
33. Hartung, G. H. 1984. Diet and Exercise in the Regulation of Plasma Lipids and Lipoproteins in Patients at Risk of Coronary Disease. *Sports Medicine* 1:413-18.
34. Castelli, W. P., et al. 1986. Incidence of Coronary Heart Disease and Lipoprotein Cholesterol Levels: The Framingham Study. *Journal of the American Medical Association* 256:2835-2838.
35. Haskell, W. L. 1984. Exercise-Induced Changes in Plasma Lipids and Lipoproteins. *Preventive Medicine* 13:23-26.
36. Leon, A. S. 1987. Age and Other Predictors of Coronary Heart Disease. *Medicine and Science in Sports and Exercise* 19:159-67.

*H*EALTH-PROMOTION ACTIVITY 6.1
Lowering the Fat Content of Your Diet

Table 6.2 gives a general picture of the amounts of dietary cholesterol and saturated and total fat in some foods. Refer to this table in answering the following questions.

In general, which foods contain little or no dietary cholesterol?

Note that margarine contains no cholesterol, but 100 percent of its Calories are from fat. Although all of the Calories in margarine come from fat, just as in butter, there is considerable difference in the percentage of fat Calories that can be attributed to saturated fat in each. Margarine has only 18 percent saturated fat Calories, and butter has 55 percent.

In general, which foods listed have very little fat?

How many servings from low-fat groups have you had today?

Which foods have you eaten in the last two days that have greater than 50 percent of their Calories as total fat?

What adjustments could you make in your diet to eat lower fat foods?

Make a meal plan for all of tomorrow's meals and incorporate some of the low-fat selections.

HEALTH-PROMOTION ACTIVITY 6.2
Eating Out: Can You Still Cut Fat?

Fast Food Delights is a new restaurant that has opened near where you live. One of your friends insists that you meet at Fast Food Delights for lunch.

FAST FOOD DELIGHTS: Menu

	Calories	Fat (grams)
Hamburger	260	11
Cheeseburger	310	15
Double cheeseburger	434	26
Bean burrito	343	12
Beef burrito	466	21
Taco	190	11
Fillet of fish	432	25
Apple pie	253	14
Hot-fudge sundae	310	11
Chocolate shake	340	11
Skim milk	90	tr

1. Select your lunch from the menu above, and write your choices below.

2. Calculate the total number of Calories and fat that your lunch contains.

_____ Calories _____ grams of fat

3. BE AWARE. Fast food is excessive in Calories and fat. It is also low in fiber, vitamin A, and vitamin C. Therefore, choose fast food only once per week. See Appendix B for the specific nutrient content of your favorite fast food.

4. Tips on ordering at a fast food restaurant:
   Avoid fried foods, such as French fries and pies.
   Split a sandwich with a friend.
   Omit the mayonnaise, special dressing, and cheese from a sandwich. Use mustard, ketchup, and taco sauce for low-fat alternatives.
   Avoid high-Calorie drinks, like milkshakes. Have water, iced tea, fruit juice, or skim milk instead.
   At the salad bar, fill up on lettuce, mushrooms, green pepper, carrots, celery, cucumber, and other vegetables. Limit the meat, cheese, nuts, seeds, croutons, and all pasta or potato salads. Use lemon wedges or a dressing made with oil and vinegar. Avoid creamy dressings (one ladle = ¼ cup = 4 tbsp = 320 to 400 Calories).
   *Bring fruit or vegetables from home as a crisp addition to your lunch.

5. If the lunch you selected from Fast Food Delights contains more than 500 Calories or 20 grams of fat, please deduct food from your selections until this goal is achieved. Pay careful attention to the tips provided in #4.

6. List four fruits or vegetables that you could easily bring from home to supplement your lunch at Fast Food Delights.

Risk Habit or Factor	Increasing Risk				
I. Smoking cigarettes	None	Up to 9 per day	10 to 24 per day	25 to 34 per day	35 or more per day
Score	0	1	2	3	4
II. Body weight	Ideal weight	Up to 9 lbs. excess	10 to 19 lbs. excess	20 to 29 lbs excess	30 lbs. or more excess
Score	0	1	2	3	4
III. Salt intake or Blood pressure upper reading (if known)	⅕ hard to achieve: no added salt, no convenience foods Less than 110	⅓ average no use of salt at table, spare use of high-salt foods 110 to 129	U.S. average salt in cooking, some salt at table 130 to 139	Above average frequent salt at table 140 to 149	Far above average frequent use of salty foods 150 or over
Score	0	1	2	3	4
IV. Saturated fat and cholesterol intake or Blood cholesterol level (if known)	⅕ average almost total vegetarian: rare egg yolk, butterfat and lean meat Less than 150	⅓ average 2 meatless days/ week, no whole milk products, lean meat only 150 to 169	½ average meat (mostly lean), eggs, cheese 12 times/ week, nonfat milk only 170 to 199	U.S. average meat, cheese, eggs, whole milk 24 times/week 200 to 219	Above average meat, cheese, eggs, whole milk over 24 times/ week 220 or over
Score	0	1	2	3	4
V. Self-rating of physical activity or Walking rating	Vigorous exercise 4 or more times/ week 20 min. each Brisk walking 5 times/week 45 min. each	Vigorous exercise 3 times/week 20 min. each Brisk walking 3 times week 30 min. each	Vigorous exercise 1 to 2 times/ week 20 min. each Brisk walking 2 times/week 30 min. each or Normal walking 4 ½ to 6 miles daily	U.S. average occasional exercise Normal walking 2½ to 4½ miles daily	Below average exercises rarely Normal walking less than 2½ miles daily
Score	0	1	2	3	4
VI. Self-rating of stress and tension	Rarely tense or anxious or Yoga, meditation, or equivalent 20 min. 2 times/ day	Calmer than average Feel tense about 3 times week	U.S. average Feel tense or anxious 2 to 3 times/day Frequent anger or hurried feelings	Quite tense Usually rushed Occasionally take tranquilizer	Extremely tense Take tranquilizer 5 times/week or more
Score	0	1	2	3	4

From J. W. Farquhar, *The American Way of Life Need Not Be Hazardous to Your Health,* © 1987 by Stanford Alumni Association. Pages 38–41. Reprinted with permission of Addison-Wesley Publishing Co., Inc., Reading, Massachusetts.

What Your Score Means

Enter your total score here _____ .

Notes:

1. Subtract 1 point if dietary fiber intake is high (almost all cereals whole grain, almost no sugar, and considerable fruit and vegetable intake).

2. Add 1 point if all exercise is competitive.

3. If you are a female taking estrogen or birth control pills, add 1 point if score is 12 or below, 2 points if risk score is 13 or above (especially if you smoke, are overweight, have high blood pressure or high blood cholesterol).

Zone	Score	
F	21–24	The probability of having a premature heart attack or stroke is about four to five times the U.S. average. Action is urgent. Try to drop four points within a month and three more points within six months.
E	17–20	Incidence of heart attack or stroke is about twice the U.S. average. Action is urgent. Try to drop four points within six months and continue reduction.
D	13–16	The U.S. average is 14. This is an uncomfortable and readily avoidable zone. Careful planning can result in a five- to six-point reduction within a year.
C	9–12	The likelihood of having a heart attack or stroke is about one-half the U.S. average. This is a zone rather easily achieved by most people

within a year if they are now in Zone D or E. Careful planning can result in a four- to six-point reduction within a year.

Zone	Score	
B	5–8	Incidence of heart attack or stroke about one-quarter of the U.S. average. This goal is achievable by many but often takes one or two years to reach.
A	0–4	Incidence of heart attack or stroke rates very low, averaging less than one-tenth the rate in the U.S. 35–65 age group. This goal requires diligent effort, considerable family support, and often takes three to four years to reach. Individuals in this range should be proud and gratified (and will often find themselves acting as models and teachers for the many who have not achieved this very low risk zone).

7

Protein

INTRODUCTION

When you think of protein, do you picture vitality, strength, muscle mass, energy, and leanness? Protein is currently enjoying a high status in our culture, one that is enhanced by the media and nurtured by family tradition. Menus revolve around the protein choice. People allot the highest percentage of their food budgets to protein foods. High-priced protein supplements entice the athletic market. Does one nutrient deserve such attention?

Indeed protein is essential for life. It is a component of every cell and has diverse physiological functions. Perhaps, though, we need to put protein in its proper perspective by taking a look at its role in our health.

Protein Structure and Function

Protein is a term used to describe thousands of different substances in the body. They are like carbohydrate and lipids in that they contain carbon, oxygen, and hydrogen, but they are unique because they also contain nitrogen. Proteins are large, complex, and diverse compounds, and it is these three attributes that enable protein to function in such various capacities. The building blocks that are used to construct this varied group have similar properties and are known as **amino acids.**

Amino Acids

Not all amino acids are the same; in fact, there are 22 different ones. The amino acids found in the food we eat are used to assemble protein in our bodies. The human body can make 13 of the 22 amino acids, so the 13 are known as **nonessential amino acids.** The other nine are considered **essential amino acids** because the body is not capable of manufacturing them (1) (see table 7.1). If a person's diet contains all nine essential amino acids, then it is possible for the body to make the other 13.

Many researchers now suggest that some of the amino acids once thought to be nonessential may become indispensable during illness or various stages of development (2, 3). For example, some authors cite only eight essential amino acids, not counting histidine, which is essential for infants. Additionally, the preterm infant needs two amino acids that are not usually considered essential—cysteine and tyrosine (3).

Figure 7.1 shows the basic structure of an amino acid. They all contain an amine group and an acid group. The R group represents a side chain of the molecule that is different for each

TABLE 7.1
The essential and nonessential amino acids

Essential Amino Acids	Nonessential Amino Acids
Histidine	Alanine
Isoleucine	Asparagine
Leucine	Aspartic acid
Lysine	Arginine
Methionine	Cysteine
Phenylalanine	Glutamic acid
Threonine	Glutamine
Tryptophane	Glycine
Valine	Hydroxyproline
	Hydroxylysine
	Proline
	Serine
	Tyrosine

of the 22 amino acids. In the amino acid glycine, the R group is simply a hydrogen molecule. Glycine represents one of the nonessential amino acids. Attaching the R group to glycine is fairly easy if the basic unit is present. Now compare the R group of glycine to that of lysine in figure 7.1. Lysine is more difficult to manufacture and is an essential amino acid.

Protein Structure

Deoxyribonucleic acid (DNA) and ribonucleic acid (RNA), materials found in the nucleus of each cell, contain the information needed to direct the assembling (synthesis) of amino acids into a specific protein (see figure 7.2). Think of DNA and RNA as a "dictionary," amino acids as "letters," and protein as the various words that can be spelled with these letters.

Using this analogy, let's say a real-estate agent wants to make three "For Sale" signs for a neighborhood. There are four of each letter,

FIGURE 7.1
Amino acids differ in their R group.

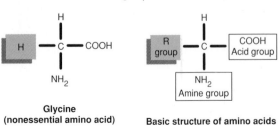

Glycine
(nonessential amino acid)

Basic structure of amino acids

Lysine
(essential amino acid)

FIGURE 7.2

The making of a protein. DNA designates the sequence in which amino acids are bonded together to form protein. Transfer RNA delivers the amino acids for assembly into a polypeptide chain. The end product is a new protein.

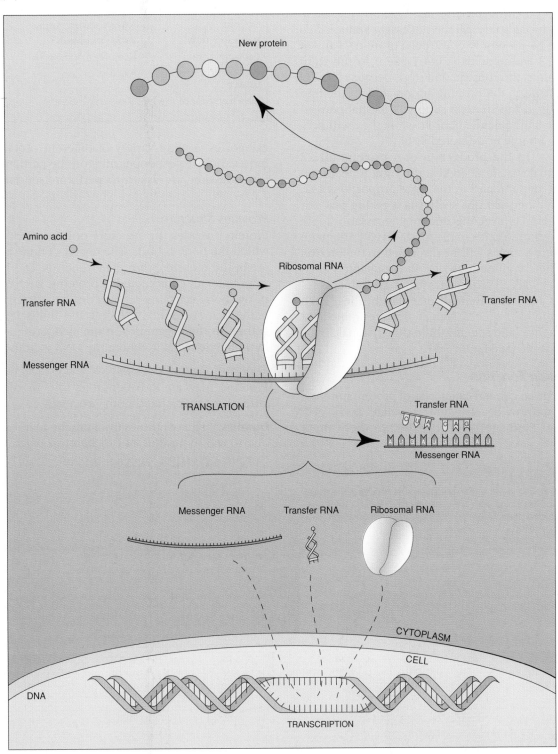

New protein

Amino acid

Transfer RNA

Ribosomal RNA

Transfer RNA

Messenger RNA

TRANSLATION

Transfer RNA

Messenger RNA

Messenger RNA

Transfer RNA

Ribosomal RNA

CYTOPLASM

CELL

DNA

TRANSCRIPTION

except there is only one "a." Despite the abundance of most of the letters needed for the signs, the person is limited to making one sign because there is only one "a." In this case no substitions are allowed.

During protein manufacture the same limitations apply. All the necessary amino acids must be present to construct a protein. If any of the 22 amino acids is not present in the right amounts, the construction stops because it is dependent on the limiting amino acid, or the one that is in the shortest supply. What happens to these amino acids then? Possibly they will produce energy or be stored as fat.

In the production of a protein, all 22 amino acids are needed at the right time, in the right amount, and in the right proportions (4). Remember that this synthesis is taking place at the cellular level; this does not necessarily apply to the amino acids in the food you eat. Adequate protein sources will be discussed in the section on dietary guidelines later in the chapter.

Three characteristics of assembled proteins influence their diverse capabilities. Each protein has a specific weight, definite amino-acid sequence, and specific three-dimensional shape as it folds (see figure 7.3).

Protein Function

The three general categories of protein function are to provide structure, regulate body processes, and supply energy. Within these three

Protein Functions	Examples
Structural components	Myosin
Enzymes	Salivary amylase; lactase
Hormones	Insulin; thyroxine
Carrier proteins	Lipoprotein; hemoglobin
Water/electrolyte balance	Albumin
Acid/base balance	

TABLE 7.2
The functions of protein

categories, a wide variety of different proteins have various roles, depending on the particular function they are asked to perform (see table 7.2).

Provides Structure
Protein provides the structure or framework on which the body is built. The matrix of bone and teeth, the muscles, skin, hair, tendons, and ligaments are all constructed of proteins. Each cell in the body contains protein: in the cell membrane that surrounds the cell and holds it together; in the organelles in the cytoplasm; and in the nucleus itself, where the DNA is housed.

Regulates Body Processes
Proteins play an indispensable role in regulating very specialized body processes.

Enzymes Life continues from minute to minute due to the thousands of biochemical reactions that are occurring. Specific proteins known as

FIGURE 7.3
The hormone insulin is one example of the structure of a small protein. The amino acids are coded by three letters. The three-dimensional shape is formed when cysteine crosslinks with other cysteines.

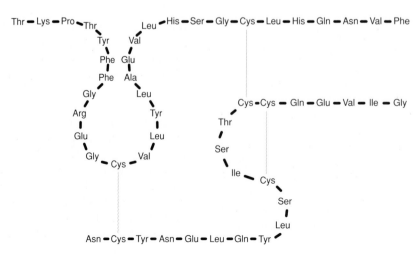

enzymes allow these reactions to take place at a fast enough pace to support life. Enzymes take part in digestion, blood clotting, muscle contraction, nerve transmission, the production of energy, growth, and many other life-sustaining activities. Lactase, for example, is an enzyme that helps to break down lactose, the carbohydrate found in milk. People who lack this enzyme can experience abdominal cramps and diarrhea if they consume milk. Other enzyme disorders may be more severe.

Hormones Hormones are internal chemical messengers and regulators of body functioning. Many hormones are proteins or parts of proteins and include insulin, growth hormone, thyroid hormone, and gastrointestinal hormones. The same protein may differ in structure between individuals, and certainly between species. Pork insulin, for example, although not identical to human insulin, is often used as a substitute for individuals with diabetes mellitus who are not producing enough of their own insulin.

Carrier Proteins Some proteins help to carry other important substances through the bloodstream to their destination. Two examples are lipoproteins (which carry triglycerides and cholesterol in the blood because they are not soluble), and hemoglobin, which transports oxygen from the lungs to all the cells of the body.

Antibodies Certain proteins known as **antibodies** recognize and attack foreign proteins (bacteria, viruses) when they enter the body. By combining with these foreign proteins, antibodies render them inactive. In many cases, once the body has encountered a particular foreign protein or antigen, it doesn't "forget" it and can quickly recall the "recipe" for the antibody. This is referred to as immunity.

Water/Electrolyte Balance Water is found throughout the body, both inside and outside the cells. A balance of this fluid is necessary for the body to function normally. Protein helps maintain this balance in two ways.

Plasma proteins (large molecules in the blood vessels), influence the movement of water from one area to another by exerting pressure, thus helping to control blood flow and circulation. Individuals with protein-deficiency disease often suffer from **edema,** an accumulation of fluid due to the shift of water into inappropriate areas because protein is not present to exert its influence.

Protein is also involved in fluid balance in an indirect way. *Electrolytes* are small, inorganic substances that have the ability (because of their small size) to pass freely through body membranes. Sodium (contained in water outside the cell), and potassium, (contained in water inside the cell), are two important electrolytes. Protein that is located in the cell membranes regulates the movement of these electrolytes. For example, these proteins transport sodium out of the cell and transport potassium into the cell. Since these electrolytes influence the movement of fluid across the cell membrane, protein also has an indirect influence on fluid balance. The presence of sodium and potassium in the appropriate locations is important for muscle contraction and nerve transmission.

Another vital function of protein in body fluids is its buffering action. Acid is a by-product of several chemical reactions that occur in the body. Normal cell functioning, such as enzyme activity, can occur only when the pH (measure of acidity) remains within a small range. Excess acid can disrupt normal body functioning and in severe cases result in coma or death. Protein buffers this acid until it can be removed from the body by the kidneys or lungs. A buffer is any agent that will bring the pH toward neutral, not acidic or alkaline.

Energy

What foods come to mind when you think of energy? Although carbohydrate and fat are most frequently associated with energy, protein can also be used to produce energy in the body. When proteins are metabolized for fuel, they yield four Calories per gram, the same as carbohydrate.

Figure 7.4 illustrates the pathways that the protein one consumes can take after entering the body. Amino acids that are not used for making specific proteins will be used to make energy or will be stored as fat for later use as energy. This may occur in several circumstances. If an insufficient supply of essential amino acids is not present, then the amino acids that are available cannot be used to make protein and may be used for fuel. Too few Calories will cause the body to use protein as an energy source until the Calorie needs of the body are met first. Also, when carbohydrate is not sufficient to meet the glucose needs of the central nervous system, certain parts of protein will be

Protein metabolism. After the digestion of protein, the amino acids that result are used to make protein and nonessential amino acids, and to supply energy. They can also be stored as fat if not immediately needed.

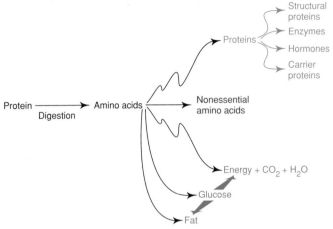

converted to supply glucose. A more common problem in America occurs when an individual consumes larger amounts of protein than needed by the body. In this instance, the excess protein is diverted to the energy pathways, or if it is above caloric needs is metabolized into fat.

Digestion, Absorption, and Transport of Protein

When foods containing protein are eaten, they are chewed, swallowed, and then proceed to the stomach for chemical processing.

The Stomach

Protein molecules are large and must be broken down into smaller components to be absorbed. Two processes occur in the stomach that aid in this dismanteling. The first process unfolds the three-dimensional structure of protein. This is known as denaturation and is accomplished by the action of hydrochloric acid in the stomach (see figure 7.5). (Protein can also be denatured outside the body by heat, acid, alcohol, and other chemicals.)

Although acid would denature many enzymes since they are proteins, pepsin, a stomach enzyme, is specially designed to function under the acid environment of the stomach. After the protein is denatured, pepsin breaks the long strands into **polypeptides** (small chains of amino acids), which are moved along to the small intestine where they will be further broken apart.

The Small Intestine

A barrage of **proteases** (protein-digesting enzymes) awaits the polypeptides in the small intestine. These have been released from the pancreas and will break the polypeptide strands into tripeptides, dipeptides, and single amino acids. Further digestion is facilitated by enzymes released from the wall of the small intestine.

Absorption and Transport

The end products of digestion are absorbed and travel through the portal vein to the liver, where they can enter the general circulation. Surprisingly, dipeptides and tripeptides are absorbed more rapidly than single amino acids.

Occasionally the system malfunctions and allows whole proteins or small subunits to slip past the barrier of the intestinal wall. Infants who have immature digestive tracts and individuals suffering from gastrointestinal illness may incur this problem (5). Such proteins will be recognized as foreign by the body and may cause a food allergy in susceptible people. (Allergies are further discussed in chapters 4 and 13.)

Once these products of protein digestion are absorbed into the body, they either are synthesized into plasma proteins by the liver or are used by individual cells to make protein. For various reasons discussed in the last section, amino acids that are not used to build protein are returned to the liver. The nitrogen portion is converted to urea and sent to the kidneys for

The three-dimensional structure of a protein is stabilized by chemical bonds. Heat, acid, or other chemicals may denature the protein.

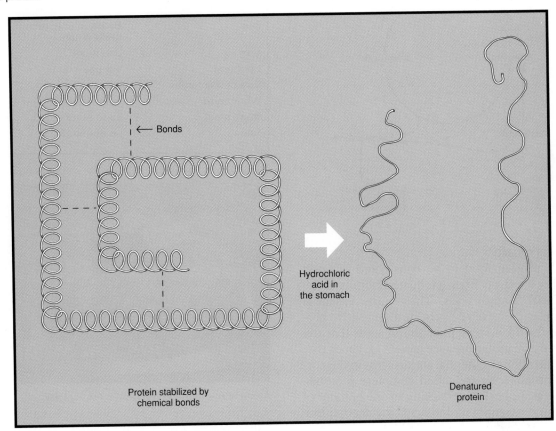

← Bonds

Hydrochloric
acid in
the stomach

Protein stabilized by
chemical bonds

Denatured
protein

excretion in the urine. The nonnitrogenous portion of the amino acid will act as either carbohydrate and provide energy or as fat and be stored as energy reserve.

The Amino Acid Pool

There is no major storage site in the body for amino acids as there are for carbohydrate and fat. The liver, however, will slightly increase in size when protein is available. There are two sources of amino acids for this "pool." The first is newly absorbed amino acids, and the second is amino acids derived from the turnover of worn-out tissue (see figure 7.6).

Fortunately, these amino acids can be recycled because about three percent of adult body proteins are replaced daily (6). This turnover is precisely balanced and very important. The greater the importance of a particular protein in the regulation of metabolism (enzymes and hormones), the faster its rate of turnover. In contrast, proteins with no regulatory role, like muscle and collagen, have a slow turnover rate (7).

One example of protein turnover takes place in the gut. As the lining of the gut wears out, it is sloughed off. The digestive tract treats these old cells just like food particles and will absorb the amino acids that result from digestion.

Of course this recycling is not 100 percent. Some of the internal proteins are broken down and excreted, and the external proteins like hair, nails, and skin cells are lost.

Dietary Guidelines for Protein Consumption

Protein Needs

As was mentioned at the beginning of this chapter, the need for protein is actually a need for essential amino acids. Both the quality and the quantity of amino acids in the diet will affect the recommendations made for protein intake.

FIGURE 7.6
The amino acid pool.

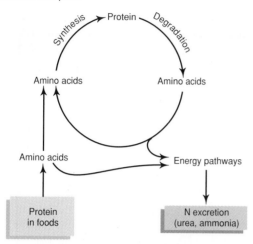

TABLE 7.3
Complementary vegetable proteins

Grains	+	Legumes
Rice		Blackeyed peas; pinto beans; or tofu
Corn		Lima beans
Cornbread		Split-pea soup
Corn or flour tortillas		Beans
Wheat bread		Peanut butter
Brown bread		Baked beans
Tofu		Lasagna noodles

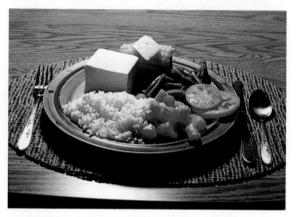

A meal of rice, tofu, and vegetables is rich in protein.

Protein Quality

For a protein food to be considered of good quality it must contain adequate amounts of the essential amino acids. These nine essential amino acids are used "as is" and are used to produce the 13 nonessential amino acids that the body can manufacture (see table 7.1). Foods that contain all nine essential amino acids in the correct proportions are called complete proteins, whereas those that are lacking in one or more of the nine essential amino acids are incomplete proteins.

When looking for sources of good-quality protein there are a few easy rules to follow. First, almost all animal sources of protein are complete. These would include meat, eggs, milk, or products made from these such as cheese. The one exception is gelatin, which lacks two of the essential amino acids.

Second, plant sources of protein are almost always incomplete. Legumes, nuts and seeds, grains, and vegetables fall into this category. This fact, however, does not mean that foods made from plant proteins are not of good quality. Proteins from different plant sources often have amino-acid patterns that compensate for each other. Grains, for example, are deficient in two amino acids, lysine and isoleucine. Combining grains with legumes, which lack tryptophan and methionine, results in a mixture containing all essential amino acids (see table 7.3). (The traditional peanut-butter-on-wheat-bread is just such a combination.) Eating two incomplete proteins at the same meal is equiva-

lent to eating a high-quality, complete protein. When two plant proteins balance one another's shortcomings, they are said to be *complementary*.

It is interesting to note that many traditional ethnic dishes combine complementary proteins: lentil curry on rice; pinto beans and corn tortillas; **tofu** (soybean curd) and rice; and corn and lima beans (succotash). Figure 7.7 introduces legumes to those who are not familiar with them.

The protein quality of one individual food is probably not of great concern in America, where most people eat a wide variety of foods daily. It is hoped that the broad selection of foods found at the dinner table will produce about the right proportions of amino acids. However, those individuals who consume only vegetable protein or very little animal protein would benefit from deliberately complementing proteins.

Protein quality can be measured in several ways. These techniques consider not only the essential amino acids that a protein source contains but also the digestibility of that food. A

FIGURE 7.7

Legumes are dried beans, peas, and lentils from pods containing one row of seeds. Most legumes need to be softened before cooking. Soak them overnight, or boil for two minutes, uncovered; then remove from heat, cover, and let stand one hour. (Lentils do not need to be softened.) After softening, legumes should be cooked as directed in recipes. Dried beans double or triple in volume as they cook, so be sure to choose a sufficiently large pan or casserole.

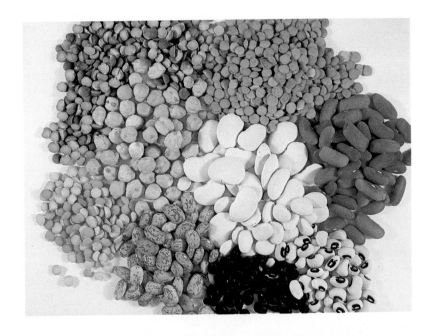

Type	Color	Size and shape	Use
Black beans	Black	Small, oval	Baked, soups, stews
Black-eyed peas	White with a black spot	Small, oval	Casseroles
Garbanzo beans (chickpeas)	Brown	Small, irregular	Dips, casseroles, salads, soups, stews
Great northern beans	White	Medium, oval	Baked, casseroles, chowder, soups, stews
Kidney beans	Red	Medium, oval	Casseroles, chili, salads, soups
Lentils	Brown or green	Small, round disk	Casseroles, salads, soups
Lima beans	White	Large, flat	Casseroles, soups
Navy beans	White	Small, round	Baked, soups
Pinto beans	Pink	Medium, oval	Baked, casseroles, soups
Red beans	Red	Small, round	Casseroles, chili
Soybeans	Tan	Small, round	Casseroles, salads
Split peas	Green or yellow	Small, round	Soups

high-quality protein source must first contain all the essential amino acids and then be able to release them so that the body can use them.

Biological value is a measurement of how well amino acids in a particular food are incorporated into new protein in the body. It does not take into account the digestibility of the protein; it only assesses the usefulness of the amino acids once they enter the body. By this standard the most perfect protein source is the egg, which is assigned the biological value score of 100.

Once egg white has been absorbed by the body, all of the protein it contains can be used to make new proteins, without any waste.

That's fine, if egg is easily digested. **Net protein utilization** (NPU) measures both the amino acid pattern and the digestibility of food. By this standard, the score of the egg white drops slightly, to 94. Although egg white is perfectly balanced in amino acid composition, it is not perfectly digestible. Not surprisingly, average

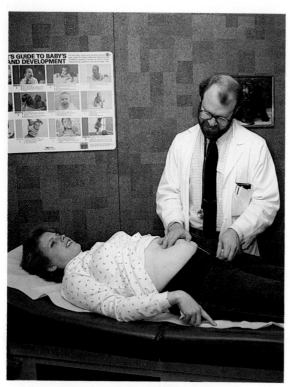
Protein needs increase during growth periods.

NPU scores for plant-derived proteins are lower (55) than those for animal-derived proteins (75). Although individual scores are important, NPU measurements of complete meals would be more representative of protein utilization in the body. Cooking methods (moist heating makes protein more digestible), accompanying nutrients, and complementary protein sources can all improve the NPU of a meal.

The **protein efficiency ratio** (PER) is yet another method used to measure protein quality, by determining the efficiency by which a protein supports growth. For example, a laboratory experiment will measure how well a growing rat will gain weight if given a fixed amount of dietary protein.

All of these measurements are used to determine recommendations for protein intake. For instance, the higher the PER or NPU of a particular food, the less an individual would need to consume. If a person's diet contains mainly low-quality (low PER) protein sources, more protein will need to be consumed.

Certainly these standards have their limitations. People do not have the same dietary requirements as rats, and Americans typically do not obtain protein from just one source.

Protein Quantity

When estimating how much protein a person needs, the two primary factors to consider are routine maintenance and growth. All of us have a basic need for amino acids in order to replace worn-out cells, produce hormones and enzymes, make antibodies, and manufacture carrier proteins. These basic maintenance needs must be met first. Additional amounts of protein are crucial for those in the growth state.

Although the term *growth* usually brings to mind the height and weight increases of the young, this category also includes pregnant and lactating females. In any of these growth periods, the total amount of protein in the body is increasing, and thus protein needs are greatly increased—far above maintenance needs.

Because protein is the only nutrient that contains nitrogen, many researchers have used the **nitrogen balance study** as a tool for measuring the body's need for protein for maintenance and growth. The amount of nitrogen taken into the body is compared to the amount eliminated, thus indicating protein usage by the body.

Measuring nitrogen intake is fairly easy. Nitrogen enters the body through the food and drink we consume, so a chemical analysis of this food and drink will reveal the nitrogen intake. Nitrogen output is more difficult to measure because nitrogen can leave the body through several routes. Hair, nails, flaked skin cells, sweat, urine, and feces all contribute to the loss of nitrogen from the body. Only the latter two, urine and feces, are commonly used to calculate nitrogen output. Fecal nitrogen is never really available for use by the body. After determining nitrogen intake and output, a simple subtraction will reveal the net gain or loss. Three results can occur.

One result is positive nitrogen balance. In this case more nitrogen is coming into the body than is leaving. (Remember that there are no significant storage sites for amino acids; they are either used to build protein or broken down to be used in the energy cycles.) In the latter case nitrogen is eliminated through the urine and would be calculated in the nitrogen output. Clearly, a positive nitrogen balance can mean only that growth is occurring.

The second result could be a case of nitrogen equilibrium. Subtracting nitrogen output from intake, the result is zero. This is the typical state of healthy adults that are not significantly increasing their lean body mass through an exercise program.

TABLE 7.4
Recommended daily allowances for protein

Age (in years)	Protein (g)
Infants	
0.0–0.5	kg × 2.2(13)
0.5–1.0	kg × 1.6(14)
Children	
1–3	16
4–6	24
7–10	28
11–14	45 (males)
	46 (females)
15–18	59 (males)
	44 (females)
Adults	
19–24	58 (males)
	46 (females)
25–51+	50 (females)
	63 (males)
	60 (pregnant females)
	65 (lactating females)

Reprinted with permission from: Food and Nutrition Board. Recommended Dietary Allowances. 10th rev. ed. 1989. Washington, DC: National Academy Press, 1989.

TABLE 7.5
The protein-packed American diet

Product	Pounds Per Year	Protein (g per day)
Red meat	150	24
Flour	112	17
Milk and milk products	310	14
Poultry	57	9
Eggs	35	6
Cheese	17	5
Potatoes	125	5
Fish	13	4
Vegetables	164	3
Peanuts	7	2
Other		3

From U.S. Department of Agriculture, Economics, Statistics, and Cooperatives Service.

A negative nitrogen balance is a third possibility. This condition occurs when more nitrogen is leaving the body than entering. Definitely not a desirable state, negative nitrogen balance means that muscle tissue and other lean tissues are being broken down to supply energy needs. Starvation or very-low-Calorie diets will cause the body to break down muscle and other protein-containing cells for energy. Energy needs have a higher priority than does body protein maintenance. Other conditions may also lead to negative nitrogen balance, such as infectious disease, chronic disease, physical stress, and emotional stress (8).

Recommended Protein Intake

Research on both quality and quantity of protein is consulted in order to establish recommendations for protein intake. The resulting guidelines are commonly presented in two ways.

Based on Weight and Age

The Recommended Daily Allowances for protein is a guideline that varies with both weight and age (see table 7.4). An adult needs 0.8 grams of protein per kilogram of body weight. Infants, because of their tremendous rate of growth, need more than double that, or 2.2 grams per kilogram of body weight. The need gradually decreases with age until adulthood is reached. Of course this is not really a change with age, but with growth requirements. In addition, the RDA allots extra allowances for protein during pregnancy (plus 10 grams) and while lactating (plus 15 grams).

The table of RDA actually recommends 63 grams of protein for a male and 50 grams for a female, this calculation being based on the reference male weighing 174 pounds (79 kilograms) and reference female weighing 149 pounds (63 kilograms). How do these figures compare to the current consumption patterns of Americans? Males between the ages of 19 and 22 take in 107 grams of protein per day, and females in the same age group consume 67 grams (9,10). Table 7.5 gives some insight as to just where this protein comes from in our diets.

Protein needs vary from individual to individual, but the RDA is generous. Meant for use with populations, the RDA recommends a protein intake that is more than that needed by 98 percent of healthy Americans.

Based on Calories

Frequently, guidelines for protein consumption are given as 10 to 12 percent of a person's caloric intake. (Again this recommendation is based on healthy adults who are not on a weight-reduction diet.) Most Americans eat far more than this. A recent food-consumption survey of nine thousand Americans reported that 16 percent of their Calories were from protein (10).

The two guidelines for protein intake, based on weight and Calories, will not necessarily produce the same recommendation. For example, physically active individuals may require large quantities of Calories. This would increase the protein guideline based on Calories but not change the recommendation based only on weight. It is useful to remember that these are just guides, not requirements.

The Athlete's Diet

No special provisions for the athlete have been made in the RDA. In the case of the endurance athlete, studies have shown that protein is used as an energy source. The actual amount of protein utilized during endurance exercise depends on the intensity and duration of the exercise. The harder and longer the exercise, the more protein will be used for energy (11,12). Unfortunately, protein is not a good fuel, and a high-carbohydrate diet that is adequate in Calories is what the body needs to discourage the use of protein as fuel. Caution should be used in the application of this information, because most Americans are not endurance athletes (which would require greater than five hours of cardiovascular exercise per week).

Weightlifters, who are actively building muscle and not just maintaining their muscle mass, may require a little more protein. Muscle-mass increase can only come from specific heavy-resistance-type exercise training (13). Eating large quantities of protein does not increase muscle mass, but protein is needed to form increased lean body weight. Under intense training a young man weighing 165 pounds (75 kilograms) could increase his lean body mass by one or two pounds (500 to 1,000 grams) per week. About 20 percent of this is an increase in pure protein (11). This requires an additional one ounce (28 grams) of protein per day. However, once the larger muscle mass is achieved, protein requirements are again reduced, without loss of muscle.

Some of the estimates available suggest that as much as 50 percent more protein may be needed for those putting on muscle mass (11,14). This would be about 1.2 grams per kilogram of body weight, or 28 grams more than the 63 grams required for the reference male.

How do athletes compare to the 91 grams that they might need? One researcher found that runners consumed a whopping 125

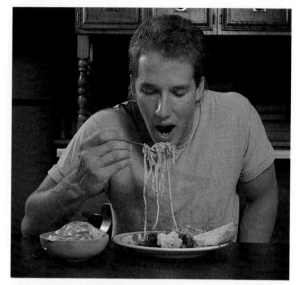

A low-fat, high-carbohydrate diet is best for athletes.

grams of protein per day, double the RDA. Protein intakes tend to be lower among endurance athletes, while some groups of power and strength athletes consume more than 20 percent of their energy as protein. Relative to body weight, protein intakes usually exceed 1.5 grams per kilogram per day, and commonly exceed 2.0 grams per kilogram per day for these athletes (15). In addition, nine percent of high school and college athletes were found to supplement their diets with protein powder (16).

Wise selections of high-quality protein foods or food combinations will provide all the protein needed for strenuous exercise training. Expensive protein supplements are not necessary for athletes, considering their large consumption of protein. Most important, all athletes should strive for a high-carbohydrate diet (58 percent of total Calories) for health as well as energy (see the Health-Promotion Insight on sports nutrition in chapter 12).

Achieving the Dietary Guidelines

Let's apply what has been learned about protein needs to some guidelines on eating.

Protein Sources

There are really two categories of protein sources: animal and plant. Animal sources of protein, with the exception of gelatin, contain all the essential amino acids. Examples of this group are beef, lamb, pork, tuna fish, salmon, eggs, cheese, yogurt, and milk.

Table 7.6
Protein sources with accompanying fat

Food	Amount	Protein (g)	Fat (%Kcal)
Frankfurter	1 (2 oz)	7	79
Peanut butter	1 tbsp	4	76
Pork chop	3 oz	21	74
Beef steak	3 oz	20	74
American cheese	1 oz	7	70
Boiled ham	1 oz	5	69
Egg	1	6	68
Milk (whole)	1 cup	8	48
Milk (2%)	1 cup	8	38
Tuna in oil (drained)	3 oz	24	37
Chicken (no skin)	3 oz	18	35
Cod, broiled	3 oz	22	15
Oatmeal	1 cup	5	14
Wheat bread	1 slice	4	14
Corn	1 cup	5	7
Lima beans	1 cup	16	<3
Lentils	1 cup	16	0

Source: J. A. T. Pennington and H. N. Church. *Food Values of Portions Commonly Used.* © 1985. J. B. Lippincott Co., Philadelphia.

Table 7.7
Leaner protein choices

Foods to Try More Often

Fish and poultry (without the skin)
Lean cuts of meat and trim off the visible fat
Skim milk or low-fat dairy products
Vegetables, legumes, and grains

Foods to Eat Less Often

Red meats (beef, lamb, pork)
Fatty luncheon meats and organ meats (liver)
Fried meats
Eggs

Ways to Prepare Food

Broil, boil, bake, roast, and stew

Table 7.8
The cost of different protein sources

Food	Serving Size	Protein (g)	Cost Per Gram of Protein ($)
Amino-acid supplements	1 pill	1.0	.120
Bacon	2 slices	3.8	.075
Milk (2%)	1 cup	8.8	.051
Beef	3 oz	24.0	.031
Corn and lima beans	1/2 cup	4.4	.031
Bologna	1 slice	3.4	.030
Flounder	3 oz	25.5	.020
American cheese	1 slice	6.6	.019
Hamburger (lean)	3 oz	23.4	.016
Tuna	3 oz	24.4	.014
Eggs	1	11.4	.012
Cottage cheese	1/2 cup	15.0	.010
Chicken	3 oz	26.8	.008
Lentils	1 cup	11.7	.004
Pinto beans	1 cup	21.0	.001

Source: J. A. T. Pennington and H. N. Church. *Food Values of Portions Commonly Used.* © 1985. J. B. Lippincott Co., Philadelphia, PA.

Animal sources are somewhat of a mixed blessing. While containing high-quality protein, some also contain high amounts of fat. (Table 7.6 compares various protein sources and the fat that they contain.) This offers a partial explanation of the high fat consumption of Americans. Many Americans eat more than double the RDA for protein, unfortunately receiving the extra fat too (see Health-Promotion Activity 7.1). Suggestions for leaner protein choices can be found in table 7.7.

Another consideration, besides the fat content, is the high price of animal protein. Table 7.8 will help you compare the cost of different protein sources. Surprisingly there is considerable variation.

Plant-derived protein, however, is not necessarily of high quality, legumes being the exception. This group includes the seeds of plants such as lima beans, pinto beans, garden peas, black-eyed peas, garbanzo beans, lentils, and soybeans. Legumes provide protein with almost as high a quality as meat, and they are also an excellent source of B-vitamins, iron, fiber, and other nutrients. Incorporating them into the week's menu can add variety and enjoyment to your meals (see figure 7.7).

The soybean is one plant source of protein that has enjoyed popularity in recent years. Several attributes have contributed to its status among legumes. This versatile bean can be made into many foods. About 18 percent of the seed contains oil, which is removed for industrial and cooking uses. The remaining soy meal contains almost 50 percent protein and is currently used to make soy milk, soy flour, isolated soy protein, and tofu.

Soy protein isolates are made by extracting the protein from the soy meal. This protein may be formed into chunks or woven into spun fibers, and it has numerous uses. Some of these uses include meat substitutes (like imitation hamburger, salami, chicken, or beef), cheese, corn chips, whipped toppings, and infant formulas. It may also be mixed with animal meat as an "extender" or filler.

For some two thousand years Asian cultures have been modifying the soybean to form tofu. Just as cheese is the curd from milk, tofu is the curd from soy milk. It has some of the same properties as cheese. Tofu is high in calcium, protein, and magnesium but is low in Calories, salt, and cholesterol.

Refined proteins are finding their way into the marketplace in a number of different foods, too. Casein (or its derivative, sodium caseinate), is a commercially isolated cow's milk protein. These may appear on the labels of frozen dessert toppings or coffee creamers. Another big market is nutritional supplements like protein powders for athletes. The majority of Americans, including athletes, don't need this additional protein, and it is usually expensive.

Table 7.8 compares the cost of plant and animal protein. Those on a tight budget or those who are interested in a low-fat, tasty alternative might try new entrees using plant protein.

Calculating Protein Intake

Three sources of information can be used to determine if you are getting adequate protein: food composition tables, food labels, and the food exchange lists. A food composition table can be found in Appendix B. The amount of protein in grams is given for every food item in the table. This table is a handy tool to use when cooking or doing a self-assessment.

Labels on food products also provide information about protein content. The actual amount of protein, in grams, will be listed first. The bottom of the label will list the percent of the U.S. RDA that the product contains. Figure 7.8 compares two food labels. Although they both contain the same amount of protein, the percent of U.S. RDA differs. This is because the U.S. RDA sets two standards for protein, based on the quality of the protein. For high-quality protein the standard is 45 grams, and for low-quality protein the standard is 65 grams. As previously discussed, a person eating high-quality

FIGURE 7.8

Both labels indicate that one serving of either nonfat milk or split-pea soup contains eight grams of protein. The U.S. RDA differs because the quality of the protein is lower in the soup.

Nonfat milk	Split pea soup
Nutrition information per serving	Nutrition information per serving
Serving size.........................1 cup	Serving size.........................1/2 cup
Servings per container................1	Servings per container.................4
Calories.........................90	Calories.........................130
Protein......................... 8 g	Protein......................... 8 g
Carbohydrate.........................13 g	Carbohydrate.........................23 g
Fat.........................0 g	Fat.........................0 g

Percentage of U.S. RDA	Percentage of U.S. RDA
Protein.........................18	Protein.........................12
Vitamin A.........................10	Vitamin A.........................*
Vitamin C.........................4	Vitamin C.........................*
Thiamin.........................8	Thiamin.........................15
Riboflavin.........................30	Riboflavin.........................8
Niacin.........................*	Niacin.........................9
Calcium.........................25	Calcium.........................3
Iron.........................*	Iron.........................6

*Contains less than 2% of the U.S RDA for these nutrients.

*Contains less than 2% of the U.S RDA for these nutrients.

protein should be able to eat less, since more of it will be utilized. Consumers, then, need not be concerned with the quality of the protein if basing their judgment on the percent of the U.S. RDA; it is already adjusted for quality.

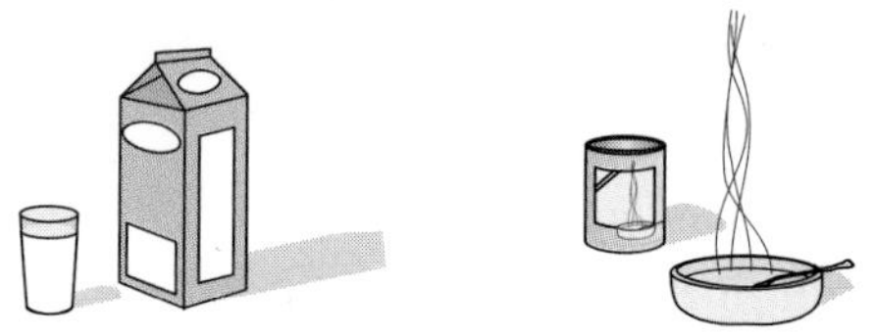

A good practical guide for estimating the amount of protein in foods is the exchange lists. The protein content for each of the six food exchanges is shown in table 7.9. These exchange lists are easily memorized and are then available for use on a daily basis, no matter where you are. As pointed out in chapter 3, exchange lists do have their shortcomings, however, and food composition tables are best for information on specific foods.

Food-exchange groups that are high in protein include the milk and protein groups. Meats, cheeses, and legumes can be found in this exchange group, providing seven grams of protein per serving. Fruits and fats generally contain no protein, with the exception of nuts. Nuts are high in fat but are a good source of protein. A two-tablespoon portion of a nut butter has from

TABLE 7.9
Exchange lists for protein

Exchange	Protein (g)	Carbohydrate (g)	Fat (g)	Calories
Milk (nonfat)	8	12	Trace	80
Vegetable	2	5	–	25
Fruit	–	10	–	40
Bread	2	15	Trace	70
Legume	9	15	1	125
Meat	7	–	3–9	55–100
Fat	–	–	5	45

From Exchange Lists for Meal Planning, 1988. American Diabetic Association.

three to eight grams of protein, depending on the type of nut. Snackers, however, need to be careful: handfuls of nuts could provide three hundred or more Calories!

Table 7.10 summarizes the protein available in a sample breakfast, lunch, and dinner. As you can see, accumulating the RDA for protein is not difficult. The reference male needs 63 grams of protein per day. Dividing this by three, say 21 grams is needed at each meal. Note that the lunch alone in table 7.10 provides 38 grams.

Now let's say that you go to a restaurant and order a large-sized portion of meat—a ten-ounce steak, for example. This alone would provide 70 grams of protein. Because this protein would not be needed immediately, and there is no significant storage, the protein would be processed in the energy cycle for energy or fat. In addition to this large quantity of protein, you would be consuming as much as 700 Calories, over 400 of which originate from fat. The section on protein excess that appears later in the chapter will discuss the health risks of eating just such a meal.

Health-Promotion Activity 7.2 will help you assess your protein intake and perhaps make some adjustments. Although the goal is not necessarily to eat the RDA for protein every day, it does provide a good guideline for assessment.

Protein for Health Promotion

In keeping with the theme of health promotion, we continue to advocate reaching and maintaining the dietary guidelines. Eating too much or too little protein does have negative effects.

TABLE 7.10
The amount of protein in a sample day's menu

Menu	Protein (g)
Breakfast	
Wheat Chex cereal (2 oz)	6
Low-fat milk (1 cup)	8
Banana (1/2 medium)	0
Grapefruit (1/2)	0
Lunch	
Whole-wheat bread (2 slices)	4
Tuna fish (3 oz)	24
Carrots (1/2 cup)	2
Apple (1 medium)	0
Low-fat milk (1 cup)	8
Dinner	
Chicken (6 oz)	36
Baked potato (1 medium)	3
Broccoli and cauliflower (1 cup)	4
Cornbread	4
Snack	
Popcorn, unbuttered (3 cups)	5
Total Protein (g) =	104

Protein Shortage

Although most Americans consume far too much protein, people in other parts of the world do not get enough. This may be the result of surviving on staples that contain too little protein or too few Calories.

Marasmus
Marasmus, a protein-deficiency disease, is actually starvation; the body is not taking in enough Calories and must use the protein that it does receive for energy. The body appears wasted because most of the muscle tissue is used to supply

FIGURE 7.9

These children are suffering from protein-Calorie malnutrition. The ones on the left have marasmus, and the one on the right has kwashiorkor.

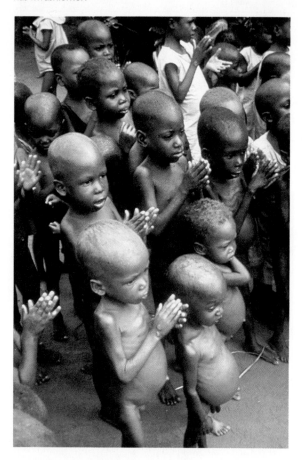

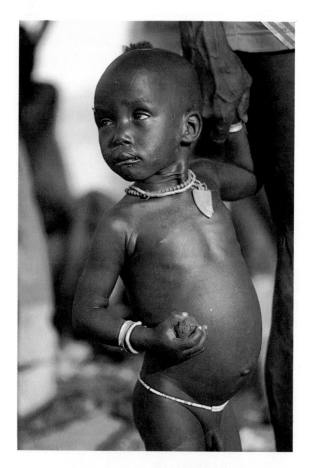

energy for just staying alive (see figure 7.9). Affecting mainly infants, marasmus deprives the body of nutrients at the time when growth is critical. Although the heads of these infants appear large for their wasted bodies, the circumference is actually small for their age. This reflects the abnormal growth of the child suffering from marasmus.

Kwashiorkor

Another protein-deficiency disease that affects mainly children under age five is **kwashiorkor.** This differs from marasmus in that caloric content may or may not be sufficient, but protein intake is too low. The body of the victim is wasted, just like those afflicted with marasmus, but it isn't as obvious. Blood proteins that normally function to maintain appropriate fluid balance are broken down and used for energy. Without the "pull" of proteins, the blood fluid moves into the tissues, causing edema (see figure

7.9). Orange-colored hair and dermatitis are other characteristics of children suffering from kwashiorkor. This disease often affects the child who is taken from the breast when the mother must begin nursing a newborn. A watery gruel nearly devoid of protein is then substituted for the protein-rich breast milk.

Both marasmus and kwashiorkor can be included under the general heading of **protein-Calorie malnutrition** (PCM). The use of expensive infant formulas has also been indicated in PCM. These formulas are improperly diluted so that they do not contain enough protein or Calories per ounce. Diarrhea may also result from unsterile preparation of these formulas, also leading to PCM.

The most pronounced effect of PCM is impaired immune function, which leaves the child vulnerable to infection and disease (17). Millions of children die each year from PCM. Some victims do survive but are permanently stunted both physically and mentally.

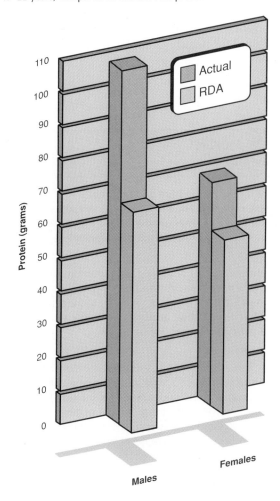

F IGURE 7.10
The intake of protein in America for males and females ages 19–22 years, compared to the RDA for protein.

Legend: Actual / RDA

Y-axis: Protein (grams), scale 0 to 110

Categories: Males, Females

Protein Excess

While protein shortages are of world concern, perhaps protein excess is of personal concern. Certainly most Americans consume much more than the RDA for protein (see figure 7.10). This section points out some of the problems associated with a high protein intake.

The Associated Fat

As previously discussed, animal sources of protein often keep bad company with fat. Chapter 6 targets animal sources of protein as a major contributor to the excess fat in the American diet. A high fat intake has been associated with heart disease, cancer, obesity, and other major killers in developed countries. Leaner protein alternatives are available and should be included in weekly menu planning. Reread the section on protein sources and see table 7.7 for a list of leaner protein choices. (See Health-Promotion Activity 7.1.)

Dehydration

Protein in excess of that needed for maintenance and growth is metabolized for energy. The breakdown of amino acids creates the waste product urea, which is excreted in the urine. In the process of excretion, large amounts of water are needed to dilute the urea as it leaves the body. For every 100 Calories of protein metabolized, the body loses 350 grams of water, whereas carbohydrate or fat use only 50 grams when metabolized (6).

High-protein regimes are particularly hazardous to the athlete, who already has difficulty remaining hydrated. Perspiration and metabolic losses can leave the athlete with too little water to function safely. A dehydrated muscle does not perform at its best either. The solution is fairly simple—consume lots of water and reduce protein intake to reasonable levels, closer to the RDA.

Calcium Loss

Some studies have shown that high protein intakes will result in a net loss of calcium from the body. Over long periods of time the loss of calcium in bone results in a debilitating disease known as **osteoporosis,** in which bone is gradually demineralized so that it becomes less dense and therefore brittle. Females especially are prone to calcium loss. Many other factors, such as physical activity, phosphorus intake, age, and hormone levels, have been implicated as risk factors. (Osteoporosis is further discussed in chapter 11.)

Recent long-term studies in which meat was the high-protein source, rather than purified proteins, did not show an increase in calcium loss (18).

High Cholesterol

Numerous studies show that diets containing animal protein induce higher cholesterol levels in subjects than do diets containing vegetable protein. The explanation seems simple: the high saturated-fat intake that usually accompanies the animal protein is responsible.

Now researchers have found that the protein itself has an effect on cholesterol. Animal proteins seem to raise blood cholesterol levels, and plant proteins have the opposite effect. Data currently available show that the protein in the diet does not change synthesis or absorption but the turnover time of cholesterol in the blood: plant proteins decrease the time that cholesterol remains in the blood. The accelerated excretion may account for its lack of accumulation in the blood (8,19,20).

High cholesterol levels are associated with atherosclerosis, heart disease, stroke, and hypertension. Further discussion on this subject can be found in chapter 6.

Obesity

An excess of Calories, no matter from what source (fat, carbohydrate, or protein), will lead to extra fat on the body. Getting Calories from the right sources and avoiding extra Calories are essential for health promotion.

---

*H*EALTH-PROMOTION INSIGHT
The Vegetarian Alternative

Vegetarians aren't a band of fanatics who go through life without indulging in fine cuisine. The fact is that vegetarians may be much healthier than nonvegetarians.

There are three categories of vegetarian, based on the animal foods left in the diet.

Vegans — "Pure" vegetarians who consume no animal products.

Lacto-vegetarians — Persons who include dairy products such as milk or cheeses in their diets but eat no other animal products.

Lacto-ovo-vegetarians — Persons who include dairy products and eggs in their diets, but no animal flesh.

People may choose to become vegetarian for economic/ecologic, health, ethical, or spiritual reasons. However, the focus of this insight is the health benefits of vegetarianism.

Health Benefits

The health benefits of a vegetarian life-style can be grouped into four categories: nutrition, disease prevention, food safety, and fitness.

Nutrition

The American Dietetic Association has now affirmed that a lacto-ovo-vegetarian diet meets the needs of all age groups (21). Even the diet of a vegan, who consumes only plant food, can be nutritionally adequate if proper food planning is practiced. This is particularly important for infants, children, and pregnant and lactating women.

The American Dietetic Association has advised that the following nutrients be considered when planning a total vegetarian diet.

Protein

Studies of both animals and plants confirm the adequacy of the vegetarian diet in meeting amino acid requirements (22,23,24,25). However, because plant foods have a lower concentration of some of the essential amino acids, a variety of unrefined plant foods is needed to assure good protein complementation. For example, meat should be replaced with legumes, seeds, and nuts; and whole grains should be used as a natural complement.

Vitamin B₁₂

No practical source of vitamin B_{12} is found in plant food (26). It must be provided as a supplement to the vegan diet or come from fortified foods such as breakfast cereals, meat analogs, or soy milk. Adults need three micrograms (μg) per day.

Vitamin D

Individuals who do not use vitamin-D-fortified milk products may require a vitamin D supplement. In some climates, daily exposure to sunshine may be adequate; however, northern climates or limited exposure to sunshine may not provide enough vitamin D. Supplements are necessary for infants whose only source of vitamin D is breast milk after four to six months of age. (See chapter 10 for more information on vitamin D.)

Calcium

More than 55 percent of the calcium Americans obtain from food comes from milk and cheese (27). When these are avoided in the diet, then leafy green vegetables, nuts, seeds, legumes, soy milk, tofu, and whole grains are good substitutes.

Iron

Iron from meat products is more easily absorbed by the body than iron from plant foods. Including vitamin C with each meal, however, helps to increase the availability of iron from plant foods. Thus vegetarians should try to include with each meal a fruit or vegetable that contains vitamin C. Adult males need an average of 10 milligrams per day, and females need 18 milligrams per day.

Zinc

Some studies suggest that due to the high fiber content of the vegetarian diet, some of the minerals, including zinc, may be less available to the body

FIGURE 7.11

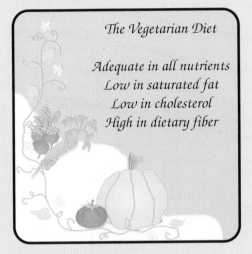

The Vegetarian Diet

Adequate in all nutrients
Low in saturated fat
Low in cholesterol
High in dietary fiber

(28,29). This is highly controversial however, and more research is needed to confirm this. Adults need 15 milligrams per day, on the average.

In addition to being nutritionally adequate, there are some distinct nutritional advantages to the vegetarian diet (see figure 7.11). For instance, in a review of the literature, dietary fiber intake was found to be 86 percent higher in vegetarians than nonvegetarians (30). Such a high fiber intake may be one reason vegetarians are leaner than nonvegetarians (31,32,33). Fewer Calories tend to be consumed when individuals eat foods high in dietary fiber.

Another advantage is that vegetarians eat less total fat, saturated fat, and cholesterol than nonvegetarians (34,35). These practices, along with the higher dietary fiber content of the diet, are greatly responsible for the lower blood-cholesterol levels of vegetarians that is reported in numerous studies (35,36,37).

Indeed, these nutritional advantages may explain the disease-prevention benefits of the vegetarian diet.

Disease Prevention

The American Dietetic Association (ADA) has published a position paper on the vegetarian diet. In this landmark paper, the ADA states that a growing body of scientific evidence supports the concept that vegetarians tend to have less heart disease, cancer, obesity, osteoporosis, and other diseases (21).

Much of the support for this connection between vegetarianism and prevention of disease comes from the Seventh-day Adventist Health Study. Seventh-day Adventists (SDA) are a unique group of people in that the majority do not smoke or drink alcohol, tea, and coffee. In addition, most do not eat meat.

Results from this twenty-year study show that vegetarian SDAs have considerably less incidence of specific diseases (see figure 7.12). Compared to the general population, SDAs show only 43 percent of the death rate for heart disease, 83 percent for breast cancer, 25 percent for lung cancer, 13 percent for cirrhosis of the liver, 49 percent for large-bowel cancers, 54 percent for uterine cancer, and 40 percent for diabetes (38). While some of this is related to the avoidance of tobacco and alcohol, evidence is increasing that restriction of meat along with the high consumption of plant foods also plays a major role.

Food Safety

Food poisoning prevention (another area of disease prevention), is certainly more acute. Recently, concern has been raised about the safety of using antibiotics in animal feed. According to the U.S. Food and Drug Administration, all turkeys, 80 percent of swine and veal, 60 percent of cattle, and 30 percent of chickens are raised on antibiotic-laced feed (39). These drugs are used to combat infection and promote growth.

This massive overuse of antibiotics on the farm is breeding strains of drug-resistant microorganisms (40,41). Several research studies have shown that commercially produced animal meats may be a path by which resistant bacteria reach humans, causing food poisoning (42,43,44). More studies are needed to confirm such a finding. However, the Food and Drug Administration is seeking to restrict the use of antibiotics in animal feed.

Fitness

Carbohydrate is the best fuel for the endurance athlete. It is present in large quantities in grains, potatoes, dried fruit, and other plant foods, but is virtually nonexistent in meat. Athletes who consume high amounts of carbohydrate have greater levels of muscle glycogen. **Glycogen** is the storage form of carbohydrate, which provides energy to the muscles. Storing greater amounts of muscle glycogen allows the athletes to exercise up to three times longer before becoming exhausted (45). For this reason, most endurance athletes today practice ''carbohydrate loading'' during hard training and before competitive events. Interestingly, eating a high-carbohydrate diet (70 percent) for the last three

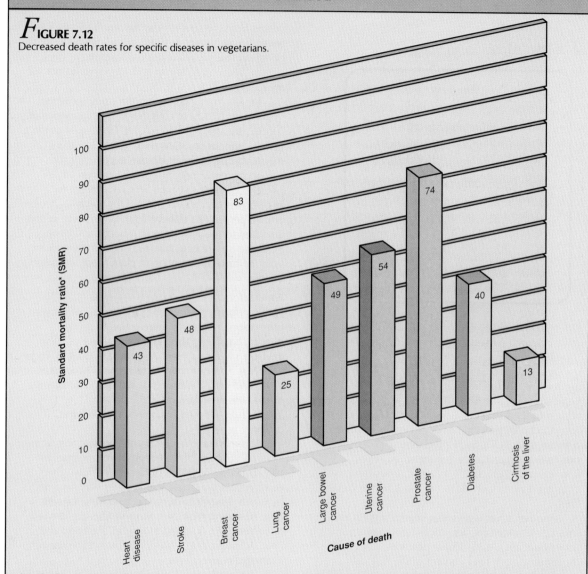

*F*IGURE 7.12

Decreased death rates for specific diseases in vegetarians.

days before an event has about the same effect. Vegetarians generally have a diet higher in complex carbohydrate than do meat eaters, which certainly does not hurt their performance (10,46).

In summary, the vegetarian diet provides all the necessary protein, minerals, and vitamins (with the exception of vitamin B_{12}) by combining a variety of wholesome foods. In addition, it also has some distinct advantages. Dietary fiber content is higher, and saturated fat, total fat, and cholesterol contents are lower than nonvegetarian diets. These qualities in part are responsible for less heart disease, cancer, obesity, diabetes, and other diseases. Furthermore, endurance performance is actually enhanced with high-carbohydrate intakes like those found in vegetarian diets. So, from a health standpoint, it may indeed be a good idea to say "please don't pass the meat" (see Health-Promotion Activity 7.3).

SUMMARY

1. Proteins are made up of 22 different amino acids, 9 of which are called essential because the body cannnot manufacture them. The other 13 are considered nonessential because the body can manufacture them if the diet contains them in adequate amounts.

2. DNA and RNA instruct the assembling of amino acids into a specific protein. However, all 22 amino acids are needed at the right time, in the right amount, and in the right proportions, or construction of a protein cannot occur.

3. The three main functions of proteins are providing structure, regulating body processes, and supplying energy.

4. Protein digestion begins in the stomach as acid denatures the three-dimensional structure of the protein and pepsin breaks the protein into polypeptides. Proteases further dismantle the polypeptides in the small intestine, where the resulting amino acids and dipeptides are absorbed into the bloodstream.

5. Once in the body, amino acids can be used to synthesize proteins, produce energy, or be stored as fat. The body must meet its energy needs first and will use protein for energy if there is not an adequate source of Calories from dietary carbohydrate or fat.

6. A protein food source is of good quality if it contains all 9 essential amino acids in the right amounts. Animal sources of protein usually do, and they are therefore considered a complete protein source. Plant protein sources are limiting in one or more of the essential amino acids and are called incomplete proteins. However, two incomplete plant proteins, like grains and legumes, can complement each other to form a complete protein.

7. Recommended protein intake for an individual can be calculated either by weight or by the percent of Calories eaten per day.

8. Although endurance athletes use some protein as fuel and muscle-building athletes need small amounts of extra protein during the initial muscle growth, a high-carbohydrate, low-fat diet is still the best nutrition for the athlete. Protein supplements and high-protein powders may cause poor performance as well as ill health.

9. Protein is readily available in the American diet. The best sources include lean animal sources such as fish, skinless chicken and turkey, and low-fat dairy products, and a wide variety of plant foods that include legumes and grains.

10. Millions of children die each year from two protein-deficiency diseases that still affect many third-world countries. Marasmus affects mainly infants who do not take in enough Calories, and kwashiorkor is caused by too little protein in the diet but adequate Calories.

11. Most Americans consume double the RDA for protein each day, which leads to several problems associated with such a high-protein intake. These include the consumption of fat that often accompanies animal sources of protein, dehydration, calcium loss, high blood-cholesterol levels, and obesity.

12. The vegetarian diet, when well planned, can meet the nutritional needs of all age groups. For vegans, vitamin B_{12} must be obtained through fortified foods or supplements. Vitamin D may also need to be supplemented for vegans who have limited exposure to sunlight.

13. A growing body of evidence suggests that vegetarians have less heart disease, diabetes, cancer, obesity, osteoporosis, and other chronic diseases.

REFERENCES

1. National Academy of Sciences (NAS). 1980. Recommended Dietary Allowances.
2. Laidlaw, S. A., and J. D. Kopple. 1987. Newer Concepts of the Indispensable Amino Acids. *American Journal of Clinical Nutrition* 46:593–605.
3. Young, V. R. 1987. Kinetics of Human Amino Acid Metabolism: Nutritional Implications and Some Lessons. 1987 McCollum Award Lecture. *American Journal of Clinical Nutrition* 46:709–25.
4. Anderson, L., et al. 1982. *Nutrition in Health and Disease*. Philadelphia: J. B. Lippincott Co.
5. Butkus, S. N., and L. K. Mahan. 1986. Food Allergies: Immunological Reactions to Food. *Journal of the American Dietetic Association* 86:601–8.
6. Worthington-Roberts, B. S. 1981. Proteins and Amino Acids. In *Contemporary Developments in Nutrition*. B. S. Worthington-Roberts, ed. St. Louis: The C. V. Mosby Co.
7. Stein, T. P. 1982. Nutrition and Protein Turnover: A Review. *Journal of Parenteral and Enteral Nutrition* 6: 444–54.
8. Young, V. R., and P. L. Pellet. 1987. Protein Intake and Requirements with Reference to Diet and Health. *American Journal of Clinical Nutrition* 45:1323–1343.
9. Pao, E. M., S. J. Mickle, and M. C. Burk. 1985. One-Day and Three-Day Nutrient Intakes by Individuals—Nationwide Food Consumption Survey Findings, Spring 1977. *Journal of the American Dietetic Association* 85 (3):313–16.
10. Pennington, J. A. T. 1986. Dietary Patterns and Practices. *Clinical Nutrition* 5:17–26.
11. Brotherhood, J. R. 1984. Nutrition and Sports Performance. *Sports Medicine* 1:350–89.
12. Lemon, P. W. R. 1987. Protein and Exercise: Update 1987. *Medicine and Science in Sports and Exercise* 19:s179–s190.
13. Williams, M. 1983. *Nutrition for Fitness and Sport*. Dubuque, Iowa: Wm. C. Brown Publishers.
14. Slavin, J. L., G. Lanners, and M. A. Engstrom. 1988. Amino Acid Supplements: Beneficial or Risky? *Physician and Sportsmedicine* 16 (3):221–24.

15. Short, S. H., and W. R. Short. 1983. Four-Year Study of University Athletes' Dietary Intake. *Journal of the American Dietetic Association* 82:632–45.
16. Parr, R. B., et al. 1984. Nutrition Knowledge and Practice of Coaches, Trainers, and Athletes. *Sports Medicine* 12:127–38.
17. Soloman, N. W. 1985. Rehabilitating the Severely Malnourished Infant and Child. *Journal of the American Dietetic Association* 85:1:28–36.
18. Spencer, H., and L. Kramer. 1986. Does a High Protein (Meat) Intake Affect Calcium Metabolism in Man? *Food and Nutrition News* 58 (2):11–13.
19. Carrol, K. K. 1985. Dietary Protein and Heart Disease. *Nutrition and the M.D.*, p. 3.
20. Kritchevsky, D. 1985. How Does Plant Protein Reduce Serum Cholesterol Levels? *Nutrition and the M.D.*, p. 3.
21. ADA Reports. 1988. Position of the American Dietetic Association: Vegetarian Diets. *Journal of the American Dietetic Association* 88 (3):351–55.
22. Crosby, W. H. 1975. Committee on Nutritional Misinformation, National Academy of Sciences. Can a Vegetarian Be Well Nourished? *Journal of the American Medical Association* 233:898.
23. Sanchez, A., J. A. Scharffenber, and U. D. Register. 1963. Nutritive Value of Selected Proteins and Protein Combinations. *American Journal of Clinical Nutrition* 13:243–49.
24. Hardinge, M. G., H. Crooks, and F. J. Stare. 1966. Nutritional Studies of Vegetarians: Proteins and Essential Amino Acids. *Journal of the American Dietetic Association* 48:25–27.
25. Register, U. D., et al. 1967. Nitrogen-Balance Studies in Human Subjects on Various Diets. *American Journal of Clinical Nutrition* 20:753–59.
26. Immerman, A. M. 1981. Vitamin B_{12} Status on a Vegetarian Diet: A Critical Review. *World Review of Nutrients in the Diet* 37:38–54.
27. Block, G., et al. 1985. Nutrient Sources in the American Diet: Quantitative Data from the NHANES II Survey. *American Journal of Epidemiology* 122:27–40.
28. Reinhold, J. G., B. Faradji, and F. Ismail-Beigi. 1975. Fiber vs. Phytate as Determinants of Availability of Calcium, Zinc, and Iron of Breadstuffs. *Nutrition Reports International* 12:75–85.
29. Oberleas, D., and B. F. Harland. 1977. Nutritional Agents Which Affect Metabolic Zinc Status. In *Zinc Metabolism. Current Aspects in Health and Disease.* A. S. Prasd, ed. New York: Alan R. Liss, Inc.
30. Calkins, B. M. 1984. The Consumption of Fiber in Vegetarians and Nonvegetarians: A Review. In *Handbook of Dietary Fiber and Nutrition.* G. Spiller, ed. Boca Raton: CRC Press.
31. Bergan, J. G., and P. T. Brown. 1980. Nutritional Status of "New" Vegetarians. *Journal of the American Dietetic Association* 76:151–55.
32. Ellis, F. R., and V. M. E. Montegriffo. 1970. Veganism, Clinical Findings and Investigations. *American Journal of Clinical Nutrition* 23:249–55.
33. Snowdon, D. A., and R. L. Phillips. 1984. Coffee Consumption and Risk of Fatal Cancer. *American Journal of Public Health* 74:820–23.
34. West, R. O., and O. B. Hayes. 1968. Diet and Serum Cholesterol Levels. *American Journal of Clinical Nutrition* 21:853–62.
35. Cooper, R., et al. 1984. Seventh-day Adventist Adolescents – Lifestyle Patterns and Cardiovascular Risk Factors. *Western Journal of Medicine* 140:471–77.
36. Kritchevsky, D., S. A. Tepper, and G. Goodman. 1984. Diet, Nutrition Intake, and Metabolism in Populations at High and Low Risk for Colon Cancer. *American Journal of Clinical Nutrition* 40:921–26.
37. Fonnebo, V. 1985. The Tromso Heart Study: Coronary Risk Factors in Seventh-day Adventists. *American Journal of Epidemiology* 122:789–93.
38. Phillips, R. L., and D. A. Snowdon. 1986. *Mortality among Seventh-day Adventists in Relation to Dietary Habits and Lifestyle. Evaluation of Plant Proteins: Application, Biologic Effect, Composition/Chemistry.* American Chemical Society.
39. Freifeld, K. 1985. Beef Stakes. *Health.* (April): 41–5.
40. Zuckerman, S. 1985. Massive Overuse of Antibiotics on the Farm. *Nutrition Action* (January/February):9–11.
41. FDA Staff. 1985. Feeding Animals Wonder Drugs and Creating Super Bugs. *FDA Consumer* (February): 14–16.
42. O'Brien, T., et al. 1982. Molecular Epidemiology of Antibiotic Resistance in Salmonella from Animals and Human Beings in the United States. *New England Journal of Medicine* 307:1–6.
43. Wells, J. G., and M. L. Cohen. 1984. Animal to Man Transmission of Antimicrobial-Resistant Salmonella: Investigations of U.S. Outbreaks, 1971–1983. *Science* 225:833–35.
44. Holmber, S., et al. 1984. Drug-Resistant Salmonella from Animals Fed Antimicrobials. *New England Journal of Medicine* 311:617.
45. Costill, D. L. 1985. Carbohydrate Nutrition Before, During, and After Exercise. *Federation Proceedings* 44:36–40.
46. Shultz, T. D., and J. E. Leklem. 1983. Dietary Status of Seventh-day Adventists and Nonvegetarians. *Journal of the American Dietetic Association* 83:27–32.

Is Fat Hiding in Your Protein?

1. List the foods that you consumed in the last 24 hours.

2. Estimate the percent of fat in the foods you ate, based on the protein sources listed in table 6.6, and write the percent next to each food. For example, if you've eaten pork chops, which are not listed, use the percent given for beef steak.

3. Now circle in your list any protein source that contains more than 50 percent of its Calories as fat.

4. Based on table 7.7, list three substitutions that you would be willing to make in a day's menu to reduce your fatty protein sources.

Are You Getting Enough or Too Much Protein?

1. Record everything you eat for one day. Make sure that you include the portion sizes. Use the food composition table in Appendix B to determine the grams of protein.

Food	Amount	Protein(g)

2. Add up your total protein intake for the day, and write it in the blank below.

_____ grams

3. How does your protein intake compare to the RDA for protein listed in table 7.4.
RDA for protein,
listed in table 7.4:

_____ grams

4. What are two disadvantages or negative consequences of your current protein consumption?

5. List two things you could do to adjust your protein intake to promote your own health.

1. In this activity your task is to create a vegetarian meal for three dinner guests. Review the chapter to see how to complement proteins, and skim some cookbooks for ideas. List the general meal plan for dinner.

2. Write a recipe for the main entree, including the grams of protein in each ingredient.

Ingredient	Amount	Protein (g)

3. Is there adequate protein in your entree? Compare the protein in your meal to one-third of your daily recommendation. How does it compare?

Protein for meal = _____ grams

$RDA \div 3 =$ _____ grams

4. Vegetarian meals can be healthier if prepared with low-fat products. Have you added eggs or whole-milk dairy products, which will increase the fat content of your vegetarian meals? If so, go back and replace them with lower-fat alternatives.

5. Name two possible vegetarian meals that you could add to your menu this week.

8

Energy Balance

INTRODUCTION

I just don't feel like I have any energy today! Energy is a commodity that we talk about quite frequently, almost as if we could go out and buy it or get it from a pill. Some foods are actually promoted as "energy foods." B-vitamins and iron are marketed for their energizing effects. However, how we feel is not necessarily the best indicator of energy balance in our bodies.

Energy balance is determined by two factors: Calories that enter the body and energy that is used by the body. This chapter provides an overview of the energy equation and the factors that influence it, as well as methods to determine imbalances in the energy equation.

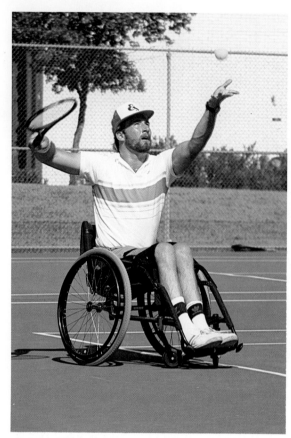

Whether physical or mental, everything humans do requires energy.

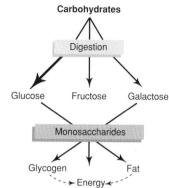

IGURE 8.1

Monosaccharides supply energy and are stored as glycogen and fat.

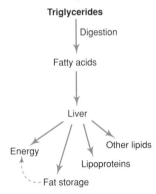

IGURE 8.2

Fatty acids can be used by the liver for energy production, stored as fat, or used to synthesize other lipids.

Food as Fuel

Everything humans do, whether physical or mental, requires energy. Humans both consume and expend energy, and this consumption and expenditure can be expressed in Calories. The major sources of these Calories are carbohydrate, fat, and protein. Let's review how these three components of food yield energy.

Carbohydrate

Carbohydrate is the main energy nutrient. During digestion, large carbohydrate molecules are broken down into monosaccharides. The predominant end product of this digestion is glucose. Glucose is absorbed into the body and then circulated through the blood supply to several locations. The first priority of newly absorbed glucose is to replenish the blood glucose, which must remain within certain stable values. (Recall that blood glucose may be depleted due to energy expenditure.)

After the blood glucose has been replenished, any excess glucose is stored as glycogen in muscle or the liver for later use. (Glycogen is converted back to glucose for energy use.) Any glucose that remains after blood glucose and glycogen stores have been filled is converted to fat for long-term energy storage (see figure 8.1).

Fat

Fat is potentially a tremendous fuel source, providing nine Calories per gram, or twice as much as either carbohydrate or protein. Triglycerides (fat) are made up of three fatty acids attached to a glycerol molecule. When fat is needed for energy, the fatty acids are broken away from the glycerol during digestion and are released into the bloodstream. All body cells use fat for fuel except those in the brain and nervous tissue, and red blood cells, which require glucose (see figure 8.2).

FIGURE 8.3

Amino acids can be used to make proteins and glucose used for energy, or stored as fat.

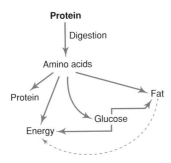

Protein

Protein, although best utilized as a building material, can also be used for energy (see figure 8.3). When glucose is not available, the body will begin to convert protein to energy. Protein used for fuel is first stripped of its nitrogen-containing amine groups. Some of the amino acids will be converted to glucose, which can be used by tissues that cannot use fatty acids for energy. Other amino acids will be broken down for energy in a manner similar to fatty acids. In either of these cases, reconversion back to protein is not possible.

The main function of protein is *not* for use as fuel for energy. However, when caloric intake is inadequate, energy needs have a higher priority, and protein will be used for energy production if necessary. If excess protein is consumed, it will be converted to fat.

Energy Resources

Carbohydrate, fat, and protein are all potential energy sources, but they are not used equally. As mentioned before, carbohydrate and fat are preferred energy sources for the body. Table 8.1 shows the amount of energy stored in various forms in the body (1).

Carbohydrate is found in the body in the form of glucose or glycogen. Glucose is the main transportation form of carbohydrate and is found in the blood. About 20 grams, or 80 Calories, of glucose can be found in the blood and interstitial fluids at any given time. Glycogen is the storage form of carbohydrate and can quickly be broken down into glucose when needed. Approximately 85 grams, or 350 Calories, of glycogen is found in the liver; 350 grams, or 1,450 Calories, of glycogen is found in muscle. This

TABLE 8.1

Substrate stores in normal male

Fuel	Weight (kg)	Energy (kcal)
Circulating Fuels		
Glucose	.020	80
Free fatty acids	.0004	4
Triglycerides	.004	40
Total		124
Tissue Stores		
Fat		
Adipose	15.0	140,000
Intramuscular	.3	2,800
Protein (muscle)	10.0	41,000
Glycogen		
Liver	.085	350
Muscle	.350	1,450
TOTAL		185,600

From D. C. Nieman, *The Sports Medicine Fitness Course.* © 1986. Bull Publishing Co., Palo Alto, CA. Reprinted by permission.

adds up to approximately 1,800 Calories of carbohydrate that is available to the body. (The actual amount depends on an individual's body size, sex, muscle mass, and current physical fitness level, as well as the type of diet consumed.)

The storage of fat is much greater than carbohydrate. The average college-age male is 15 percent body fat, and the average college-age female is 25 percent body fat. This means that a 160-pound male, for example, would be carrying about 24 pounds of fat. Since human fat tissue has 3,500 Calories per pound, this male would have 84,000 Calories of fat in storage. In that the average male expends 100 Calories per mile of running, this would represent enough energy from fat to run 840 miles!

Protein, as was already explained, does not significantly contribute to the energy supply unless carbohydrate and fat are unavailable. The body does contain about 15 percent of its weight as protein.

Metabolic processes in the body must transform the chemical energy that is stored in food sources into other forms that the body needs to perform its work. Some of the energy released by these processes is used to produce **adenosine triphosphate (ATP),** which in turn is broken down to release energy needed by all the cells in the body. ATP is a complex compound that is held together by high-energy bonds. When these bonds are broken, energy is released rapidly for body processes like muscle

Formation of ATP in anaerobic glycolysis. Only small amounts of ATP can be generated without oxygen.

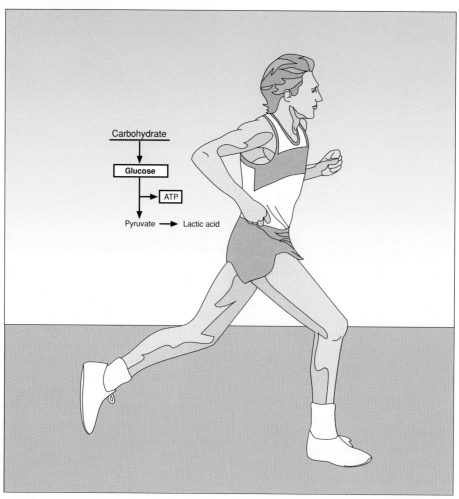

contraction. ATP can be used up very quickly (within seconds), which is why it is important to have adequate energy stores available to produce more ATP. ATP can be formed from carbohydrate, fat, or protein.

Energy Production

Metabolism is the collective term for all the processes in the body that involve energy transformation. There are two types of metabolic processes that produce energy.

The first of these is the **anaerobic system,** or **anaerobic glycolysis** (see figure 8.4). In this process, glucose or glycogen is broken down through a series of reactions to form lactic acid. Energy in the form of ATP is

produced. The advantage of this system is that it can occur without oxygen. For instance, the energy needed to sprint a short distance is usually derived from this system.

Only about five percent of the total ATP production occurs through this pathway; thus its capacity is limited. Moreover, lactic acid quickly builds up in muscles during anaerobic glycolysis, leading to fatigue. The increased acidity of the lactic acid may also inhibit the enzymes that normally function in muscle cells.

The **aerobic system,** or **oxygen system,** is the other pathway that yields energy for body processes. In the presence of oxygen, glycogen, blood glucose, triglycerides, and amino acids may all be ultimate sources of ATP

FIGURE 8.5

Formation of ATP from fat, carbohydrate, and protein via the aerobic system of metabolism.

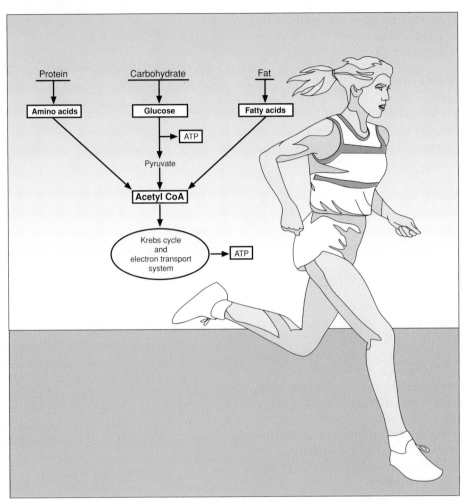

production in the aerobic system. The major advantage of this system is that large quantities of ATP can be produced from energy sources in the body. This system is depicted in figure 8.5.

Glucose may enter the aerobic system through **aerobic glycolysis.** In this pathway glucose is broken down to form pyruvate, which is then converted to acetyl CoA. Next, acetyl CoA enters **Krebs cycle,** a series of events in oxidative energy production that yield large quantities of ATP. The waste products of this system are water and carbon dioxide (which is expired during respiration).

Triglycerides and amino acids can also enter Krebs cycle, but they must use other metabolic pathways before they are in the appropriate form to enter. Triglycerides, in particular,

are an enormous source of stored energy that can be metabolized in Krebs cycle. However, when triglycerides are utilized in Krebs cycle, small amounts of carbohydrate must accompany them, or serious complications may result. For instance, diets that are very low in carbohydrate do not contain sufficient amounts of carbohydrate to assist in the metabolism of triglycerides in the Krebs cycle. This results in the incomplete metabolism of these triglycerides in which triglyceride (fat) fragments known as ketone bodies are produced.

Normally, small amounts of ketone bodies are removed from the body in urine. If the ketone bodies accumulate, however, a condition known as **ketoacidosis,** or ketosis, will result. Ketoacidosis can lead to dehydration when the body tries to eliminate the excess ketones by increasing urine output. In addition, ketoacidosis causes the body fluids to become more acidic, and can be fatal. Individuals on diets with less than 100 grams of carbohydrate per day are prone to ketosis.

Energy Value of Foods

There are four nutrients that can be used to produce energy. Carbohydrate and protein each supply four Calories per gram; fat supplies nine Calories per gram; and alcohol supplies seven Calories per gram. Other nutrients, such as vitamins and minerals, help the body to extract energy but do not provide Calories. The Calories in food represent a form of potential energy that our bodies can use to produce heat and work.

Factors Affecting Energy Input

Many external and internal factors affect energy input. Let's examine three: hunger, appetite, and choice of food.

Hunger

Hunger, or internal regulation, is one of the most basic physiological reasons for eating. There are two major theories about what controls hunger. One theory states that the brain has centers that detect the levels of circulating nutrients, hormones, and neurotransmitters, and that these centers respond by making a person feel either hunger or satisfaction. The second theory suggests that the liver is responsible for monitoring circulating nutrients and metabolites and for triggering nerve impulses that stimulate or depress hunger.

Several other mechanisms are related to the control of hunger. Stomach distension, or **satiety,** the feeling of fullness and satisfaction, seems to decrease hunger. High-fiber diets create such a sensation and induce satiety at lower energy intakes (2). Physical activity also plays a role in the regulation of food intake (3). For example, walking briskly for an hour will actually decrease a person's appetite.

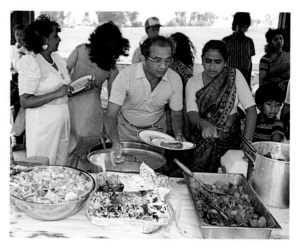
Tempting foods can influence an individual's energy intake.

Appetite

Appetite is the term used for the nonphysiological, or external, regulation of eating. External influences that shape our eating behavior include psychological factors, environmental factors, food accessibility, and food characteristics. These were thoroughly discussed in chapter 1. Although it may seem odd, the same factors that cause some people to lose their appetite will cause an increase in appetite for others. For example, tension and stress lead some individuals to eat or drink, whereas others may feel sick and not care to eat at all. Some experts believe that these nonphysiological factors may have more impact on what and when we eat than does hunger itself (4). (See Health Promotion Activity 8.1.)

Choice of Food

What people choose to eat has an impact on their energy input. For instance, foods that are high in fiber and water tend to have less Calories per unit than foods that are high in fat. This concept is known as the Caloric density of foods. Foods that have a low Caloric density will usually be more filling than high Caloric density foods (see Health-Promotion Activity 8.2).

Factors Affecting Energy Output

The amount of energy the body uses each day is dependent on three factors: basal metabolic rate, physical activity, and thermogenesis (5).

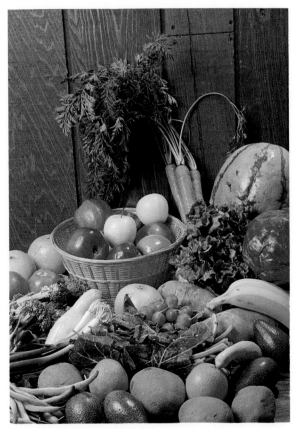
Increase your consumption of low-Calorie density foods, which are low in Calories and high in nutrients.

Basal Metabolic Rate

The **basal metabolic rate (BMR)** represents the energy expended by the body to maintain life and normal body functions. This includes the maintenance-level functioning of the heart, lungs, brain, liver, kidney, and nervous system. It is measured with an instrument called a respirometer, which measures the amount of oxygen consumed and carbon dioxide expired from the lungs of an individual who is lying down quietly. The amount of oxygen consumed is proportional to the energy being used.

Numerous factors influence BMR (6). Males tend to have higher rates than females of the same age and size; those with greater muscle mass have a higher BMR; as body temperature increases, BMR increases; and as levels of certain hormones like thyroxine, epinephrine, or growth hormone increase, so does BMR. Aging actually decreases BMR by about two percent per decade after age 20. This decrease is mostly attributable to the loss of lean body mass due to declining activity patterns as people age.

Surprisingly, BMR accounts for the largest number of Calories expended by an individual each day. A 154-pound male uses 60–75 percent of his total daily energy expenditure on BMR—that's 1,500 Calories per day. An individual's BMR is roughly equivalent to one Calorie of energy per kilogram of body weight per hour. For a 50 kg female that would be 1 Calorie times 50 kg times 24 hours, or 1,200 Calories per day. (See Health Promotion Activity 8.3.)

Physical Activity

While most people expend the majority of their Calories on BMR, physical activity also contributes to the total daily energy expenditure. Just how many Calories are expended on activity can vary greatly (see table 8.2). The average sedentary person expends only about 25 percent of his or her total Caloric intake on physical activity, or only about 500 to 800 Calories in one day! Top athletes, on the other hand, may use as much as 1,500 Calories per day for physical activity in addition to BMR.

Note in table 8.2 that **aerobic activities** (using large muscle groups in continuous exercise for long periods), tend to use more energy. Aerobic activities include jogging, bicycling, aerobic dancing, and cross-country skiing. (See the Health-Promotion Insight at the end of the chapter for help with designing an aerobic exercise program.)

Conversely, anaerobic activities, such as weight lifting, do not use as much energy as aerobic activities. Spontaneous activity is emerging as an important factor in the energy balance equation. This includes activities like climbing the stairs, walking to work, and mowing the lawn with a human-powered lawn mower, which may account for up to 900 Calories of energy per day (5).

Thermogenesis

In addition to using energy for BMR and physical activity, the body also uses energy for thermogenesis. Thermogenesis is the production of body heat in response to food intake and in the nonshivering response to cold.

Heat is produced when the food we eat is digested, absorbed, transported, metabolized, and stored. This is known as diet-induced thermogenesis (DIT), or the **thermic effect of food (TEF).** Between 6–10 percent of the energy a person consumes will be used in this manner (6).

TABLE 8.2

Activities that rate high in cardiovascular-respiratory benefits and their approximate energy expenditures

Summarized below are some of the better cardiovascular-respiratory exercises and the number of kcal expended per hour of the exercise. An important concept is to select several of these activities that are enjoyable, and to use them in such a way that scheduled exercise sessions are looked forward to, not dreaded.

Activity	Kcal per Hour
Badminton, competitive singles	480
Basketball	360–660
Bicycling	
10 mph	420
11 mph	480
12 mph	600
13 mph	660
Calisthenics, heavy	600
Handball, competitive	660
Rope skipping, vigorous	800
Rowing machine	840
Running	
5 mph	600
6 mph	750
7 mph	870
8 mph	1,020
9 mph	1,130
10 mph	1,285
Skating, ice or roller, rapid	700
Skiing, downhill, vigorous	600
Skiing, cross-country	
2.5 mph	560
4 mph	600
5 mph	700
8 mph	1,020
Swimming, 25–50 yards per min.	360–750
Walking	
Level road, 4 mph (fast)	420
Upstairs	600–1,080
Uphill, 3.5 mph	480–900
Gardening, much lifting, stooping, digging	500
Mowing, pushing hand mower	450
Sawing hardwood	600
Shoveling, heavy	660
Wood chopping	560

Caloric consumption is based on a 150-pound person. There is a ten percent increase in caloric consumption for each fifteen pounds over this weight, and a ten percent decrease for each fifteen pounds under.

From D. C. Nieman, *The Sports Medicine Fitness Course.* © 1986. Bull Publishing Co., Palo Alto, CA. Reprinted by permission.

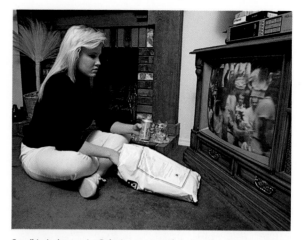

Small imbalances in Calories can result in weight changes. Just a twelve-ounce soft drink per day at 100 Calories may result in a ten-pound gain in weight over a one-year period if energy output remained the same.

The body also produces heat in response to cold. For example, hibernating animals maintain their body temperature despite the cold environment. Human infants are also able to do this, although to a much lesser extent. This ability may be due to the presence of brown fat. Brown fat differs from the usual yellow fat in that it contains more mitochondria, the energy-producing bodies of the cell. These extra mitochondria generate more heat by burning more fuel, thus keeping the body warm. The extent to which adults have brown fat, if any, is still being studied (7).

The Balancing Act

In order for most individuals to maintain a certain weight over a period of time, energy input must equal energy output. This sounds simple, but actually it is quite complex because small imbalances can lead to large weight gains or losses over time. For example, suppose a person drinks one extra soft drink per day for a year. Assuming that energy expenditure stays constant and the soft drink contains 100 Calories, the person will gain about ten pounds in the course of the year.

$$\begin{array}{r} 100 \text{ Calories} \\ \times\, 365 \text{ days per year} \\ \hline 36{,}500 \text{ Calories per year} \end{array}$$

$$3{,}500 \text{ Calories} = 1 \text{ pound}$$

$$\frac{36{,}500 \text{ Calories/year}}{3{,}500 \text{ Calories/pound}} = 10.4 \text{ pounds}$$

Body composition of a reference male and female.

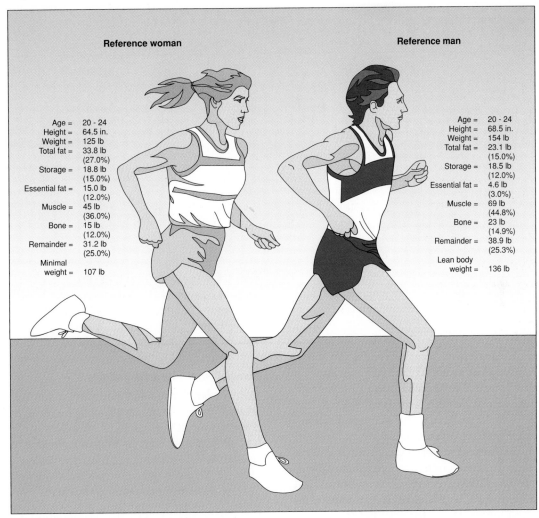

Reference woman		Reference man	
Age =	20 - 24	Age =	20 - 24
Height =	64.5 in.	Height =	68.5 in.
Weight =	125 lb	Weight =	154 lb
Total fat =	33.8 lb (27.0%)	Total fat =	23.1 lb (15.0%)
Storage =	18.8 lb (15.0%)	Storage =	18.5 lb (12.0%)
Essential fat =	15.0 lb (12.0%)	Essential fat =	4.6 lb (3.0%)
Muscle =	45 lb (36.0%)	Muscle =	69 lb (44.8%)
Bone =	15 lb (12.0%)	Bone =	23 lb (14.9%)
Remainder =	31.2 lb (25.0%)	Remainder =	38.9 lb (25.3%)
Minimal weight =	107 lb	Lean body weight =	136 lb

Most people measure these imbalances by differences in their weight over time. This method is useful, but other methods of determining energy balance are better in relation to health.

Body Composition Assessment

Body composition refers to body fat and lean body mass. Body fat consists of essential fat (which is necessary in the structure of various cells and for protection of some internal organs), and storage fat (a depot for excess Calories). Lean body mass consists of all tissues other than fat, including bone, teeth, muscle, heart, liver, and other organs (see figure 8.6).

Body weight is often confused with body fat. For example, a valuable player from a West-Coast pro football team suffered needlessly because his coach confused weight with fatness. The player was 5′10″ and weighed 285 pounds, and he was being fined for being overweight, in accordance with team policy. Because this particular player was relatively short, his coach assumed that he weighed too much for that height. For about a year the distraught player tried unsuccessfully to lose weight. Finally, a university that was carrying on a research program on the relationship of fat and physical performance analyzed the body fat content of each team member. A sophisticated method, underwater weighing, was used.

TABLE 8.3
1983 Metropolitan height and weight tables

Height Feet	Inches	Men Small Frame	Medium Frame	Large Frame
5	1	123–129	126–136	133–145
5	2	125–131	128–138	135–148
5	3	127–133	130–140	137–151
5	4	129–135	132–143	139–155
5	5	131–137	134–146	141–159
5	6	133–140	137–149	144–163
5	7	135–143	140–152	147–167
5	8	137–146	143–155	150–171
5	9	139–149	146–158	153–175
5	10	141–152	149–161	156–179
5	11	144–155	152–165	159–183
6	0	147–159	155–169	163–187
6	1	150–163	159–173	167–192
6	2	153–167	162–177	171–197
6	3	157–171	166–182	176–202

To the utter amazement of everyone, it was determined that the 285-pound player was only two percent fat! This is an astonishingly low amount, considering that the average college-age male is fifteen percent fat. His coach stopped fining him, the player stopped dieting, and with the advice of researchers, he gained weight to 325 pounds. This gave him a more normal fat content, and he found that he felt stronger and performed better on the football field.

Although low body fat is more the exception than the norm in the U.S., this incident does show the importance of looking at the quality (body composition) of weight, not just the quantity. A variety of methods have been developed to assess body composition, some relatively simple and others rather complex. Theoretically, all techniques are designed to measure the amount of fat mass on an individual's body, relative to the amount of lean body weight. The simpler techniques give a rough estimation of body fatness, whereas more sophisticated methods give an accurate body-fat percent.

Height and Weight Tables

Many organizations have established height and weight tables from large sample sizes of our population. In table 8.3 are examples of the typical height and weight charts from the Metropolitan Life Insurance Company. Released in 1983, these were derived from data of more than four million people from 26 insurance companies. Note that the table is divided into small, medium, and large frame sizes. While it is tempting for everyone to claim to have a large frame, only about 25 percent of the population have a large frame. Twenty-five percent have a small frame, and 50 percent have a medium frame (8). A method to estimate frame size, which involves measuring elbow width, can be found in table 8.4.

A number of limitations in using the 1983 Metropolitan Life Insurance Tables should be noted. The weights for height in the 1983 tables are 2–13 percent higher than in the tables published by the same company in 1959 (9). The upward revisions are not uniformly distributed through the height categories, however, with the largest increases being for shorter men and women. Also, these tables lead one to believe it is healthy or desirable to be in the weight range

| Height | | Women | | |
Feet	Inches	Small Frame	Medium Frame	Large Frame
4	9	98–108	106–118	115–128
4	10	100–110	108–120	117–131
4	11	101–112	110–123	119–134
5	0	103–115	112–126	122–137
5	1	105–118	115–129	125–140
5	2	108–121	118–132	128–141
5	3	111–124	121–135	131–148
5	4	114–127	124–138	134–152
5	5	117–130	127–141	137–156
5	6	120–133	130–144	140–160
5	7	123–136	133–147	143–164
5	8	126–139	136–150	146–167
5	9	129–142	139–153	149–170
5	10	132–145	142–156	152–173
5	11	133–148	145–159	155–176

These weight ranges show weights in pounds at ages 25–29 based on lowest mortality.
Tables have been adjusted to represent weight without clothes and height without shoes.

From 1983 Metropolitan weight tables. Courtesy of the Metropolitan Life Insurance Company.

of a stated category, when actually the tables are just average weights for a particular group of Americans. Americans happen to be among the most overweight people in the world, so it is not necessarily healthy to weigh what an average American weighs!

The height and weight tables are also based on a very specific population–those who purchased nongroup life insurance (10). Minorities are underrepresented, as are the elderly and those with low incomes. Therefore, it is difficult to apply this data to the general population. Furthermore, although the table is divided into frame sizes, they were not actually measured in the population originally studied. Basing tables solely on mortality also ignores the nonfatal risks of increased weight, such as decreased mobility, difficulty in breathing, and social stigmas (9).

Finally, there are individual differences in muscularity, for which the charts do not make provision. (Our football-player friend would be about 100 pounds "overweight," according to the tables, yet he is perfectly healthy considering how little fat he actually has.) On the other hand, many people with small muscle mass can step on the scale and be "underweight" according to the charts, and yet they have too much fat.

TABLE 8.4
How to determine body frame by elbow breadth

	Height	Elbow Breadth
Men	61–62''	2½–2⅞
	63–66	2⅝–2⅞
	67–70	2¾–3
	71–74	2¾–3⅛
	75	2⅞–3¼
Women	57–58''	2¼–2½
	59–62	2¼–2½
	63–66	2⅜–2⅝
	67–70	2⅜–2⅝
	71	2½–2¾

To measure elbow breadth, extend the arm, and then bend the forearm upwards at a 90 degree angle, fingers straight up, palm turned toward the body. Measure with a sliding caliper the width between the two prominent bones on either side of the elbow (measure the widest point). Make sure the arm is positioned correctly, and that the upper arm is parallel to the ground. The elbow breadth frame gauge is available from: Metropolitan Life Insurance Company, Health and Safety Education Division, One Madison Avenue, New York, NY 10160 ($5).

Basic data from I. Hanes. Courtesy of the Metropolitan Life Insurance Company.

As you can see, the charts are at best a rough guideline for desirable weights. What really matters is an individual's body composition.

FIGURE 8.7

Nomogram for body mass index (kg/m²). Weights and heights are without clothing. The ratio weight height² (metric units) is read from the central scale after a straight edge is placed between height and body weight.

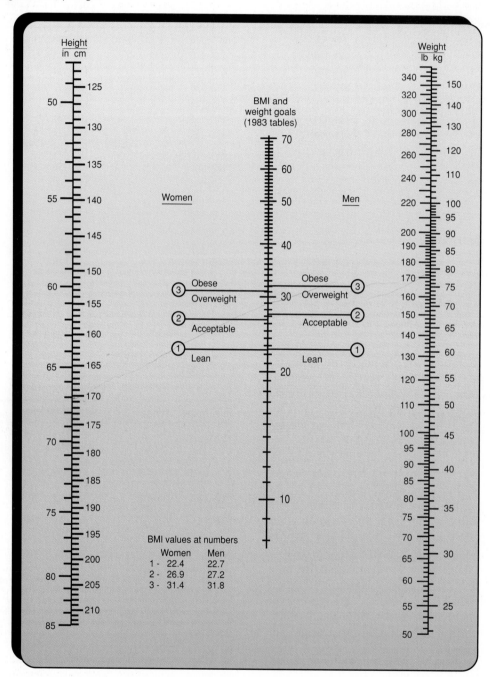

Body Mass Index

Scientists have suggested several ratios between height and weight as possible standards for ideal weight. One of these, the **Body Mass Index (BMI),** correlates well with more sophisticated measures of body fat (12). BMI is body weight in kilograms divided by height in meters squared (13). Figure 8.7 shows a special chart, called a nomogram, which converts an individual's height and weight to BMI and compares BMI to population data.

Tape Measurements

Often, the first indication that a person has put on some extra fat is that clothes begin to fit more snugly or that an extra notch is needed in the belt. As individuals gain fat, however, they may weigh the same amount. Fat is not as compact as muscle; it "fits" more loosely, so a person may gain inches but not weight.

A tape measure can be used for a more precise measure of body fat than clothes or belts. The procedure is to measure the circumference of selected sites on the body. The tape measure is also useful to measure changes in fat with either weight loss or gain. A tape measure will often reveal changes in body composition before the scale indicates any change. Tape measures, however, are still a crude measure of body fat percentage.

Skinfold Measurements

The most widely used method for determining obesity is based on the thickness of skinfolds. The calipers used to determine skinfold thickness are fairly inexpensive, and the measurements are obtained quickly, accurately, and easily (13).

Approximately one-half of the body's fat is stored beneath the skin and is called subcutaneous fat. The skinfold caliper measures the thickness of the subcutaneous fat layer at various sites on the body (12,13). These measurements are then used to estimate total body fat. The skin and fat are pulled away from the muscle by firmly grasping the thumb and forefinger, and the caliper is placed over the middle portion of that fold to measure the thickness.

Figure 8.8 demonstrates the technique on the triceps. The triceps measurement is taken midway between the top of the shoulder and the elbow, on the back of the arm. The arm is relaxed and held vertically, with the fold being measured running parallel to the length of the arm. New norms have been developed to help in the interpretation of the one-site triceps measurement (see table 8.5). Two measurements should be taken on the right arm, and if they are the same, this is satisfactory.

FIGURE 8.8

Body composition testing (triceps). The skinfolds should be firmly grasped by thumb and forefinger and pulled away from the body. Each site should first be measured and then marked with a black, felt-tip pen. The location of triceps is midway between the acromion and olecranon processes. The measurement of triceps skinfold is the vertical fold on the posterior midline. Each site should be measured two to five times until a consistent reading within one millimeter is obtained. Keep the caliper heads slightly away from the thumb and forefinger. Measure a true double fold of skin, avoiding the "flare." All measurements are on the right side (for reliability).

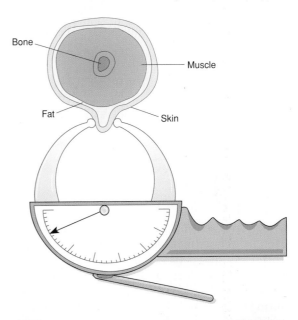

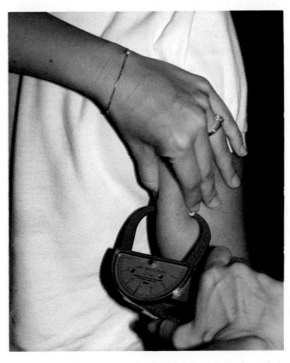

TABLE 8.5
Triceps skinfold norms (percentiles of triceps skinfold thicknesses [mm] by age group and sex)

Males					
Percentiles	*5*	*15*	*50*	*85*	*95*
Age group					
18–24	4	5	8	13	16
25–34	4	6	10	15	17
35–44	5	6	11	15	18
45–54	5	7	10	15	18
55–64	5	7	10	15	17
65–74	4	6	10	14	16
Females					
Percentiles	*5*	*15*	*50*	*85*	*95*
Age group					
18–24	9	11	17	23	26
25–34	10	13	20	26	29
35–44	12	15	22	29	32
45–54	12	16	24	31	33
55–64	12	16	24	31	33
65–74	11	15	22	29	31

From D. C. Nieman, *The Sports Medicine Fitness Course*, © 1986. Bull Publishing Co., Palo Alto, CA. Reprinted by permission.

Underwater Weighing

Underwater weighing is one of the most widely used laboratory methods of measuring body fat. This technique is based on the fact that muscle and bones are more dense than water, whereas fat is less dense. No one wants to be a "floater" during this test, because muscles and bones sink, and fat rises to the top of the water. Therefore, the more a person weighs under water, the leaner he or she is. Weight under water reflects density, and this measurement is used in a mathematical equation to estimate body fat (14).

Underwater weighing is one of the most accurate ways to measure body fat, but it is also expensive. A pool, autopsy scale, and underwater chair are needed (see figure 8.9).

Bioelectrical Impedance

Several articles have appeared in the literature evaluating the effectiveness of bioelectrical impedance in assessing body fat. The equipment is portable, computerized, rapid, safe,

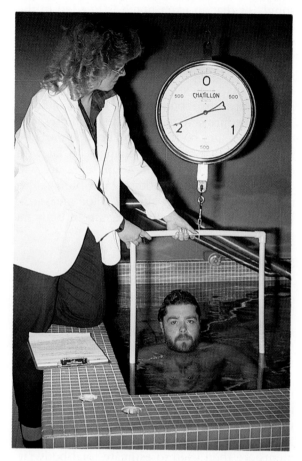

FIGURE 8.9
Underwater weighing is a sophisticated method of assessing body fat.

noninvasive, and convenient to use (15). The subject lies on a table, with the limbs not touching the body. Current-injector electrodes are placed on the right hand and right foot. A harmless electric current is generated and passed through the subject.

The water compartment of the body is a conductor of electricity, whereas fat does not conduct electricity. The total body water is detected as shifts in electrical conductance or impedance. Once total body water is known, various formulas can be used to calculate lean and fat weights. Bioelectrical impedance appears promising as a method of body fat measurement for overall accuracy, cost, and simplicity (16,17).

TABLE 8.6
Percent body-fat norms

Classification	Male	Female
Lean	<8%	<15%
Healthy	8–15%	15–22%
Plump	16–19%	23–27%
Fat	20–24%	28–33%
Obese (overfat)	>24%	>33%

Note: Average college male = 12–15%; average college female = 22–25%

From D. C. Nieman, *The Sports Medicine Fitness Course.* © 1986. Bull Publishing Co., Palo Alto, CA. Reprinted by permission.

TABLE 8.7
Athletic norms for body-fat percent

Type of Athlete	Male	Female
Elite runners	4–9%	6–15%
Wrestlers	4–10%	–
Gymnasts	4–10%	10–17%
Body builders	6–10%	10–17%
Elite swimmers	5–11%	14–24%
Basketball	7–11%	18–27%
Canoers/kayakers	11–15%	18–24%
Tennis	14–17%	19–22%

From D. C. Nieman, *The Sports Medicine Fitness Course.* © 1986. Bull Publishing Co., Palo Alto, CA. Reprinted by permission.

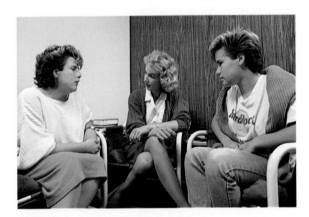

Classification

Many research studies have been conducted to find the average body-fat percentage of Americans. Once again, the aim is for an optimal body fat, *not* just average. Table 8.6 classifies the percent body fat from lean to obese. For men, a body fat less than 15 percent is considered healthy, and above 24 percent is obese. Women are allowed more fat because they carry more essential fat in breast tissue and other organs that have reproductive function. For females, up to 22 percent body fat is considered healthy, and above 33 percent is obese. Averages and athletic norms have been included in table 8.7 for comparison purposes (18,19).

After assessing an individual's body-fat content, the formula in figure 8.10 can help to determine a desirable weight. Chapter 9 suggests methods to change body composition.

FIGURE 8.10

Counseling for a Healthy Body Composition

To determine desirable weight, use this formula:

$$\text{Desired weight} = \frac{\text{Present lean body weight}}{100\% - \text{Desired fat }\%}$$

Example:

$$\frac{108}{100\% - 20\%} = \frac{108}{.8} = 135$$

For example:
Woman - Age = 35
Height = 5'8"
Weight = 150 lbs

1. Data
Body fat % = 28%
Fat weight = 42 lbs
Lean body weight = 108 lbs
Classification = fat (see table 8.6)

2. Discuss previous history of weight, successes, trends, failures, what she likes for herself. Determine a fat %, based on this history, that she desires. This woman desired 20 - 22%, which in the above formula worked out to be 135 - 138.5 lbs. Needed to lose 11 - 15 lbs of fat (not weight).

3. Discuss what it takes to lose fat. Help them set realistic eating and exercising habits (see chapter 9).

The Fitness Explosion

Since the publication of Dr. Kenneth H. Cooper's book *Aerobics* in 1968, more than sixty million Americans have started running, swimming, cycling, and walking their way to better health (15). Despite this fact, only 20 percent of the U.S. adult population are exercising appropriately; 40 percent are completely sedentary (20). People of lower socioeconomic status, Southerners, people in cities and the country (as opposed to people in the suburbs), and the elderly are all underrepresented in the exercising population (21). Thus, the basic criteria for designing an effective cardiovascular or aerobic exercise program will be discussed. Aerobic exercise is beneficial in two ways: it increases the ability to take in oxygen and use the oxygen efficiently, and it improves the quality of body composition (12).

Designing an Aerobic Exercise Program

Generally increasing any type of activity, whether walking to the store, gardening, or taking the stairs rather than the elevator, is beneficial for increasing energy output. However, aerobic-type activities are particularly good for this purpose.

Aerobic activities are those that involve the major muscle groups being in continuous movement for sufficient periods of time. Examples are running, jogging, swimming, cross-country skiing, and bicycling. (Activities during which you stop, such as tennis or basketball, are not considered to be aerobic.) The American College of Sports Medicine has designed guidelines for aerobic programs, which include the prescription for frequency, intensity, and time of an aerobic exercise. These are called the FIT guidelines (see figure 8.11).

*F*IGURE 8.11

Guidelines for Aerobic Exercise Prescription

Factor (Think fit)		Low	Average	High
F	Frequency (days/wk)	3	3–4	5 +
I	Intensity			

Age range	10 - second pulse count
20–24	27
25–29	26
30–34	25–26
35–39	25
40–44	25
45–49	24–25
50–54	24
55–59	23–24
60–64	23
65–69	22–23

		Low	Average	High
T	Time (continuous min./workout)	20	30–45	30–60
	Mode examples (plus other continuous, rhythmical activities like swimming, cycling, skating, skiiing, etc.)	Brisk walking	Walk/jog	Running

Days/time you plan to exercise
(allow 1 hour for warmup, exercise, cool down, and calisthenics)

Sun.	Mon.	Tues.	Wed.	Thurs.	Fri.	Sat.
___ AM/PM	___ AM/PM	___ AM/PM	___ AM/PM	___ AM/PM	___ AM/PM	___ AM/PM

Frequency

The first FIT guideline is for frequency. The minimum frequency to be considered aerobic activity is three days per week. Some people will choose to exercise every day, but this may increase the likelihood of injury. For individuals who choose to exercise only three days per week, there should be no more than two days of rest between exercise periods. More than this will reduce the conditioning effect.

Intensity

The next FIT guideline is intensity. This refers to how hard you are exercising. By no means does aerobic exercise imply that you must be out of breath; in fact, it means you should be breathing hard but at a level at which you could still carry on a conversation as you exercise.

Heart rate can reveal whether a person is working at the right level of intensity. Determine the heart rate that you should achieve while exercising from figure 8.11. Pulse should be taken about five minutes into an exercise, and activity adjusted accordingly.

Time

The last FIT guideline is time. Each exercise session must start out with three to five minutes of warm-up. This prepares your heart, blood pressure, muscles, and joints to exercise without damage. Warming up involves performing whatever activity you are about to partake in at a slower speed. For example, if you are going to jog, warm up by walking.

Next bring your heart rate into target range for a minimum of 20 minutes. A key concept is continuous activity at target heart rate for a minimum of 20 minutes. At the end of your aerobic session, remember to take time to cool down by continuing the same motion but at a much slower pace, or simply by walking. This is crucial because it allows the heart rate and blood pressure to decrease slowly and reduces the risk of fainting.

Now, if the activity you are planning follows the FIT guidelines, you can be sure it is aerobic. A word of caution though: always listen to your body and take it easy if necessary. It takes years to get out of shape, so expect that it will take about three months to start feeling the benefits of exercise. If you are over age 35 or have any medical problems or questions, consult your physician before starting an exercise program.

Benefits of Aerobic Exercise

Aerobic exercise provides both physiological and psychological benefits, including the following (12).

1. Decreases stress levels
2. Decreases physiological decline due to aging
3. Improves quality of sleep
4. Improves lower back pain
5. Reduces heart disease risk factors
6. Builds heart, lungs, blood vessels, muscles
7. Decreases body fat and increases lean body weight
8. Increases basal metabolic rate
9. Improves respiratory function
10. Elevates mood

Despite the many benefits of aerobic exercise, many people don't exercise. By far the most common excuse given for not exercising is lack of time (47 percent of the people in a survey conducted by Louis Harris and Associates, Inc.). Interestingly enough, many of these same people have an average of 25 hours per week of leisure time. Unfortunately, most Americans equate leisure with inactivity and then claim they have no time for exercise. Take a second look at the benefits. Can you afford not to exercise?

Plan to Succeed in an Exercise Program

When planning an aerobic exercise program, consider several factors that have been associated with improved compliance (22,23,24,25).

1. Establish realistic goals based on a formal health, medical, and fitness assessment.
2. Monitor yourself daily and record results in a log book.
3. Include significant others for reinforcement.
4. Start and progress slowly.
5. Emphasize feeling good, better health, social contacts.
6. Have fun.
7. Partake in a variety of aerobic exercises.
8. Plan rewards (T-shirts, pins, cups, attention, recognition, friendship, encouragement, monetary).

SUMMARY

1. Glucose, the main product of carbohydrate digestion, is distributed first to the blood. When blood glucose has been replenished, additional glucose is stored as glycogen; any excess glucose is converted to fat for long-term storage.
2. Triglycerides from the diet can also be used for energy or stored as fat.
3. Protein is used for fuel only during starvation or other times of Caloric deficit. Its main function is as a building material.
4. Fat is the greatest energy resource in the body. Human fat tissue has 3,500 Calories per pound.
5. ATP is the form of energy in the body available for immediate use. ATP can be formed through a series of biochemical reactions in the body from carbohydrate, fat, or protein.
6. There are two major metabolic pathways that yield ATP. Anaerobic glycolysis is a system that can produce energy without oxygen for a limited time. The aerobic system yields large amounts of ATP from glucose, glycogen, triglycerides, or amino acids.
7. Four nutrients can produce energy. Carbohydrate and protein each supply four Calories per gram. Fat supplies nine Calories per gram, and alcohol provides seven Calories per gram.
8. Energy input is affected by hunger, appetite, and choice of food. Psychological factors, environmental factors, food accessibility, and food characteristics all influence appetite.
9. Three factors affect energy output: basal metabolic rate (BMR), physical activity, and thermogenesis. BMR accounts for the largest number of Calories expended by an individual each day.
10. The number of Calories a person spends on physical activity each day is highly variable, contributing from 25 percent of the total energy output in a sedentary person to over 50 percent in a top athlete.
11. Small imbalances in the energy equation over long periods of time may lead to weight gain or loss.
12. Body composition refers to body fat and lean body mass. A variety of methods have been developed to assess body composition, some crude and others more sophisticated.
13. Height and weight charts provide a rough guideline for desirable weights but do not measure body fat. Ratios of weight to height, such as the body mass index, are better correlated with body fat measurements.
14. Circumference measurements with the tape measure are an estimate of body fat.
15. Skinfold measurements are the most widely used method for determining obesity. The calipers used to determine skinfolds are fairly inexpensive, and measurements are obtained quickly and accurately.
16. Underwater weighing is a standard laboratory procedure for measuring body fat. The measurement is based on the principle that lean body tissue is more dense than water, while fat tissue is less dense than water.
17. Bioelectrical impedance represents a good method of body fat assessment for overall accuracy, cost, and simplicity.
18. Body fat percentages are classified from lean to obese. A healthy body-fat percentage is 15 percent for males and 22 percent for females.
19. Guidelines for aerobic exercise include suggested criteria for frequency, intensity, and time. Aerobic exercise has several physiological and psychological benefits.

REFERENCES

1. Williams, M. H. 1983. *Nutrition for Fitness and Sport.* Dubuque, Iowa: Wm. C. Brown Publishers.
2. Duncan, K. H., J. A. Bacon, and R. L. Weinsier. 1983. The Effects of High and Low Energy Density Diets on Satiety, Energy Intake, and Eating Time of Obese and Nonobese Subjects. *American Journal of Clinical Nutrition* 37:763–67.
3. Brotherhood, J. R. 1984. Nutrition and Sports Performance. *Sports Medicine* 1:350–89.
4. Drenowski, A. 1983. Cognitive Structure in Obesity and Dieting. In *Obesity,* volume 4 of *Contemporary Issues in Clinical Nutrition.* M. R. C. Feenwood, ed. New York: Churchill Livingstone.
5. Sims, E. A. H., and E. Danforth. 1987. Expenditure and Storage of Energy in Man. *Journal of Clinical Investigation* 79:1019–1025.
6. Horton, E. S. 1983. Introduction: An Overview of the Assessment and Regulation of Energy Balance in Humans. *American Journal of Clinical Nutrition* 38:972–77.
7. Schultz, L. O. 1987. Brown Adipose Tissue: Regulation of Thermogenesis and Implications for Obesity. *Journal of the American Dietetic Association* 87:761–64.
8. Weigley, E. S. 1984. Average? Ideal? Desirable? A Brief Overview of Height-Weight Tables in the United States. *Journal of the American Dietetic Association* 84:417.
9. Robinette-Weiss, N., et al. 1984. The Metropolitan Height-Weight Tables: Perspective for Use. *Journal of the American Dietetic Association* 84:1480–1481.
10. National Institutes of Health. 1985. Consensus Development Conference Statement. Health Implications of Obesity, February 11–13, 1985. *Annals of Internal Medicine* 103:981–1077.
11. Revicki, D. A., and R. G. Israel. 1986. Relationship between Body Mass Indices and Measures of Body Adiposity. *American Journal of Public Health* 76:992–94.
12. Pollock, M. L., J. H. Wilmore, and S. M. Fox. 1984. *Exercise in Health and Disease.* Philadelphia: W. B. Saunders Co.
13. Jackson, A. S., and M. L. Pollock. 1985. Practical Assessment of Body Composition. *Physician and Sports Medicine* 13:76–90.

14. AAHPERD. 1985. Technical Manual: Health-Related Physical Fitness. Reston, Virginia: AAHPERD.
15. Nieman, D. C. 1986. *The Sports Medicine Fitness Course.* Palo Alto, CA: Bull Publishing Co.
16. Segal, K. R., et al. 1985. Estimation of Human Body Composition by Electrical Impedance Methods: A Comparative Study. *Journal of Applied Physiology* 58:1565–1571.
17. Lukaski, H. C. 1987. Methods for the Assessment of Human Body Composition: Traditional and New. *American Journal of Clinical Nutrition* 46:537–56.
18. Fleck, S. J. 1983. Body Composition of Elite American Athletes. *American Journal of Sports Medicine* 11:398.
19. Wilmore, J. H. 1982. *The Physiological Basis of the Conditioning Process.* Boston: Allyn and Bacon, Inc.
20. Stephens, T., D. R. Jacobs, and C. C. White. 1985. A Descriptive Epidemiology of Leisure-Time Physical Activity. Public Health Report 100:147–58.
21. Levitsky, D. 1983. Exercising within Several Hours of Eating Can Burn More Kilocalories. *Journal of the American Dietetic Association* 83:290.
22. Shephard, R. J. 1985. Motivation: The Key to Fitness Compliance. *Physical and Sports Medicine* 13:88–101.
23. Shephard, R. J. 1985. Factors Influencing the Exercise Behavior of Patients. *Sports Medicine* 2:348–66.
24. Sallis, J. F., et al. 1986. Predictors of Adoption and Maintenance of Physical Activity in a Community Sample. *Preventive Medicine* 15:311–341.
25. Franklin, B. A. 1988. Program Factors That Influence Exercise Adherence: Practical Adherence Skills for the Clinical Staff. In *Exercise Adherence.* R. K. Dishman, ed. Champaign, IL: Human Kinetics Books.

*H*EALTH-PROMOTION ACTIVITY 8.1
Eliminating the Excuses for Overeating

Thoughtfully answer the following questions.

1. How often have you used exercise as an excuse for overeating?

   ☐ Never

   ☐ Sometimes

   ☐ Quite often

2. What other reasons (excuses?) do you find yourself using for overeating? List them.

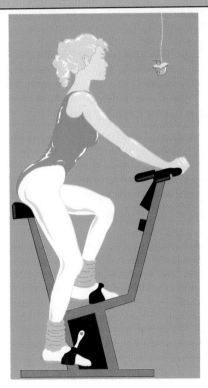

3. Which of these reasons (excuses) would it be easiest to eliminate? Put a check mark (✓) in #2 above.

4. How willing are you to give up the reasons (excuses) you have been using for overeating?

   ☐ Very willing

   ☐ Somewhat willing

   ☐ I'll have to think about it.

List thirteen desserts you have enjoyed in the past.

Put the numbers of those desserts **in the doughnut** which you now know to be empty and refined Calories.

Put the numbers of those desserts **in the doughnut hole** which you now know to be unrefined and nutritious Calories.

Now pick three desserts which you can easily cross off your list, given them up, won't eat them again. Draw a line through those three.

Now pick three desserts which you will hang onto until the bitter (sweet!) end. You always want them on your list, even if only occasionally.

Now write in the names of three desserts you could add to your meals, which would be nutritious Calories. Add these names **in the doughnut hole.**

What have you learned from this activity?

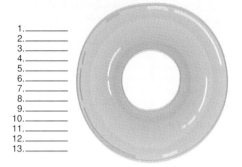

1._____
2._____
3._____
4._____
5._____
6._____
7._____
8._____
9._____
10._____
11._____
12._____
13._____

*H*EALTH-PROMOTION ACTIVITY 8.3
Determining Your Energy Expenditure

Estimating Basal Metabolic Rate (BMR)

1. Determine your ideal body weight in kilograms. (Convert pounds to kilograms by dividing your weight in pounds by 2.2 pounds per kilogram.)
2. Multiply your ideal weight in kilograms by 24 kcal/kg/day. The product will be your BMR.

Estimating Energy Expenditure from Physical Activity

1. Determine your activity level from the following chart.

Activity Level	Percent of BMR
Not very active	30–40 percent
Moderately active	40–50 percent
Very active	50–100 percent

2. Multiply your BMR by the percentage you found in the table. This will approximate the Calories you expend on physical activity.

Estimating Energy Expenditure from Thermogenesis

1. Add together your BMR and the energy you expend in activity.
2. Multiply this number by eight percent, which represents thermogenesis.

Estimating Total Energy Expenditure

1. Add together BMR + energy expended for activity + thermogenesis = Total energy expenditure.

How does your energy expenditure compare with the amount of Calories you take in daily? Are you willing to adjust the balance? Table 8.2 can help you choose an activity that can increase your Caloric expenditure.

9

Weight Management

INTRODUCTION

Thin is in, yet as we shall see in this chapter, Americans are among the fattest people in the world. Despite our "thin" standards of beauty, society promotes "fat" ways of living and a sedentary life-style.

What are the disadvantages of being overweight? Why are so many Americans obese? What can be done to both prevent and treat this problem? And what about the opposite end of the spectrum, in which people decrease their food intake to dangerously low levels? In this chapter we will explore these issues and others. The practical summary near the end of this chapter will help you put all the information of this chapter into proper perspective.

Percentage of overweight Americans by gender and race from 1960 to 1980. Although the percentage of the various subgroups shows little change during this 20-year period, there are dramatic differences among subgroups. The percentage figures are much higher for black female adults than other subgroups.

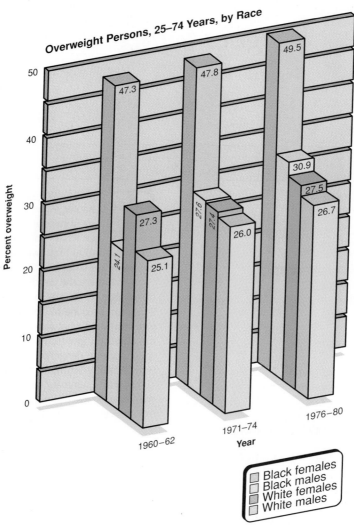

Definitions/Statistics

In the previous chapter, we defined **obesity** as the condition of having too much body fat (1). For practical purposes, obesity is usually associated with weighing more than 20 percent above one's ideal weight. For example, if a woman's ideal weight is 120 pounds but she weighs 144 pounds, she would be considered obese.

National studies of Americans during the last 30 years show that many are overweight and obese. Twenty-four percent of adult men and 26.5 percent of adult women are considered obese (2). As you can see in figure 9.1, the figures are much higher for black women. Among the population of U.S. adults over 40 years of age, 80 percent of men and 70 percent of women are more than 10 percent overweight (3).

The U.S. Census Bureau has submitted figures showing that the average U.S. female is now 64 inches tall and weighs 142 pounds. This is 16 pounds above the recommended weight. The average U.S. male is 69.5 inches tall and weighs 173 pounds, 12 pounds above the recommended weight (see figure 9.2).

Some people suggest that America no longer be called "the land of the free" but instead "the land of the fat." A recent study has

FIGURE 9.2

Average height and weight for U.S. males and females. The average male weighs 12 pounds more than recommended, and the average female carries 16 extra pounds.

AVERAGE
U.S. MALE ADULT

AVERAGE
U.S. FEMALE ADULT

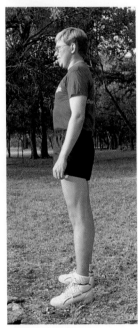
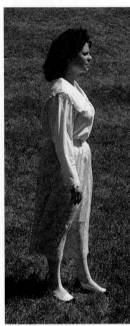

HEIGHT = 69.5''
WEIGHT = 173 lb.
IDEAL WEIGHT
FOR HEIGHT = 161 lb.

HEIGHT = 64''
WEIGHT = 142 lb.
IDEAL WEIGHT
FOR HEIGHT = 126 lb.

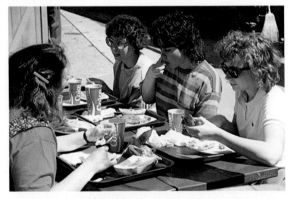

The increase in obesity among our children and youth is partly related to the types of food available today.

shown that the U.S. tends to have a greater percentage of overweight males and females than Canada or Britain (4) (see figure 9.3).

National surveys also reveal that a large number of our children and teenagers are obese (5). Among American children and youth aged 6 to 17 years, 28.9 percent of the boys and 25.2 percent of the girls are considered obese. When

FIGURE 9.3

Prevalence of excessive body weight (BMI>25), (a) males aged 20-64, and (b) females aged 20-64, Britain (1980), Canada (1981), United States (1976-1980). Note: BMI = Body mass index, which is the weight in kilograms divided by the height in meters squared (Kg/m²).

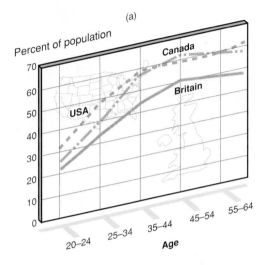
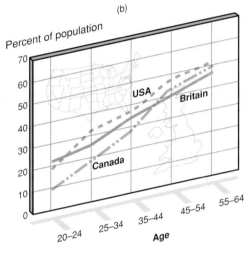

comparing figures with those from 1963, the percentage of children 6 to 11 years who are obese today is approximately 54 percent higher, and among youth 12 to 17 years of age it is 39 percent higher (see figure 9.4).

Disadvantages of Obesity

The National Institutes of Health has summarized the large number of health problems associated with obesity (1). Some health experts feel that obesity deserves to be termed our nation's "number-one health problem." There are at least seven health problems associated with obesity.

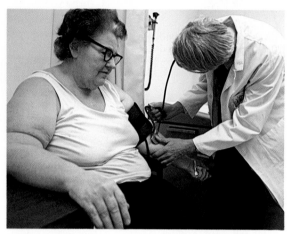

There are many disadvantages associated with obesity, ranging from psychological burdens to various diseases.

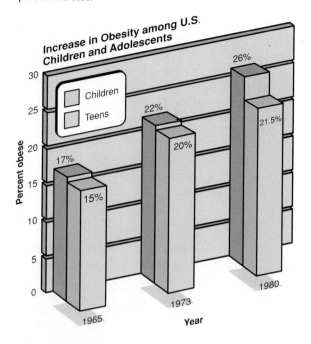

FIGURE 9.4
Percentage of overweight children and adolescents in the U.S. For children 6–11 years of age, there has been a 54 percent increase in obesity since 1965, and for adolescents a 39 percent increase.

1. *A psychological burden.* In America, we have thin standards of beauty but fat ways of living. Some have called our era the "age of caloric anxiety." Because of the strong pressures from society to be thin, obese people often suffer feelings of guilt, depression, anxiety, and low self-worth. This burden may be the greatest negative effect of obesity.

2. *Increased high blood pressure.* National survey results reveal that high blood pressure in the obese is three time more common than in normal-weight subjects.

3. *Increased high levels of cholesterol in the blood.* U.S. adults who are obese are more likely to have high blood-cholesterol levels than normal-weight subjects (double the risk).

4. *Increased diabetes.* The prevalence of diabetes is nearly three times higher in obese than nonobese people.

5. *Increased cancer.* The American Cancer Society study involving one million men and women showed that obese males had a higher mortality rate from cancer of the colon, rectum, and prostate. Obese females had a higher mortality rate from cancer of the gallbladder, bile ducts, breast, uterus, and ovaries.

6. *Increased early death.* Hippocrates, the ancient Greek physician, once noted that "sudden death is more common in those who are naturally fat than in the lean." Several modern studies have confirmed the wisdom of Hippocrates. For example,

in the American Cancer Society study, the lowest death rates were seen among healthy men who weighed 5 to 10 percent below average, and among healthy women who weighed 10 to 20 percent below average. The highest death rates were found in those who were the heaviest. In other words, obesity is a real life-shortener.

7. *Increased heart disease.* Not only do obese people have more of the typical risk factors for heart disease (high blood pressure and cholesterol); they also experience more deaths from this cause.

Recent information is showing that *where* the excess fat is deposited has much to do with the medical complications of obesity (6). Obese subjects most vulnerable to heart disease, high blood pressure and cholesterol, diabetes, and early death tend to have more of their fat deposited in abdominal areas rather than the hip and thigh areas.

In other words, health risks are greater for those who have most of their body fat in the upper body. This can be determined by looking at the ratio of waist-to-hip circumferences. A high ratio predicts elevated complications from obesity. In males, risk increases greatly when the

TABLE 9.1
Desirable weight ranges for men — ages 25 and over[a]

Height (ft in)	Weight Range	Weight[b] MRW = 100 Average Desirable	Weight[c] MRW = 110 10% Overweight	Weight MRW = 120 20% Overweight
5 1	105–134	117	129	140
5 2	108–137	120	132	144
5 3	111–141	123	135	148
5 4	114–145	126	139	151
5 5	117–149	129	142	155
5 6	121–154	133	146	160
5 7	125–159	138	152	166
5 8	129–163	142	156	170
5 9	133–167	146	161	175
5 10	137–172	150	165	180
5 11	141–177	155	170	186
6 0	145–182	159	175	191
6 1	149–187	164	180	197
6 2	153–192	169	186	203
6 3	157–197	174	191	209

[a]Adapted from the 1959 Metropolitan Desirable Weight Table. (Weight, in pounds, without clothing; height without shoes.)
[b]Midpoint of medium frame range — used to compute MRW: MRW = [(Actual weight)/(Midpoint of medium frame range)] × 100.
[c]In the US adult population over 40 years of age, 80% of men and 70% of women have weights that exceed MRW = 110, and, consequently, are at increased risk for cardiovascular disease.
The average weight of the adult US population is above MRW = 120; an individual with a weight over MRW = 120 is "obese."

waist/hip ratio rises above 1.0, and in females when it rises above 0.8. For example, if a male has a waist circumference of 40 inches and a hip circumference of 37 inches, the waist/hip ratio is 1.08 (40/37 = 1.08), putting him at risk for the medical complications listed previously. If a female has a waist circumference of 35 inches and a hip circumference of 40, the waist/hip ratio is 0.88 (35/40 = 0.88), putting her at risk.

In general, the weight associated with optimal health tends to be at least 10 percent below the average weight of the average American (7). Look at tables 9.1 or 9.2 to see if your weight is optimal for your height. If you are very muscular, you should be at the higher end of the weight range for your height. If you have low muscle mass, your weight should be at the lower end of the weight range for your height. For people with normal musculature, the midpoint value of the range is recommended. The midpoint value of the medium frame range is listed in tables 9.1 and 9.2, with calculated body weights representing both 10 percent and 20 percent overweight. Eighty percent of men and 70 percent of women in the United States have weights that are 10 percent above this recommended average weight.

Theories of Obesity

Explanations of why so many Americans weigh more than they should have been a source of confusion for both researchers and the public. Currently, most theories of obesity are in one of three categories (see figure 9.5): genetic and parental influences, dietary factors, or insufficient energy expenditure.

Genetic and Parental Influences

In 1965, Dr. Jean Mayer reported that 80 percent of the children with two obese parents became obese when reaching adulthood, compared with only 14 percent of the children with two normal-weight parents (8). Since then, many other studies have shown that hereditary factors are very important in explaining why some people find it so hard to avoid obesity.

A recent study comparing fraternal and identical twins found that the body weights of the identical twins were much more similar than the body weights of fraternal twins, upon reaching adulthood (9). A study of adults who

TABLE 9.2
Desirable weight ranges for women — ages 25 and over[a]

Height (ft in)	Weight Range	Weight[b] MRW = 100 Average Desirable	Weight[c] MRW = 110 10% Overweight	Weight MRW = 120 20% Overweight
4 9	90–118	100	110	120
4 10	92–121	103	113	124
4 11	95–124	106	117	127
5 0	98–127	109	120	131
5 1	101–130	112	124	134
5 2	104–134	116	128	139
5 3	107–138	120	132	144
5 4	110–142	124	136	149
5 5	114–146	128	141	154
5 6	118–150	132	145	158
5 7	122–154	136	150	163
5 8	126–159	140	154	168
5 9	130–164	144	158	173
5 10	134–169	148	163	177

[a]Adapted from the 1959 Metropolitan Desirable Weight Table. (Weight, in pounds, without clothing; height without shoes.)
[b]Midpoint of medium frame range — used to compute MRW: MRW = [(Actual weight)/(Midpoint of medium frame range)] × 100.
[c]In the US adult population over 40 years of age, 80% of men and 70% of women have weights that exceed MRW = 110, and, consequently, are at increased risk for cardiovascular disease.
The average weight of the adult US population is above MRW = 120; an individual with a weight over MRW = 120 is "obese."
Note: For women between the ages of 18–25 years, subtract one pound for each year under 25.

FIGURE 9.5
Most theories explaining obesity center around these three factors.

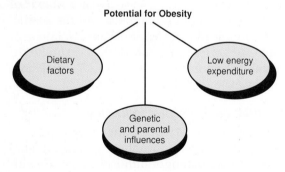

had been adopted before the age of one revealed that despite being raised by adoptive parents, their body weights were still very similar to that of their birth parents (10).

These studies demonstrate that some people are more prone than others to obesity due to genetic factors. Such people have to be unusually careful about their dietary and exercise habits to counteract these inherited tendencies.

Another factor related to genetic influences is the number of fat cells one has. According to the **fat-cell theory,** fat-cell number can increase to two or three times normal if an individual ingests too many Calories (11). And once formed, the extra fat cells cannot be removed by the body. This can happen anytime during the life span of an individual but appears to be particularly important during infancy, when fat cells are still dividing. Infants who form extra fat cells when overnourished tend to remain overfat as children (12), and obese children and teenagers can remain obese as adults. According to one study, 36 percent of obese adults had been over heavy as infants. Twice as many obese women as nonobese women are reported to have been obese as children.

One theory states that a mother who breast-feeds her baby may help prevent formation of extra fat cells; another states that if solid food is introduced after nine months, this may help prevent infant obesity. At the present time, however, most studies do not support these theories (13). Nonetheless, preventing infant and child obesity appears to be vitally important in reducing risk of adult obesity. Future studies will need to determine what life-style factors are most important in preventing infant and child obesity.

The presence of extra fat cells has several important implications. Some obese people are likely to be heavy just because of the extra fat-cell mass, even when the fat cells contain only normal amounts of fat. In addition, obese people with extra fat cells are going to find weight loss very difficult because of biological pressures to keep the extra cells supplied with fat. The only way such a person could attain society's "ideal" weight would be to reduce each cell to much smaller than normal size, which would involve sensations akin to the feelings of constant starvation.

It makes sense to give more attention to preventing obesity than to spend huge amounts of money researching methods to treat obesity. In addition, obese people who have extra fat cells and have been obese since early in life may have to accept higher weight standards. Despite vigorous efforts to eat and exercise healthfully, body-fat levels in such people may still be higher than desirable.

Dietary Factors

There is some evidence that obese people tend to consume more Calories than normal-weight individuals (14), choosing larger portions of rich foods that are high in fats and sugars. In one study, nearly half of obese women were found to have a serious problem with **binge eating,** compared with only 10 to 15 percent of normal-weight women (15). Binge eating is defined as the consumption of large quantities of rich foods within short periods of time.

There is good reason to believe that the abundance of tasty, Calorie-rich foods, especially those high in fat, is the primary reason why so many Americans are fat. The average American consumes 40 percent of Calories as fat, much higher than the 25 to 30 percent recommended. In the laboratory, much evidence has accumulated from studies of rats and other animals that this amount of dietary fat is too high if obesity is to be prevented.

The most commonly used dietary means of inducing obesity in rats is to feed them a high-fat diet (11). When the fat content of the rat diet (which in standard chows is two to six percent) is increased to 30–60 percent, rats typically become obese. The rats appear to enjoy the extra dietary fat so much that they consume more Cal-

Dietary fat versus carbohydrate in body fat formation. When extra fat Calories are consumed, the body expends very few Calories to fill fat cells with fat (triglycerides). However, seven times more Calories are used to change dietary carbohydrate to fat.

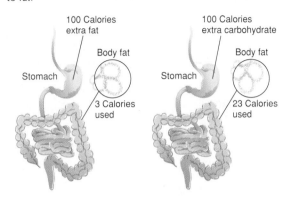

ories than normal. Obesity can also be produced in rats by feeding them "supermarket diets," which includes such foods as chocolate chip cookies, salami, cheese, marshmallows, milk chocolate, peanut butter, and sweetened whole milk. Rats become very obese on such diets.

With humans, most studies have shown that naturally lean subjects have a very difficult time gaining weight on a low-fat regimen. However, weight is easily gained when the diet is high in fat (16,17).

One explanation of why dietary fat promotes obesity so easily in both rats and humans is that the body uses less Calories to store dietary fat as body fat than it does for dietary carbohydrate. Figure 9.6 shows that if an individual consumes 100 extra Calories from dietary fat (for example, one tablespoon of butter), then only three Calories are used by the body to transform the butter into body fat. However, 100 extra Calories of carbohydrate require 23 Calories to make the transformation. In other words, excess dietary fat is more fattening than excess carbohydrate.

Another study has shown that when obese women are given 2,000 Calories of carbohydrate all at once (one huge meal), only 20 Calories are actually stored as fat (18). It is difficult for the body to turn the carbohydrate into fat, and when it does, the majority of the fat is used for metabolism. This is vitally important information: the message is that pasta, potatoes, and bread do not make you fat nearly as much as the high-fat sauce, sour cream, and margarine used with them!

A high-fiber, low-fat diet prolongs eating time, increases the
quality of food, and reduces Calories.

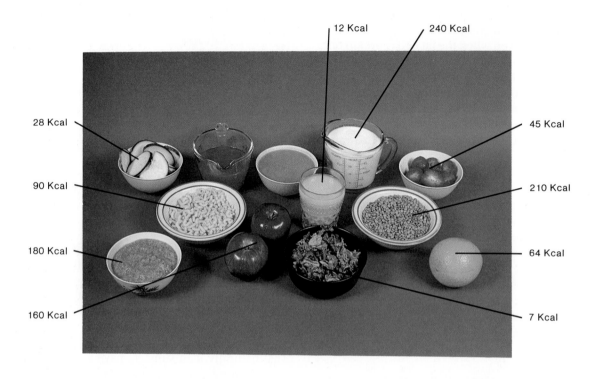

12 Kcal   240 Kcal

28 Kcal   45 Kcal

90 Kcal   210 Kcal

180 Kcal   64 Kcal

160 Kcal   7 Kcal

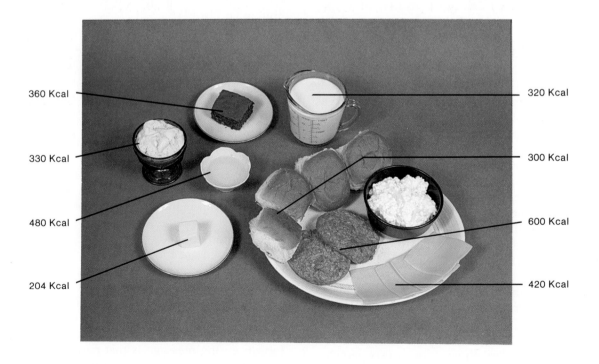

360 Kcal   320 Kcal

330 Kcal   300 Kcal

480 Kcal   600 Kcal

204 Kcal   420 Kcal

The importance of a low-fat, high carbohydrate, high-fiber diet for both prevention and treatment of obesity cannot be emphasized enough. In one study, subjects were allowed to eat until satisfied under two different conditions. In phase one of the study, only low-Calorie, high-carbohydrate, high-fiber foods were offered. In phase two, only high-Calorie, high-fat, low-fiber foods were allowed. Researchers found that when both obese and non-obese subjects were in phase one of the diet (whole grains, vegetables, salads, fruits, low-fat dairy products), eating time was prolonged 33 percent, but subjects felt satisfied after consuming only 1,570 Calories per day. During phase two, subjects felt satisfied only after consuming 3,000 Calories per day. Apparently the human body can avoid obesity only if the fat content of the diet is low (see figure 9.7).

Insufficient Energy Expenditure

During a 24-hour period, all humans expend energy in three ways: through the resting metabolic rate, physical activity and exercise, and in digesting and metabolizing food (thermic effect of food) (17) (see figure 9.8).

Most people (except for athletes who train several hours a day) expend the largest number of Calories per day through the **resting metabolic rate (RMR).** This represents the energy expended by the body to maintain life and normal body functions, such as respiration and circulation. In the average 154-pound male, the resting metabolic rate amounts to approximately 1,500 Calories per day, or 60 to 75 percent of the total daily energy expenditure. This is a lot of energy, equivalent to walking 15 miles! No wonder some people feel tired even if they sit all day!

Surprisingly, the obese individual actually has a higher RMR than a normal-weight person. This is because the RMR is closely tied to the amount of lean body weight (nonfat tissue, such as muscle and bone) an individual has. Obese people, because of the extra weight they carry, have more lean body weight than lean persons. This results in a higher RMR.

All **physical activity,** all muscular movement, expends Calories. The average sedentary person usually expends only 500–800 Calories beyond the resting metabolic rate in physical activity, most of this from informal, unplanned types of movement. The top athletes in the world usually match their resting metabolic rate energy expenditure in hard, intense exercise. Most physical-fitness experts recommend burning at least 200 to 400 Calories during planned exercise sessions to improve health.

Table 9.3 outlines the average recommended energy intakes for different groups of people, and table 9.4 shows the amount of physical activity needed (figures include RMR) to match these energy intakes. Notice that most Americans fall far short of being this active. Health-Promotion Activity 9.1 will help you determine how many Calories you expend each day.

Most studies show that both obese children and adults are less active than normal-weight people (11). Some researchers have shown that when swimming, obese adolescent girls spend less time actually moving their arms and legs and more time floating than do normal-weight girls. Obese girls have been found to be inactive 77 percent of the time while playing tennis, compared with 56 percent of the time for normal-weight girls. Obese men informally walk an average of four miles per day, compared to six miles per day for those of normal weight; obese women walk two miles per day, versus five miles per day for normal-weight women.

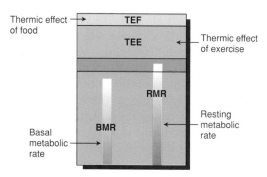

FIGURE 9.8

The three major categories of energy expenditure by the human body.

Thermic effect of food — TEF

TEE — Thermic effect of exercise

RMR

Basal metabolic rate — BMR

Resting metabolic rate

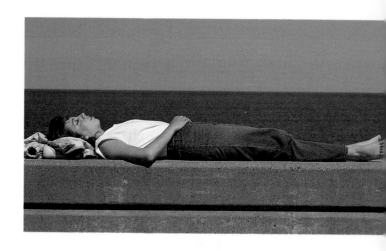

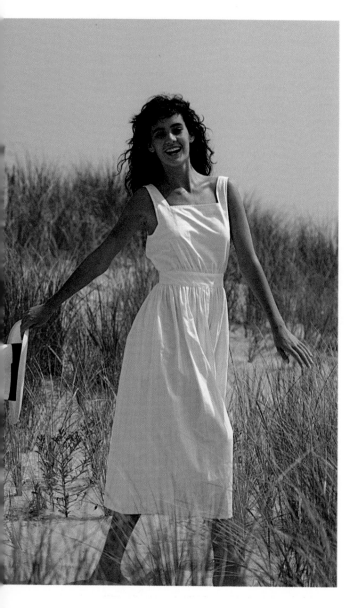

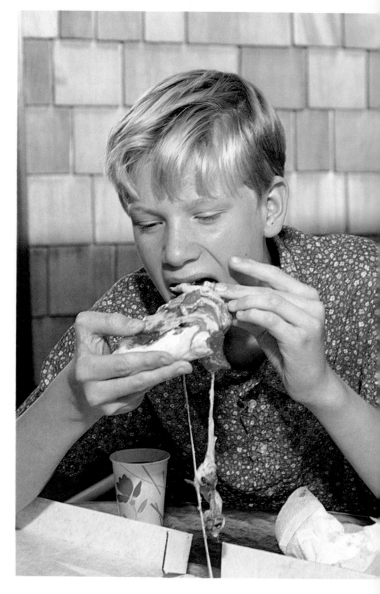

TABLE 9.3
Median heights and weights and recommended energy intake

Category	Age (years) or condition	Weight (kg)	Weight (lb)	Height (cm)	Height (in)	REE[a] (kcal/day)	Average Energy Allowance (kcal)[b] Multiples of REE	Average Energy Allowance (kcal)[b] Per kg	Average Energy Allowance (kcal)[b] Per day
Infants	0.0–0.5	6	13	60	24	320		108	650
	0.5–1.0	9	20	71	28	500		98	850
Children	1–3	13	29	90	35	740		102	1,300
	4–6	20	44	112	44	950		90	1,800
	7–10	28	62	132	52	1,130		70	2,000
Males	11–14	45	99	157	62	1,440	1.70	55	2,500
	15–18	66	145	176	69	1,760	1.67	45	3,000
	19–24	72	160	177	70	1,780	1.67	40	2,900
	25–50	79	174	176	70	1,800	1.60	37	2,900
	51+	77	170	173	68	1,530	1.50	30	2,300
Females	11–14	46	101	157	62	1,310	1.67	47	2,200
	15–18	55	120	163	64	1,370	1.60	40	2,200
	19–24	58	128	164	65	1,350	1.60	38	2,200
	25–50	63	138	163	64	1,380	1.55	36	2,200
	51+	65	143	160	63	1,280	1.50	30	1,900
Pregnant	1st trimester								+0
	2nd trimester								+300
	3rd trimester								+300
Lactating	1st 6 months								+500
	2nd 6 months								+500

[a]Calculation based on FAO equations, then rounded.
[b]In the range of light to moderate activity, the coefficient of variation is ± 20%.
[c]Figure is rounded.

Reprinted with permission from: Food and Nutrition Board. Recommended Dietary Allowances. 10th rev. ed. 1989. Washington, DC: National Academy Press, 1989.

TABLE 9.4
Examples of daily energy expenditures of mature women and men in light occupations

Activity Category	Time (hr)	Man, 70 kg Rate (kcal/min)	Man, 70 kg Total kcal	Woman, 58 kg Rate (kcal/min)	Woman, 58 kg Total kcal
Sleeping, reclining	8	1.0–1.2	540	0.9–1.1	440
Very light: Seated and standing activities, painting trades, auto and truck driving, laboratory work, typing, playing musical instruments, sewing, ironing	12	up to 2.5	1,300	up to 2.0	900
Light: Walking on level, 2.5–3 mph, tailoring, pressing, garage work, electrical trades, carpentry, restaurant trades, cannery workers, washing clothes, shopping with light load, golf, sailing, table tennis, volleyball	3	2.5–4.9	600	2.0–3.9	450
Moderate: Walking 3.5–4 mph, weeding and hoeing, loading and stacking bales, scrubbing floors, shopping with heavy load, cycling, skiiing, tennis, dancing	1	5.0–7.4	300	4.0–5.9	240
Heavy: Walking with load uphill, tree felling, work with pick and shovel, basketball, swimming, climbing, football	0	7.5–12.0		6.0–10.0	
Total	24		2,740		2,030

From Recommended Dietary Allowances, 9th ed., 1980. Food and Nutrition Board, National Academy of Sciences.

FIGURE 9.9

The prevalence of obesity among teenagers rises sharply with hours of TV watched per day.

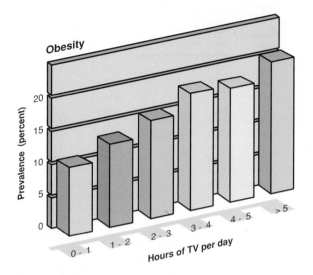

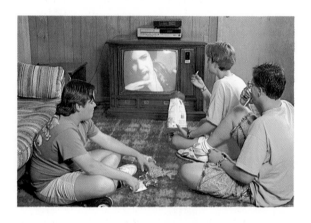

FIGURE 9.10

After a meal, the body expends extra Calories to digest and metabolize the meal. This thermic effect of food will last for several hours.

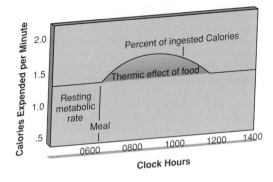

In one national study, twice as many teens who watched more than five hours of television per day were obese, compared to teens who watched less than one hour per day (19) (see figure 9.9). The researchers suggested that TV watching decreased the opportunity for exercise and prompted more snacking because of all the food advertisements. Children 4 to 8 years of age have been found to have increased body fat levels if daytime activity is less than normal.

Thus it appears that obese people tend to be less physically active than normal-weight people (20). However, because the obese weigh more, more Calories are expended when they *do* engage in physical activity. For this reason, most experts feel that overeating, not inactivity, explains the large number of obese people in this country.

The **thermic effect of food** (TEF) is the increase in energy expenditure above the RMR that can be measured for several hours after a meal (see figure 9.10). In other words, as your body digests, absorbs, transports, metabolizes, and stores the food you eat, energy is required (17). The TEF is higher after carbohydrate and protein meals than after fat meals. The average person's TEF is about seven to ten percent of total ingested Calories, about 120 to 170 Calories per day for women and about 180 to 260 Calories per day for men (21). For example, if you eat a meal containing 800 Calories, your body uses 56 to 80 Calories just to process the meal.

TEF has been found to be higher when people consume larger meals. In normal individuals, TEF raises the energy expenditure of the body 43 percent over RMR one hour after a 1,500 kcal meal; after a 1,000 kcal meal, there is a 25 percent increase over RMR. As you can see in figure 9.10, TEF peaks about 60–90 minutes following a meal and lasts for four to six hours (11). Because TEF is related to the size of the meal, there may be an advantage in consuming food at two or three set meals instead of indulging in constant nibbling.

Most researchers have concluded that there is a slight decrease in the TEF in obese persons, especially diabetic obese patients. However, the difference is too small in terms of actual Calories to be important. In addition, most obese people have higher RMR's due to their increased muscle mass, more than making up for the small decrease in TEF (22).

Although still somewhat controversial, new evidence shows that moderate exercise, like walking, both before and after meals increases

_T_ABLE 9.5
Treatment for obesity

Type	Mild	Moderate	Severe
		Classification of Obesity	
	Mild	**Moderate**	**Severe**
% overweight	20–40%	41–100%	>100%
Sample weights for 140-lb ideal	168–196 lb	197–280 lb	>280 lb
Prevalence	90.5%	9.0%	0.5%
Treatment	Behavior therapy (diet, exercise, behavior modification)	VLCD and behavior therapy**	Gastric surgery

** Very-low-Calorie diet under medical supervision only

From A. J. Stunkard, _Eating and Its Disorders_. © 1984. Raven Press, New York. Used with permission.

the TEF above and beyond normal levels (17). Because people are more active during the day, some are suggesting that heavier meals should be eaten at breakfast and lunch and that the evening meal should be light. Walking before and after high-carbohydrate, high-fiber meals may help some people lose extra weight.

Treatment of Obesity

Weight loss has proven to be very difficult for most overweight and obese individuals. Most studies show that the majority of people entering weight-management programs return to their starting weight within two years (23). It's been said that obesity is harder to treat than alcoholism. We can live without alcohol, and for many alcoholics it is easier to stay off alcohol completely than to drink moderate amounts. We all need food to live, however, and so we do not have the option of complete abstinence. Thus the obese person is faced with the difficulty of learning to consume food in moderate amounts.

Table 9.5 outlines the three classifications of obesity and the basic type of treatment now recommended for each. Notice that the large majority of obese people are "mildly obese." For this reason, most of the discussion will focus on this classification. First, however, we will review treatment schemes for "severe" and "moderate" obesity.

Severe Obesity

As noted in table 9.5, **severe obesity** is defined as the condition of weighing more than double the ideal weight. Severe obesity is associated with serious medical complications.

Until recently, severely obese people were rarely able to lose weight and keep it off. The advent of surgical treatments for obesity nearly 30 years ago has dramatically changed this picture. Large amounts of weight (up to 200 pounds) can now be lost and maintained by severely obese patients. The surgery involves radically reducing the volume of the stomach to less than 50 millileters. This is called "gastric stapling" or "gastric restriction procedures" (24) (see figure 9.11).

Only certain people are allowed to undergo this type of surgery. For example, the patient must show a history of repeated failures to lose weight by acceptable nonsurgical methods, be severely obese (more than 100 percent overweight for at least three to five years), and be experiencing some medical complications from the obesity. There must be a commitment by the patient, surgeon, and hospital for lifelong follow-up (25). Complications occur in five to ten percent of cases, with mortality from zero to three percent.

Weight reduction by this method is dramatic and long-term, with an expected weight loss of 55 percent of excess weight. Patients go through drastic forced changes in eating habits. The 50-millileter stomach volume requires people to eat less during each meal, to eat more often, and to eliminate any liquids at mealtime.

*F*IGURE 9.11

When all else fails, severely obese people may need to reduce the size of their stomachs to avoid early death. In gastric reduction surgery, or gastric stapling, the surgeon sews together the top part of the stomach.

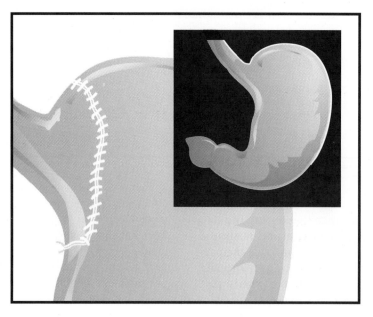

Moderate Obesity

Moderate obesity, defined as the condition of being 41–100 percent overweight, is present in about nine percent of the obese population (11). The amount of body-fat tissue is high enough to demand special efforts under medical supervision. Treatment for moderate obesity consists of a special diet with behavior modification in medical clinics.

Moderately obese people have at least 50 pounds of excess fat tissue. This high amount of body fat demands the fastest weight loss that can be tolerated with safety and comfort. Fasting is attractive to some patients, but this method can be unsafe, uncomfortable, and ineffective. In fasting, 40 to 50 percent of the weight loss comes from the lean body weight, compromising health and personal appearance. Also, conventional reducing diets of 1,200–1,500 Calories produce too slow a weight loss to be practical.

A compromise between the two, the very-low-Calorie diet, has recently proven very effective and safe (26). Also called the protein-sparing modified fast, the **very-low-Calorie diet** provides 400–700 Calories per day. Eating protein is emphasized, to help avoid loss of muscle tissue. Patients can use either special-formula beverages or natural foods such as fish, fowl, or lean meat (along with mineral and vitamin supplements).

In contrast to the liquid protein diets of the recent past, which were associated with a number of fatalities, very-low-Calorie diets appear to be safe *when administered under careful medical supervision* for periods of up to three months (11). The importance of medical supervision needs to be underscored. The Cambridge Diet is a good example of a very-low-Calorie diet (330 Calories/day) that has been offered directly to the public, with no provision for adequate medical supervision (27). (Most manufacturers of other types of very-low-Calorie diets have been reluctant to furnish them directly to the public, instead limiting distribution to physicians, hospitals, and clinics to ensure proper supervision.) Within two years, five million Americans used the Cambridge Diet, and at least six people died. During rapid weight loss, sudden death from various complications can occur. For this reason, very-low-Calorie diets should be used only by moderately obese people under the supervision of a physician, hospital, or clinic actively engaged in the study and use of such diets. When VLCD are administered this way, they are generally safe (28).

Patients tend to lose three to five pounds a week on the VLCD. Unfortunately, losses are poorly maintained unless unusual effort is expended by the patient and a team of dietitians, psychologists, exercise physiologists, and medical personnel for years following the initial program.

Mild Obesity

Mild obesity, defined as the condition of being 20–40 percent overweight, is by far the most common form of obesity, afflicting 90.5 percent of obese people (11). For most mildly obese individuals, a weight loss of about one percent total body weight per week is optimal. For example, if a person weighs 150 pounds, the goal should be to lose no more than 1.5 pounds each week. Another goal is to lose primarily fat tissue and to protect the lean body weight.

As we will further discuss later, one pound of body fat is equal to 3,500 Calories. To lose 1.5 pounds of body fat, 5,250 Calories must be lost from the body, which amounts to 750 Calories a day for one week. We will see that a combination of both diet and exercise is necessary to achieve this healthfully.

Conservative treatment for mild obesity involves three elements (29).

1. **Diet:** The caloric intake should be reduced, preferably by reducing the fat content of the diet; intake of complex carbohydrate should be increased.
2. **Exercise:** Energy expenditure should be increased by 200 to 400 Calories per day by increasing all forms of physical activity.
3. **Behavioral modification:** Several techniques should be employed, including:
   a. Self-monitoring. Diet diaries are kept, emphasizing recording of food amounts consumed and circumstances surrounding the eating episode (see Health-Promotion Activity 9.2).
   b. Control of the events that precede eating. Identification of the circumstances that elicit eating and overeating.

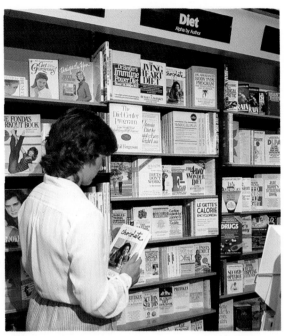

Every year, 27 percent of males and 46 percent of females in the U.S. try to lose weight.

   c. Development of techniques to control the act of eating. Typical behavioral modification techniques are used (see table 9.9).
   d. Reinforcement through use of rewards. A system of formal rewards facilitates progress.

Diet

Very-low-Calorie diets are not recommended for the mildly obese. When the daily caloric intake falls below 1,200, the diet usually contains insufficient amounts of the various vitamins and minerals (30). Thus, as a person loses body weight, the overall nutritional status of the individual is compromised. In addition, diets containing less than 1,200 Calories per day result in high amounts of muscle-tissue loss and, without medical supervision, can result in life-threatening complications.

At any given time, 2.5 million Americans are estimated to be dieting to lose weight (31). The U.S. government has estimated that every year, 27 percent of males and 46 percent of females in this country are trying to lose weight, the majority by altering their diets without an increase in physical activity (32). Other surveys show that the majority of American women want to lose weight but have a hard time doing so.

TABLE 9.6
Criteria for evaluating weight-loss programs

NCAHF disparages commercial weight-loss or control programs that:

1. promise or imply dramatic, rapid, weight loss (i.e., substantially more than one percent of total body weight per week);

2. promote diets that are extremely low in Calories (i.e., below 800 Calories per day; 1,200 Calories per day diets are preferred) unless under the supervision of competent medical experts;

3. attempt to make clients dependent upon special products rather than teaching how to make good choices from the conventional food supply (this does not condemn the marketing of low-Calorie convenience foods that may be chosen by consumers);

4. do not encourage permanent, realistic life-style changes, including regular exercise and the behavioral aspects of eating wherein food may be used as a coping device (i.e., programs should focus upon changing the *causes* of overweight rather than simply the *effects*, which is the overweight itself);

5. misrepresent salespeople as "counselors" supposedly qualified to give guidance in nutrition and/or general health. Even if adequately trained, such counselors would still be objectionable because of the obvious conflict of interest that exists when providers profit directly from the products they recommend and sell;

6. require large sums of money at the start or require that clients sign contracts for expensive, long-term programs. Such practices too often have been abused as salespeople focus attention upon signing up new people rather than delivering continuing, satisfactory service to consumers. Programs should be on a pay-as-you-go basis;

7. fail to inform clients about the risks associated with weight-loss in general, or the specific program being promoted;

8. promote unproven or spurious weight-loss aids, such as human chorionic gonadotrophin hormone, starch blockers, diuretics, sauna belts, body wraps, passive exercise, ear stapling, acupuncture, electric muscle stimulating devices, spirulina, amino acid supplements (e.g., arginine, ornithine), and glucomannan;

9. claim that "cellulite" exists in the body;

10. claim that use of an appetite suppressant or methylcellulose (a "bulking agent") enables a person to lose body fat without restricting accustomed Caloric intake; and

11. claim that a weight-control product contains a unique ingredient or component unless it is unavailable in other weight-control products.

From National Council Against Health Fraud. NCAHF Guidelines for Evaluating Commercial Weight-Loss Promotions. *NCAHF Newsletter* (March/April):1, 1987. Used with permission.

In response, a $10-billion industry dedicated to providing "quick and easy" weight-loss methods has sprung up. A proliferation of diet books and products utilizing false and misleading concepts is now available. Table 9.6 outlines eleven criteria that the National Council Against Health Fraud recommends in using to evaluate the validity and effectiveness of weight-loss programs. It is an excellent guide that you should study carefully.

The Journal of the American Dietetic Association has published an in-depth analysis of some of the most common published diets in America (33). Based on this article and other information, diets were rated either excellent, good, fair, or poor (see figure 9.12). Of the diets, those with an excellent rating conform to the U.S. Dietary Goals and Recommended Dietary Allowances. These diets are recommended because they follow principles advocated for a healthy life-style. Diets with a poor rating tend to be either too high in fat and cholesterol or deficient in several important minerals and vitamins. Some of the poor diets are also based on unproven and misleading information. These "novelty" diets promote certain nutrients, foods, or combinations of foods as having unique, magical, or previously undiscovered qualities that promote fat loss.

The whole concept of dieting can be criticized on psychological grounds, for going on a diet implies eventually going off it and resuming old eating habits (11). For this reason, one can argue that the most effective diet is not a diet at all but rather a gradual change in eating patterns and a shift to foods that the person can continue to eat indefinitely. This means increasing the intake of complex carbohydrates, particularly in fruits, vegetables, legumes, and cereals, and decreasing the intake of fats and refined sugars. This course of action probably gives

Diet books can be excellent sources of information, or they can give misleading or false ideas about how to lose weight.

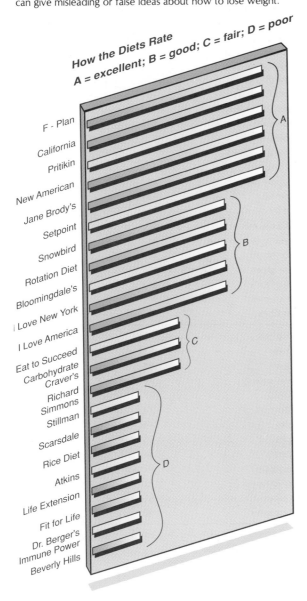

How the Diets Rate
A = excellent; B = good; C = fair; D = poor

- F - Plan
- California
- Pritikin
- New American
- Jane Brody's
- Setpoint
- Snowbird
- Rotation Diet
- Bloomingdale's
- I Love New York
- I Love America
- Eat to Succeed
- Carbohydrate Craver's
- Richard Simmons
- Stillman
- Scarsdale
- Rice Diet
- Atkins
- Life Extension
- Fit for Life
- Dr. Berger's Immune Power
- Beverly Hills

A
B
C
D

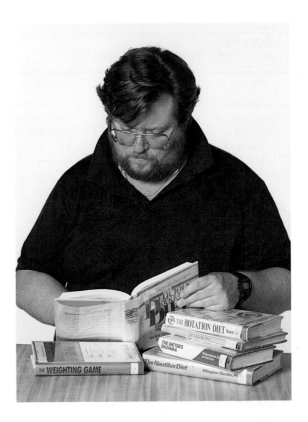

the best chance of maintaining the weight that is lost, and it is an eminently safe one. One should never lose weight by any method that cannot be permanently included in a healthy lifestyle.

In other words, the same diet that is being recommended for the treatment and prevention of heart disease, cancer, and diabetes is the same diet that should be used in preventing and treating obesity. This diet is high in carbohydrate but low in fat. Complex carbohydrate found in whole grains, vegetables, and fruits are emphasized, and only low-fat meats and dairy products are used.

In light of current evidence, then, the most important dietary habit to feature in both preventing and treating obesity is a strong emphasis on *low-caloric density foods high in carbohydrate and dietary fiber.* Table 9.7 shows that when comparing the amount of Calories per cup of food, vegetables and fruits have the lowest number of Calories, whereas high-fat and sugar foods contain the most. As stated previously, obese people tend to take in less Calories when consuming high-fiber, high-carbohydrate foods, and still tend to feel satisfied. The dietary fiber and water in the fruits and vegetables take up room in the stomach, apparently helping to decrease hunger drive when the stomach contents reach a certain level.

TABLE 9.7
Calories found in one-cup portions of food

Food	Calories per Cup	Ranking	Food	Calories per Cup	Ranking
Vegetable oils	1,927	Very high in Calories (fats)	Macaroni (cooked)	190	Moderately low (juices, soups, cereals, milk)
Shortening	1,812		Whole-wheat cereal (cooked)	180	
Margarine	1,616				
Butter	1,600		Wheat Chex	169	
Mayonnaise	1,582		Tomato soup (with milk)	160	
Peanut butter	1,520		Grape juice	155	
Salad dressing, blue cheese	1,234		Whole milk	150	
Honey	1,040		Oatmeal (cooked)	145	
Cake icing	1,035		Plain yogurt	144	
			Pineapple juice	139	
Nuts, macadamia	940	High (nuts, seeds and sugar)	Crabmeat	135	
Jams/preserves	880		Corn (cooked)	134	
Chocolate candy	860		Peas (cooked)	126	
Peanuts, oil roasted	840		Low-fat milk	121	
Sunflower seeds	821		White bread	120	
Cashews	787		Apple juice	116	
Almonds	766		Orange juice	112	
White sugar	720		Rice Krispies	112	
Granola	595		Corn Chex	111	
Sour cream	493	Moderately high (dried fruit, cheese, flour)	Nonfat milk	86	Low (non-fat milk, fruits)
Dates	489		Oranges	85	
Walnuts	486		Pumpkin	83	
Dried pears	472		Winter squash	79	
Coconut	466		Pineapple	77	
Cheddar cheese	455		Blackberries	74	
Raisins	434		Apples	64	
Flour (wheat, enriched)	420		Grapes	58	
Grape-Nuts	407		Onions	58	
Corned beef hash	400		Cantaloupe	57	
Prunes	385		Beets (cooked)	52	
Ice cream (16% fat)	349		V-8 juice	51	
			Watermelon	50	
Sweet potato	344	Moderate (legumes, some dairy products, rice)	Carrots	48	Very low (vegetables)
Pork (lean, roasted)	341		Broccoli (cooked)	46	
Ricotta cheese (skim milk)	340		Strawberries	45	
Ice cream (10% fat)	269		Green beans	44	
Turkey	262		Kale (cooked)	41	
Ham (roasted)	249		Kohlrabi (raw)	38	
Soybeans (cooked)	234		Summer squash (cooked)	36	
Brown rice (cooked)	232		Sprouted mung beans	32	
Cottage cheese (4%, large curd)	232		Zucchini (cooked)	28	
Yogurt (fruit-flavored)	231		Collards (cooked)	27	
Red kidney beans (cooked)	230		Cauliflower (raw)	24	
Spanish rice	213		Cabbage (raw)	22	
Lentils (cooked)	210		Celery	18	
			Mushrooms (raw)	18	
			Cucumber	14	
			Spinach (raw)	12	
			Romaine lettuce	8	
			Iceberg lettuce	7	
			Swiss chard (raw)	6	

Data from U.S. Department of Agriculture Food Consumption Tables (Handbook No. 8 series).

The Wrong Way to Lose Weight Various other substances have been advocated for weight reduction, but none of these is recommended for those seeking permanent weight loss. As you read the following list, compare them with the principles in table 9.6 to learn why most experts describe these substances as being in the realm of quackery (34).

1. **Starch blockers:** This enzyme inhibitor is supposed to block the digestion and absorption of ingested carbohydrate. Several studies have now shown these not only to be ineffective but also a possible risk to health; several federal courts have declared them illegal because they are unapproved new drugs. In addition, starch blockers tie into that common American myth that carbohydrates are responsible for obesity. As we have discussed already, dietary fat is the culprit, not dietary carbohydrate.

2. **Bulk producers:** These are substances like methycellulose (found in Metamucil) and glucomannan, which absorb liquid in the stomach and create a feeling of fullness. Glucomannan is chemically extracted from konjac tubers (underground vegetables from Japan), and is supposed to absorb liquid, forming a high-fiber gel that produces a feeling of fullness to help stop the hunger drive. There is no scientific evidence that such bulk-producing products effectively cause weight loss or do anything other than create the feeling of fullness of ordinary bulky foods such as whole grains, apples, carrots, and other fruits and vegetables.

3. **Spirulina:** This is a dark green powder or pill derived from algae, and it has been promoted as a weight-loss product. Claims have been made that phenylalanine, an amino acid found in spirulina (and in most other protein sources), "acts on the brain's appetite center to switch off your hunger pangs. . . ." The Food and Drug Administration (FDA) is not aware of any evidence that phenylalanine is safe and effective as an appetite suppressant.

4. **Benzocaine:** This is the active ingredient in dietetic candy, lozenges, and gum. Benzocaine is a topical anesthetic said to work by "numbing" the tongue, reducing the ability to taste foods. According to the AMA Drug Evaluations, "there are no conclusive data to support benzocaine's effectiveness as an anorexiant."

5. **Phenylpropanolamine (PPA):** This is the active ingredient in most nonprescription weight-control products, such as Dexatrim, Appedrine, Control, Dietac, Prolamine, and Adrinex. PPA is related to amphetamines and has similar side effects, including nervousness, insomnia, headaches, nausea, tinnitus (ringing in the ears), and elevated blood pressure. Although PPA may be somewhat effective for short-term weight control, the long-term effect of PPA and other weight-control drugs is seriously questioned and may be associated with harmful side effects.

6. **Growth hormone releasers:** Various products such as Lipogene-GH, Nite Diet, Dream Away, Nite Time Diet, and HGH-3X are all sold with the claim that if they are taken at bedtime, weight loss will occur overnight due to the increased release of growth hormone from the amino acids arginine and ornithine contained in the products. In other words, these amino acids stimulate human growth hormone, causing the user to "burn fat" overnight. However, research has suggested that a person's weight does not seem to be related to the level of growth hormone in the system. This erroneous idea was submitted by Pearson and Shaw in their book *Life Extension.*

7. **Cholecystokinin (CCK):** CCK is a hormone involved in digestion (especially of fat). Producers of CCK claim that this substance will reduce hunger and cause sudden and dramatic weight loss. No CCK product has been approved by the FDA for public sale for any purpose.

8. **DHEA:** This unapproved drug is derived from human urine and other sources. Manufacturers tout DHEA as a "natural" weight-loss product. DHEA is known chemically as dehydroepiandrosterone or dehydroandrosterone. FDA has ordered manufacturers to stop selling this unapproved drug. The FDA has not received any data to substantiate the claims for DHEA.

9. **Grapefruit pills:** For several decades, grapefruit has been promoted by various people as having special fat-burning properties. Grapefruit pills contain grapefruit extract, diuretics, and bulk-forming agents. Some contain phenylpropanolamine (PPA), along with herbs or other ingredients. FDA has not approved the sale of these products and is unaware of any valid medical evidence that such products are safe or effective. The U.S. Postal Service has taken action to bar use of the mails by one grapefruit-pill supplier, Citrus Industries, marketer of the Grapefruit Super Pill.

10. **Herbalife:** Herbalife sells items described as "herbal-based" health, nutrition, weight-control, and skin-care products, marketing them through a multilevel program. Herbalife International in 1987 agreed to pay $850,000 to settle a suit brought by the California Attorney General. The suit charged Herbalife with the following:

    —misrepresenting that the firm's Cell-U-Loss product directs weight loss to particular portions of the body;

    —misrepresenting that the firm's Slim and Trim diet products will allow users to experience a typical weight loss of 10–29 pounds per month;

    —making unapproved drug and herbal claims for some of the products;

    —failing to disclose that the active ingredient in one product, N.R.G., is caffeine; and

    —using an illegal pyramid scheme for the sale of its products.

Exercise

As we will see in this section, in the "battle of the bulge," two weapons are needed—both diet and exercise. However, research tends to support control of caloric intake as being much more powerful than exercise with respect to weight loss.

As stated previously, obese people are generally less active than others. There are several important benefits of exercise for the obese.

1. Expenditure of extra Calories from the exercise itself

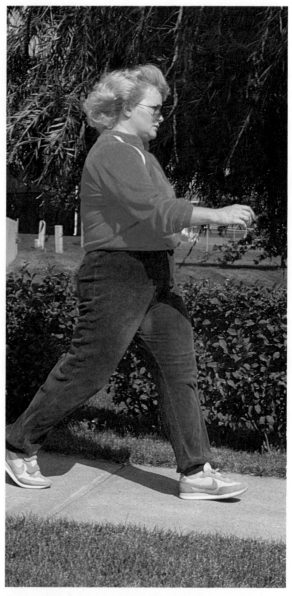

There are several important benefits of regular exercise for obese people.

2. Elevation of the resting metabolic rate following the exercise bout
3. Protection of the lean body weight
4. Better appetite control
5. Decrease in risk of various diseases common to obesity
6. Improved psychological well-being

Expenditure of Extra Calories from the Exercise Bout Table 9.8 shows the number of Calories burned per hour during various types of physical activity. Notice that a rule of thumb, a 150-pound person burns about 100 to 120 Calories for every mile walked or run. A person wishing to lose the equivalent of one pound of body fat (3,500 Calories) would have to walk nearly 35 miles. Because the body is so efficient in its energy expenditure, most researchers today are showing that adding two to five miles of daily walking to a weight reduction diet (typically 1,200 to 1,500 Calories) does not add significantly to the amount of weight lost (35).

For example, one study in Dallas, Texas, compared the effects of a 1,200 Calorie diet alone and the effects of the same diet plus 30 minutes of brisk walking, five days per week (36). In addition to a control group that did not exercise or diet, an exercise-only group was formed. Figure 9.13 shows that the diet and exercise group lost the most weight over the twelve weeks of the study. Notice, however, that the diet-only group lost nearly the same amount of weight, whereas the exercise-only group fared little better than the control group. Most researchers have concluded that controlling dietary intake has the greatest effect on weight loss.

Elevation of Resting Metabolic Rate Although the issue remains controversial, there is evidence that the effects of physical activity on metabolism can last for a number of hours after the exercise is completed, thus adding to the caloric deficit. One researcher has summarized that for every 100 Calories burned during exercise, approximately 15 more Calories are burned during the following 12 hours (37). The longer and more intense the exercise, the greater the number of Calories burned after the exercise session is over.

Protection of Lean Body Weight Although exercising may not accelerate the loss of total body weight when a person is dieting, various researchers have shown that exercise does result in more of the weight loss coming from fat and less from the lean body weight (30,38).

In one study of moderately obese women, all were given an 800-Calorie, liquid-formula diet for five weeks. Half of the subjects exercised by walking two to three miles per day, and the other half remained sedentary. Figure 9.14 shows that the walking group did not lose more total weight than the group that did not exercise. However, loss from fat was greater in the exercise group (74 percent of total weight lost) than in the nonexercise group (57 percent of total weight lost).

TABLE 9.8
Activities that rate high in cardiovascular-respiratory benefits and their approximate energy expenditures

Summarized are some of the better cardiovascular-respiratory exercises and the number of kcal expended per hour of the exercise. An important concept is to select several of these activities that are enjoyable, and to use them in such a way that scheduled exercise sessions are looked forward to, not dreaded.

Caloric expenditure is based on a 150-lb person. There is a 10% increase in caloric expenditure for each 15 lbs over this weight and a 10% decrease for each 15 lbs under.

Activity	Kcal per Hour
Badminton, competitive singles	480
Basketball	360–660
Bicycling	
10 mph	420
11 mph	480
12 mph	600
13 mph	660
Calisthenics, heavy	600
Handball, competitive	660
Rope skipping, vigorous	800
Rowing machine	840
Running	
5 mph	600
6 mph	750
7 mph	870
8 mph	1,020
9 mph	1,130
10 mph	1,285
Skating, ice or roller, rapid	700
Skiing, downhill, vigorous	600
Skiing, cross-country	
2.5 mph	560
4 mph	600
5 mph	700
8 mph	1,020
Swimming, 25–50 yards per min.	360–750
Walking	
Level road, 4 mph (fast)	420
Upstairs	600–1,080
Uphill, 3.5 mph	480–900
Gardening, much lifting, stooping, digging	500
Mowing, pushing hand mower	450
Sawing hardwood	600
Shoveling, heavy	660
Wood chopping	560

From E. L. Wynder, *The Book of Health: The American Health Foundation.* © 1981 Franklin Watts, Inc., New York. Used with permission.

*F*IGURE 9.13

Percentage changes in body weight in males and females according to treatment effects of diet and exercise (DE), diet (D), exercise (E), and control (C). Notice that although diet and exercise together promote the best weight loss, most of this comes from eating less, not exercising more.

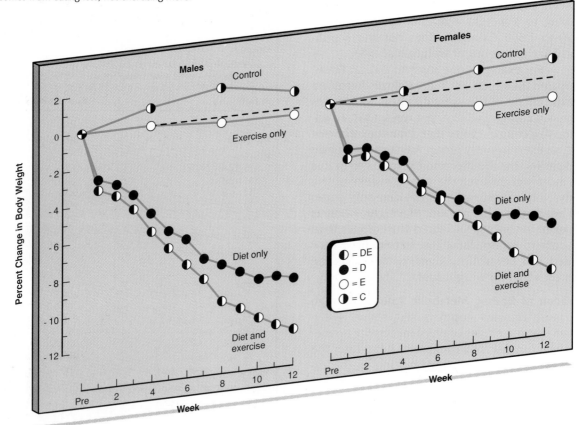

*F*IGURE 9.14

During a weight-loss program, exercise may not help individuals lose more total body weight but can promote greater loss of fat weight while protecting the lean body weight.

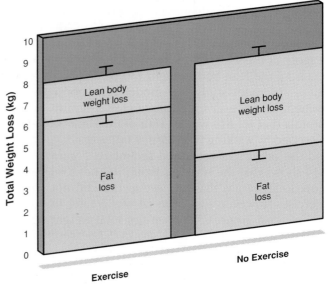

Thus, exercise is beneficial when coupled with food restriction because it promotes loss of body fat and preserves the lean body weight. As discussed previously, the resting metabolic rate is higher in people with higher lean body weights. Therefore, over a long time period, regular physical activity may indirectly result in a large number of Calories being consumed because of the increased lean body mass.

The issue of "spot reducing" needs clarification. The concept of spot reduction is based on the widely held belief that it is possible to selectively "burn off" fat from specific areas of the body by exercising nearby muscles. For example, some people believe that doing sit-ups burns abdominal fat. Research, however, has shown that the concept of spot reduction is false. In one study, subjects performed a total of 5,000 sit-ups over a 27-day period. Fat-tissue biopsies revealed that sit-ups did not selectively reduce fat-cell size in the abdominal area to a greater extent than at other body-fat sites (39). Specific calisthenics may help tone the muscles in a certain area, but they do not help melt away the fat, primarily because very few calories are expended (40). If spot reducing really worked, then fat people who chew gum would have thin faces!

So in conclusion, the success of a weight-loss program should be measured by the type of weight lost and the overall health status of the individual, rather than just the total amount of weight lost. Optimal body-composition changes occur with a combination of Calorie restriction (balanced, healthful diet) and exercise. This combination promotes loss of fat weight while sparing the lean body weight.

Better Appetite Control Most researchers have reported that active people eat more but are leaner than sedentary people. In other words, for moderately active humans, long-term exercise promotes increased caloric intake, but leaner bodies. In a careful, one-year study at Stanford University, involving 81 middle-aged males, those who did the most jogging lost the most body fat and showed the biggest increase in food Calories (41).

In contrast, a review of the literature shows that a single bout of exercise appears to depress the appetite. The effect of exercise in the short term is to decrease food intake immediately after exercise. In a 14-day study of military cadets, food intake was depressed on exercise days and increased on rest days (42).

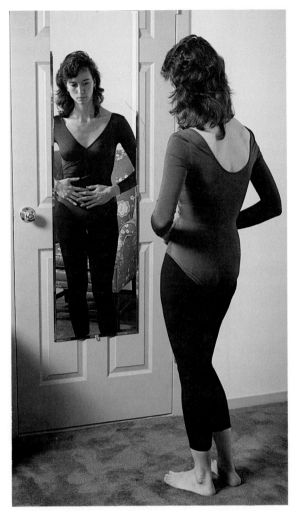

Individuals with anorexia nervosa claim to "feel fat" even when extremely thin.

In summary, the immediate response of humans to exercise is to decrease food intake, but the long-term response is to eat more but stay leaner than sedentary controls. It is possible that a certain level of physical activity is necessary before the body can precisely control food intake to match energy expenditure. In other words, exercise may help "fine tune" the appetite.

Decrease in Risk of Various Diseases As discussed at the beginning of this chapter, obesity is associated with many health problems, such as heart disease, diabetes, high blood pressure, and high blood-cholesterol levels. Although a thorough discussion of these health problems is beyond the scope of this textbook, it should be noted that there is now strong evidence that exercise can help to counter each of these complications (43). For this reason alone, the obese would do well to exercise.

Improved Psychological and Social Support In addition to the physiological benefits, exercise is also associated with feelings of well-being, reduction in anxiety and depression, and an increase in self-concept and elevated mood (44). The strong, increasing evidence of this provides additional support for including exercise in weight-loss programs. During weight loss, many people experience feelings of depression and irritability, and exercise can help counter these.

Fad Products Countless fraudulent exercise devices are available (45), including the following:

Mechanical vibration and fat loss: Passive exercise devices include roller machines, oscillating tables, passive-motion tables, and massagers that do all the work—shaking, rolling, and moving body parts. Such gadgets have been hailed as effortless exercise devices that take off or redistribute fat. Studies indicate, however, that mechanically vibrating body fat is similar to massaging and shaking several pounds of beef fat in a plastic bag—the fat is still all there after the shaking stops. A pound of fat contains 3,500 Calories, and these must be burned by the body, not massaged.

Weight-reducing clothing: Special weight-reducing clothing, including heated belts, rubberized suits, and oilskins rely chiefly on dehydration and localized pressure. Although circumference measures or scale weight may temporarily decrease, these losses are not associated with decreased body fat. Rubberized suits are potentially dangerous because they block body heat loss and sweat evaporation.

Cellulite cures: **Cellulite** is the term used to describe unsightly fat tissue that causes the overlying skin to appear dimpled like an orange peel. Supposedly, 80 percent of all women and 10 percent of all men have cellulite deposits located primarily in the thigh, buttock, and knee areas. Proponents of cellulite cures claim that cellulite fat is trapped fat in abnormal and chronically inflamed connective tissue, with impeded blood and lymph access. High-protein diets, massage, sauna, special skin creams, body

wrappings, or pseudoelectric devices are claimed to "break up or reduce cellulite deposits." Exorbitant fees are often charged for these unfounded cures. Most medical and nutrition authorities contend that cellulite is simply subcutaneous fat, packaged somewhat differently in normal connective tissue. The only real cure is fat loss through regular aerobic exercise and improved diet.

Electrical muscle stimulators (EMS): EMS devices are claimed to provide "all the figure-toning of 3,000 sit-ups without moving an inch." In addition, other benefits include face lifts without surgery, slimming and trimming, weight loss, bust development, spot reducing, and removal of cellulite. The Food and Drug Administration considers claims for EMS devices promoted for such purposes to be misbranded and fraudulent.

Behavior Modification

Behavior modification is one of the most widely used treatments for obesity (11). More than 100 studies have tested the effectiveness of behavior modification, and it has proven to be more effective than any other treatment with which it has been compared. Behavior modification takes into consideration the details of the eating behavior to be changed, the events that trigger eating, and the consequences of eating (feelings, procedures to provide rewards) (46).

The primary behavior to be changed is eating, and a number of exercises are designed to slow the rate of eating and allow body signals indicating satisfaction to exert their effect. The focus is on events that trigger eating, such as shopping for food or keeping high-fat foods in the house. Patients are taught to remove from their environment the various stimuli that prompt eating. Rewards are provided for carrying out the proper behaviors. Table 9.9 outlines some of the more common techniques (47). (See Health-Promotion Activity 9.2 for a typical behavioral modification exercise.)

A Practical Summary

Suppose that you are going to help a friend of yours, who should weigh 120 pounds but weighs 144 pounds instead, to lose weight. The 24 extra pounds of weight means that she is considered mildly obese. Of these 24 pounds, 75 percent (or 18 pounds) is probably excess body fat, and 25 percent is extra lean body weight. (Remember that obese people tend to have higher lean body weights because of the extra muscle that is built up from carrying around the excess weight.)

Before counseling your friend to make various life-style changes, you might first have her keep a diet diary (see Health-Promotion Activity 9.2). By identifying the circumstances surrounding her eating and her feelings about them, you can help her decide how to control some of these circumstances. In addition, you can set up a reward system.

For example, if you find that your friend's primary problem is eating snacks high in fats (for example, potato chips or salted nuts), perhaps low-Calorie snacks such as fresh fruit pieces could be substituted. In addition, if the snacking stems from anxiety over schoolwork, for example, a brisk, ten-minute walk before each study session might help reduce this anxiety. If she accomplishes these two changes in behavior (low-Calorie snacks and brisk walking), on a weekly basis she might decide to reward herself by buying a new music tape or a special outfit.

In addition to these changes, her overall exercise and dietary life-style will need to be permanently altered (48). A practical approach would be to first determine a time frame for achieving ideal weight. Because your friend has 18 pounds of excess fat, she will need to expend 63,000 Calories to lose it. (As stated previously, each pound of body fat contains 3,500 Calories.) An important principle to remember is that mildly obese individuals should not lose more than one percent of their body weight per week. A weight-loss graph as shown in table 9.10 can be used to help ensure that weight loss is steady but gradual. Weight losses greater than one percent of body weight are poorly maintained and may cause mental depression and decreased motivation. A rapid loss of weight is too stressful to the human mind and body.

Based on your friend's weight, then, losing one percent of that per week would mean losing no more than 1–1½ pounds of body weight per week. To lose one pound of body fat per week, she would have to lose 500 Calories from her body each day (500 Calories × 7 = 3,500 Calories). If she would start walking 2½ miles every day, this would represent close to 250 Calories. Then by removing the equivalent of 2½ tablespoons of fat from her diet

TABLE 9.9
Behavioral principles of weight control

Stimulus Control	
Shopping	Shop for food after eating; shop from a list; avoid ready-to-eat foods; don't carry more cash than is needed for list.
Plans	Plan to limit food intake; substitute exercise for snacking; eat meals at scheduled times; don't accept food offered by others.
Activities	Store food out of sight; eat all food in the same place; remove food from inappropriate home storage areas; keep serving dishes off the table; use smaller dishes and utensils; avoid being the food server; leave the table immediately after eating.
Holidays, Parties	Plan eating habits before parties; eat a low-calorie snack before parties; practice polite ways to decline food.
Eating Behavior	Put fork down between mouthfuls; chew thoroughly before swallowing; pause in the middle of the meal; do nothing else while eating (reading, TV).
Reward	Solicit help from family and friends (praise); use self-monitoring records as basis for rewards; plan specific rewards for specific behaviors.
Self-Monitoring	Keep diet diary that includes time and place of eating, type and amount of food, who is present, and how you feel.
Nutrition Education	Use diet diary to identify problem areas; make small changes that you can continue; learn nutritional values of foods; decrease fat intake; increase complex carbohydrate.
Physical Activity	
Informal Activity	Increase routine, informal activity; increase use of stairs in particular; keep a record of distance walked/day.
Formal Exercise	Begin a moderate exercise program; keep a formal record; increase the exercise gradually.
Cognitive Restructuring	Avoid setting unreasonable goals; think about progress, not shortcomings; avoid imperatives like "always" and "never;" counter negative thoughts with reason; set weight goals that are reasonable; realize that when any event takes place, the mind has the power to decide what reaction should take place (negative reactions can be controlled).

From A. J. Stunkard, "What Is Behavior Therapy? A Very Short Description of Behavior Weight Control." *American Journal of Clinical Nutrition* 41: 821–23, 1985. © American Society for Clinical Nutrition. Used with permission.

Weight-loss record   Name _____

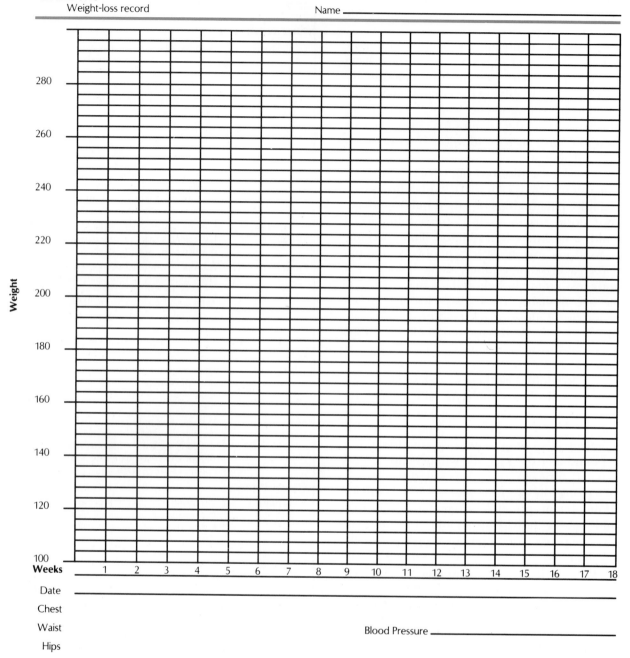

Date _____

Chest

Waist   Blood Pressure _____

Hips

each day, she would decrease her caloric consumption by 250 Calories (one tablespoon of fat has 100 Calories). She could accomplish this by using low-fat or nonfat dairy products and only lean cuts of meats, by reducing use of visible fats (margarines, salad dressing, mayonnaise, oil, sour cream, etc.) and by substituting other types of low-Calorie spreads (low-fat yogurts, low-Calorie fruit jams, low-fat cheese spreads, etc.). She should also eat more fruits, salads, steamed vegetables, and whole-grain products.

Thus, the net result would be 500 Calories "negative caloric balance," and in one week, close to one pound of fat would be lost.

Because the walking helps protect the lean body weight, only a little water and muscle would be lost. After 18 weeks, if she continued to exercise and eat a low-fat diet, the 18 pounds of excess body fat and lean body weight (6 pounds) should be gone—permanently.

The primary weapons in this battle of the bulge—daily exercise and a low-fat diet—will also help her to feel better and aid in the prevention of other health problems as well.

HEALTH-PROMOTION INSIGHT
Eating Disorders-Bulimia and Anorexia Nervosa

Our unresolved paradox is this: our food-laden, sedentary society holds the thin and beautiful in high esteem. On the one hand our magazine covers, movie stars, and athletic heroes advance the concept that thin is in. But on the other hand we are led, through advertising, to believe that technological labor-saving devices and sumptuous foods rich in fats and sugars are benefits associated with high-class living.

Out of this quandary has emerged a sector of our population with extremely disordered eating habits: the bulimics and anorexics.

Bulimia has several characteristics.

1. There are recurrent episodes of binge eating (rapid consumption of a large amount of food in a short period of time, often less than two hours).
2. During the eating binges there is a feeling of lack of control over the eating behavior.
3. The individual regularly engages in either self-induced vomiting, use of laxatives, or rigorous dieting or fasting in order to counteract the effects of the binge eating.
4. There is a minimum average of two binge-eating episodes per week for at least three months.

Anorexia nervosa can be characterized as follows.

1. There is an intense fear of becoming obese, even when underweight.
2. There is a disturbance in the way in which one's body weight, size, or shape is perceived. For example, one claims to "feel fat" even when extremely thin or believes that one area of the body is "too fat" even when obviously underweight.
3. There is a refusal to maintain body weight over a minimal normal weight for age and height. For example, weight loss is more than 15 percent below normal. In a growing child, there is a failure to make expected weight gains, leading to body weights 15 percent below expected.
4. With females, there is an absence of at least three consecutive menstrual cycles when otherwise expected to occur. This is called amenorrhea.

Among college students, four percent of the women and 0.4 percent of the men are classified as bulimic (49). However, an alarming number of college students have symptoms of bulimia and anorexia, such as binge eating, vomiting excess food, and an extreme fear of gaining weight. For example, in one study, 23 percent of college women and 14 percent of college men reported episodes of binge eating at least once a week on the average. In addition, 28 percent of the women and 7 percent of the men stated that they were "often" to "always" terrified of gaining weight.

A startling number of adolescents are engaging in unhealthful behaviors to regulate their body weight. In one study of tenth-grade students, 13 percent reported use of vomiting, laxatives, or diuretics to control their weight. These students expressed an abnormal concern with their weight, frequently dieted, and experienced guilt following periods of excessive eating.

There are many published reports of the abnormal weight-control behaviors of athletes, especially ballet dancers, gymnasts, runners, and swimmers. At one competitive swimming camp, researchers found that of the 900 swimmers aged 9 to 18, 15.4 percent of the girls and 3.6 percent of the boys used a variety of abnormal weight-loss techniques to meet the demands of their sport (51). Girls in particular were likely to misperceive themselves as overweight.

Binge eating and the various forms of purging behavior (vomiting, laxative and diuretic use) can cause serious medical problems (50). Included are stomach dilation and rupture, infection of the lung from vomitus, low body levels of chloride and potassium ions, infection and rupture of the esophagus, enlargement of the salivary glands, and tooth erosion and loss.

Furthermore, death is common among anorexics who refuse to stop their low intake of food (52). Karen Carpenter, a famous pop singer of the 1970s, died from complications related to her battles with anorexia.

Bulimic symptoms are more likely to arise in individuals who have a history of weight problems. In addition, 30 to 50 percent of anorexics develop bulimia (53). One of the main features of anorexia nervosa, the morbid fear of becoming fat, is also central to bulimia.

What can be done to help the anorexic or bulimic? Most experts feel that such individuals should be referred to eating-disorder clinics. These clinics usually have a staff of professionals, including physicians, psychologists, dietitians, and nurses, to meet the varied needs of people with eating disorders (54). Often bulimics and anorexics have very deep-seated emotional problems at the foundation of their eating problems. Long-term, professional care is necessary, which is provided by eating-disorder clinics that have been established in many hospitals.

*S*UMMARY

1. The majority of American adults weigh more than they should, and approximately one-fourth of all children, youth, and adults are obese.
2. There are many disadvantages associated with obesity, including diseases such as cancer, diabetes, and heart disease. Obesity is also associated with early death.
3. Three major theories of obesity were discussed, with emphasis placed on the importance of genetic and parental influences, dietary factors (especially excess dietary fat), and insufficient energy expenditure.
4. Some people are more prone to obesity than others, due to genetic factors, and need to be unusually careful in their dietary and exercise habits.
5. When humans eat diets high in fat, excess body fat is formed more easily than with a high-carbohydrate, high-fiber diet. Including more fruits, vegetables, legumes, and whole grains in the diet, and moderating high-fat, low-fiber foods such as oils, margarine, butter, cheese, and fatty meats, is probably the most important measure for controlling obesity.
6. Although obese people have higher resting metabolic rates than normal-weight people because of their extra lean body weight, they tend to exercise less than lean people. However, most studies have found that overeating, rather than underexercising, causes obesity.
7. Following a meal, energy is expended by the body to process the food. This is called the thermic effect of food. Some obese people may have a slightly lower thermic effect of food, but this does not appear to be a major factor explaining why people gain weight.
8. Obesity is very difficult to treat. There are three classifications of obesity, and each requires a different approach.
9. Severe obesity is the condition of weighing more than double the ideal weight. In certain cases, gastric stapling is the recommended treatment.
10. Moderate obesity is the condition of being 41–100 percent overweight. Because of the high amounts of excess body fat, the very-low-Calorie diet is recommended, but only under medical supervision.
11. The majority of obese people are mildly obese (20–40 percent overweight). For most of these individuals, a weight loss of about one percent total body weight per week is optimal, through a combination of improved diet, increased exercise, and appropriate behavioral modification.
12. To lose one pound of fat, one must expend 3,500 Calories.
13. The caloric intake should be reduced, preferably by reducing the fat content of the diet and increasing the intake of complex carbohydrates. Weight-watchers must beware of the many ``quick and easy'' weight-loss methods that are available.
14. There are several important benefits of exercise for the obese, including expenditure of extra Calories, protection of the lean body weight, better appetite control, and decrease in risk of various diseases common to obesity.
15. Behavior modification consists of various procedures to help one change eating behavior, events that trigger the eating, and the various consequences.
16. Bulimia and anorexia nervosa are eating disorders that have many harmful effects on health, and even life itself. Bulimics consume large amounts of food during short periods of time, and then engage in various purging techniques. People with anorexia nervosa have disturbed perceptions of their body images, leading to excessive loss of weight. Long-term professional care is necessary.

REFERENCES

1. National Institutes of Health. 1985. Consensus Development Conference Statement. Health Implications of Obesity. February 11-13, 1985. *Annals of Internal Medicine* 103:981-1077.
2. National Center for Health Statistics: Health, United States, 1987. DHHS Pub. No. (PHS) 88-1232. March, 1988. Public Health Service. Washington, D.C.: U.S. Government Printing Office.
3. Simopoulos, A. P. 1986. Obesity and Body Weight Standards. *Annual Review of Public Health* 7:481-92.
4. Millar, W. J., and T. Stephens. 1987. The Prevalence of Overweight and Obesity in Britain, Canada, and United States. *American Journal of Public Health* 77:38-41.
5. Gortmaker, S. L., et al. 1987. Increasing Pediatric Obesity in the United States. *American Journal of Diseases in Children* 141:535-40.
6. Jéquier, E. 1987. Energy, Obesity, and Body Weight Standards. *American Journal of Clinical Nutrition* 45:1035-1047.
7. Manson, J. E., et al. 1987. Body Weight and Longevity: A Reassessment. *Journal of the American Medical Association* 257:353-58.
8. Mayer, J. 1965. Genetic Factors in Human Obesity. *Annals of New York Academy of Sciences* 131:412-21.
9. Stunkard, A. J., T. T. Foch, and Z. Hrubec. 1986. A Twin Study of Human Obesity. *Journal of the American Medical Association* 256:51-54.
10. Stunkard, A. J., et al. 1986. An Adoption Study of Human Obesity. *New England Journal of Medicine* 314:193-98.
11. Stunkard, A. J. 1984. *Eating and Its Disorders.* New York: Raven Press.
12. Freedman, D. S., et al. 1987. Persistence of Juvenile-Onset Obesity over Eight Years: The Bogalusa Heart Study. *American Journal of Public Health* 77:588-92.
13. Patterson, R. E., et al. 1986. Factors Related to Obesity in Preschool Children. *Journal of the American Dietetic Association* 86:1376-1381.
14. de Boer, J. O., et al. 1987. Energy Requirements and Energy Expenditure of Lean and Overweight Women, Measured by Indirect Calorimetry. *American Journal of Clinical Nutrition* 46:13-21.
15. Marcus, M. D., R. R. Wing, and D. M. Lamparski. 1985. Binge Eating and Dietary Restraint in Obese Patients. *Addictive Behaviors* 10:163-68.
16. Danforth, E. 1985. Diet and Obesity. *American Journal of Clinical Nutrition* 41:1132-1145.
17. Sims, E. A. H., and E. Danforth. 1987. Expenditure and Storage of Energy in Man. *Journal of Clinical Investigation* 79:1019-1025.
18. Acheson, K. J., et al. 1987. Carbohydrate Metabolism and De Novo Lipogenesis in Human Obesity. *American Journal of Clinical Nutrition* 45:78-85.
19. Dietz, W. H., and S. L. Gortmaker. 1985. Do We Fatten Our Children at the Television Set? Obesity and Television Viewing in Children and Adolescents. *Pediatrics* 75:807-12.
20. Tyron, W. W. 1987. Activity as a Function of Body Weight. *American Journal of Clinical Nutrition* 46:451-55.
21. Ravussin, E., et al. 1986. Determinants of 24-hour Energy Expenditure in Man. *Journal of Clinical Investigation* 78:1568-1578.
22. Nair, K. S., J. Webster, and J. S. Garrow. 1986. Effect of Impaired Glucose Tolerance and Type II Diabetes on Resting Metabolic Rate and Thermic Response to a Glucose Meal in Obese Women. *Metabolism* 35:640-44.
23. Brownell, K. D. 1984. The Psychology and Physiology of Obesity: Implications for Screening and Treatment. *Journal of the American Dietetic Association* 406-14.
24. Priddy, M. L. B. 1985. Gastric Reduction Surgery: A Dietitian's Experience and Perspective. *Journal of the American Dietetic Association* 85:455-58.
25. Van Itallie, T. B., et al. 1985. Guidelines for Morbid Obesity. *American Journal of Clinical Nutrition* 42:904-5.
26. Lockwood, D. H., and J. M. Amatruda. 1984. Very Low Calorie Diets in the Management of Obesity. *Annual Review of Medicine* 35:373-81.
27. Wadden, T. A., et al. 1983. The Cambridge Diet: More Mayhem? *Journal of the American Medical Association* 250:2833-2834.
28. Wadden, T. A., A. J. Stunkard, and K. D. Brownell. 1983. Very Low Calorie Diets: Their Efficacy, Safety, and Future. *Annals of Internal Medicine* 99:675-83.
29. Stunkard, A. J. 1987. Conservative Treatments for Obesity. *American Journal of Clinical Nutrition* 45:1142-1154.
30. Belko, A. Z., et al. 1987. Diet, Exercise, Weight Loss, and Energy Expenditure in Moderately Overweight Women. *International Journal of Obesity* 11:93-104.
31. Arrington, R., J. Bonner, and K. R. Stitt. 1985. Weight Reduction Methods of College Women. *Journal of the American Dietetic Association* 85:483-84.
32. National Center for Health Statistics. 1986. Health, United States, 1986. DHHS Pub. No. (PHS) 87-1232. Public Health Service. Washington, D.C.: U.S. Government Printing Office.
33. Fisher, M. C., and P. A. Lachance. 1985. Nutrition Evaluation of Published Weight-Reducing Diets. *Journal of the American Dietetic Association* 85:450-54.
34. Willis, J. 1985. The Fad-Free Diet: How to Take Weight Off (and Keep It Off) Without Getting Ripped Off. *FDA Consumer* (July/August):26-29.
35. Van Dale, D., et al. 1987. Does Exercise Give An Additional Effect in Weight Reduction Regimens? *International Journal of Obesity* 11:367-75.
36. Hagan, R. D., et al. 1986. The Effects of Aerobic Conditioning and/or Caloric Restriction in Overweight Men and Women. *Medicine and Science in Sports and Exercise* 18:87-94.
37. Bahr, R., et al. 1987. Effect of Duration of Exercise on Excess Postexercise O_2 Consumption. *Journal of Applied Physiology* 62:485-90.
38. Hill, J. O., et al. 1987. Effects of Exercise and Food Restriction on Body Composition and Metabolic Rate in Obese Women. *American Journal of Clinical Nutrition* 46:622-30.
39. Katch, F. I., et al. 1984. Effects of Sit Up Exercise Training on Adipose Cell Size and Adiposity. *Research Quarterly Exercise Sport* 55:242-47.
40. Despres, J. P., et al. 1985. Effects of Aerobic Training on Fat Distribution in Male Subjects. *Medicine and Science in Sports and Exercise* 17:113-18.
41. Brotherhood, J. R. 1984. Nutrition and Sports Performance. *Sports Medicine* 1:350-89.
42. Wilmore, J. H. 1983. Appetite and Body Composition Consequent to Physical Activity. *Research Quarterly Exercise Sport* 54:415-25.
43. Pollock, M. L., J. H. Wilmore, and S. M. Fox. 1984. *Exercise in Health and Disease.* Philadelphia: W. B. Saunders Co.
44. Nieman, D. C. 1986. *The Sports Medicine Fitness Course.* Palo Alto, CA: Bull Publishing Company.
45. Franklin, B. A. 1984. Myths and Misconceptions in Exercise for Weight Control. In *Nutrition and Exercise in Obesity Management.* J. Storlie and H. A. Jordan, eds. New York: SP Medical & Scientific Books.
46. Bray, G. A. 1983. In *Nutritional Support of Medical Practice.* H. A. Schneider, ed. Philadelphia: Harper and Row.
47. Stunkard, A. J., et al. 1985. What Is Behavior Therapy? A Very Short Description of Behavioral Weight Control. *American Journal of Clinical Nutrition* 41:821-23.

48. American College of Sports Medicine. 1984. Position Statement on Proper and Improper Weight Loss Programs. *Medicine and Science in Sports and Exercise* 17.
49. Zuckerman, D. M., et al. 1986. The Prevalence of Bulimia Among College Students. *American Journal of Public Health* 76:1135–1137.
50. Killen, J. D., et al. 1986. Self-Induced Vomiting and Laxative and Diuretic Use Among Teenagers. *Journal of the American Medical Association* 255:1447–1449.

51. Dummer, G. M., et al. 1987. Pathogenic Weight-Control Behaviors of Young Competitive Swimmers. *Physician Sportsmedicine* 15(5):75–86.
52. Casper, R. C. 1986. The Pathophysiology of Anorexia Nervosa and Bulimia Nervosa. *Annual Review of Nutrition* 6:299–316.
53. Swift, W. J., et al. 1987. A Follow-Up Study of Thirty Hospitalized Bulimics. *Psychosomatic Medicine* 49:45.
54. Position of The American Dietetic Association. 1988. Nutrition Intervention in the Treatment of Anorexia Nervosa and Bulimia Nervosa. *Journal of the American Dietetic Association* 88:68–71.

HEALTH-PROMOTION ACTIVITY 9.1
Calculating Energy Expenditure

In this activity you will be calculating the number of Calories you expend per day on the average. Remember from your study of this chapter that during any given 24-hour period, the majority of your energy expenditure (if you are no more than moderately active) comes from the resting metabolic rate, with smaller amounts from physical activity and the energy used in digesting and metabolizing your food.

Table 9.11 outlines a method to determine the amount of Calories burned in one day, combining both RMR and physical activity. Notice that Category 1 represents the energy you expend during sleeping or resting in bed, or in other words, your resting metabolic rate. Categories 2 through 9 represent different forms of physical activity, with Category 9 being the most intense.

Table 9.11

Calculating Energy Expenditure

Category Value	Average #Hr/Day		Calories/kg per hr	Body wt (kg)		Calories per Category
1	———	x	1.04	x ———	=	———
2	———	x	1.52	x ———	=	———
3	———	x	2.28	x ———	=	———
4	———	x	2.76	x ———	=	———
5	———	x	3.36	x ———	=	———
6	———	x	4.80	x ———	=	———
7	———	x	5.60	x ———	=	———
8	———	x	6.00	x ———	=	———
9	———	x	8.00	x ———	=	———

Directions: Estimate total hours in each category. Multiply as indicated.

Total 24 hour kcal = ——— Calories expended

Category 1 = Sleeping; resting in bed.

Category 2 = Sitting; eating; listening; writing; etc.

Category 3 = Light activity while standing; washing, shaving, combing, cooking.

Category 4 = Slow walk, driving, dressing, showering.

Category 5 = Light manual work: floor sweeping, window washing, driving a truck, painting, waiting on tables, nursing chores, several house chores, electrician, walking at moderate speed.

Category 6 = Leisure activities and sports in a recreational environment; baseball, golf, volleyball, canoeing or rowing, archery, bowling, slow cycling, table tennis, etc.

Category 7 = Manual work at moderate pace: mining, carpentry, house building, snow shoveling, loading and unloading goods, etc.

Category 8 = Leisure and sport activities of higher intensity (not competitive): canoeing, bicycling (less than 10 mph), dancing, skiing, badminton, gymnastics, moderate swimming, tennis, walking, etc.

Category 9 = Intense manual work, high-intensity sport activities or sport competition: tree cutting, carrying heavy loads, jogging and running (faster than 12 minutes per mile), racquetball, swimming, cross country skiing, mountain hiking, etc.

Adapted from C. Bouchard, "A Method to Assess Energy Expenditure in Children and Adults." *American Journal of Clinical Nutrition* 37:461, 1983. © American Society for Clinical Nutrition. Used with permission.

The average female in the United States burns only 1,700 to 2,000 total Calories per day, and the average male 2,500 to 3,000 Calories per day. Individuals spending more time doing activities in categories 6 through 9 will burn more than these amounts.

First estimate the number of Calories you burn in a given day by averaging the number of hours you spend doing activities in each category. (Make sure that your total number of hours is 24!) Review table 9.4 to help you estimate the number of hours you might spend doing activities in each category.

Next, multiply the number of hours by the Calories/kg factor and then your weight (kilograms). The final step is to total the Calories you have estimated in the final column. Your final result should be the estimated amount of Calories you consume each day.

HEALTH-PROMOTION ACTIVITY 9.2
Monitoring Dietary Habits

In this health promotion activity you will keep a food diary (see table 9.12).

Follow the instructions listed for filling out the food diary, and do this for at least one day. One of the first things you will notice is that keeping an accurate diary will make you unusually aware of everything you eat and why.

Instructions for Filling Out the Food Diary

Time: starting time for a meal or snack.

Minutes spent eating: length of the eating episode in minutes.

M/S: meal or snack: indicate type of eating by the appropriate letter, "M" or "S".

H: hunger on a scale of 0 to 3. 0 = no hunger, 3 = extreme hunger.

Body position: 1 — walking; 2 — standing; 3 — sitting; 4 — lying down.

Activity while eating: Record any activity you carry out while eating, such as watching television, reading, or sweeping the floor.

Location of eating: Record each place you eat; for example, your car, kitchen table, or living room couch.

Food type and quantity: Indicate the content of your meal or snack by kind of food and quantity. Choose units of measurement that you will be able to reproduce from week to week. Accuracy is not as important as consistency.

Eating with whom: Indicate with whom you are eating, or if you are eating that meal or snack alone.

Feelings before and during eating: Record your feelings or mood immediately before or during eating. Typical feelings are angry, bored, confused, depressed, frustrated, sad, etc. Many times you will have no feelings associated with eating. In this case, write down "none."

When you are finished filling out the food diary for one day, answer the following questions:

1. Did you eat food only during mealtimes, or did you tend to snack?
2. How many total minutes did you spend eating? Did you eat too quickly, gulping your food?
3. Did you tend to eat in response to hunger or habit?
4. What body position were you usually in during eating?
5. What other activities did you engage in during eating? Did these activities cause you to eat more than you should?
6. Did you have a set place to eat, or did you eat just about anywhere?
7. How would you rate the quality of your diet? Was it too high in fat and sugar?
8. Did you usually eat with another person? Did eating with this other person cause you to eat too much?
9. How would you rate your usual feelings both before and after eating? Did you tend to eat in response to depression or anxiety? Did you feel good about yourself after the meal was over?

Table 9.12

Food Diary

Day of Week _____   Name _____

Time	Minutes Spent Eating	M/S	H	Body Position	Activity While Eating	Location of Eating	Food Type and Quantity	Eating with Whom	Feeling While Eating
6:00									
11:00									
4:00									
9:00									

From J. M. Ferguson, *Learning to Eat.* © 1975. Bull Publishing Co., Palo Alto, CA. Used with permission.

*H*EALTH-PROMOTION ACTIVITY 9.3
Weight-Management Counseling

In this activity you will review your ability to determine appropriate weight-loss goals for mildly obese individuals. Before answering the questions below, you should review the practical summary one more time.

The subject we will consider weighs 224 pounds; his ideal weight is 166 pounds. He needs to lose 58 pounds, which means that he is 35 percent overweight (mildly obese). Of these 58 pounds, 75 percent is excess body fat (43.5 pounds). The other 25 percent (14.5 pounds) is excess lean body weight, mainly muscle from carrying around his 224 pounds.

1. If he has 43.5 extra pounds of body fat, how many excess Calories does he have stored in his body?

   _____ Calories

2. What is the maximum amount of weight this subject should lose per week?

   _____ pounds per week

3. This represents how many Calories of exercise and/ or less food per week?

   _____ Calories per week

4. Based on the practical summary at the end of this chapter, outline below your dietary and exercise recommendations.

   Exercise: How many miles of walking per day? (Use table 9.8 and adjust for his body weight.)

   _____ miles of walking per day

   Diet: How many Calories less dietary fat per day?

   _____ Calories of fat per day less
   Other Recommendations?

Vitamins, Minerals, Water, and Your Health

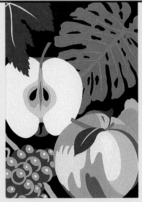

Vitamins are nutrients that are essential for life itself. In fact, the word vitamin comes from the Latin "vita," which means "life." The body uses these organic substances to accomplish much of its work. Vitamins do not supply energy, but they do help release energy from carbohydrate, fats, and proteins. They also play a vital role in chemical reactions throughout the body. There are two types of vitamins: fat-soluble and water-soluble. In chapter 10, a complete review of the 13 vitamins will be given.

Like vitamins, minerals are needed in small amounts by the body, and their major function is regulating body processes. Minerals are inorganic substances that are important components of both plant and animal tissues. If a human body is cremated, the remaining material, equivalent to about five pounds of residue, is mineral or ash. Minerals altogether make up about four percent of our body. Chapter 11 reviews the important role minerals play in our bodies.

Water is needed by all humans for life. Our bodies contain more water than any other substance or chemical, representing approximately 60 percent of adult human body weight. Chapter 12 reviews the role of water and other beverages, such as coffee and alcohol, in health.

10

Vitamins

OUTLINE

INTRODUCTION

*T*here is probably no other aspect of nutrition about which more misconception and misinformation abounds than with vitamins. The public has been led to believe that a normal diet does not contain sufficient amounts of vitamins and that use of vitamin pills is necessary to make up the deficit.

In this chapter, the four fat-soluble and nine water-soluble vitamins will be reviewed. Each has a major role to play in the human body, and these will be discussed.

Vitamins are found in a wide variety of foods, and tables outlining the most common food sources will be given. Vitamins can be easily lost from fruits and vegetables, depending on how they are prepared. You will learn how to preserve the vitamins in the foods you eat.

Popular reasons often given for vitamin supplementation will be reviewed, as well as the reasons why special groups of people may benefit from vitamin supplementation. Finally, the type of diet associated with low cancer risk will be described; that is, a diet high in vitamin-rich fruits and vegetables.

FIGURE 10.1

College students in the U.S. consume more than the RDA for vitamins, except vitamin B$_6$.

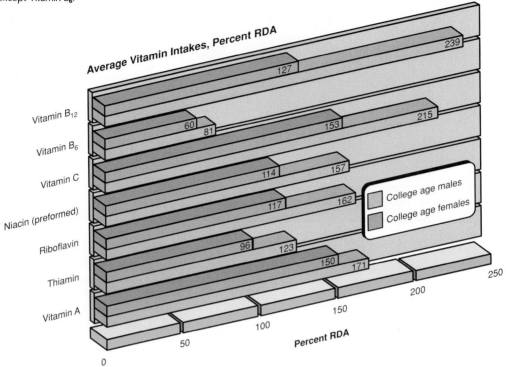

Overview

"If a little is good, more must be better" is the popular belief today among many health-seekers when it comes to vitamins and minerals. More than sixty million people, 39 percent of the United States adult population, take vitamin supplements, supplied by a $3-billion industry. The number of people taking extremely large doses—in the belief that this will provide extra energy, health, and protection from disease—is not known, but the number must be considerable. Each year more than 4,000 cases of vitamin poisoning are reported in the United States alone. A survey of United States adults showed that eight percent take potentially toxic doses of vitamin A, eleven percent take potentially harmful doses of vitamin C, and sixteen percent take excessive doses of vitamin E.

High intakes of vitamins and minerals beyond body needs are not beneficial. Our bodies closely follow the law of **homeostasis,** or balance. Too much or too little of any one of the nutrients can lead to various health problems. With respect to the body, moderation is always a virtue. And as we will see, this moderation is best achieved by eating a variety of wholesome foods.

Figure 10.1 shows that according to national surveys (1,2), college students are obtaining more than 100 percent of the Recommended Dietary Allowance (RDA) for all of the major vitamins except vitamin B$_6$. Even though college students are not always regarded as the most healthful eaters, they appear to eat sufficient good food to obtain more than enough vitamins. In other words, there is no need to use vitamin supplement pills. But what about vitamin B$_6$? As reviewed in chapter 3, the RDA are set to meet the needs of practically all healthy individuals and exceed the needs of a considerable proportion of the population. Therefore, nutrient intakes below RDA cannot be interpreted to mean that individuals are malnourished or should take supplements to increase

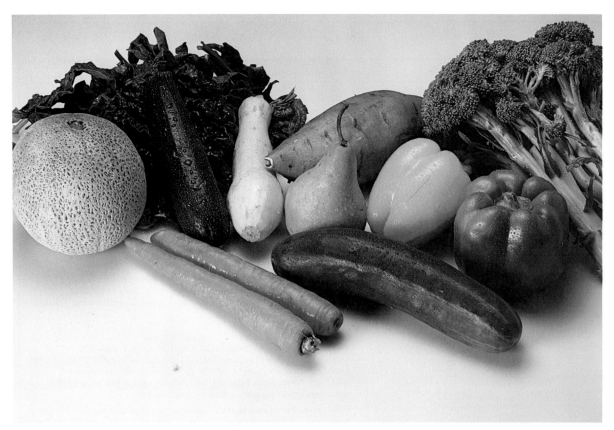

Vitamin A is concentrated primarily in fruits and vegetables that are yellow-orange and dark green.

intake. However, fruits and vegetables are major sources of vitamin B$_6$, and college students, for a variety of healthful reasons, would do well to increase their intake.

Vitamins are nutrients that are essential for life itself. The body uses these organic substances to accomplish much of its work. Vitamins do not supply energy, but they do help release energy from carbohydrate, fats, and proteins. They also play a vital role in chemical reactions throughout the body. There are two types of vitamins: **fat-soluble vitamins** (A,D,E, and K), and **water-soluble vitamins** (eight B-complex and vitamin C). Thirteen vitamins have been discovered, the most recent in 1948. Despite more than 40 years of additional research, no new vitamins have been discovered. It is unlikely that more will ever be found. Table 10.1 outlines the true facts about vitamins.

Let's explore the different vitamins and minerals, their functions, amounts needed by the body, and good food sources for each. Although we will be discussing deficiency diseases and/ or symptoms for each vitamin, please realize that these diseases are relatively rare in the United States, being more commonly found in developing countries that do not have the benefit of a high-quality food supply.

Fat-Soluble Vitamins

Vitamin A

Long before **vitamin A** was discovered, the cure for its deficiency was known. Night blindness is one of the first symptoms of low vitamin A stores. As a cure, early Egyptians recommended eating roasted ox liver. It wasn't until 1915 that McCollum and Davis discovered and described "fat-soluble A" as an essential growth-promoting factor. Thirty years later, chemists synthesized pure vitamin A.

Recommended Intake

Active preformed vitamin A is called **retinol,** while the precursor form is called **carotene,** or provitamin A. Carotene, which is found in plant foods, converts to active vitamin A in the intestinal wall.

TABLE 10.1
Vitamins: A condensed summary

Vitamins	Adult RDA	Role in Body and Good Food Sources
Fat soluble		
Vitamin A	800–1,000 μg R.E.	Assists in the formation and maintenance of healthy skin, hair, and mucous membranes; aids in the ability to see in dim light (night vision); essential for proper bone growth, tooth development, and reproduction. **Food:** deep yellow/orange and dark green vegetables and fruits (carrots, broccoli, spinach, cantaloupe, sweet potatoes); cheese, milk, and fortified margarines.
Vitamin D	5–10 μg	Aids in the formation and maintenance of bones and teeth; assists in the absorption and use of calcium and phosphorus. **Food:** milks fortified with vitamin D; tuna, salmon, or cod liver oil. Also made in the skin when exposed to sunlight.
Vitamin E	8–10 mg α-TE	Protects vitamin A and essential fatty acids from oxidation; prevents cell membrane damage. **Food:** vegetable oils and margarine, nuts, wheat germ and whole grain breads and cereals, green leafy vegetables.
Vitamin K	60–80 μg	Aids in synthesis of substances needed for clotting of blood; helps maintain normal bone metabolism. **Food:** green leafy vegetables, cabbage, and cauliflower. Also made by bacteria in intestines of humans, except for newborns.
Water Soluble		
Vitamin C	60 mg	Important in forming collagen, a protein that gives structure to bones, cartilage, muscle, and vascular tissue; helps maintain capillaries, bones, and teeth; aids in absorption of iron; helps protect other vitamins from oxidation. **Food:** citrus fruits, berries, melons, dark green vegetables, tomatoes, green peppers, cabbage, and potatoes.
Thiamin	1.1–1.5 mg	Helps in release of energy from carbohydrates; promotes normal functioning of nervous system. **Food:** whole-grain products, dried beans and peas, sunflower seeds, nuts.
Riboflavin	1.3–1.7 mg	Helps body transform carbohydrate, protein, and fat into energy. **Food:** nuts, yogurt, milk, whole-grain products, cheese, poultry, leafy green vegetables.
Niacin	15–19 mg N.E.	Helps body transform carbohydrate, protein, and fat into energy. **Food:** nuts, poultry, fish, whole-grain products, dried fruit, leafy greens, beans. Can be formed in the body from tryptophan, an essential amino acid found in protein.
Vitamin B$_6$	1.6–2.0 mg	Aids in the use of fats and amino acids; aids in the formation of protein. **Food:** sunflower seeds, beans, poultry, nuts, leafy green vegetables, bananas, dried fruit.
Folic acid	180–200 μg	Aids in the formation of hemoglobin in red blood cells; aids in the formation of genetic material. **Food:** dark green leafy vegetables, nuts, beans, whole-grain products, fruit juices.
Pantothenic acid	4–7 mg	Aids in the formation of hormones and certain nerve-regulating substances; helps in the metabolism of carbohydrate, protein, and fat. **Food:** nuts, beans, seeds, dark green leafy vegetables, poultry, dried fruit, milk.
Biotin	30–100 μg	Aids in the formation of fatty acids; helps in the release of energy from carbohydrate. **Food:** occurs widely in foods, especially eggs. Made by bacteria in the human intestine.
Vitamin B$_{12}$	2.0 μg	Aids in the formation of red blood cells and genetic material; helps the functioning of the nervous system. **Food:** milk, yogurt, cheese, fish, poultry, and eggs. Not found in plant foods unless fortified (such as in some breakfast cereals).

Vitamin A in one-cup portions of food

Food	Vitamin A per Cup of Food (R.E.)
Carrot juice	6,335
Sweet potato (cooked)	5,594
Pumpkin (canned)	5,404
Carrots (raw)	3,094
Spinach (cooked)	1,474
Crabmeat, steamed	1,009
Kale (cooked)	962
Dried apricots	941
Margarine, corn, soft	744
Winter squash (cooked)	729
Sour cream	546
Cantaloupe	516
Apricot nectar	330
Prunes	320
Ricotta cheese, skim milk	319
Tomato (raw)	272
Broccoli (cooked)	220
Cabbage (raw)	210
Lettuce, romaine	146
Nectarines	133
Chard (raw)	119
Green peas (cooked)	107

Adult RDA for males and females is 1,000 and 800 R.E., respectively.

Note: foods are compared on an equal-value basis (one cup) instead of using generally accepted standard portion sizes. Studies have shown that selected portions of food by men and women vary considerably. For this reason, foods in the tables of this chapter are compared on an equal-value basis so that you can better determine where the nutrients are concentrated. Then you can choose the amount of food you want to eat based on this information. Some of the foods will not be consumed in quantities as large as one cup.

Sources of Vitamin A

Sources of carotene include fruits and vegetables that are yellow-orange and dark green (see table 10.2). Carrots, sweet potatoes, spinach, cantaloupe, winter squash, apricots, and broccoli are rich sources. In the dark green vegetables, the green color of chlorophyll conceals the yellow-orange of the carotene.

Individuals with exceptionally high intakes of carotene, for example, those who drink very large quantities of carrot juice, may experience a change of skin color as yellow pigment is deposited beneath the surface. This effect, however, is not toxic because conversion to the active form of vitamin A occurs rather slowly. Skin color returns to normal as the carotene intake decreases to more typical levels.

Animal foods contain vitamin A in the form of retinol rather than carotene. Primary sources include fish liver oil, liver, egg yolk, milk, cheese, fish, and ice cream. Unfortunately, many of these foods are also high in cholesterol and saturated fats (see chapter 6).

Losses during Food Preparation

Vitamin A (carotene or retinol) is fairly stable to heat from cooking but is susceptible to breakdown from exposure to oxygen and to sunlight. In other words, steaming broccoli will affect the carotene levels very little, but letting the broccoli sit on the counter, exposed to room air and sunlight, will decrease the carotene substantially. (*Note:* see Sidebar 10.1 for a summary of nutrient-saving tips.)

Recommended Dietary Allowance

The Recommended Dietary Allowance (RDA) of vitamin A is now given in **retinol equivalents (R.E.).** Previously, vitamin A content in foods was expressed in **international units (I.U.).** Both measurements are widely found today in charts, graphs, and food labels. To convert, one retinol equivalent equals 3.33 I.U. of retinol or 10 I.U. of carotene. The adult RDA is 1,000 R.E. for men and 800 R.E. for women. Data from national surveys indicate that the average college male is consuming 5,629 I.U. (approximately 1,690 R.E) and the average college female 3,951 I.U. (approximately 1,186 R.E.) per day, which is more than adequate (1). Children require less, whereas pregnant and lactating women should strive for 800 and 1,300 R.E., respectively (see chapters 13 and 14). In certain disease states that involve fat malabsorption, or when mineral oil is used in large quantities as a laxative, the body's ability to absorb vitamin A decreases.

Role in Body

The role of vitamin A in the body is to help the eyes readjust to light changes, prevent thickening of the cornea, keep the skin and mucosal linings healthy, aid in bone and teeth formation, and assist in the reproductive process. Carotene may inhibit certain types of cancers (see Health-Promotion Insight).

Nutrient-Saving Tips

Vegetables

1. Trimming

The outer leaves of lettuce and cabbage, and the leafy parts of collard greens, turnip greens, and kale have higher values of vitamins and minerals than the inner, tender leaves or stems and midribs.

2. Storing

Vegetables, especially the leafy, dark green variety, need to be refrigerated promptly in the vegetable crisper or in moisture-proof bags to stay fresh. Their nutrients keep best at temperatures near freezing, at high humidity, and away from exposure to air. Unripe tomatoes keep their nutrients best if they are ripened away from sunlight at temperatures from 60–75 degrees Fahrenheit. Cover them with a cloth to ripen. Don't put them on a hot windowsill or in the refrigerator (they'll get soft and watery).

3. Cooking

To retain the high levels of nutrients in vegetables, microwave cooking, steaming, or using a pan or wok with very small amounts of water and a tight-fitting lid are best. The less contact with water, the more nutrients retained. A good nutrition practice is to save any water used to cook vegetables and use it as a base for soup. Carrots, sweet potatoes, and potatoes are best prepared in their skins in either the microwave or the oven (baking).

Microwave cooking helps to retain the nutrients present in food. Analysis of thiamin, riboflavin, vitamin B_6, folacin, and vitamin C content showed that microwave cooking was comparable to or better than conventional cooking methods. Using minimal water and cooking times yields the highest nutrient values.

4. Holding and Reheating

Cooked vegetables reheated after two or three days in the refrigerator have only one-third to one-half as much vitamin C as when prepared while fresh. Although cooking enough food for later meals may save time, this is at the expense of nutrients. The microwave has made vegetable preparation easy and quick so that bulk cooking is no longer necessary. In addition, using a microwave is an excellent way to preserve nutrients.

Fruits and Fruit Juices

1. Vitamin A value is high in yellow-orange fruits such as apricots, peaches, cantaloupes, mangoes, and papayas.
2. Vitamin C is well retained in citrus fruits and juices, which can be canned or frozen with little loss of this vitamin. Orange juice can be kept in the refrigerator for several days before any vitamin C is lost.
3. Whole citrus fruits keep their nutrients well for several days at room temperature.

Frozen Foods

1. Frozen vegetables and fruits are often better than supermarket "fresh" in total nutrition. This is because such foods are often frozen immediately after harvesting. "Fresh" food often lingers in grocery stores or at home for a while before they're eaten.
2. Thawing and refreezing food should be avoided because nutrients, flavor, and quality are negatively affected.

Canned Foods

1. In general, the longer the storage period and the higher the storage temperature, the greater the loss of nutrients.
2. When canned fruits or vegetables are stored for a year at 65 degrees Fahrenheit, only about 10 percent of the vitamin C is lost. Canned tomato juice shows virtually no loss of vitamin A in storage.
3. To get the full nutritive value from canned vegetables, serve any liquid packed with the vegetable. This can be used in soup. To reduce the salt content that can often be high in the liquid, look for the newer, low-sodium canned varieties.

Milk

1. Keep milk cold, covered, and away from strong light. Riboflavin may be lost in direct light.
2. The calcium and protein values stay about the same whether the milk is whole, skim (nonfat), or low-fat.
3. Pasteurization of raw milk does not destroy the principal nutrients. Raw milk is an unsafe food because of the bacteria that are present.

Cereals

1. Whole-grain cereals are those with the germ and outer layers retained. That's where the B vitamins and minerals are concentrated. Brown rice, whole-wheat products, dark rye flour, and oatmeal are all whole grains.
2. Enriched cereals are milled cereals to which iron, thiamin, riboflavin, and niacin have been added. However, fiber and many other nutrients are not added back. Whole-grain products are best.

Night blindness occurs if there is insufficient vitamin A available
to resupply the visual pigment, rhodopsin.

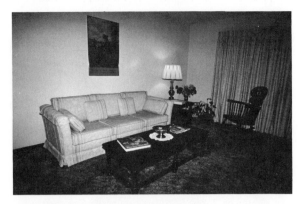

In dim light, you can make out the
details in this room.

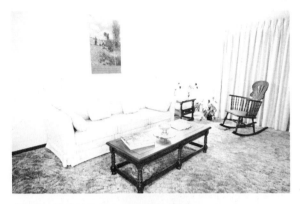

A flash of bright light momentarily blinds
you as the visual purple in the retina is
bleached.

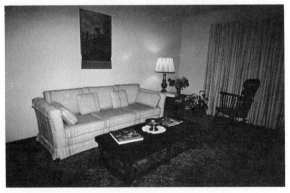

You quickly recover, and can see the
details again in a few seconds.

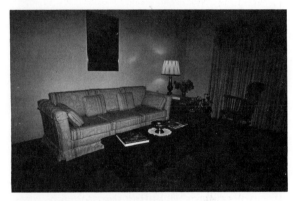

With inadequate vitamin A, you do not
recover but remain blind for many
seconds; this is night blindness.

Low Intake

Night Blindness Night blindness occurs if
there is insufficient vitamin A available to resupply the visual pigment, **rhodopsin.** As light
strikes the eyes, the rhodopsin bleaches, triggering nerve impulses to the brain and allowing
interpretation of the scenery. Then, amazingly
enough, clear sight does not resume until the
rhodopsin is regenerated with vitamin A. If vitamin A stores are low, there will be a delay. In
dimly lit settings (night driving, movie theaters,
etc.), this delayed sight recovery is called night
blindness (see figure 10.2). Thus, because vitamin A stores are slowly used up in this process, daily dietary replenishment is necessary.

Xerophthalmia Xerophthalmia is a disease of
the eye, proceeding through different stages.
With severe vitamin A deficiency, **xerosis,** or
drying of the conjunctiva, occurs. The conjunctiva is the mucous membrane lining the eyelids.

Xerosis of the cornea may follow. In this serious
development, the cornea becomes opaque and
distorted. Proper treatment, including vitamin A
supplementation, is urgently needed to prevent
the advanced state of keratomalacia (softening
of the cornea) and subsequent blindness. Young,
malnourished children are at high risk for rapid
onset of this devastating disease (see figure
10.3). It is estimated that 500,000 people, mostly
children in developing countries, become blind
each year due to xerophthalmia (3) (see figure
10.4). More than five million others show signs
of moderate vitamin A deficiency, which makes
them more vulnerable to infectious diseases. Intermittent high-dose supplementation of vitamin A, fortification of common foods, increased
production of foods rich in vitamin A, and nutrition education are prevention measures commonly used to prevent this disease in areas of
the world where it is prevalent.

*F*IGURE 10.3

Xerophthalmia is a disease of the eye, proceeding through different stages, resulting from vitamin-A deficiency. (*a*) Normal cornea. (*b*) In vitamin-A deficiency, the cornea becomes thickened. Eventually, sight is lost.

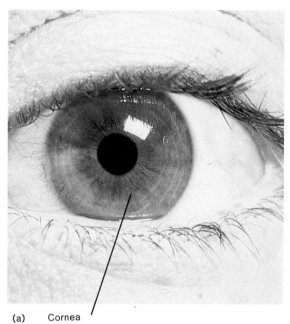

(a)   Cornea

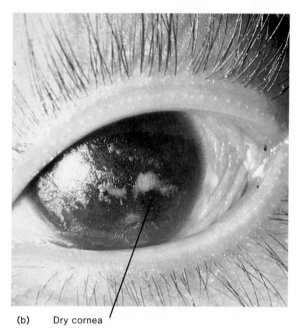

(b)   Dry cornea

Keratinization of the Epithelial Tissues   Low vitamin A stores can also cause drying of other body tissues. The **epithelial tissue** is particularly vulnerable. This tissue forms the epidermis of the skin, mucous membranes, and the lining of various organs including the stomach, intestines, bladder, mouth, nose, throat, and lungs. During extended periods of low vitamin A intake, **keratin** (a tough, protein substance normally found in hair and nails) is produced instead of normal epithelial cells. The development of keratin (keratinization) leaves the skin and membranes cracked and hard. As a result, bacteria and viruses can easily enter and cause increased infectious diseases. Often infection and complications in the respiratory system, gastrointestinal tract, and genito-urinary tract develop. Taste and smell sensitivity decreases as the epithelial cells degenerate, resulting in loss of appetite.

Impaired Bone and Tooth Development   Bone growth and tooth development depend on sufficient vitamin A intake. In the deficiency state, bones fail to grow in length. Normally, growing bones undergo a remodeling sequence of degradation and renewal, resulting in longer bones.

This process is hindered if inadequate vitamin A is consumed. Tooth spacing in the jawbone is also dependent on adequate vitamin A intake.

Cancer Incidence   Current research indicates a link between low vitamin A stores and onset of skin, lung, esophageal, larynx, and bladder cancers. For this reason, the American Cancer Society and the National Cancer Institute recommend an emphasis of carotene-rich foods in the diet (see Health-Promotion Insight at the end of this chapter).

High Intake

Vitamin A is stored in the liver and released into the body at a steady level for use by the body tissues. When excessive amounts are consumed, beyond the liver's capacity for storage, blood levels dramatically increase.

Symptoms of Excess Vitamin A   Loss of appetite, dry skin, hair loss, bone pain, cessation of menstruation, nausea, enlarged liver and spleen, abnormal skin pigmentation, headaches, and hyperirritability are among the symptoms of vitamin A toxicity. During pregnancy, high doses of vitamin A are associated with miscarriages, growth retardation, and birth defects (4,5).

FIGURE 10.4

Geographic distribution of vitamin-A deficiency and xerophthalmia. Nearly five million people worldwide suffer from vitamin-A deficiency. Most of them are children.

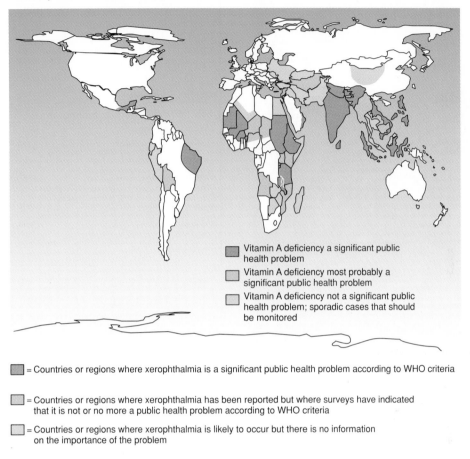

Vitamin A deficiency a significant public health problem

Vitamin A deficiency most probably a significant public health problem

Vitamin A deficiency not a significant public health problem; sporadic cases that should be monitored

= Countries or regions where xerophthalmia is a significant public health problem according to WHO criteria

= Countries or regions where xerophthalmia has been reported but where surveys have indicated that it is not or no more a public health problem according to WHO criteria

= Countries or regions where xerophthalmia is likely to occur but there is no information on the importance of the problem

Vitamin A toxicity is the result of supplementation with vitamin A pills. Food alone, with the exception of liver, cannot induce vitamin A poisoning. Early accounts of arctic explorers consuming large amounts of polar bear or dog livers in their attempts to survive indicate symptoms of vitamin A toxicity (6). Reports from these explorers describe feelings of drowsiness, irritability, severe headaches, nausea, loss of skin (which they reported peeling off in sheets), and anorexia. Very high levels of vitamin A (retinol) are concentrated in liver.

Case Study   Most people would never consider sitting down to a plate of cooked polar bear liver, but popping a few vitamins in the mouth is often a routine practice. Vitamin A, as well as all other fat-soluble vitamins, is easily concentrated in the body during high-intake periods, leading to potential toxicity. Some health-food faddists urge consumers to take vitamins in quantities several times higher than the RDA. However, this practice is especially dangerous with fat-soluble vitamins. Vitamin A toxicity symptoms have been reported with daily doses of 7,500 R.E. (seven to eight times the RDA for males, or nine to ten for females) taken over a prolonged period of time.

In one case, a woman took 7,500 R.E. daily for three years (7). Blurred vision, with intermittent flashes of bright lights, plagued her. Examination revealed swelling near the optic nerves, bleeding behind the right eye, and abnormally high brain- and spinal-fluid pressure. After six months with no supplementation, her eyes returned to normal.

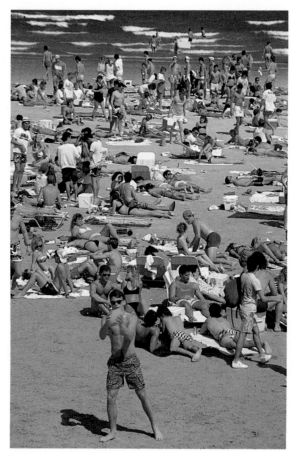

Vitamin D₃ is formed in the skin when the skin is exposed to sunlight.

TABLE 10.3
Vitamin D in one-cup portions of food

Food	Vitamin D per Cup (µg)
Margarine, corn (soft)	18.00
Cereal — Product 19 (fortified)	5.90
Cereal — Grape Nuts (fortified)	5.03
Egg white	3.5
Milk, 2% fat (low-fat)	2.55
Milk, 4% fat (whole)	2.55
Mayonnaise (low calorie)	2.25
Butter (regular)	1.68
Cereal — Raisin Bran	1.68
Ham (extra lean)	1.68
Cereal — Rice Krispies	1.25
Sour cream	.48
Oysters	.30

The adult RDA is 5–10 µg.

Vitamin D

As with vitamin A, the cure for vitamin D deficiency was known for many years prior to discovery. Cod liver oil was originally discovered to cure bone abnormalities caused by rickets in children. Research in the early 1900s showed that skeletal structure was affected by a fat-soluble substance in the diet. Pure vitamin D in crystalline form was isolated by 1930.

Recommended Intake

Vitamin D occurs in two major forms, vitamin D₂ **(ergocalciferol)** and vitamin D₃ **(cholecalciferol).** (For your information, the label D₁ was improperly given to an impure mixture of sterols.) Vitamin D₃ is a natural substance occurring in animal cells and formed by the action of sunlight on a cholesterol derivative in the skin. The activity of vitamin D₃ is actually similar to that of a hormone, since it is formed in the skin and then travels through the blood to act on a distance target organ. (For example, the hormone insulin is secreted by the pancreas and then travels through the blood to the various body cells to help in the transport of glucose into the cell.) Synthetic vitamin D₂ is formed when ergosterol found in plants is exposed to ultraviolet light.

Sources of Vitamin D

Sunlight exposure is an important means of obtaining sufficient vitamin D. The amount of sunlight needed depends on the amount of skin pigmentation one has. People with darker skin tend to block out much of the ultraviolet light from sunlight. On the other hand, some people with lighter skin live in areas of the world where sunlight is limited for many months of the year (Russians in Siberia, for example). As a result, food sources become more important for such people (see table 10.3). For lighter-skinned people, about 30 minutes of sunshine per day enables sufficient vitamin D formation (8). Window glass, dust, smoke, and clothing are all barriers preventing ultraviolet rays reaching the skin.

High levels of vitamin D do not naturally occur in foods, and none is found in plant foods. Egg yolks, liver, fatty fish (herring, sardines, tuna, salmon), cream, and butter contain small quantities of vitamin D. Years ago the

American Medical Association made arrangements for vitamin D to be added to milk. Today, the 10 micrograms (400 I.U.) of vitamin D added to each quart of milk is a vital source for much of the population, especially children. Breakfast cereals are often fortified with vitamin D (see table 10.3).

Vegans, people who avoid all animal and dairy products, need to be conscientious in being exposed to sunlight in a regular fashion (see Health-Promotion Insight, chapter 7).

Losses during Food Preparation
Vitamin D is fairly stable to heat and oxidation. Because the major source of vitamin D in humans is through the action of sunlight on the skin, few precautionary methods during food preparation need to be taken to conserve vitamin D.

Recommended Dietary Allowance
Recently, the accepted unit for measuring vitamin D became the microgram (μg). International units (I.U.) were previously used and are still found on food labels. For conversion to micrograms, one I.U. is equal to 0.025 μg (or 2.5 μg are equal to 100 I.U.). The RDA is 10 μg (400 I.U.) for infants, children, and adolescents to ensure proper skeletal growth. Young adults (ages 19–24) have an RDA of 10 μg (400 I.U.). Individuals older than 24 have an RDA of 5 μg (200 I.U.). During pregnancy and lactation, the RDA is increased to 10 μg (400 I.U.).

Because vitamin D is fat-soluble, the fatty tissues of the human body can build up large amounts of this vitamin. Intakes above the RDA are thus potentially dangerous and strongly discouraged.

Role in Body
Vitamin D is needed for bone growth and regulation of blood-calcium and phosphorus levels. Active vitamin D functions at three major sites, controlling the blood levels of calcium and phosphorus. The first site is the small intestine, where vitamin D aids in calcium and phosphorus absorption, increasing blood-concentration levels. The second site of control is in the bones themselves. When the blood level of calcium and phosphorus drops, vitamin D and parathyroid hormone (from the parathyroid glands in the neck) work together to pull calcium and phosphorus out of the bone into the bloodstream. Blood calcium levels can also be increased by the action of vitamin D at the third

*F*IGURE 10.5
Rickets is a childhood disease caused by inadequate deposits of calcium and phosphorus into the bones because of inadequate vitamin D.

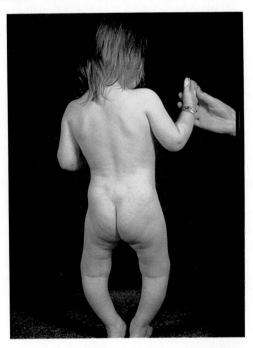

site, the kidneys. By decreasing the amount of calcium excreted in the urine, more calcium can be recycled back into the blood supply (see chapter 11, on minerals).

Low Intake

Rickets Rickets is a childhood disease caused by inadequate deposits of calcium and phosphorus into the bones. When there isn't enough vitamin D to regulate and maintain the blood supply of calcium and phosphorus, then soft bones, unable to withstand weight-bearing stress, develop. Children living in northern climates, in smoggy cities, and with darker skin are more susceptible to vitamin D deficiency. In the cities, the shade from tall buildings can block out the sunlight. Without sufficient sunlight exposure, the child is dependent on dietary sources of vitamin D, especially fortified milk.

The characteristics of rickets include bowing of the legs, projection of the sternum, failure of the fontanel (soft spots on the top of infant's heads) of the skull to close, knock-knees, poor muscle tone, and bulging of the forehead (see figure 10.5). Teeth may be slow to appear, poorly formed, and prone to decay. Unfortunately, rickets is a worldwide problem, including in the United States. Recently reported cases include inner-city black children, infants breast-fed for a long time without receiving vitamin D supplements, and children on very restricted diets (9).

Rickets must be treated with physician-prescribed doses of vitamin D to prevent permanent skeletal abnormalities and to guard against toxicity.

Osteomalacia   **Osteomalacia** has been called "adult rickets." This disease also involves soft bones. Women who have undergone multiple pregnancies, eaten a marginal diet, and avoided sun exposure are at risk. Fat malabsorption, with its consequent decrease in vitamin D and calcium absorption, may also cause osteomalacia. Monitored supplementation with small doses of the active form of vitamin D helps to correct osteomalacia. (*Note:* see chapter 15 for a description of osteoporosis, or "bone-thinning disease," which is different from osteomalacia.)

High Intake
Of the thirteen vitamins, vitamin D is the most toxic. Excess amounts are stored in fat tissue, the liver, and other sites. Vitamin D is slowly excreted through the bile. When intake vastly exceeds the body's actual needs, excess vitamin D causes **hypercalcemia** (high levels of calcium in the blood) and calcification of the soft tissues. The heart, blood vessels, bronchi, kidney tubules, and stomach may develop calcium deposits. Damage can be irreversible and fatal if hypercalcemia is prolonged. The symptoms accompanying hypercalcemia include anorexia, nausea, weight loss, excessive urination, and urea in the blood. Children may experience growth retardation as well. Toxicity does not occur by the natural routes of vitamin D intake (sunlight conversion and food sources). Once again, supplementation with vitamin pills or high doses of fish liver oil is the cause.

Case Study   Vitamin poisoning often occurs when individuals subscribe to the theory that a little is fine, but more is better. Unfortunately, there are quite a few reports of cases in which high vitamin D ingestion proved disastrous. In-

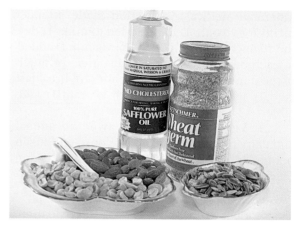

Although the major source of vitamin E is plant oil, moderate amounts of vitamin E are widely distributed.

fants and children have frequently been the victims. In one sad case, a bright, active three-year-old boy was prescribed 100,000 I.U. of vitamin D per day (7). His family doctor had diagnosed borderline rickets. The child's parents were alarmed, so, unknown to the physician, they also gave their son two tablespoons of cod liver oil and multivitamin drops. An average of 150,000 I.U. was given daily for the next two and one-half years. This toxic level caused nausea, limb stiffness, restlessness, insomnia, and irritability. Hypercalcemia was diagnosed, along with abnormal bone growth and calcium deposits. The child's kidney function was impaired, resulting in high blood pressure and heart damage. Although vitamin D supplementation was finally terminated, the damage proved irreversible. He died at age seven.

Vitamin E
Vitamin E is a family of eight naturally occurring compounds called **tocopherols** and **tocotrienols.** The vitamin was discovered by Evans, Bishop, and associates in the early 1920s. Early research was conducted on rats and showed that sterility and abnormal fetal development occurred in the deficiency state. Later research, however, showed that these vitamin E deficiency symptoms do not occur in humans.

Recommended Intake
The most active form of vitamin E is alpha-tocopherol. All other forms are expressed as alpha-tocopherol equivalents.

TABLE 10.4
Vitamin E in one-cup portions of food

Food	Vitamin E per Cup (mg α-TE)
Vegetable oil (safflower)	74.2
Sunflower seeds	71.7
Almonds (chopped)	31.1
Vegetable oil (corn)	31.1
Wheat germ	15.9
Peanuts	11.4
Kale (boiled)	10.4
Yams (cooked)	6.2
Blackberries	5.0
Asparagus tips (cooked)	3.6
Oatmeal (cooked)	3.5
Spinach (boiled)	3.4
Pecans	3.3
Sesame seeds	3.3
Swiss chard (boiled)	2.6
Whole-wheat cereal	2.6
Cabbage (boiled)	2.4
Ricotta cheese (skim milk)	1.6
Cottage cheese (2% low-fat)	1.5
Brown rice (cooked)	1.3

The adult male and female RDA are 10 and 8 mg α-TE, respectively.

Sources of Vitamin E
Moderate amounts of vitamin E are widely distributed. The major food sources of vitamin E are vegetable oils, especially wheat germ oil. Margarine, whole grains, dark green leafy vegetables, nuts, seeds, and legumes also contribute to vitamin E intake. Other plant foods contain smaller quantities, with foods of animal origin providing even less (see table 10.4).

Losses during Food Preparation
Milling grains, bleaching flours, freezing, boiling, and frying diminish the vitamin E content of foods.

Recommended Dietary Allowance
The RDA, as expressed in alpha-tocopherol equivalents (α-TE), is 10 mg α-TE for boys and men (15 I.U.), and 8 mg α-TE for girls and women (12 I.U.). During pregnancy and lactation, the RDA increases to 10 mg and 12 mg α-TE, respectively. People whose diets are higher in polyunsaturated fatty acids (plant oils) or omega-3 fatty acids (fish oils) need more vitamin E to inhibit oxidation. In some animal studies, when fish oil capsules are included in the diet, vitamin E deficiency develops.

Role in Body
In humans, the principle role of vitamin E seems to be as an **antioxidant.** The vitamin prevents oxidation of unsaturated fatty acids, phospholipids, and vitamins A and C by accepting the oxygen that would damage them. Selenium aids vitamin E in this noble exercise. There is increasing evidence that vitamin E is essential for normal neurological function.

Low Intake
Unlike the other vitamins, a deficiency of vitamin E does not produce its own unique disease. It is actually difficult for humans to develop a deficiency state. Most of the few cases on record coincide with fat malabsorption in adults and inadequate intake in premature infants (10,11). These individuals experienced increased red blood cell breakdown. Adults had increased excretion of creatinine (a sign of muscle breakdown) and pigmentation in small intestinal muscles. Far more is known about vitamin E deficiency in animals, but these results do not seem to parallel human metabolism.

In rats, vitamin E deficiency causes female infertility and low sperm counts in males. In guinea pigs, rabbits, and monkeys, deficiency symptoms mimic the symptoms of muscular dystrophy in humans. Research has shown that vitamin E supplementation does not stop or reverse the muscle wasting of this disease in humans. Animal studies indicate that vitamin E shortage increases red blood cell breakdown and may also result in yellow pigment deposited in the fat. More research is needed to further understand the relationship between animal and human vitamin E deficiency.

High Intake
Rumor has it that vitamin E increases sexual potency and enhances sexual performance. This rumor is false. Animal studies linking vitamin E deficiency to infertility have nothing to do with

human virility. Myths have also flourished regarding the ability of vitamin E to prevent heart attacks. High-dose supplementation of vitamin E is totally unwarranted and may be detrimental for some people.

Recent reports have also linked vitamin E to prevention of cancer, through its role as an antioxidant (see Health-Promotion Insight at the end of this chapter). The publicity given these reports of cancer prevention will probably increase self-supplementation. It is therefore necessary to understand the limits of such supplementation to avoid harmful side effects.

Although excess vitamin E is by no means as toxic as vitamins A and D, it does accumulate in the body and is associated with several negative conditions. In one controlled study lasting four weeks, one group took 400 mg α-TE daily, while the other group took a placebo (12). Triglyceride levels increased in the women taking vitamin E, and thyroid hormone decreased in both men and women taking vitamin E. In another experiment lasting two months, 2,135 mg α-TE of vitamin E were given to 18 patients with heart trouble (13). Another matched group of 18 was given a placebo. Three of the patients receiving the vitamin E experienced severe diarrhea, which subsided when the dosage was lowered, but returned when the original dose was reinstated. Other reports of vitamin E supplementation above 265 mg α-TE per day list an assortment of side effects, including nausea, headaches, fatigue, blurred vision, muscle weakness, sudden sweating, increased pulse, and impaired blood clotting (14,15). In general, daily supplementation of adults with about 200 mg of α-TE has not been shown to be harmful, but the effects of more than 800 mg a day have not been studied sufficiently (16). There is no evidence that more than the RDA is needed by humans.

Vitamin K

Vitamin K was the last of the four fat-soluble vitamins to be discovered. Its absence in a special formulated chicken diet led to hemorrhaging. For this reason, Dr. Dam of Denmark named it vitamin K, the "koagulation vitamin."

TABLE 10.5
Vitamin K in one-cup portions of food

Food	Vitamin K per Cup (μg)
Green peas (boiled)	377
Green beans (boiled)	363
Broccoli (boiled)	310
Cabbage (boiled)	181
Spinach (boiled)	160
Vegetable oil (corn)	131
Asparagus tips (boiled)	103
Iceberg lettuce (raw)	62
Tomato (raw)	55
Wheat germ (toasted)	44
Bean sprouts (mung, raw)	34
Strawberries	21
Carrot (raw, shredded)	14
Milk (skim, low-fat, whole)	10
Orange sections (raw)	9
Baked potato (with skin)	7
Mushrooms (raw, chopped)	6
Cucumber (raw, sliced)	5
Apple slices (raw, unpeeled)	3

The adult safe and adequate daily dietary range is 60–80 μg.

Recommended Intake
There are several related forms of vitamin K known as **quinones.** Each form originates from a different source such as alfalfa, fishmeal, and bacteria.

Sources of Vitamin K
Small amounts of vitamin K are found in a wide variety of foods. Dark green and deep yellow vegetables are the richest sources, especially green peas, broccoli, spinach, and other greens. Significant amounts are also present in milk and dairy products, cereals, fruits, and other vegetables (see table 10.5).

Losses during Food Preparation
Vitamin K is stable to heat but sensitive to light and oxidizing agents such as acid, alkali, and alcohol.

Recommended Dietary Allowance
Not only is vitamin K found in different foods, but it is also synthesized in the human intestinal tract, specifically the jejunum and ileum. Studies

FIGURE 10.6

When you cut your skin, a series of steps is activated to form a blood clot, ending the bleeding. Vitamin K is essential in the process.

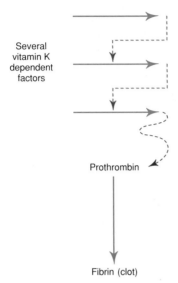

Several vitamin K dependent factors

Prothrombin

Fibrin (clot)

show that approximately 50 percent of the daily requirement for vitamin K is supplied by intestinal bacteria. The RDA for males and females ages 19-24 years is 70 μg and 60 μg, respectively. For adult men over 24 years of age, the RDA is 80 μg. For all women over the age of 24, including pregnant and lactating women, the RDA is 65 μg.

Role in Body

When a cut in your skin occurs, a whole series of steps is activated to form a blood clot, ending the bleeding. An essential ingredient in this process is **prothrombin,** the formation of which is dependent on adequate stores of vitamin K. Vitamin K is also essential for the production of at least three other protein factors involved in the clotting process (17). Without vitamin K, normal clotting ability is altered, and bleeding cannot be stopped (see figure 10.6).

In hospital patients undergoing surgery, blood clotting time is measured in advance. If the blood is very slow to clot, treatment that includes vitamin K may be given before surgery. This precautionary screening is vital to prevent possible death from internal and external bleeding.

Low Intake

Since vitamin K is normally produced in the intestines and is widely distributed in different foods, deficiency states are rare. As with the other fat-soluble vitamins, deficiency can occur when fat is not absorbed properly in the small intestine. Liver disorders can also interfere with the role of vitamin K.

One group at higher risk, however, is newborn infants. Vitamin K doesn't transfer easily through the placenta, and newborns do not yet have vitamin-K producing bacteria in their intestines. In addition, breast milk contains little vitamin K. This can result in low vitamin K stores. To prevent bleeding problems, newborns are routinely given a vitamin K injection immediately after birth.

With prolonged antibiotic therapy, the intestinal bacteria that produce vitamin K may be destroyed. If this coincides with a deficient diet, vitamin K stores will become depleted within several months.

High Intake

Some people are at risk for blood clots circulating in the bloodstream, which can lead to coronary heart attacks or strokes (cerebrovascular disease). To help prevent this from happening, anticoagulant drugs are often prescribed. Anticoagulants such as Dicumarol and Coumadin slow the clotting process, having the opposite effect of vitamin K. To allow the drug to function properly, it is recommended that excess vitamin K in foods be avoided.

Two forms of vitamin K are quite toxic when consumed in large doses. Since 1963, these toxic forms have been removed from the market. The toxic symptoms reported included vomiting, liver damage, anemia, skin spots, kidney damage, and bleeding (7). Today, therapeutic amounts of vitamin K are generally given only under the care of a physician.

Water-Soluble Vitamins

Thiamin

The disease **beriberi** sparked research eventually leading to the discovery of **thiamin** in the 1930s. Fifty years earlier, one researcher concerned with the high incidence of beriberi among Japanese sailors noted that the addition of meat and milk to the diet seemed to prevent the disease. Shortly thereafter, another researcher observed that chickens fed polished

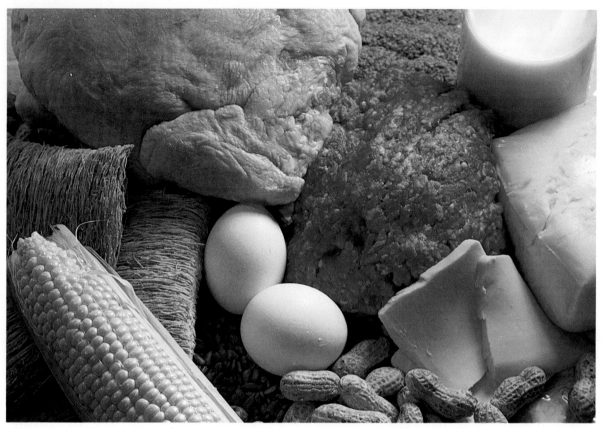

Whole grains, poultry, nuts, seeds, and lentils are high in the B-vitamins.

rice developed symptoms similar to patients with beriberi. He experimented and found that feeding the chickens brown rice or rice bran eliminated the disease symptoms. In both cases, the original diets were deficient in thiamin, and the addition of thiamin-rich foods alleviated the problem.

Recommended Intake

Because thiamin cannot be stored in the body, an adequate daily intake is important. To compensate for low intakes, the urinary excretion of thiamin can decrease to conserve the body's supply.

Sources of Thiamin

Thiamin is lost in the refining of wheat and rice. Enrichment procedures for breads and cereal products replace the thiamin content. The best sources of thiamin include seeds, nuts, pork (preferably lean, to reduce saturated-fat intake), whole and enriched grains, legumes, wheat germ, and fish. Many foods contain at least a small amount of thiamin (see table 10.6).

TABLE 10.6
Thiamin in one-cup portions of food

Food	Thiamin per Cup (mg)
Sunflower seeds (raw)	3.3
Wheat germ (toasted)	1.9
Grape Nuts cereal	1.5
All Bran cereal	1.1
Peanuts	1.0
Lean pork	1.0
Pecans	.9
Whole-wheat flour	.7
Raisin Bran cereal	.5
Mixed grain bread	.4
Acorn squash (baked)	.3
Cashews, walnuts, almonds	.3
Dried beans (cooked)	.3
Oatmeal (cooked)	.3
Bran muffin	.3
Broiled fish (bass)	.2
Rice (cooked)	.2
Raisins	.2

The adult male and female RDA are 1.5 mg and 1.1 mg, respectively.

Losses during Food Preparation

Cooking vegetables, cereal, rice, pasta, and meat with excessive water and then discarding it results in the loss of thiamin from these foods. Rinsing pasta and rice before or after cooking is unnecessary and also diminishes thiamin content. Both the addition of baking soda to make cooked vegetables look bright green and the addition of sulfite to dried fruit lowers thiamin content. High temperatures and exposure to oxygen destroy thiamin as well. Heavy intake of tea, coffee, or alcohol decreases the intestinal absorption of thiamin.

Recommended Dietary Allowance

The body's need for thiamin is proportional to the caloric intake. For every 1,000 kilocalories consumed, 0.5 mg of thiamin is recommended. Thus athletes, especially runners, swimmers, and other endurance athletes, need more thiamin. Because athletes tend to eat more than sedentary people, however, more than enough of the extra thiamin is ingested, with no supplementation being necessary.

The RDA for the average man is 1.5 mg, and for the average woman, 1.1 mg. Pregnant women need 1.5 mg of thiamin, and lactating women an additional 1.6 mg. The average college male and female consume 1.84 mg and 1.06 mg thiamin per day, respectively (1).

Role in Body

Thiamin is an essential part of a coenzyme, thiamin pyrophosphate (TPP), that releases energy from carbohydrate. Thiamin, therefore, is not an energy source itself but helps in the process of activating the energy in food. Thiamin is also needed for nerve transmission and heart muscle tone. Deficiency of thiamin affects the nervous system, cardiovascular system, and gastrointestinal function. Initial deficiency symptoms include fatigue, loss of appetite, nausea, irritability, depression, constipation, indigestion, headaches, and insomnia.

Low Intake

Beriberi As the severity of symptoms from thiamin deficiency increases, the disease beriberi occurs. The legs feel heavy and weak, calf muscles cramp, and feet feel hot and numb. Severe weight loss is sometimes masked by fluid retention (edema). Walking becomes impaired, and heartbeat irregularities are experienced. Unless treatment is initiated, beriberi is fatal.

FIGURE 10.7

Cracks at the corners of the mouth (stomatitis) may indicate a B-vitamin deficiency.

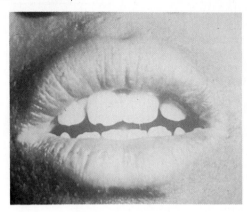

Cases of beriberi still occur in developing countries where people consume a high refined-carbohydrate diet (e.g., unenriched white rice). Infants breast-fed by thiamin-deficient mothers can rapidly develop the acute symptoms of beriberi and die within a few hours (see figure 10.7).

Wernicke-Korsokoff Syndrome In alcoholics, thiamin deficiency may lead to **Wernicke-Korsakoff Syndrome.** Excessive alcohol consumption increases thiamin requirements but often leads people to eat less food than normal, thereby decreasing thiamin intake. This syndrome is characterized by weakness of eye movements, poor muscle coordination, memory loss, confusion, and short attention span. Immediate treatment is essential to prevent brain damage and heart failure.

High Intake

Since thiamin cannot be stored in the body, it appears that any amount above 5 mg will not be absorbed (18). It is possible that high doses may interfere with riboflavin and vitamin B_6 intestinal absorption (19). The abundance of B-complex "stress tablets" on the market, containing from 5 to 15 mg of thiamin (three to fifteen times the RDA), is totally inappropriate for routine use. Excess absorbed thiamin is excreted in the urine.

Riboflavin

Discovery of **riboflavin** followed the discovery of thiamin. Research on the disease beriberi showed that high temperatures destroyed thiamin but didn't affect a certain growth-promoting property in food. Analysis revealed

TABLE 10.7
Riboflavin in one-cup portions of food

Food	Riboflavin per Cup (mg)
Grape Nuts cereal	1.7
All Bran cereal	1.3
Almonds (chopped)	1.0
Wheat germ (toasted)	.9
Raisin Bran cereal	.6
Plain yogurt (low-fat)	.5
Mozzarella cheese (skim milk)	.5
Ricotta cheese (skim milk)	.5
Spinach (boiled)	.4
Fish—Mackerel	.4
Cottage cheese (low-fat)	.4
Milk (nonfat, low-fat, whole)	.4
Fruit-flavored yogurt	.4
Mixed-grain bread	.4
Sunflower seeds	.4
Turkey—Dark meat—no skin	.4
Broccoli (cooked)	.3
Mushrooms (raw, chopped)	.3
Granola	.3

The adult male and female RDA are 1.7 and 1.3 mg, respectively.

this to be a second B-vitamin, now known as riboflavin. Although there is no deficiency disease associated with riboflavin, such as beriberi or rickets, there are symptoms (reviewed below) resulting from an insufficient intake.

Recommended Intake
Body stores of riboflavin are located in the liver, heart, and kidneys. Urinary excretion of riboflavin varies, depending on the limited storage capacity and the intake level.

Sources of Riboflavin
Milk and milk products are the most abundant sources of riboflavin, providing almost half of daily needs. Whole-grain or enriched breads and cereals contain high amounts of riboflavin. Dark green leafy vegetables, nuts and seeds, and organ meats are also rich in riboflavin (but organ meats are also high in cholesterol). Poultry and fish contain smaller amounts (see table 10.7). (*Note:* see Sidebar 10.2 for a discussion of nutrition scoreboards, which utilizes riboflavin and other nutrients in rating foods.) Individuals on low-calorie diets with limited amounts of dairy products may not be getting enough riboflavin.

Losses during Food Preparation
Riboflavin is fairly resistant to heat and oxidation but is rapidly destroyed by light. For this reason, milk is no longer sold in clear glass containers. Plastic jugs and waxed cardboard containers protect the riboflavin content of milk. As is the case with thiamin, adding baking soda to vegetables during cooking destroys riboflavin.

Recommended Dietary Allowance
The RDA for men is 1.7 mg, and for women, 1.3 mg. With pregnancy the RDA is 1.6 mg, and with lactation, it increases 1.8 mg. The average college male and female obtain 2.76 mg and 1.52 mg, respectively, from the diet (1).

Role in Body
Riboflavin is a component of two vital coenzymes that help release energy from food. Tissue repair, cellular respiration, fatty-acid oxidation, and amino-acid breakdown are all dependent on riboflavin. Because of riboflavin's important role in the "energy schema," some athletes believe that supplementation of riboflavin will improve performance. However, there is no evidence to support this claim. Riboflavin is also necessary for normal growth and healthy eyes.

Low Intake
Tissue damage, growth failure, and eye problems occur when riboflavin is lacking in the diet. Skin inflammation near the nose and eyes, cracks on the lips and corners of the mouth, swelling of the tongue, eye strain, and headaches are among the symptoms reported. Riboflavin deficiency often accompanies other B-complex vitamin deficiencies. Alcoholics, oral contraceptive users who also have a marginal diet, the elderly, the poor, and newborn infants with jaundice treated with phototherapy are at risk for deficiency.

High Intake
Pure riboflavin is yellow-orange in color. No storage sites are availabe, so when taken in excess, it is excreted into the urine, turning it a bright yellow. No cases of riboflavin toxicity are known.

Niacin
Niacin was discovered in 1867, but its importance to the body wasn't measured until much later. **Pellagra,** which means "rough skin" in Italian, was a new disease occurring in impoverished sections of Europe and the southern United States. The disease seemed to be linked

Nutrition Scoreboard of Foods

What foods rank highest, nutritionally? Would you like to be able to walk into a store and pick out the foods that are just brimming with nutrients?

The Center for Science in the Public Interest has published such data. In this book, foods are given nutrition points based on a formula that ranks foods according to its nutritional value. Positive ratings are given for protein, unsaturated fat, complex carbohydrate,

four vitamins (A, riboflavin, niacin, C), and two minerals (iron and calcium). A food loses points for total fat content, saturated and monounsaturated fatty acids, cholesterol, sodium, and added sugars. The information is listed in the tables that follow. Notice that foods with the very highest scores are dark green and yellow vegetables, melons, legumes, tuna, and low-fat dairy products.

Sidebar 10.2 Table
Nutritional Scoreboard

	Score		Score		Score
Dairy Products		Green pepper	44	Pineapple, fresh	18
Yogurt, low-fat, plain	64	Sweet corn, fresh	41	Cherries	17
Skim milk	55	Cauliflower, fresh	36	Pomegranate	14
Buttermilk, 1% fat	46	Cabbage, chopped	36	Plum, red	12
Low-fat milk, 2% fat	43	Artichoke, fresh	23	Grapes	10
Soy milk	33	Green beans, fresh	22		
Cottage cheese, 1% fat	30	Summer squash	22	**Miscellaneous**	
Whole milk	28	Turnips	21	Black beans	93
Chocolate milk, 2% fat	27	Bean sprouts	18	Chickpeas (garbanzo beans)	90
Ricotta cheese, part skim	26	Eggplant	18	Tuna, waterpack	75
Low fat American cheese	26	Romaine lettuce	17	Whole-wheat pita bread	73
Mozzarella cheese, part skim	19	Onion, chopped	12	Chicken, roasted, skinless	68
Cottage cheese, 4% fat	17	Mushrooms, fresh	9	Salmon, pink, fillet	67
Yogurt, low-fat, fruit	10	Cucumber	6	Turkey, roasted	62
Ricotta cheese, whole milk	− 1			Lentils	57
Cheddar cheese	− 10	**Fruits**		Kidney beans	56
Cream cheese	− 11			Whole-wheat bread	55
American cheese	− 18	Watermelon	68	Brown rice	47
		Papaya	60	Orange juice	47
Vegetables		Cantaloupe	60	Tomato juice	36
Spinach	93	Mango	52	Apple juice	23
Collard greens, fresh	90	Orange	49	Sirloin steak	17
Sweet potato	82	Grapefruit	42	Potato chips	15
Potato	71	Banana	36	Egg	− 7
Kale, fresh	71	Honeydew melon	35	Tang	− 9
Winter squash	70	Strawberries	34	Butter	− 13
Broccoli, fresh	68	Pear	29	Hawaiian Punch	− 13
Asparagus, fresh	67	Raspberries	27	Hot dog	− 20
Mixed vegetables, frozen	63	Peach	26	Vanilla ice cream	− 22
Brussels sprouts, fresh	58	Prunes	26	Luncheon meat	− 33
Tomato	56	Tangerine	26	Hershey's Milk Chocolate	− 42
Carrot	48	Apple	23	Sodas	− 55
Green peas, frozen	45	Blueberries	21		

Excerpts from *Eater's Digest* by Michael F. Jacobson. © 1972, 1976 by Michael F. Jacobson. Reprinted by permission of Doubleday, a division of Bantam, Doubleday, Dell Publishing Group, Inc.

to diets based on refined corn. In 1913, pellagra reached epidemic proportions in the southern United States, with over 200,000 cases reported. In 1915, Dr. Goldberger conducted an experiment on twelve prisoners, promising them early release for their cooperation (20). The group was fed a Southern-style diet of cornbread, sweet potatoes, cabbage, white rice, corn mush, corn grits, gravy, biscuits, syrup, and black coffee. After about five months, the symptoms of pellagra appeared, leading Dr. Goldberger to conclude that a pellagra-preventing factor related to the B-vitamins was missing from the diet. He recommended more meat and milk. Years later, in animal research, niacin was able to cure pellagra-like symptoms in dogs. Finally the role of niacin in preventing pellagra and contributing to a healthy diet was known.

Recommended Intake

Niacin is a generic term that includes two similar compounds, nicotinic acid and niacinamide. They have equal biologic activity, although nicotinic acid taken alone causes temporary skin flushing. Nicotine from tobacco is unrelated to all forms of niacin.

Sources of Niacin

The body can acquire niacin in two ways. The first is from foods rich in niacin, such as lean meat, poultry, fish, nuts, and whole grains and enriched cereal products (see table 10.8).

The second way to obtain niacin is from foods rich in tryptophan, an amino acid (see chapter 7). In the presence of other B-vitamins, tryptophan can be converted into niacin. Each 60 mg of tryptophan can make one milligram of niacin. Thus the protein content of the diet influences the body's niacin status. The typical pellagra-producing diet is low in both niacin and tryptophan. Corn, for example, is low in tryptophan, and part of its niacin is bound to a substance that makes it unavailable to the human body. Without consuming other foods rich in niacin or tryptophan, a corn-based diet is thus inadequate. Fortunately, the practice of using lime in corn tortilla dough releases niacin from its bound form. Otherwise, some Mexican, Central American, and South American cultures would be at risk for pellagra.

Niacin- and tryptophan-rich foods include yeast, nuts, whole grains, fish, seeds, poultry, and lean pork. To accurately assess a

TABLE 10.8
Preformed niacin in one-cup portions of food

Food	Niacin per Cup (mg N.E.)
Peanuts	20.7
Grape Nuts cereal	20.1
Roasted chicken breast (no skin)	19.2
Tuna (canned in water)	17.0
All Bran cereal	15.0
Wheat Chex cereal	8.1
Turkey (no skin)	7.6
Raisin Bran cereal	6.7
Sunflower seeds	6.5
Mixed nuts (roasted)	6.4
Wheat germ (toasted)	6.3
Whole-wheat flour	5.2
Almonds (chopped)	4.4
Mixed-grain bread	4.2
Chopped dates	3.9
Dried apricots	3.9
Broiled fish (trout, flounder, bass)	3.9
Prunes	3.2
Bran muffin	3.2
Baked potato	2.8
Brown rice (cooked)	2.7

The adult male and female RDA are 19 and 15 mg N.E., respectively.

food's contribution to the body's niacin supply, a unit of measurement called **niacin equivalents (N.E.)** is used. This unit takes into account the milligrams of niacin a food actually contains and the amount of niacin that can be made from tryptophan. One milligram of niacin equals one niacin equivalent. For example, one cup of milk contains 0.2 mg of actual niacin, and through tryptophan conversion, another 1.3 mg of niacin can be obtained. Altogether, one cup of milk has 1.5 N.E.

Losses during Food Preparation

Niacin is fairly stable to heat, light, and oxidation. Some niacin does escape in cooking liquid.

Recommended Daily Allowance

The RDA for niacin is 19 mg N.E. and 15 mg N.E. for adult men and women, respectively. Pregnant women need 17 mg N.E. per day, and lactating women need 20 mg N.E. The average college male and female ingests 29.76 mg and 15.89 mg of preformed niacin per day, respectively (1).

Role in Body

Niacin is a vital part of coenzymes needed to release energy from carbohydrates, protein, and fat. Thiamin, riboflavin, and niacin each work together in the "energy schema" of human cells, helping to release energy from the food you eat. Niacin is essential for growth, the production of energy in cells, and hormone synthesis.

Low Intake

Pellagra Early deficiency symptoms include weakness, fatigue, loss of appetite, and indigestion. As months pass, the signs of pellagra will begin to appear. Inflammation of the tongue and mouth (extending throughout the gastrointestinal tract), anemia, and vomiting are followed by four well-known final stages of this disease. These are known as the four D's: dermatitis, diarrhea, dementia, and finally death. In the first stage, dermatitis, the skin becomes red and swollen, then rough and cracked. The second stage is severe diarrhea. The third stage is dementia, which includes confusion, dizziness, memory loss, and hallucinations. Unless treatment is given, the last stage is inevitably death (see figure 10.8).

High Intake

Many people have the impression that water-soluble vitamins are not toxic. They believe that any excess amount taken will simply be excreted by the kidneys into the urine if the body cannot use it. This is not the case with niacin. Nicotinic acid is toxic when taken in high doses, with symptoms including headaches, visual disturbances, skin itching and peeling, gastrointestinal upset, irregular heartbeats, and possible liver damage. Individuals taking niacin as a prescribed drug to lower their serum-cholesterol level should be aware of possible side effects. The combination of niacin and cholesterol-lowering drugs such as Colestipol seems to successfully decrease the amount of harmful cholesterol in the blood (21).

Vitamin B₆

Discovered in 1934, **vitamin B₆** is in demand throughout the body. Over 60 enzyme systems depend on vitamin B₆. Its absence produces a myriad of symptoms but no specific disease.

Recommended Intake

Vitamin B₆ comes in three forms: **pyridoxine, pyridoxal,** and **pyridoxamine.** These forms convert from one to the other, and are all active in protein metabolism.

FIGURE 10.8
Deficiency of niacin leads to the disease pellagra.

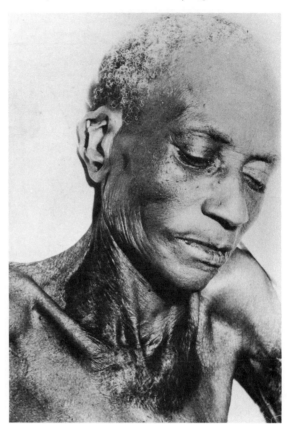

Sources of Vitamin B₆

Small quantities of vitamin B₆ are in a wide variety of food. Legumes, dried fruit, seeds and nuts, bananas, rice, and many vegetables are good sources of vitamin B₆ (see table 10.9).

Losses during Food Preparation

The availability of vitamin B₆ decreases with light exposure, oxidation, extremely high temperatures, milling of grains, and certain binding agents.

Recommended Dietary Allowance

For men and women, the RDA for vitamin B₆ is 2.0 mg and 1.6 mg, respectively. During pregnancy, 2.2 mg is recommended, with an extra 2.1 mg recommended during lactation. The average college male and female obtain 1.77 mg and 1.19 mg of vitamin B₆ per day, respectively, from the diet (2). Although this intake is below the RDA, as indicated in the introduction, nutrient intakes below the RDA cannot be interpreted to mean individuals are malnourished.

TABLE 10.9
Vitamin B$_6$ in one-cup portions of food

Food	Vitamin B$_6$ per Cup (mg)
Grape Nuts cereal	2.1
Sunflower seeds	1.8
All Bran cereal	1.5
Lentils (cooked)	1.2
Wheat germ (toasted)	1.1
Dried beans (cooked)	1.0
Banana	1.0
Rice (enriched, cooked)	.9
Roasted chicken breast (no skin)	.8
Raisin Bran cereal	.7
Turkey (no skin)	.6
Baked potato	.6
Tuna (canned in water)	.5
Spinach (cooked)	.4
Prunes, raisins, dates	.4
Whole-wheat flour	.4
Mixed nuts (dry roasted)	.4
Acorn squash (baked)	.4
Yams (baked)	.3
Broccoli (cooked)	.3
Brussels sprouts (cooked)	.3
Bran muffin	.3
Chopped onions	.3

The adult male and female RDA are 2.0 and 1.6 mg, respectively.

Role in Body
Vitamin B$_6$, in its various forms, works in enzyme systems to build and dismantle proteins. It is also an important participant in the conversion process of tryptophan to niacin, the manufacture of hormones and bile acids, central nervous system control, and the synthesis of hemoglobin.

Low Intake
For adults, deficiency symptoms include muscular weakness, nervousness, insomnia, and a facial skin disorder. A type of anemia may also develop.

The need for vitamin B$_6$ in the diet of infants was dramatically illustrated 30 years ago. By mistake, a commercial infant formula was overheated, destroying the vitamin B$_6$. Hundreds of babies developed symptoms, including irritability, weight loss, vomiting, weakness, anemia, and even convulsions. Once the cause was determined, the problems quickly cleared up when vitamin B$_6$ was supplied.

Individuals at elevated risk of B$_6$ deficiency include women taking oral contraceptive agents, the elderly, chronic alcoholics, and people on high-protein diets (high-protein diets require higher vitamin B$_6$ intakes). In addition, individuals using certain medications such as isonicotinic acid hydrazide (INH) (a drug used for tuberculosis) or penicillamine (used for rheumatoid arthritis) are at risk because these drugs are B$_6$ antagonists. Most physicians recommend B$_6$ supplements to people using these drugs.

High Intake
One must take exceptionally large doses of vitamin B$_6$ to experience side effects. Intakes of 100 mg (about 50 times the RDA) up to 2,000 mg have resulted in restlessness, insomnia, unsteadiness, and numbness of the hands and feet (7). The body might also become dependent on the higher intake of the vitamin.

Recently, individuals have been advocating vitamin B$_6$ supplements to help relieve the symptoms of **premenstrual syndrome.** Recent research reports have been unable to find any evidence supporting this (22). (In addition to vitamin B$_6$, zinc, magnesium, and vitamins E and A were found to be unrelated to premenstrual syndrome.)

Folate

Searching for a cure for **megaloblastic anemia** (presence of large, abnormal red blood cells in the blood) led to the discovery of **folate.** While none of the known vitamins could cure this type of anemia, a special yeast preparation seemed to help. It turned out that a new vitamin, folate, was the antianemic factor in the yeast.

Recommended Intake
The term folate describes *folic acid,* along with its many related compounds. Folate in the diet cannot be utilized until the body converts it to active forms. The liver is the storage site for folate, generally containing a four- to five-month supply.

TABLE 10.10
Folate in one-cup portions of food

Food	Folate per Cup (μg)
Grape Nuts cereal	402
Wheat germ (toasted)	398
All Bran cereal	301
Spinach (cooked)	262
Asparagus tips (cooked)	176
Peanuts	147
Orange juice	136
Raisin Bran cereal	133
Broccoli (cooked)	107
Granola cereal	99
Cashews	95
Brussels sprouts, beets (cooked)	92
Almonds	76
Lentils, dried beans (cooked)	70
Mixed-grain bread	65
Cauliflower (cooked)	63
Pineapple juice	58
Orange sections	55
Bran muffin	42
Green beans, squash (cooked)	39
Corn (cooked)	33
Bananas	32

The adult male and female RDA are 200 and 180 μg, respectively.

Sources of Folate

Good sources of folate are green leafy vegetables, nuts and seeds, legumes, fortified breakfast cereals, whole grains, and citrus fruits and their juices (see table 10.10). The presence of vitamin C seems to protect folate from destruction. Although folate is present in many foods, only 25 percent is ready for immediate absorption. The other 75 percent must be converted by enzymes in the digestive tract.

Losses during Food Preparation

Folate is very sensitive to prolonged heat, storage, and food processing methods. In some cases, more than half the folate content is lost during food preparation. Therefore, raw salads, for example, are an excellent source of folate.

Recommended Dietary Allowance

The RDA for folate for men is 200 μg and for women is 180 μg. Pregnant women have an RDA of 400 μg, and lactating women require 280 μg.

Role in Body

After absorption, folate is used to build a family of coenzymes that work closely with vitamin B_{12}. DNA and RNA synthesis, blood-cell synthesis and maturation, and rapid cell division are vital functions dependent on folate and vitamin B_{12}.

Low Intake

Folate deficiency is not uncommon. Inadequate dietary intake due to poor food choices, improper food-preparation techniques, and poor intestinal absorption contribute to low stores. Vitamin B_{12} deficiency, alcoholism, pregnancy, certain medications (such as oral contraceptive agents, aspirin, and anticonvulsants), certain diseases (such as Hodgkin's disease, leukemia, and tropical sprue) also contribute to reduced folate activity.

Anemia When the folate level decreases, changes occur in the production of red blood cells in the bone marrow. The number of cells decreases, and the size dramatically increases. Although large in size, these newly released red blood cells are immature, resulting in a decrease in the total **hemoglobin** (iron-containing pigment) concentration in the blood. White blood cells and platelet levels also decrease. The result is macrocytic or megaloblastic (large cell) anemia. When left untreated, the symptoms include tiredness, diarrhea, sore tongue, irritability, forgetfulness, and shortness of breath (dyspnea). When treated with folate supplements, these symptoms quickly disappear. A serious complication can result, however, if the anemia was actually caused by vitamin B_{12} deficiency (see next section). If this is the case, then folate supplements provide only a partial remission of the anemia symptoms. Meanwhile, dangerous neurological disturbances worsen. For this reason, the exact cause of megaloblastic anemia must be uncovered before treatment begins. This is also why folate supplements are regulated by the Food and Drug Administration (FDA), so that only low dosages are available without a prescription.

High Intake

As mentioned, an excessive intake of folate could conceal anemia actually caused by a lack of vitamin B_{12}. Meanwhile, severe and sometimes irreversible nerve damage could continue unchecked.

Other consequences of high folate intake involve its interference with prescribed medications, especially anticonvulsants (23). Taking excess folate cancels the benefits of such drugs, and convulsions may then result.

If taken during pregnancy, folate supplements may reduce zinc absorption, potentially retarding fetal growth (24). This is another example of that paramount of all health principles—moderation is the best policy. Too much of a good thing becomes a definite harm in the human organism, which operates on the principle of homeostasis (balance).

Vitamin B₁₂

Vitamin B₁₂ is a very large, complex molecule. Scientists took decades to understand the structure of vitamin B₁₂ and its role in the human body. As with many of the other vitamins, a deficiency causes a specific disease. **Pernicious anemia** (of which large red blood cells is one of the symptoms) occurs when vitamin B₁₂ is not properly absorbed. Absorption of vitamin B₁₂ is dependent on a special substance secreted in the stomach, known as **intrinsic factor.** Without intrinsic factor (IF), vitamin B₁₂ deficiency develops. Years ago, the only cure for pernicious anemia was to eat a pound of liver every day, enabling a fraction of the vitamin B₁₂ to be absorbed into the patient's bloodstream. Today, vitamin B₁₂ injections are regularly given to individuals unable to produce enough IF.

Recommended Intake

An atom of cobalt is located in the middle of vitamin B₁₂, which explains why the term cobalamins is often used to describe vitamin B₁₂. There are many different forms of the vitamin.

Sources of Vitamin B₁₂

Vitamin B₁₂ has the distinction of being present only in foods of animal origin—none is found in plant foods. All meat and dairy products contain vitamin B₁₂ (see table 10.11). Vitamin B₁₂ is often added to breakfast cereals, soy milk, and meat-substitute preparations (meat analogs). When a vitamin is added to a food that it is not normally present in, this is called fortification. Some breakfast cereals are fortified with vitamin B₁₂.

TABLE 10.11
Vitamin B₁₂ in one-cup portions of food

Food	Vitamin B₁₂ per Cup (μg)
Oysters	43.2
Crabmeat	13.5
Grape Nuts cereal	6.0
C. W. Post/Raisins cereal	5.5
Wheat Chex cereal	2.4
Low-fat cottage cheese	1.6
Pork (lean)	1.2
Cheerios cereal	1.2
Low-fat, plain yogurt	1.3
Cheddar cheese	0.9
Milk (all varieties)	0.9
Ricotta cheese (skim milk)	0.7
Ice cream (16% fat)	0.5
Turkey	0.5

The adult RDA is 2 μg.

Recommended Dietary Allowance

Vitamin B₁₂ is the most potent vitamin known; therefore, the RDA is quite low. For all adults, the RDA is 2 μg. During pregnancy and lactation, the RDA is 2.2 and 2.6 μg, respectively. With the exception of vegans (people who avoid all meat and dairy products), most people easily obtain the RDA. The average college male and female obtain 7.18 μg and 5.02 μg, respectively, from the diet daily (2).

Role in Body

Coenzymes with vitamin B₁₂ are essential for the formation of DNA, maintenance of the protective myelin sheath surrounding nerves, and the production of red blood cells. Vitamin B₁₂ works closely with folate in these functions (24). This makes diagnosing a deficiency of one or the other a bit difficult. Treating a vitamin B₁₂ deficiency with folate can have disastrous results, leading to permanent nerve damage.

Low Intake

Unlike the other B-vitamins, the body is able to store enough vitamin B₁₂ to last five to seven years (25). Since only a minute amount of vitamin B₁₂ stores is lost daily, a deficiency from an inadequate dietary intake takes years to develop. Also, the body seems to adapt to lower intakes by absorbing a higher than normal percentage from the vitamin B_{12} present in the diet.

Vegans who strictly avoid all meat and dairy products must obtain vitamin B_{12} from fortified foods or through supplements because plant foods do not contain vitamin B_{12}. Some vegans have reportedly lived more than 13 years without obtaining vitamin B_{12} from their food, and yet appear healthy. Researchers are still trying to determine from where these vegans are obtaining vitamin B_{12}. The bacteria in the large intestine produce vitamin B_{12}. This source has been thought to be unavailable to humans, however, because the necessary intrinsic factor is secreted by the stomach and then absorbed in the small intestine before it can reach the colon. Thus the vitamin B_{12} in the colon cannot be absorbed. However, vegans may have developed some mechanism of making colonic vitamin B_{12} available to their systems. More research is needed to explore this theory.

Pernicious Anemia Pernicious anemia is characterized by the release of large, immature red blood cells from the bone marrow into the bloodstream. The symptoms include weakness, paleness, loss of appetite, shortness of breath, weight loss, depression, confusion, and unsteadiness. Inability to produce the intrinsic factor that enables vitamin B_{12} absorption is the cause of most pernicious anemia. However, some vegans who have avoided all animal products for many years, and who also have gastrointestinal problems, can develop pernicious anemia. Deficiency of intrinsic factor is a rare defect and is most likely genetically induced, occuring in most cases after age sixty.

Stomach surgery, intestinal infection or surgery, and malabsorption syndromes can also block vitamin B_{12} absorption. Most patients with pernicious anemia must undergo regular vitamin B_{12} injections. These are generally given monthly, and they eliminate the need for intrinsic factors by sending vitamin B_{12} directly into the bloodstream.

High Intake

Vitamin B_{12} toxicity has not been associated with daily doses as high as 100 μg (24). In a few rare cases, vitamin B_{12} injections have caused adverse reactions. Segments of the population have the mistaken view that vitamin B_{12} injections will provide them with extra vitality and energy. Some

TABLE 10.12
Biotin in one-cup portions of food

Food	Biotin per Cup (μg)
Peanuts	102
Walnuts (chopped)	46
Almonds (chopped)	26
Lentils (cooked)	26
Cauliflower (cooked)	21
Green peas (cooked)	13
Spinach (cooked)	11
Corn (cooked)	10
Tomato	10
Raisins	7
Bananas	7
Watermelon	6
Rice (enriched, cooked)	6
Whole-grain bread	6
Yams (baked)	5
Grapefruit	5
Oatmeal (cooked)	5
Milk (nonfat, low-fat)	5
Cantaloupe	5
Cottage cheese (low-fat)	5

The adult safe and adequate recommended range is 30–100 μg.

endurance athletes believe that vitamin B_{12} injections will enhance performance by building up their red blood cell supply. There is absolutely no evidence to support this. Vitamin B_{12} injections benefit only those rare individuals who have a deficiency of the vitamin to begin with.

Biotin

Biotin was discovered in the 1930s, when a diet rich in raw egg whites induced a deficiency disease in rats. A substance present in egg whites, avidin, binds to biotin, preventing its absorption in the small intestine. Since one must consume over two dozen raw egg whites daily to produce a deficiency, avidin binding of biotin is not a problem in the typical human diet.

Recommended Intake and Food Sources

Biotin is widely present in many foods, especially many vegetables, legumes, nuts, whole grains, fruits, and milk (see table 10.12). In addition to dietary sources, biotin is also produced in the intestines. The exact contribution from intestinal synthesis is unknown.

Since uncertainty exists over how much biotin comes from the diet and how much is produced in the body, an RDA has not been established. A safe and adequate dietary recommended range of 30–100 µg per day has been developed.

Role in Body
Biotin is very active in many of the body's enzyme systems, especially those involving carbohydrate and fat metabolism. Only small amounts are stored in the body.

Low Intake
Biotin deficiency is a very rare occurrence. Several reports of people consuming incredible amounts of raw egg whites exist. Hospitalized patients fed biotin-deficient formulas have been reported to develop biotin deficiency. Infants with a certain type of rash (seborrheic dermatitis) have been reported to be relieved by biotin supplements.

The symptoms of biotin deficiency include skin rash, fatigue, paleness, muscle pains, nausea, hair loss, and increased serum cholesterol. There are three contributors to biotin deficiency: poor dietary intake, consumption of avidin from raw egg whites, and decreased intestinal synthesis due to drug interactions. Because these factors are now known, few cases of biotin deficiency occur.

High Intake
There are no known cases of toxicity from excessive biotin intake.

Pantothenic Acid

Discovered in 1938, **pantothenic acid** was named after the Greek word *pantos,* meaning "everywhere." This vitamin is widely available in all types of food. There is no deficiency disease associated with pantothenic acid.

Recommended Intake
Pantothenic acid is in legumes, nuts, many vegetables, poultry, dried fruits, whole grains, yogurt, and many fresh fruits (see table 10.13). Milling of grains removes substantial amounts of pantothenic acid. Although there is no established RDA for pantothenic acid, the safe and adequate daily intake is 4 to 7 mg for adults. Most people easily obtain this level.

TABLE 10.13
Pantothenic acid in one-cup portions of food

Food	Pantothenic Acid per Cup (mg)
Peanuts	6.8
Lentils (cooked)	2.7
Sunflower seeds	2.0
Rice (enriched, cooked)	1.8
Pecans, cashews	1.7
Wheat germ (toasted)	1.6
Mushrooms (chopped, raw)	1.5
All Bran cereal	1.5
Chopped dates	1.4
Dried beans (cooked)	1.4
Roasted chicken breast (no skin)	1.3
Low-fat yogurt	1.2
Sweet potato	1.1
Green peas	1.1
Grape Nuts cereal	1.1
Baked potato	.9
Milk (nonfat, low-fat, whole)	.8

The adult safe and adequate recommended range is 4–7 mg.

Low Intake
Just as pantothenic acid is widely available in the diet, it is also found throughout the body as part of an enzyme essential to fat, carbohydrate, and protein metabolism. Pantothenic acid deficiency is virtually unknown, except in combination with other B-vitamin deficiencies. With chronic alcoholism and severe malnutrition, multiple B-vitamin deficiencies are likely to occur with overlapping symptoms. Some researchers suggest that symptoms unique to pantothenic acid deficiency may include weakness, cramping, vomiting, insomnia, and a prickling numbness of the extremities, all of which quickly disappear when pantothenic acid intake is normalized.

In animals with dark fur, pantothenic acid deficiency causes graying and loss of hair. This development does not occur in humans. Some entrepreneurs have promoted products containing pantothenic acid to help people prevent hair loss or graying. There is no evidence to support the claim that this can help.

High Intake
High doses of pantothenic acid do not appear to cause toxic reactions.

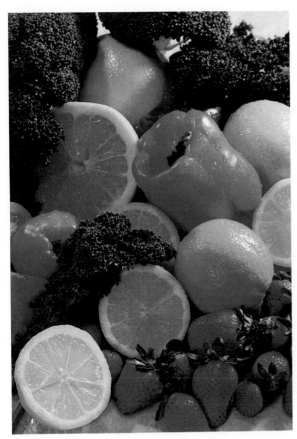

Many fruits and vegetables are high in vitamin C.

TABLE 10.14
Vitamin C in one-cup portions of food

Food	Vitamin C per Cup (mg)
Broccoli (cooked)	98
Orange juice	97
Oranges	96
Strawberries	85
Grapefruit juice	72
Cauliflower (raw)	72
Tomato soup	68
Cantaloupe	68
Sweet potato (cooked)	56
Kale (cooked)	53
V-8 juice	53
Cabbage (raw)	43
Blackberries	30
Pineapple	24
Winter squash (cooked)	20
Collards (cooked)	19
Green peas (cooked)	16
Watermelon	15
Onions (raw)	14

The adult RDA is 60 mg.

Vitamin C

Scurvy, the vitamin C deficiency disease, caused countless deaths until the mid-1500s, when an association with diet was finally discovered. Canadian Indians told explorers to drink an extract from the white cedar tree to prevent or cure scurvy. Later, several British reports recommended that sailors include citrus fruits in their diet as a preventative measure. By 1795, the British Navy adopted this practice, and sailors became known as "limeys" because of their regular intake of lemon and lime juice. The results were dramatic. Whereas before ships would return to port with only half of their crew alive, the new practice of drinking citrus juices virtually eliminated the disease. **Vitamin C** was eventually discovered to be the chemical responsible for preventing scurvy and was given the name ascorbic ("without scurvy") acid.

Recommended Intake
Most animals are capable of producing their own supply of vitamin C. Humans, monkeys, guinea pigs, and a few other species must rely on dietary sources.

Sources of Vitamin C
The fruit and vegetable group supplies the highest concentration of vitamin C. Broccoli, citrus fruits and their juices, strawberries, melons, cauliflower, tomatoes, and potatoes are all rich sources (see table 10.14). Foods from animal sources, such as milk, eggs, meat, poultry, and fish, are largely devoid of vitamin C.

Losses during Food Preparation
Care must be taken during food preparation to preserve vitamin C. Excess heat over a prolonged period, air exposure to cut surfaces, large amounts of cooking water, and exposure to baking soda reduces the level of vitamin C. Figure 10.9 demonstrates that vegetables can lose up to half their vitamin C content if they are cut and stored in the refrigerator for a day, then steamed for three minutes, and finally stored in a heated cabinet for 30 minutes (26).

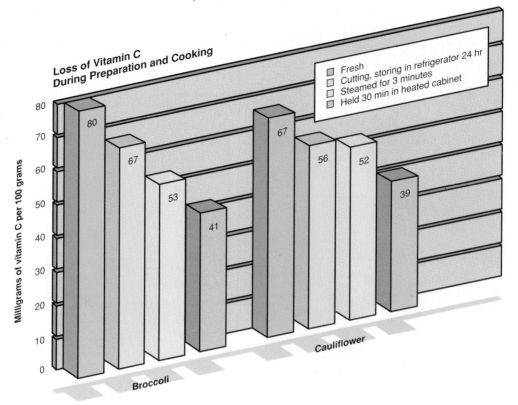

FIGURE 10.9
Preparation of vegetables (cutting, washing, storing, and cooking), decreases the vitamin-C content dramatically.

Loss of Vitamin C During Preparation and Cooking

Milligrams of vitamin C per 100 grams

- ☐ Fresh
- ☐ Cutting, storing in refrigerator 24 hr
- ☐ Steamed for 3 minutes
- ☐ Held 30 min in heated cabinet

Broccoli: 80, 67, 53, 41

Cauliflower: 67, 56, 52, 39

Recommended Dietary Allowance
The RDA for men and women is 60 mg of vitamin C. Pregnant women need 70 mg and lactating women 95 mg. Figure 10.1 shows that college students consume vitamin C at levels of 50–100 percent above the RDA.

Role in Body
Vitamin C has multiple roles in the body. Important functions include synthesis of collagen in the connective tissues of bones, teeth, and tendons; synthesis of hormones; wound healing; promotion of iron absorption; protection of vitamins A and E from oxidation; and protection against injury and infection.

Low Intake
Scurvy   Although rarely seen today, occasional cases of scurvy occur in infants, alcoholics, and the elderly (see figure 10.10). Infants fed regular cow's milk instead of infant formula or breast milk will not obtain enough vitamin C. After several months, if no other food or supplements are given, the symptoms of scurvy will develop. Weakening of the collagen causes most of the problems. Collagen is a protein substance that forms the basis of connective tissue. The connective tissue then becomes the building material for bones, cartilage, teeth, tendons, ligaments, skin, and blood vessels. Without vitamin C, collagen cannot be synthesized, and consequently many body systems deteriorate. Infants with scurvy have pain and swelling of their thighs and legs. They become irritable, pale, feverish, nauseated, and prone to weight loss. Teeth and gums are often swollen and tender. Bones develop abnormally. Prompt treatment with vitamin C will reverse the symptoms.

In adults deprived of vitamin C for several months, the symptoms of scurvy are similar as described above for infants. Fatigue, swelling of gums, tooth loosening, skin discoloration from bruising, anemia, leg tenderness, and muscle and cartilage structure degeneration develop. The disease is very responsive to vitamin C therapy.

FIGURE 10.10

Vitamin-C deficiency leads to the disease scurvy.

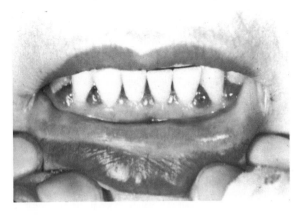

TABLE 10.15

Nutritional supplement use among specific populations

Population Surveyed	Location of Study	Percent Supplement Users
Children	Kansas	33
Adolescents	8 southern states	21
College students	Minnesota	32
Athletes	Not specified	72
Registered nurses	10 large states	38
Dietitians	Washington	37
Lactating women	Indiana/ Pennsylvania	80
Vegetarians	Oregon	55
Western adults	7 western states	67
Elderly	California	97

High Intake

Of all the vitamins, vitamin C is the one most often taken as a supplement to the diet. Despite scientific evidence to the contrary, many people attribute almost magical qualities to vitamin C. Ever since Dr. Linus Pauling began advancing the concept that massive doses of vitamin C could prevent and cure both the common cold and cancer, millions of people have dosed themselves with high quantities of vitamin C. Pauling has advised people to consume 1,000 to 10,000 mg of vitamin C daily, 17 to 167 times the RDA. More than 15 other researchers have been unable to confirm Dr. Pauling's recommendations. It appears that Dr. Pauling's original study on the role of vitamin C in preventing the common cold was flawed in both its design and implementation. Recent research by the Mayo Clinic, using a double blind placebo design, has also not been able to show any benefit of massive vitamin C doses in curing cancer, contrary to Dr. Pauling's research findings.

Vitamin C is not highly toxic, but very high doses can cause problems. Rebound scurvy can occur in individuals who suddenly stop their massive vitamin C doses. Apparently the body becomes adapted to the high vitamin C intake, and when intake returns to more normal levels, symptoms of scurvy can occur. To avoid rebound scurvy, individuals who are using high amounts of vitamin C supplements should reduce their intake gradually.

Other complications from vitamin C megadosing include diarrhea, decreased copper absorption, and increased uric acid excretion leading to gout and kidney stones. The tooth enamel can be damaged if large amounts of chewable tablets are ingested.

The Supplementation Issue

Most reputable nutritionists state that vitamin or mineral **supplementation** is unwarranted for people eating a balanced diet. Consuming a variety of foods from the four basic food groups is the best approach (see chapter 3). Misinformation and confusing advertisements have blurred the truth about vitamin and mineral supplementation.

According to a survey conducted by the Food and Drug Administration, 40 percent of adult Americans take some form of vitamin or mineral supplement. Some groups of people report even higher levels of supplementation. Table 10.15 outlines a few of the surveys taken on this topic (27).

Vitamin Supplementation Myths

Vitamin deficiency diseases have not been encountered in the major health and nutrition surveys done recently in the U.S. In fact such diseases now occur so rarely in this country as to be medical curiosities. Nevertheless, large numbers of apparently healthy people take vitamin supplements. Americans spend almost $3 billion each year on their vitamin and mineral pills.

TABLE 10.16
Myths and facts about vitamin supplementation

Myth	Fact
Vitamin supplements prevent colds and other illnesses.	If a vitamin is missing from the diet, then taking that vitamin can prevent or cure the deficiency disease; however, taking extra doses of vitamins does not prevent or cure other illnesses.
Vitamin supplements protect against harmful chemicals and pollution.	Vitamins do not have magical abilities to ward off harmful agents.
Vitamin supplements provide a hedge against an undesirable diet.	The nutritional consequences of consuming a poor diet high in fat, salt, and sugar, with little fiber, cannot be reversed with vitamins.
Vitamin supplements are necessary because the soil is so depleted today.	Crops can't grow in depleted soil. If a nutrient is low, the yield will be low, but the vitamin content will be normal.
Some people need very high intakes of vitamins to be healthy.	A multitude of studies have shown that it is extremely rare for anyone to need amounts higher than the RDA.
Vitamin pills from natural sources are always safe and are much better than synthetic ones.	There is no difference between natural and synthetic vitamin pills except the price. Most vitamins labeled ''natural'' are actuallly synthetic, and both kinds can be toxic if taken in excess.
Vitamin supplements give extra energy, especially during times of stress.	Only carbohydrates, fats, and proteins provide the body with energy (kilocalories). Vitamins only assist in releasing this energy. The rate of this energy release is not affected by high vitamin intakes.
Vitamin supplements are harmless, so taking extra amounts will just give extra benefits and security.	Excess doses can be toxic and can interfere with the absorption and function of other vitamins and minerals.

Why are so many people taking so many pills? Some of the reasons given include the following (views encouraged by nutrition supplement companies):

1. to prevent colds and other illnesses,
2. to make up for what is missing in food, and
3. to give extra energy during times of stress.

In reality, however, these reasons are based on misinformation. Specific vitamins cannot prevent colds, viruses, or flus. Disease prevention involves more than taking a pill. A balanced diet, sufficient rest, and avoiding or limiting exposure to infectious agents are more successful practices.

It is also a misconception to think that swallowing a vitamin pill will make up for a poor diet. Getting a good diet means more than just obtaining all the recommended amounts of vitamins. There are many other nonvitamin aspects of the diet that comprise good nutrition, such as consuming optimal amounts of dietary fiber and complex carbohydrate while moderating dietary fat. To justify a poor diet by taking vitamin pills is a misguided practice.

Some people take supplements advertised as "stress tablets," hoping to reverse feelings of depression, low energy, or malaise during times of high stress. Unfortunately, vitamins do not provide energy. They enable the energy in food to be released, but this energy is provided by optimal amounts of dietary carbohydrate and fats.

Some people use vitamin supplements because they feel the soil is depleted, thereby reducing the nutrients in foods. Estimates of the nutrient content of our food supply by the U.S. Department of Agriculture indicate that the amounts of most nutrients available to the consumer have increased during this century. Other mistaken beliefs include the thought that vitamin pills protect against harmful chemicals and pollution and the exaggerated idea that megadoses of vitamins multiply the reported benefits of normal vitamin intake. All of these views are unsubstantiated (see table 10.16). There is no evidence in the scientific literature that Americans generally require vitamin supplements (28).

Vitamin pills are not harmless extractions from food. When taken in high doses, vitamins are similar to drugs. Almost every vitamin is capable of producing toxic reactions in the body (see table 10.17) (29). The fat-soluble vitamins are especially dangerous. As shown in table 10.17, as little as 5 to 10 times the RDA for vitamin A can cause toxic reactions in some

TABLE 10.17
Vitamin safety index

Vitamin	RDA (males)	Minimum Toxic Dose	Vitamin Safety Index*
Vitamin A	1,000 μg R.E.	5,000–10,000 μg R.E.	5–10
Vitamin D	5 μg	25–50 μg	5–10
Vitamin E	10 μg α-TE	400 μg α-TE	40
Vitamin C	60 mg	2,000–5,000 mg	33–83
Thiamin	1.5 mg	280 mg	187
Riboflavin	1.7 mg	1,000 mg	588
Niacin	19 mg N.E.	1,000 mg N.E.	53
Pyridoxine (B$_6$)	2.0 mg	200 mg	100
Folacin	200 μg	15 mg	75
Biotin	30–100 μg	50 mg	500–1,667
Pantothenic acid	4–7 mg	10,000 mg	1,430–2,500

*The vitamin safety index equals the minimum toxic dose divided by the RDA.

people. In addition to the direct effects, vitamins also interfere with each other and with various minerals during intestinal absorption. For example, excessive vitamin C decreases copper absorption, high levels of folic acid decrease zinc absorption, and large amounts of niacin can counteract vitamin B$_6$ absorption.

On April 8, 1987, four prominent scientific groups joined forces to warn the American public about the unsafe use of vitamin and mineral supplements. The American Dietetic Association, the American Institute of Nutrition, the American Society for Clinical Nutrition, and the National Council Against Health Fraud issued the following joint statement (30): Healthy children and adults should obtain adequate nutrient intakes from dietary sources. Meeting nutrient needs by choosing a variety of foods in moderation, rather than by supplementation, reduces the potential risk for both nutrient deficiencies and nutrient excesses. Individual recommendations regarding supplements and diets should come from physicians and registered dietitians.

Supplement usage may be indicated in some circumstances, including:

1. women with excessive menstrual bleeding (may need iron);
2. women who are pregnant or are breast-feeding (need more of some nutrients such as iron, folic acid, calcium);
3. people with very low calorie intakes;
4. some vegetarians who are highly restrictive in their diets;
5. newborns may need vitamin K to prevent abnormal bleeding (under direction of a physician).

Certain disorders and some medications may interfere with nutrient intake, digestion, absorption, metabolism, or excretion and thus change requirements.

Nutrients are potentially toxic when ingested in sufficiently large amounts. In addition, high-dosage vitamin and mineral supplements can interfere with the normal metabolism of other nutrients and with the therapeutic effects of certain drugs.

The Recommended Dietary Allowances represent the best currently available assessment of safe and adequate intakes. There are no demonstrated benefits of self-supplementation beyond these allowances.

In a statement released from the American Medical Association (31), it was emphasized that sound dietary practices should eliminate any need for supplemental vitamins after infancy in essentially all healthy children. Healthy adult men and women and healthy nonpregnant, nonlactating women consuming a usual, varied diet do not need vitamin supplements. All health practitioners should emphasize repeatedly that properly selected diets are the primary basis for good nutrition.

The news about cancer is getting better, and the best news is about cancer prevention.

There are many things you can do to help protect yourself from cancer. In fact, some researchers are saying that 90 percent of all cancers are related to the environment and to things we eat, drink, and smoke. In this Health Promotion Insight, we'll discuss the type of life-style that is associated with low cancer risk.

What is Cancer?

Cancer, in simple terms, is a group of diseases in which abnormal cells grow out of control and can spread throughout the body. Normally, the cells of your body reproduce themselves in an orderly manner so that regular body functions can continue. Occasionally, certain cells undergo an abnormal change and begin a process of uncontrolled growth. These cells may grow into masses of cells called tumors.

In the beginning, cancer cells usually remain at the original site. Later, however, some of the cancer cells may invade neighboring organs or tissues (metastasis). If the cancer is left untreated, it can spread throughout the body, resulting in death. This is why early detection is so important. Aids to early detection include the Seven Warning Signals of cancer (32). These are

1. a change in bowel or bladder habits,
2. a sore that does not heal,
3. unusual bleeding or discharge,
4. a thickening or lump in the breast or elsewhere,
5. indigestion or difficulty in swallowing,
6. an obvious change in a wart or mole, and
7. a nagging cough or hoarseness.

There are other ways to detect cancer early. Colorectal and pap tests and regular breast exams are recommended by the American Cancer Society (32). The breasts should be examined monthly as a routine good-health habit. For women between the ages of 20–40, a doctor should examine the breasts every three years, and women over the age of 40 should have this done yearly. The doctor should also conduct mammograms for women over the age of 40 on a periodic basis.

Statistics

Cancer can strike at any age. It kills more children aged 3 to 14 than any other disease. And cancer strikes more frequently with advancing age. About 75 million (30 percent) Americans now living will eventually have cancer. Over the years, cancer will strike in approximately three out of four families. In any given year about 985,000 people will be diagnosed as having cancer (with 500,000 more with nonmelanoma skin cancer). Every year, close to 494,000 will die of cancer (1,350 per day). Of every five deaths in the U.S., one is from cancer. Unfortunately, cancer death rates are not going down, like those of cardiovascular disease. There has been a steady rise in the age-adjusted national death rate, mainly due to lung cancer.

Figure 10.11 from the American Cancer Society (32) shows the progress of cancer from 1930 to 1985. Notice the dramatic increase in lung cancer. Figure 10.12 shows that the number-one cancer killer for men and women is lung cancer. Cigarette smoking is responsible for 85 percent of lung-cancer cases among men and 75 percent among women (83 percent overall). Close to 139,000 people die every year from lung cancer.

The number-two cancer killer for men and the number-three cancer killer for women is colon cancer. Nearly 60,000 people die every year from colon cancer. The leading cancer killer for women is breast cancer, with 42,300 annual deaths. Prostate cancer overall is the third leading cancer killer among men.

Cancer Prevention

As stated previously, the majority of cancers are now thought to be preventable. The National Cancer Institute estimates that diet is responsible for 35 percent of all cancers, more than any other cause. Their estimate for tobacco is 30 percent, with viruses, occupational hazards, alcohol, excess sunshine, environmental pollution, various medical procedures, and food additives responsible for the rest.

The National Cancer Institute (NCI) has set a goal of reducing the 1985 cancer mortality rate by 50 percent by the year 2000 (33). Based on various practical considerations, the NCI has estimated that a 50 percent reduction in cancer incidence and mortality is possible by the year 2000 if the following prevention, screening, and treatment activities are enacted.

1. reduce percentage of adults who smoke to 15 percent or less (now presently 30 percent)
2. reduce average consumption of fat to 25 percent or less of total calories (presently 40 percent)

*F*IGURE 10.11

Cancer deaths from 1930 to 1985 have increased primarily because of the dramatic rise in lung-cancer deaths. *Note:* Rates are for both sexes combined, except breast and uterus for female population only, and prostate for male population only.

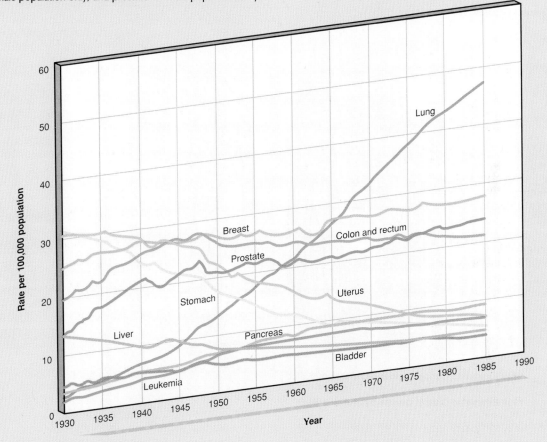

3. double the average consumption of fiber to 20–30 g per day

4. increase the percentage of women aged 50-70 who have annual physical breast exam and mammography to 80 percent for each

5. increase the percentage of women who have a Pap smear every three years to 90 percent for ages 20–39 and to 80 percent for ages 40-70

6. increase adoption of state-of-the-art treatment

The American Cancer Society, along with several other organizations, has submitted nutrition guidelines to help Americans prevent cancer. This is in response to the increasing evidence that nutrition plays a major role in both causing and preventing cancer. Although much more research needs to be done to totally confirm these relationships, the American Cancer Society has felt that enough is known to warrant broad public recommendations. These include the following.

1. *Avoid obesity.* Individuals 40 percent or more overweight increase their risk of colon, breast, prostate, gallbladder, ovary, and uterine cancers. Women who are obese have a 55 percent greater risk, and men have a 33 percent greater risk of cancer than those of normal weight. (See chapter 9 for a discussion of obesity and how to achieve or maintain normal weight.)

FIGURE 10.12

Cancer incidence and deaths by site and sex, 1988 estimate. Lung cancer is now the number-one cancer killer in both men and women.

Cancer statistics, 1989

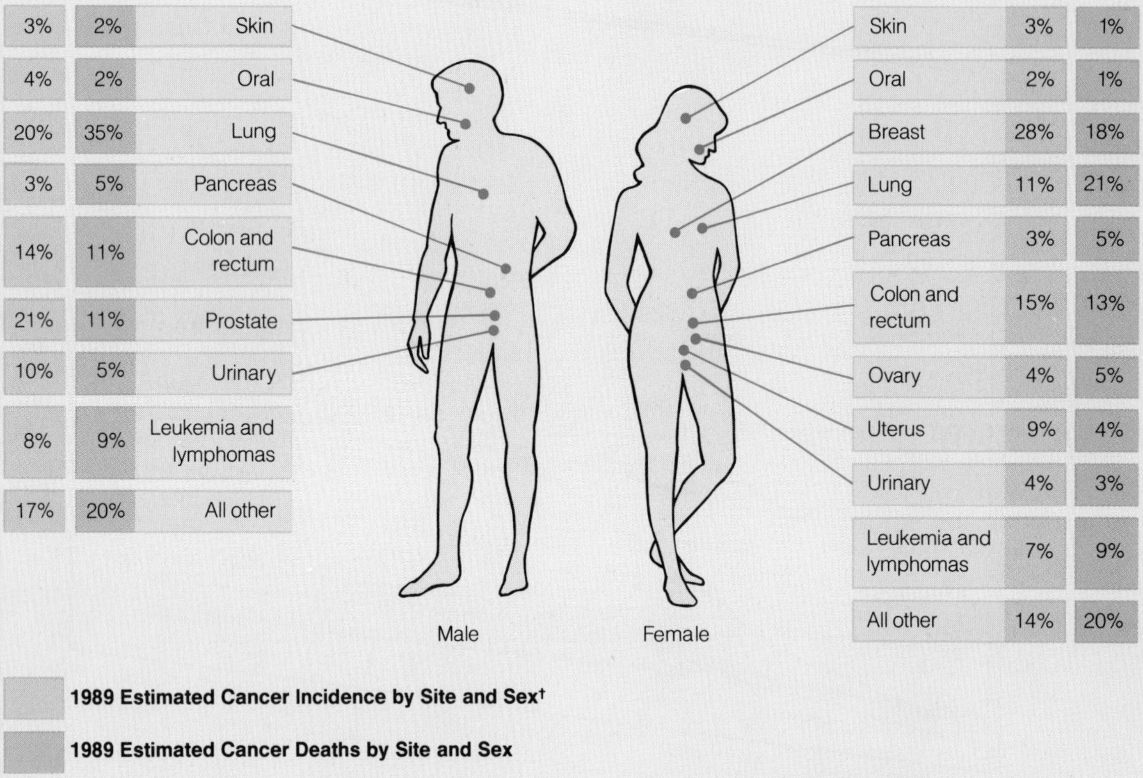

		Male	Female		
3%	2%	Skin	Skin	3%	1%
4%	2%	Oral	Oral	2%	1%
			Breast	28%	18%
20%	35%	Lung	Lung	11%	21%
3%	5%	Pancreas	Pancreas	3%	5%
14%	11%	Colon and rectum	Colon and rectum	15%	13%
21%	11%	Prostate	Ovary	4%	5%
10%	5%	Urinary	Uterus	9%	4%
8%	9%	Leukemia and lymphomas	Urinary	4%	3%
17%	20%	All other	Leukemia and lymphomas	7%	9%
			All other	14%	20%

1989 Estimated Cancer Incidence by Site and Sex†

1989 Estimated Cancer Deaths by Site and Sex

†Excluding nonmelanoma skin cancer and carcinoma in situ.

2. *Cut down on total fat intake.* A diet high in fat may be a factor in the development of certain cancers, particularly breast, colon, and prostate. In addition, by restricting fatty foods, people are better able to control body weight. (See chapter 6 for a discussion of foods that are high in fat.)

3. *Eat more high-fiber foods such as whole-grain cereals, fruits, and vegetables.* Some studies suggest that diets high in fiber may help to reduce the risk of colon cancer. Americans now eat only about 10–15 grams of dietary fiber a day. Populations that consume diets containing twice this amount have a lower rate of cancers of the colon and rectum. The data suggest that if dietary fiber is increased to a per capita figure of 20–30 grams per day, a 50 percent reduction in cancer of the colon and rectum is possible. In addition, foods high in fiber are a good substitute for foods high in fat.

Fiber is a term used for the plant components that are not readily digested in the human intestinal tract. Whole-grain cereal products, unskinned fruits and vegetables, legumes (dry beans), and nuts all have dietary fiber. However, foods from animal sources (meat, cheese, eggs, milk, etc.), do not have any fiber at all. Be aware that fiber supplements are not the answer. All studies to date that show cancer-protective effects are associated with fiber-rich foods. (See chapter 5 for a discussion of foods high in dietary fiber.)

Recent studies have shown that the following foods are most commonly used by Americans.

Coffee, tea: 80% (of all American adults)
White bread, rolls, crackers: 77%
Margarine: 42%
Whole milk: 41%
Doughnuts, cookies, cake: 41%
Sugar: 41%
Green salad: 40%
Regular soft drinks: 39%
Cheeses: 33%
Eggs: 31%
Mayonnaise, salad dressings: 31%
Hot dogs, ham, lunch meats: 30%
Alcoholic beverages: 27%
Hamburgers, cheeseburgers, meat loaf: 26%

As you can see, nearly all of these foods, except for green salad, can be characterized as very low in fiber. Many of them are also high in fat. Fiberless foods such as meats and dairy products provide almost half of all the fat eaten by Americans.

4. *Include foods rich in vitamins A and C in the daily diet.* Vitamin A and its precursor, beta-carotene, appear to be particularly valuable in cancer prevention, and vitamins E and C may be protective to a lesser degree (34, 35). About 20 studies in various parts of the world suggest an inverse association between eating foods containing vitamin A or beta-carotene and various types of human cancer, with risk reduced 30–50%. These studies have shown that eating such foods (especially dark green and orange vegetables and various fruits) may lower the risk of cancers of the larynx, esophagus, and lung. Beta-carotene is capable of quenching singlet oxygen and peroxides that are formed in the body. (Carcinogens such as radiation may have their effect through singlet oxygen and peroxides.) Retinoids may inhibit formation of key enzymes that enhance tumor promotion. As you have seen in table 10.2, high amounts of vitamin A can be found in many foods. Supplementation is therefore unnecessary, and in high amounts it can be harmful because of its toxicity. Vitamin A is a fat-soluble vitamin, and in excess amounts will build up to toxic levels in the body because it is not easily eliminated.

Vitamins C and E appear to prevent the formation of **nitrosamines,** potential carcinogens resulting from metabolic reactions in the human digestive tract of nitrates, nitrites, and substances readily found in foods (especially processed or smoked meats, and nitrate salts used in food processing). Nitrates react with amines or amides in the digestive tract to form nitrosamines and nitrosamides, respectively. Vitamins C and E compete with the amine or amide for the nitrosating agent. Epidemiologic studies suggest that fruits and vegetables containing vitamin C may offer specific protection for the upper digestive tract. Adults should try to get at least 60 mg of vitamin C each day. Vegetarians, who have low cancer risk, often get more than 200 mg a day. Table 10.14 outlines foods high in vitamin C.

5. *Include cruciferous vegetables in your diet.* **Cruciferous vegetables** include cabbage, broccoli, Brussels sprouts, kohlrabi, and cauliflower. Some studies have suggested that consumption of these vegetables may reduce the risk of cancer, particularly of the gastrointestinal and respiratory tracts.

6. *Be moderate in consumption of alcoholic beverages.* Heavy drinkers of alcohol, especially those who are also cigarette smokers, are at unusually high risk for cancers of the oral cavity, larynx, and esophagus.

7. *Be moderate in consumption of salt-cured, smoked, and nitrite-cured foods.* Smoked foods such as hams, some varieties of sausages, fish, etc., absorb some of the tars that come from incomplete combustion. These tars contain cancer-causing chemicals, similar to those of cigarette smoke. Evidence shows that salt-cured or pickled foods may increase the risk of stomach and esophageal cancer. Nitrites are used with meats to help protect against food poisoning (botulism), and to improve color and flavor. These lead to the formation of nitrosamines, which are powerful cancer-causing chemicals. The American meat industry is working on reducing its use of nitrites.

Of the seven recommendations that we have just discussed, how many do you already practice? If you follow all seven and do not smoke, your chance of cancer is greatly reduced.

SUMMARY

1. There are four fat-soluble vitamins (vitamins A, D, E, and K) and nine water-soluble vitamins (thiamin, riboflavin, niacin, vitamin B_6, folate, vitamin B_{12}, pantothenic acid, biotin, and vitamin C).

2. According to national surveys, college students obtain more than 100 percent RDA for all vitamins except for vitamin B_6 (which is still at adequate levels). Most reputable nutritionists promote that vitamin or mineral supplementation is unwarranted for people eating balanced diets. Vitamin supplements are not recommended because toxicity and disturbance of normal nutrient absorption can occur with high doses.

3. Fruits and vegetables that are yellow-orange and dark green are excellent sources of vitamins A and K. Sunlight exposure is an important means of obtaining sufficient vitamin D. Vitamin E is found in vegetable oils, whole grains, nuts, seeds, and other plant foods. Legumes, nuts, seeds, whole grains, and roasted poultry are excellent sources of the B-complex vitamins. Vitamin C is found in a wide variety of fruits and vegetables.

4. Various food-preparation techniques can help protect the vitamin content of foods. Reducing trimming, decreasing storage and cooking time, and avoiding use of large quantities of water during cooking are helpful. Microwave cooking, steaming, or using a pan or wok with very small amounts of water and a tight-fitting lid are the best cooking methods.

5. Well-defined deficiency diseases exist for most of the vitamins. Although these are rare in developed countries like the U.S., people in many countries of the world suffer from these diseases.

6. Nearly 40 percent of adult Americans use vitamin supplements. Although people give various reasons for supplementation, these reasons are usually based on misinformation. However, supplement usage is indicated in some circumstances, including women with excessive menstrual bleeding, women who are pregnant or breast-feeding, people with very low caloric intakes, vegetarians who are very restrictive in their diets, and newborns who may need vitamin K to prevent abnormal bleeding.

7. The majority of cancers are now thought to be preventable. The National Cancer Institute estimates that diet is responsible for 35 percent of all cancers. Specific dietary recommendations to prevent cancer include reducing the average consumption of fat to 25 percent or less of total calories, doubling the average consumption of fiber to 20–30 grams per day, controlling obesity, and consuming foods rich in vitamins A, C, and E. Cruciferous vegetables and citrus fruits are highly recommended.

REFERENCES

1. National Center for Health Statistics. Dietary Intake Source Data, by M. D. Carroll, S. Abraham, and C. M. Dresser. United States 1976–80, Second National Health and Nutrition Examination Survey. Vital and Health Statistics. Series II-No. 231. DHHS Pub. No. (PHS) 83-1681. Public Health Service. Washington, D.C.: U.S. Government Printing Office, March 1983.

2. Nutrient Intakes: Individuals in 48 States, Year 1977–78. Consumer Nutrition Division, Human Nutrition Information Service, U.S. Department of Agriculture, Hyattsville, Maryland 20782. Nationwide Food Consumption Survey 1977–78, Report No. I-2, May 1984.

3. Bauernfeind, J. C. 1988 Vitamin A Deficiency: A Staggering Problem of Health and Sight. *Nutrition Today* (March/April).

4. Stänge, L., K. Carlstrom, and M. Eriksson. 1978. Hypervitaminosis A in Early Human Pregnancy and Malformations of the Central Nervous System. *Acta Obstêtrics Gynecology Scandanavia* 57:289–91.

5. Lammer, E. J., et al. 1985. Retinoid Acid Embryopathy. *New England Journal of Medicine* 313:837–41.

6. Nater, J. P., and H. M. G. Doeglas. 1970. *Acta Dermatovenen* (Stockholm), English ed., 50:109.

7. Marshall, C. W. 1985. *Vitamins and Minerals: Help or Harm?* Philadelphia: George Stickley Co.

8. Reid, I. R., D. J. Gallagher, and J. Bosworth. 1986. Prophylaxis against Vitamin D Deficiency in the Elderly by Regular Sunlight Exposure. *Age Ageing* 15(1):35–40.

9. Anonymous. 1980. Vitamin D Deficiency Rickets, Revisited. *Nutrition Review* 38:116.

10. Horwitt, M. K., B. Century, and A. Zeman. 1963. Erythrocyte Survival Time and Reticulocyte Levels after Tocopherol Depletion in Man. *American Journal of Clinical Nutrition* 12:99–106.

11. Binder, H. J., and H. Spiro. 1967. Tocopherol Deficiency in Man. *American Journal of Clinical Nutrition* 20:594–601.

12. Tsai, A. C., et al. 1978. Study on the Effect of Megavitamin E Supplementation in Man. *American Journal of Clinical Nutrition* 31:831–37.

13. Anderson, T. W., and D. B. W. Reid. 1974. A Double-Blind Trial of Vitamin E in Angina Pectoris. *American Journal of Clinical Nutrition* 27:1174–1178.

14. Committee on Safety, Toxicity, and Misuse of Vitamins and Trace Minerals, National Nutrition Consortium, Inc. 1978. Vitamin-Mineral Safety, Toxicity, and Misuse. Chicago: American Dietetic Association.

15. Bieri, J. G. 1983. Medical Uses of Vitamin E. *New England Journal of Medicine* 308:1063–1071.

16. Horwitt, M. K. 1986. The Promotion of Vitamin E. *Journal of Nutrition* 116:1371–1377.

17. Suttie, J. W., et al. 1988. Vitamin K Deficiency from Dietary Vitamin K Restriction in Humans. *American Journal of Clinical Nutrition* 47:475–80.

18. Hayes, K. C., and D. M. Hegsted. 1973. *Toxicity of Vitamins in Toxicants Occurring Naturally in Foods,* Washington, D.C:: Food and Nutrition Board, National Academy of Sciences.

19. Ostwald, R., and G. Briggs. 1966. *Toxicity of Vitamins in Toxicants Occurring Naturally in Foods.* Washington D.C.: Food and Nutrition Board, National Academy of Sciences.

20. Goldberger, J. 1915. The Prevention of Pellagra: A Test Diet among Institutional Inmates. Public Health Report 30:3117–3131.

21. Blankenhorn, D. H., et al. 1987. Beneficial Effects of Combined Colestipol-Niacin Therapy on Coronary Atherosclerosis and Coronary Venous Bypass Grafts. *Journal of the American Medical Association* 257:3233–3240.

22. Mira, M., P. M. Stewart, and S. F. Abraham. 1988. Vitamin and Trace Element Status in Premenstrual Syndrome. *American Journal of Clinical Nutrition* 47:636–41.

23. Herbert, V. 1987. Recommended Dietary Intakes of Folate in Humans. *American Journal of Clinical Nutrition* 45:661–70.

24. Simmer, K., et al. 1987. Are Iron-Folate Supplements Harmful? *American Journal of Clinical Nutrition* 45:122–25.

25. Herbert, V. 1987. Recommended Dietary Intake (RDI) of Vitamin B_{12} in Humans. *American Journal of Clinical Nutrition* 45:671–78.

26. Carlson, B. L., and M. H. Tabacchi. 1988. Loss of Vitamin C in Vegetables during the Foodservice Cycle. *Journal of the American Dietetic Association* 88:65–67.

27. McDonald, J. T. 1986. Vitamin and Mineral Supplement Use in the United States. *Clinical Nutrition* 5:27–33.

28. Harper, A. E. 1987. ``Nutrition Insurance'' — A Skeptical View. *Nutrition Forum* 4(5):33–37.

29. Hathcock, J. N. 1985. Quantitative Evaluation of Vitamin Safety. *Pharmacy Times* (May): 104–13.

30. Anonymous. Scientific Groups Warn against Vitamin Misuse. 1987. *Nutrition Forum* 4(5):40.

31. The American Medical Association Council on Scientific Affairs. 1987. Vitamin Preparations as Dietary Supplements and as Therapeutic Agents. *Journal of the American Medical Association* 257:1927–1936.

32. American Cancer Society. 1988. Cancer Facts & Figures — 1988. New York: American Cancer Society.

33. Greenwald, P., and E. Sondik. 1986. Diet and Chemoprevention in NCI's Research Strategy to Achieve National Cancer Control Objectives. *Annual Review of Public Health* 7:267–91.

34. Olson, J. A. 1986. Carotenoids, Vitamin A, and Cancer. *Journal of Nutrition* 116:1127–1130.

35. Watson, R. R., and T. K. Leonard. 1986. Selenium and Vitamins A, E, and C: Nutrients with Cancer Prevention Properties. *Journal of the American Dietetic Association* 86:505–10.

*H*EALTH-PROMOTION ACTIVITY 10.1
Are You Ingesting More Than the RDA for Vitamin C?

As we have discussed in this chapter, vitamin C plays many important roles in the body, including cancer prevention.

In this activity, you will calculate the vitamin C content of your diet. Below, list all of the foods you ate yesterday. This may require some careful recall. This method is called the 24-hour recall and is used in many large-population diet studies. The major advantage of this method is that by recalling what you ate yesterday, you have not had an opportunity to alter your diet. The major problem with this method is that what you ate yesterday may not be typical of your usual intake.

After listing all the foods you ate yesterday, use the dietary information found in appendix B and write down the vitamin C value for each food. Be sure that you carefully note portion sizes and make the appropriate adjustments in your figures. Total the vitamin C figures, and then compare your one-day total with the RDA (60 mg). Did you meet the RDA? What foods do you need to include more of to increase your vitamin C intake?

24-Hour Vitamin C Intake

Foods Eaten Yesterday	Portion Size	Vitamin C Value	Foods Eaten Yesterday	Portion Size	Vitamin C Value

HEALTH PROMOTION ACTIVITY 10.2
Foods to Improve the Vitamin Content of Your Diet

As you have learned, most people do not need to supplement their diets if the quality of their diet is appropriate. In this Health-Promotion Activity, you will review the quality of your diet to determine what foods you can either add or substitute for others to improve the vitamin content of your diet.

Review the 13 vitamin tables in this chapter. Below list ten foods that you are willing to add to your diet to improve your vitamin intake. Try to emphasize foods that are ranked high in each table, and select a wide variety of foods.

Foods High in Vitamin Content

1.

2.

3.

4.

5.

6.

7.

7.

8.

9.

10.

HEALTH PROMOTION ACTIVITY 10.3
Problems and Risks of Using Vitamin Supplements in High Doses

This chapter emphasized that when vitamin supplements are used in quantities far exceeding the RDA, various health problems can arise. In this activity, you will review the chapter and list seven of these problems associated with vitamin megadosing.

List below seven problems or risks involved when large quantities of vitamins are used in supplement form. Try to list more than three types of vitamins.

Vitamin	Megadosing Side Effects
1.	
2.	
3.	
4.	
5.	
6.	
7.	

11

Minerals

INTRODUCTION

*M*ore than one-third of the dietary nutrients you need to maintain life are minerals. These minerals play very important roles in the human body and are also related to such diseases as cancer and high blood pressure. In this chapter, you will be introduced to sixteen minerals, learning why they are important to your life and health and how to make sure your diet contains sufficient amounts of each.

We've been hearing a lot about sodium lately. Information from this chapter will guide you in moderating your intake and finding appropriate substitutes to keep your diet tasteful. The Health-Promotion Insight will review the most current information on minerals and high blood pressure, with special attention given to sodium.

Although mineral supplementation is usually unnecessary if one consumes a wide variety of wholesome foods, improper food processing and preparation techniques can decrease the mineral quality of food. Techniques to avoid this problem will also be reviewed.

TABLE 11.1
Mineral composition of an adult human body

Element	Grams/70-kg Male
Calcium	1,160
Phosphorus	670
Potassium	150
Sulfur	112
Chlorine	85
Sodium	63
Magnesium	21
Iron	4.5
Zinc	2.0
Iodine	0.02

Of the nearly 45 dietary nutrients known to be necessary for human life, 17 are **minerals,** and of the 92 chemical elements found on this earth, at least 50 are found in the human body. Of these elements, oxygen, hydrogen, carbon, and nitrogen account for 96 percent of body weight, primarily in the form of water. The remaining four percent of body weight represents minerals (1). Table 11.1 summarizes the major minerals of which humans are composed (2).

Although mineral elements represent only a very small fraction of human body weight, they play very important roles in all areas of the body. They help form hard tissues such as bones and teeth, aid in normal muscle and nerve activity, act as catalysts in many enzyme systems, help control body water levels, and are integral parts of organic compounds in the body, like hemoglobin and the hormone thyroxine. Evidence is also growing that certain minerals like calcium and selenium may help prevent cancer. Deficiencies of zinc may decrease the ability of the immune system to function. Excess sodium may elevate blood pressure in susceptible individuals. These concepts and others will be discussed in this chapter. You may find that minerals are much more important for your health and well-being than you had previously realized. Only in the last 30 years have scientists themselves begun to understand how integral minerals are in human health. Table 11.2 summarizes the functions, food sources, and recommended dietary intakes of minerals.

Minerals that the body must have from the diet can be categorized as follows:

1. **Major Minerals.** These are minerals needed in amounts greater than 100 mg/day, and include calcium, phosphorus, magnesium, sodium, chloride, potassium, and sulfur. Three of these—sodium, chloride, and potassium—are also known as the three body electrolytes. Sulfur is a component of the essential amino acid, methionine. Sulfur is easily obtained by eating adequate protein. For this reason, we will not be discussing sulfur further in this chapter.

2. **Minor Minerals.** These are trace elements needed in amounts no more than a few mg/day, and include iron, zinc, iodine, fluoride, copper, selenium, chromium, cobalt, manganese, and molybdenum. Of these, only four—iron, zinc, selenium, and iodine—have been studied sufficiently to establish required dietary amounts (RDA). For five of the other six (all except cobalt), "safe and adequate" daily ranges have been estimated by the Food and Nutrition Board of the National Academy of Sciences (3) (see table 11.2).

There are several other minerals that may be essential for humans, but research has not yet established their importance. These include tin, nickel, silicon, and vanadium. More than a dozen other minerals are also found in the human body, but these are regarded as contaminants. These include lead, mercury, arsenic, aluminum, silver, cadmium, barium, strontium, and others. Many experts feel that the body would do well not to have these minerals and that excesses can harm human health. We'll discuss three of these—lead, mercury, and aluminum—later in the chapter.

Figure 11.1 summarizes the average daily intake of minerals by male and female adults, ages 25 to 30 (4). The percent RDA for copper and manganese were calculated by using the midpoint values of the "estimated safe and adequate" daily dietary intakes recommended by the Food and Nutrition Board (3). Notice that copper is very low for both sexes, while females have less than optimal intakes (less than 67 percent RDA) for manganese. In this chapter we will

TABLE 11.2
Minerals: a condensed summary

	RDA Adults*		What It Does and Major Food Sources
Major Minerals	M	F	
Calcium	800 mg	800 mg	Used for building bones and teeth and maintaining bone strength; also involved in muscle contraction, blood clotting, and maintenance of cell membranes. *Food:* all dairy products, dark green leafy vegetables, beans, nuts, sunflower seeds, dried fruit, molasses, canned fish.
Phosphorus	800 mg	800 mg	Used to build bones and teeth; release energy from carbohydrate, proteins, and fats; and form genetic material, cell membranes, and many enzymes. *Food:* beans, sunflower seeds, milk, cheese, nuts, poultry, fish, lean meats.
Magnesium	350 mg	280 mg	Used to build bones, produce proteins, release energy from muscle carbohydrate stores (glycogen), and regulate body temperature. *Food:* sunflower and pumpkin seeds, nuts, whole-grain products, beans, dark green vegetables, dried fruit, lean meats.
Sodium	500 mg		Regulates body-fluid volume and blood acidity; aids in transmission of nerve impulses. *Food:* most of the sodium in the American diet is added to food as salt (sodium chloride) in cooking, at the table, or in commercial processing. Animal products contain some natural sodium.
Chloride	750 mg		Is a component of gastric juice and aids in acid-base balance. *Food:* table salt, seafood, milk, eggs, meats.
Potassium	2000 mg		Assists in muscle contraction, the maintenance of fluid and electrolyte balance in the cells, and the transmission of nerve impulses. Also aids in the release of energy from carbohydrate, proteins, and fats. *Food:* widely distributed in foods, especially fruits and vegetables, beans, nuts, seeds, and lean meats.
Minor Minerals			
Iron	10 mg	15 mg	Involved in the formation of hemoglobin in the red blood cells of the blood and myoglobin in muscles. Also a part of several enzymes and proteins. *Food:* molasses, seeds, whole-grain products, fortified breakfast cereals, nuts, dried fruits, beans, poultry, fish, lean meats.
Zinc	15 mg	12 mg	Involved in the formation of protein (growth of all tissues), wound healing, and prevention of anemia. A component of many enzymes. *Food:* whole-grain products, seeds, nuts, poultry, fish, beans, lean meats.
Iodine	150 μg	150 μg	Integral component of thyroid hormones. *Food:* table salt (fortified), dairy products, shellfish, and fish.
Fluoride	1.5–4.0 mg		Maintenance of bone and tooth structure. *Food:* fluoridated drinking water is the best source. Also found in tea, fish, wheat germ, kale, cottage cheese, soybeans, almonds, onions, milk.
Copper	1.5–3.0 mg		Vital to enzyme systems and in manufacturing red blood cells. Needed for utilization of iron. *Food:* nuts, oysters, seeds, crab, wheat germ, dried fruit, whole grains, legumes.
Selenium	55–70 μg		Functions in association with vitamin E and may assist in protecting tissues and cell membranes from oxidative damage. May also aid in preventing cancer. *Food:* nuts, whole grains, lean pork, cottage cheese, milk, molasses, squash.
Chromium	50–200 μg		Required for maintaining normal glucose metabolism. May assist insulin function. *Food:* nuts, prunes, vegetable oils, green peas, corn, whole grains, orange juice, dark green vegetables, legumes.
Manganese	2.0–5.0 mg		Needed for normal bone structure, reproduction, and the normal functioning of the central nervous system. Is a component of many enzyme systems. *Food:* whole grains, nuts, seeds, pineapple, berries, legumes, dark green vegetables, tea.
Molybdenum	75–250 μg		Component of enzymes and may help prevent dental caries. *Food:* tomatoes, wheat germ, lean pork, legumes, whole grains, strawberries, winter squash, milk, dark green vegetables, carrots.

* Instead of RDA, "safe and adequate" daily dietary intake range is given for fluoride, copper, chromium, manganese, and molybdenum. Estimated minimum requirements are given for sodium, chloride, and potassium. It is recommended that sodium intake be limited to 2,400 mg per day.

FIGURE 11.1

Intake of most minerals is adequate for young American adults, although some are lower than the recommended level (at least 67 percent RDA is desirable). Females in particular need to emphasize foods high in minerals in their diets.

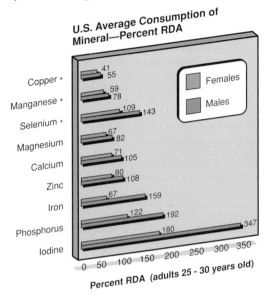

U.S. Average Consumption of Mineral—Percent RDA

Mineral	Females	Males
Copper *	41	55
Manganese *	59	78
Selenium *	109	143
Magnesium	67	82
Calcium	71	105
Zinc	80	108
Iron	67	159
Phosphorus	122	192
Iodine	180	347

Percent RDA (adults 25 - 30 years old)

FIGURE 11.2

Nearly all of the calcium in the human body is in the bones.

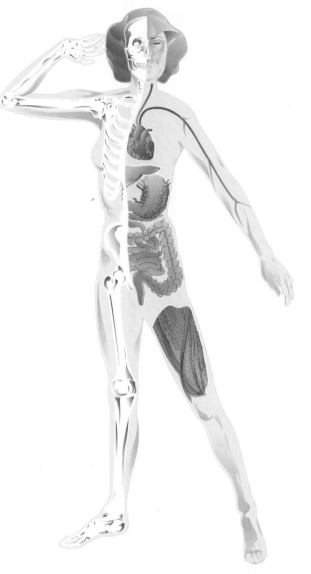

99 percent in bones and teeth

1 percent in blood, other body fluids, and various soft tissues

review recommendations for improving intakes of these and other minerals. In general, a greater intake of legumes, dark green vegetables, nuts, seeds, lean meats, and dried fruit is recommended.

Major Minerals

Calcium

Calcium is not only the most abundant mineral in the human body but also the most popular. Americans have been urged to consume more calcium (offered now in everything from high-calcium bread to high-calcium soft drinks) to help prevent weak bones, high blood pressure, and bowel cancer. In the clamor for more calcium, Americans have dramatically increased their consumption of calcium supplements. Are supplements necessary? Let's review the facts.

Recommended Intake

The body of an adult male contains between 950 and 1,300 grams of calcium. The adult female, because of her smaller size, contains between 770 and 920 grams of calcium. Figure 11.2 shows that 99 percent of this calcium is in the bones and skeleton; only one percent is in body fluids and soft tissues. However, as we will see in the next section, the body calcium found outside the bones serves many highly important biochemical functions (3).

Most researchers have found that to maintain these body calcium stores, about 500 mg of calcium per day need to be consumed in

FIGURE 11.3

American female adults tend to consume less calcium than recommended. Considerable controversy exists as to whether this is harmful for bone health.

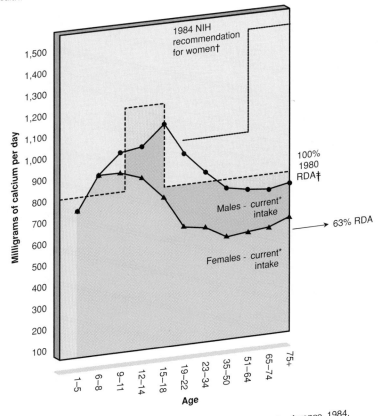

†National Institutes of Health Consensus Development Conference, 1984.
†Recommended Dietary Allowances, National Academy of Sciences, 1980. The RDA for pregnant and lactating women is 1,200 mg.
* USDA National Food Consumption Survey, 1977–78.

the diet (5). The Recommended Dietary Allowance (RDA) for adults has been set at 800 mg/day, and for teenagers, pregnant, and lactating women, 1,200 mg/day (3). As discussed in chapter 3, the RDA are estimated to exceed the requirements of most people. The Food and Agriculture Organization of the United Nations has stated that only 400 to 500 mg of calcium are needed each day (1).

Figure 11.3 shows the average calcium intakes of U.S. males and females over the different age groups in comparison to the RDA (6). Notice that females in some age groups are below the RDA but are still obtaining the 500 mg/day that is needed to maintain body calcium balance. Figure 11.4 illustrates that most Americans obtain their calcium from milk products, with four of the top five contributors coming

from this food group. Various grain products are also an important calcium source for Americans.

Figure 11.3 also shows that the National Institutes of Health (NIH) recommend that women, to help prevent **osteoporosis,** need 1,000 mg/day before menopause and up to 1,500 mg/day after menopause (7). The NIH recommendations have stirred much controversy. *Osteoporosis* is defined as an age-related disorder, characterized by decreased bone mineral content and increased risk of fractures. Women, and to a lesser extent men, have been urged to increase their consumption of calcium-rich foods to decrease their risk of osteoporosis. Some studies have shown that high calcium intake helps retard or prevent the progress of osteoporosis. Other studies have shown little benefit

FIGURE 11.4

This graph shows that Americans get the majority of their calcium from dairy products. Although skim and low-fat milk have the same amount of calcium as whole milk, Americans use such large quantities of whole milk that it contributes more to their diets.

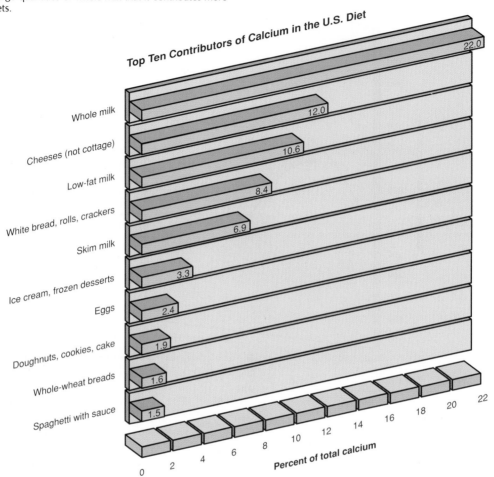

Top Ten Contributors of Calcium in the U.S. Diet

Food	Percent of total calcium
Whole milk	22.0
Cheeses (not cottage)	12.0
Low-fat milk	10.6
White bread, rolls, crackers	8.4
Skim milk	6.9
Ice cream, frozen desserts	3.3
Eggs	2.4
Doughnuts, cookies, cake	1.9
Whole-wheat breads	1.6
Spaghetti with sauce	1.5

in calcium intakes above 500 mg/day (8). Other factors such as adequate estrogen or physical activity may be more important. Chapter 15 will discuss osteoporosis in much more detail.

The food tables in this chapter need explanation. Foods are compared on an equal-volume basis (one cup) instead of using generally accepted, standard portion sizes. Studies have shown that selected portions of food by men and women vary considerably and often are larger than some nutritionists deem as "normal." For this reason, foods in the tables of this and the previous chapter are compared on an equal-volume basis so that you can better understand where the nutrients are concentrated. You can then choose the amount of food you want to eat based on this information.

As you can see in table 11.3, one cup of low-fat milk has just under 300 mg of calcium. To obtain the RDA for calcium (800 mg/day), one must consume the equivalent of 2.7 cups of milk. By comparison, the RDA for calcium is also found in 1.9 cups of yogurt, 2.3 cups of almonds, 4.5 cups of broccoli, and 5.2 cups of cottage cheese. Milk products are the richest source of calcium, but nuts, mackerel (canned) and oysters, dark green vegetables, seeds, and legumes are also good sources.

For postmenopausal women, the equivalent of five cups or 1.25 quarts of milk are recommended to obtain 1,500 mg of calcium per

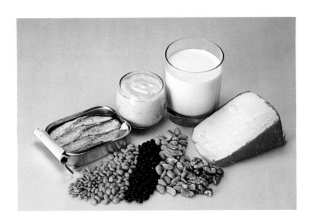

TABLE 11.3
Calcium in one-cup portions of food

Food	Calcium in One-Cup Portions (mg)
Sesame seeds	1,404
Mozzarella cheese, skim milk	980
Cheddar cheese	815
Ricotta cheese, skim milk	669
Plain yogurt, low-fat	415
Fish, mackerel (canned)	388
Almonds	346
Fish, brook trout	338
Low-fat milk	297
Lobster	286
Dried figs	286
Brazil nuts	246
Oysters	226
Filbert nuts	216
Macaroni and cheese	199
Broccoli, cooked	178
Sunflower seeds	168
Soup — cream of potato with milk	166
Cottage cheese (low-fat)	155
Soybeans (cooked)	131
Peanuts, roasted	125

The RDA for adults is 800 mg/day.
Note: Information for all of the tables in this chapter derived from U.S.D.A. Handbook No. 8, using the Nutritionist III software program (N-Squared Computing, Silverton, Oregon.)

day. Some people find that consuming this amount of milk or other high-calcium foods is prohibitive and have sought appropriate calcium supplements.

First, consuming more than 800 mg of calcium per day to prevent bone loss is not recommended by all experts. Second, even the NIH highly recommends that the calcium be obtained from foods high in calcium, especially low-fat dairy products. Third, as we will see later in this section, high intakes of calcium can cause health problems in some people. For these reasons, calcium supplements should not be used unless a physician prescribes them for various medical reasons or because dairy products cannot be consumed.

Some individuals cannot digest the lactose (milk sugar) present in dairy products. This is called **lactose intolerance.** Milk has 11 grams of lactose per cup, cottage cheese has 6 grams per cup, and ice milk has 10 grams per cup (10). Cheese has less than one gram of lactose per

ounce. Approximately 10 percent of Caucasians and up to 90 percent of Orientals and Blacks lack the enzyme lactase that digests the lactose. Lactose then passes undigested into the colon, where the bacteria ferment the sugar, causing gas, bloating, diarrhea, and the formation of volatile free fatty acids (see figure 11.5). Some dairy products such as yogurt can be used by lactose-intolerant individuals because the lactase enzyme is found in the yogurt (9). Also, one brand of milk (Lactaid's Calci-Milk) is pretreated with the lactase enzyme so that 70 percent of the lactose is broken down to glucose and galactose. This type of milk tastes slightly sweeter.

Lactose-intolerant people may need to use a mild calcium supplement if yogurt or Calci-Milk is unacceptable to them. Several forms of calcium supplements are available, with the amount of calcium they contain varying widely. Calcium carbonate or gluconate or lactate are all acceptable, with calcium carbonate being the least expensive. The actual number of milligrams of calcium contained per pill should be checked, because each combination is not 100 percent pure calcium. Bone meal and dolomite are not acceptable sources of calcium because they may contain harmful amounts of lead, arsenic, mercury, and other potentially toxic metals.

Role in Body
The major minerals in bones are calcium and phosphorus (see next section). There is twice as much calcium in bones as there is phosphorus (10). Together, these minerals form deposits of calcium phosphate, which are held within the skeleton by soft, fibrous, organic materials.

FIGURE 11.5

Some individuals cannot digest the lactose (milk sugar) present in milk products because they have a deficiency of the enzyme lactase.

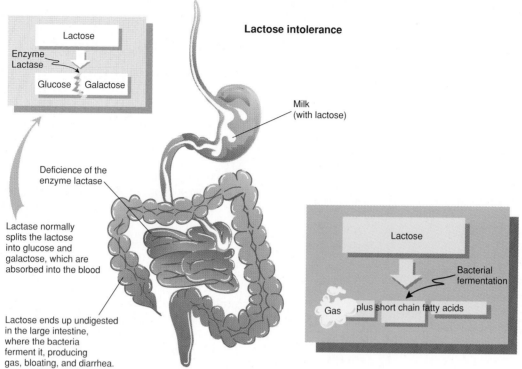

Lactose intolerance

Lactose

Enzyme Lactase

Glucose   Galactose

Milk (with lactose)

Deficience of the enzyme lactase

Lactase normally splits the lactose into glucose and galactose, which are absorbed into the blood

Lactose

Bacterial fermentation

Gas   plus short chain fatty acids

Lactose ends up undigested in the large intestine, where the bacteria ferment it, producing gas, bloating, and diarrhea.

Bones are constantly being reformed, with approximately 700 mg of calcium entering and leaving the bones each day (3). This calcium comes from both body stores and diet. The turnover of bone calcium varies with age. Infants turn over their bone calcium so rapidly that by age one, they have entirely new bones! This process slows down so that by adulthood, bones take approximately 25 years to be "remodeled" (10). As adults get older, however, the bones begin to lose calcium, and bone mass begins to decrease. In certain individuals, this leads to osteoporosis (see chapter 15).

The small amount of calcium outside your bones plays a vital role in nerve and muscle function. Every time you blink your eye, throw a baseball, or do a push-up, calcium is used as the nerve sends impulses to the muscles, and finally as calcium helps the muscle cells to contract. If for some medical reason the amount of calcium in the blood is reduced to below-normal levels, tetany or spasmotic contractions of the muscles can occur (11). The amount of calcium in the blood is normally under precise hormonal regulation, varying only three percent.

Calcium is also important for blood clotting, normal functioning of heart muscle cells, activation of certain enzymes and hormone secretion, and for the integrity of cell substances (1).

There is some evidence that calcium may help prevent high blood pressure. The Health-Promotion Insight at the end of this chapter reviews this in further detail. Some researchers have also suggested that calcium can help prevent bowel cancer (12). Calcium may bind bile salts in the colon, thus increasing their passage out of the large intestine with the stool. Excess bile salts in the colon have been associated with increased risk of colon cancer.

Low Intake

Calcium deficiency can result from three factors (11):

1. extremely low calcium in the diet;
2. deficiency of vitamin D, which is needed for calcium absorption;
3. interference with absorption of calcium in the intestines.

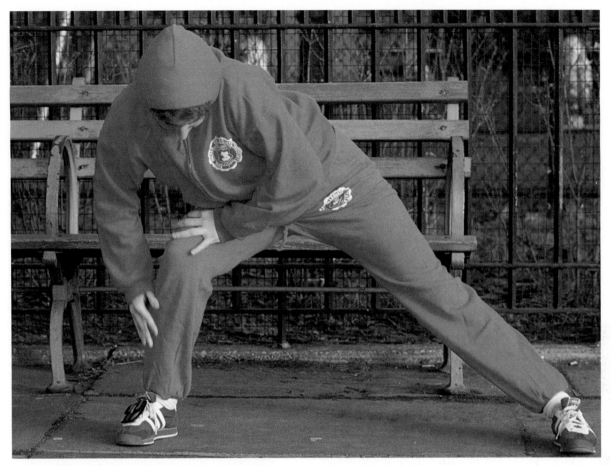

A small amount of calcium is important for body functions.

Some studies have shown that humans can maintain calcium balance on intakes as low as 200–400 mg/day (the equivalent of about one cup of milk). However, such a low calcium intake is not recommended (3). Intakes below 500–800 mg/day may lead to osteoporosis in later life (see chapter 15).

As reviewed in chapter 10, vitamin D deficiency leads to a decrease in calcium absorption from the intestine, causing rickets in children and osteomalacia (bone softening) in adults.

Normally, only about 30 to 60 percent of ingested calcium is actually absorbed through the small intestine into the bloodstream (10). The rest goes into the large intestine, where it passes out of the body with the stool. Some dietary factors decrease the ability of your small intestine to absorb the calcium.

Most dark green vegetables are good sources of calcium. However, spinach, chard, beet greens, and rhubarb contain oxalic acid, which can bind the calcium in the small intestine, and make it unavailable to the body. For example, six times more calcium is absorbed from milk than from spinach. Generally, when the diet contains sufficient calcium, the calcium-binding effect of oxalic acid does not appear to be a cause for concern.

Modern diets, which are rich in animal proteins and phosphorus, may promote the loss of calcium in the urine (10). This has led to the concept of the Ca/P ratio. If the Ca/P ratio is low (low calcium, high phosphorus intake), more than the normal amount of calcium may be lost in the urine, decreasing the calcium level in bones. Table 11.4 outlines the Ca/P ratios of many foods. This will be discussed in further detail in the phosphorus section.

Lactose from milk, some types of amino acids, and vitamin D enhance calcium absorption (2).

TABLE 11.4
Calcium/phosphorus ratio of selected foods

Food	Calcium/Phosphorus Ratio	
Collards, cooked	7.79	
Papayas	4.71	
Dandelion greens, cooked	3.34	
Oranges	2.88	
Beet greens, cooked	2.84	Excellent
Kale, cooked	2.61	
Spinach, raw, chopped	2.44	
Broccoli, cooked	2.41	
Blackberries	1.53	
Ricotta cheese, skim milk	1.49	
Grapes	1.44	
Celery	1.38	
Milk, low-fat	1.28	Good
Yogurt, low-fat and plain	1.27	
Snap green beans	1.26	
Boysenberries	1.00	
Pineapple	1.00	
Onions	0.86	
Dates, chopped	0.83	
Grape juice	0.81	
Sweet potato	0.80	
Strawberries	0.75	
Pumpkin	0.75	
Summer squash	0.70	
Fish, mackerel, canned	0.68	Fair
Prunes	0.65	
Brussels sprouts	0.64	
Lobster	0.64	
Cauliflower	0.63	
Carrots	0.63	
Almonds	0.51	
Raisins	0.51	
Cottage cheese, low-fat	0.46	
Soybeans	0.41	
Brazil nuts	0.29	
Kidney beans	0.27	
Crabmeat	0.25	
Chocolate candy	0.20	Poor—be
Corned beef hash	0.20	careful
Cola-type soda	0.18	unless
Peanuts	0.17	food is
Beer	0.17	good for
Turkey	0.16	other
Grape Nuts	0.15	reasons.
Whole-wheat cereal	0.13	
Cashews	0.09	
Deviled ham	0.08	
Chicken liver	0.05	
Pork	0.03	

TABLE 11.5
Minimum toxic doses of minerals

Mineral	Recommended Adult Intake	Minimum Toxic Dose (MTD)	Mineral Safety Index (MSI)
Calcium	1,200 mg	12,000 mg	10
Phosphorus	1,200 mg	12,000 mg	10
Magnesium	400 mg	6,000 mg	15
Iron	15 mg	100 mg	6.7
Zinc	15 mg	500 mg	33
Copper	3 mg	100 mg	33
		< 3 mg	< 1
Fluoride	4 mg	20 mg	5
		4 mg	1
Iodine	150 μg	2000 μg	13
Selenium	70 μg	1000 μg	14

Calcium and phosphorus intakes are based on the U.S. RDA.

Data from J. N. Hathcock, "Quantitive Evaluation of Vitamin Safety," *Pharmacy Times.* (May, 1985):pp. 104–113. Used with permission.

High Intake

There is some evidence that calcium intakes, especially from regular use of calcium supplements, may be associated with increased risk of kidney stones (13). Humans can usually tolerate calcium intakes ranging from 1,000 to 2,500 mg per day without ill results. Larger amounts can result in abnormally high levels of calcium in the blood, decreasing normal kidney function.

Calcium supplements are not advised in amounts greater than 500–800 mg per day. The minimum toxic dose is 12,000 mg, or ten times the U.S. RDA (see table 11.5) (14). As mentioned previously, some "health-food" enthusiasts feel that generous daily supplements of bone meal are important for health. Lead poisioning from bone-meal ingestion has been reported. Significant amounts of lead have also been found in dolomite, a form of limestone also marketed as a calcium supplement.

Phosphorus

Phosphorus represents one percent of the human body weight, and after calcium it is the most common mineral found in the body. Phosphorus teams with calcium in many of its roles.

*F*IGURE 11.6

Dairy products also contribute most of the phosphorus Americans consume.

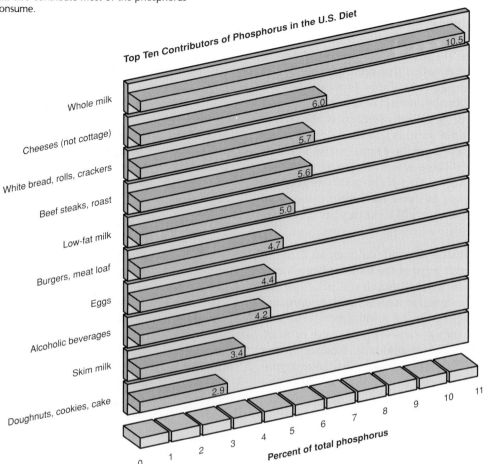

Top Ten Contributors of Phosphorus in the U.S. Diet

Food	Percent
Whole milk	10.5
Cheeses (not cottage)	6.0
White bread, rolls, crackers	5.7
Beef steaks, roast	5.6
Low-fat milk	5.0
Burgers, meat loaf	4.7
Eggs	4.4
Alcoholic beverages	4.2
Skim milk	3.4
Doughnuts, cookies, cake	2.9

Percent of total phosphorus

Recommended Intake

The average American takes in nearly twice as much phosphorus as calcium (see figure 11.3). Although the RDA for phosphorus is 800 mg/day, much more than this is consumed. For example, the average American female adult, ages 25–30 years, ingests 977 mg of phosphorus per day, well above the 564 mg/day of calcium that is consumed. American males of the same age take in 1,532 mg of phosphorus per day, nearly double their intake of calcium of 836 mg/day.

Phosphorus is found in many types of foods. Figure 11.6 illustrates that the top ten contributors of phosphorus in the American diet are primarily of dairy-product origin, with cereal products and meats also contributing (6). Notice that whole milk is by far the number-one source of phosphorus in the United States. Because one cup of whole milk contains two pats of butter, Americans would do well to substitute low-fat milk or other low-fat dairy products to decrease saturated fat intake. Other than dairy products, phosphorus is also found in seeds and nuts, fish, grain products, lean meats, and legumes. Vegetables and fruits do not contain high amounts of phosphorus.

Phosphorus-rich diets that are low in calcium have been associated with increased loss of calcium in the bones (10). In animals, a Ca/P ratio above two (twice as much calcium as phosphorus) helps to increase the absorption of calcium in the small intestine. This may help increase the calcium content of bones. Much more research on humans is needed to verify the optimal Ca/P ratio.

Some researchers are advising Americans to eat more foods that are high in calcium but low in phosphorus. Table 11.4 outlines the calcium to phosphorus ratio of some foods. Food is considered "good" if the ratio is above one and "poor" if the ratio is less than 0.50. U.S. females have an average Ca/P ratio of 0.58, and U.S. males of 0.55. These are much lower than they should be. Notice that leafy green vegetables steal the show. Are you including enough of these nutritious types of food in your diet?

Role in Body

Phosphorus teams up with calcium in forming bones and teeth. Most of the body's phosphorus, 85 percent, is in the skeleton (10). The remainder is contained in muscle, skin, nerves, and other organs. Phosphate is involved in the metabolism of carbohydrate, lipids, and protein, helps to regulate the acid-base balance in the body, and functions as a cofactor in many enzyme systems. Phosphorus also enters into all of the high-energy systems that possess very high-energy phosphate bonds. These bonds capture and then release vital energy in the cells of many tissues, especially those involved in muscle contractions.

About 60–70 percent of dietary phosphate is absorbed by the small intestine, being absorbed to a greater extent than is calcium.

Low Intake

The widespread distribution of phosphorus in the U.S. food supply makes phosphorus deficiency a very rare phenomenon. Different types of diseases can lead to phosphorus depletion, but these are also rare. Symptoms of phosphorus depletion include weakness, lack of appetite, general tiredness, and muscle pains.

High Intake

Phosphorus supplements are rarely used by Americans, so risk of unusually high intakes is low. Table 11.5 shows that the minimum toxic dose for phosphorus is the same as for calcium—12,000 mg, or ten times the U.S. RDA.

The chief concern is that Americans are consuming more phosphorus than calcium, as discussed previously. In general, if Americans would increase their consumption of fruits and vegetables and decrease intake of animal meat, a much more favorable balance between calcium and phosphorus intake would result (see table 11.4).

Magnesium

Magnesium is the most abundant ion in plant cells, the second most common ion in the oceans, the third most common on land, and the fourth most abundant metal in living organisms (15).

Recommended Intake

Both U.S. males and females consume less magnesium than recommended (14). Males and females 25–30 years of age average 288 and 187 mg per day, respectively, which is below the RDA of 350 and 280 mg per day. Table 11.6 shows that magnesium-rich foods include seeds and nuts, whole-grain cereals, dark green vegetables, legumes, and dried fruits—foods that Americans do not typically consume (see chapter 2). National surveys show that only 25 percent of Americans equal or exceed the RDA for magnesium.

Role in Body

The adult human body contains about 25 grams of magnesium. Sixty percent of this is in the skeleton, 20 percent is in the skeletal muscle, 19 percent is in other body cells, and only one percent is in different body fluids (15).

Magnesium is required for more than 300 different enzyme systems of the body and is therefore involved in many important activities. In particular, magnesium is indispensible in the formation and use of high-energy phosphate bonds (ATP). The use and storage of carbohydrate, fat, and protein in the body involves many reactions that are magnesium-dependent (2). It is also essential in nerve and muscle activity.

TABLE 11.6 Magnesium in one-cup portions of food	
Food	**One-Cup Portion (mg)**
Pumpkin seeds	738
Sunflower seeds	509
Almonds	385
Wheat germ	362
Cashews	356
Peanuts	273
Spinach, cooked	157
Swiss chard, cooked	150
Granola, homemade	141
Lima beans, cooked	126
Dried figs	118
Hot cereal, Roman Meal	109
Broccoli (cooked)	94
Whole-wheat bread	93
Acorn squash, baked	87
Blackeye peas (cooked)	85
Cereal, Grape Nuts	76
Prunes	73
Fish, bass, broiled	67
Cereal, Raisin Bran	64
Dates	63
Beets (cooked)	62
Cooked oatmeal	56
Raisins	48

The RDA for adult males and females is 350 mg/day and 280 mg/day, respectively.

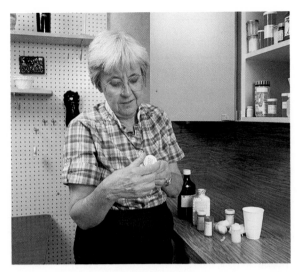

Some medications can cause side effects.

Some researchers have suggested that low magnesium intakes may contribute to heart disease and high blood pressure (17). Magnesium deficiency in animals does produce heart and blood vessel damage, and high blood pressure (see Health-Promotion Insight at the end of this chapter).

High Intake

There is no evidence that large intakes of magnesium are harmful to people with normal kidney function. Table 11.5 indicates that the minimum toxic dose is more than 15 times the U.S. RDA.

What if a person has poor kidney function, as do many of the elderly? There is concern that excessive blood-magnesium levels can develop in the elderly when given high amounts of laxatives (11). Many laxatives contain high amounts of magnesium. For example, just one-half tablespoon of milk of magnesia contains 1,000 mg of magnesium. Some elderly persons with poor kidney function who heavily rely on such laxatives can develop symptoms of magnesium "intoxication," which include slurring of speech, unsteadiness, lethargy, profuse sweating, abnormal heart rhythms and drowsiness.

Low Intake

Magnesium deficiency is very rare and is almost impossible to induce in humans through restricted diets. Even during prolonged fasting, magnesium levels in the blood stay normal (15). The human body has a remarkable capacity to conserve magnesium.

Magnesium deficiency can develop, however, during some disease states, including kidney diseases, hormonal imbalances, or intestinal disorders. During magnesium deficiency, people have many central nervous system symptoms, including confusion, depression, hallucinations, memory loss, and a decreased ability to concentrate (15). Other symptoms include numbness, cramps, muscular weakness, shaking, and muscle twitching.

TABLE 11.7
Sodium in one-cup portions of food

Food	One-Cup Portion (mg)	Food	One-Cup Portion (mg)
Soy sauce	16,464	Green pea soup (milk)	1,048
Salad dressing, blue cheese	2,672	Cereal, All Bran	961
Deviled ham, canned	2,560	Low-fat cottage cheese	918
Tomato catsup	2,496	Beef broth	782
Salad dressing, thousand island, low-cal	2,448	Macaroni and cheese	729
Margarine	2,434	Mozzarella cheese, skim milk	707
Barbecue sauce	2,032	Cheddar cheese	701
Parmesan cheese, grated	1,862	Whole-wheat bread	636
Ham, lean, roasted	1,858	Mashed potatoes	619
Butter	1,856	Crab, steamed	572
Salad dressing, thousand island	1,744	Tuna fish, canned in water	525
Tomato sauce	1,481	Tuna salad	434
Mayonnaise	1,254	Cereal, Total	409
Peanut butter	1,200	Cereal, Product 19	378
Corned beef hash, canned	1,188	Cereal, Rice Krispies	340
Pork and beans	1,180	Cereal, Frosted Flakes	284
Cream of mushroom soup (milk)	1,076	Buttermilk	257
		Yogurt, plain, low-fat	159

The estimated minimum requirement is 500 mg per day, with a recommendation not to exceed 2,400 mg.

The Electrolytes: Sodium, Potassium, and Chloride

Sodium is the major cation (positive ion) of fluids outside the body cells. Scientists call minerals like sodium, **chloride,** and **potassium** **"electrolytes"** because in water they can conduct electrical currents. Sodium and potassium ions carry positive charges, whereas chloride ions are negatively charged. Sodium chloride, or table salt, is 60 percent chloride and 40 percent sodium. One teaspoon of salt weighs 5 grams and contains 2 grams (or 2,000 mg) of sodium.

Recommended Intake
No RDA for the three electrolytes has been established, because all three are plentiful and widespread in the American diet. The Food and Nutrition Board has, however, established estimated minimum requirements for each. For sodium, chloride, and potassium, respectively, the amounts are 500, 750, and 2,000 mg.

Of concern is the sodium to potassium ratio (Na/K). For U.S. males, ages 25–30 years, the Na/K ratio equals 3,097 mg Na/2,889 mg K, or 1.07; for U.S. females, 2,016 mg Na/1,938 mg K, or 1.04 (4). In the Health-Promotion Activity at the end of this chapter, we will discuss that for prevention of high blood pressure, a Na/K ratio of 0.60 is recommended. In other words, Americans should consume 40 percent more potassium than sodium to help keep blood pressure levels normal. At present, Americans are actually consuming more sodium than potassium, which may partially explain the fact that nearly one out of three Americans has high blood pressure.

Table 11.7 compares the sodium content of one-cup portions of foods. Notice that fresh fruits, vegetables, and unsalted nuts are not on this list because of their very low sodium

Among Americans, concerns about the amount of salt in the
diet are greater than for other ingredients.

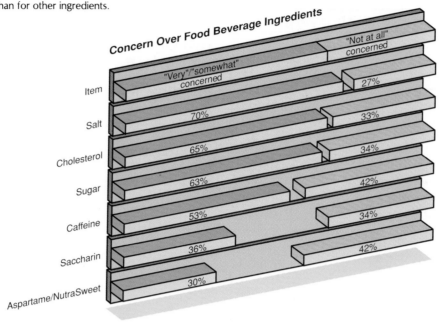

Concern Over Food Beverage Ingredients

"Very"/"somewhat" concerned | "Not at all" concerned

Item

Salt — 70% / 27%

Cholesterol — 65% / 33%

Sugar — 63% / 34%

Caffeine — 53% / 42%

Saccharin — 36% / 34%

Aspartame/NutraSweet — 30% / 42%

*T*ABLE 11.8

Low-Sodium, High-Potassium Foods	
Food Category	**Examples**
Fruits and Fruit Juices	Pineapple, grapefruit, pears, strawberries, watermelon, raisins, bananas, apricots, oranges
Low-Sodium Cereals	Oatmeal (unsalted), Roman Meal hot cereal, Shredded Wheat
Nuts (unsalted)	Hazel nuts, macadamia nuts, almonds, peanuts, cashews, coconut
Vegetables	Summer squash, zucchini, eggplant, cucumber, onions, lettuce, green beans, broccoli
Beans (dry, cooked)	Great North, lentils, lima beans, red kidney beans
High-Sodium, Low-Potassium Foods	
Food Category	**Examples**
Fats	Butter, margarine, salad dressings
Soups	Onion, mushroom, chicken noodle, tomato, split pea
Breakfast Cereals	Corn flakes, Product 19, Wheaties, Total, Nutri-Grain
Breads	Most varieties
Processed Meats	Most varieties
Cheeses	Most varieties

levels. Processed foods such as soy sauce, salad dressings, lunch meats, condiments, margarine and butter, sauces and soups, and cheese are all very high in sodium. Table 11.8 shows that low-sodium, high-potassium foods include fruits and fruit juices, low-sodium cereals, unsalted nuts, vegetables, and legumes.

Figure 11.7 shows the result of a recent national poll conducted by the Roper Organization (19). Asked which of six food items people were concerned about for health reasons, 70 percent indicated they were "very" or "somewhat" concerned about the amount of salt in their diet. Cholesterol, sugar, caffeine, saccharin, and aspartame/NutraSweet followed, in that order.

There is reason for concern, because sodium is hidden in many different types of foods and beverages. In fact, two-thirds of the sodium Americans ingest comes from commercial food products with sodium already added. Only one-third comes from salt or condiments added during cooking or eating. Table 11.9 shows that some brands of mineral water have more than 100 mg per cup. Even drinking water can supply

TABLE 11.9
Sodium in mineral water (values for 8 fl oz servings)

Very Low (0–5 mg)	Low (6–35 mg)	Medium (36–65 mg)	High (over 100 mg)
Bel-Air Mineral Water	S. Pellegrino	á Santé Mineral Water	Appolinaris Natural Mineral Water (135 mg)*
Black Mountain Spring Water	Crystal Geyser Sparkling Mineral Water	Calistoga Mineral Water	Calso (100–110 mg)
Canada Dry Seltzer		Canada Dry Club Soda	Vichy Saint-Yorre Royale Mineral Water (397 mg)*
Cragmont Club Soda Sodium Free		Cragmont Club Soda	
Forest Lake Natural Spring Water		Mendocino Mineral Water	
Lady Lee Sparkling Water		Napa Valley Springs Mineral Water	
Perrier		Saratoga Original Vichy Water*	
Poland Spring Sparkling Water		Schweppes Club Soda	
Saratoga Naturally Sparkling Mineral Water*			
Schweppes Seltzer			
Seagrams Seltzer			
White Rock Sparkling Mineral Water*			

Most of the sodium figures given are from the manufacturer's formulations. *Indicates values reprinted with permission from the New York Times Co., 1983. Additional sodium may be present depending on the water supply available to local bottlers.

Data from *HeartBriefs*, American Heart Association, Alameda County Chapter, Oakland, CA. © 1985. Used with permission.

more than you might expect. One out of four U.S. water supplies contains more than 50 mg of sodium per quart. Including water used in cooking and for beverages, more than 100 mg of sodium can end up coming from your water faucet (18). Many food additives also contain sodium (see chapter 4).

Coinciding with public concerns over excess sodium in food and beverages, a new Food and Drug Administration (FDA) policy requires that food manufacturers state the sodium content on food labels in milligrams per serving whenever nutrition labeling is required or provided voluntarily (see chapter 4 for a description of terms used).

Grain products contain nearly 25 percent of all sodium consumed by Americans. Figure 11.8 shows that white breads, rolls, and crackers are the number-one source of sodium,

being added by food manufacturers during preparation. Table 11.10 illustrates that large amounts of salt in cereal products is not necessary. Breakfast cereals such as Nabisco Shredded Wheat and Puffed Wheat contain less than 5 mg of sodium per serving. Others, like Bran Chex, Corn Chex, Product 19, and Wheaties contain more than 300 mg per serving.

Combination foods, like soups, gravies, entrees, and sauces, supply 20 percent of the sodium in the American diet. The meat group supplies 19 percent. Figure 11.8 shows that processed meats such as hot dogs, ham, and lunch meats are the second highest source of sodium. Many companies, however, have now provided lower-sodium versions of their products to meet the growing public demand for less sodium in its foods.

The dairy group accounts for 13 percent of all sodium consumed in the U.S. Although cheese doesn't always taste salty, many brands

FIGURE 11.8

Grain products are the number-one source of sodium in the American diet, followed by processed meats. Sodium is added to these products during processing.

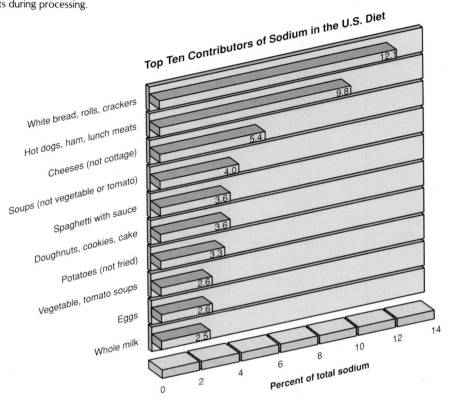

Top Ten Contributors of Sodium in the U.S. Diet

Food	Percent of total sodium
White bread, rolls, crackers	12.1
Hot dogs, ham, lunch meats	9.8
Cheeses (not cottage)	5.4
Soups (not vegetable or tomato)	4.0
Spaghetti with sauce	3.6
Doughnuts, cookies, cake	3.6
Potatoes (not fried)	3.3
Vegetable, tomato soups	2.6
Eggs	2.6
Whole milk	2.5

TABLE 11.10

Comparison of popular cereals

No-Sodium Breakfast Cereals		Comparatively High-Sodium Cereals	
The following cereals contain less than 5 mg sodium per serving.		*Ready-to-Eat Cereals*	*Sodium per serving (mg)*
Ready-to-Eat Cereals		Cheerios (General Mills)	250
Shredded Wheat (Nabisco)	Puffed Rice (Nabisco)	Wheaties (General Mills)	270
Puffed Wheat (Nabisco)	Raisin Squares (Kellogg's)	Kix (General Mills)	290
Hot Cereals		Rice Krispies (Kellogg's)	290
Corn Grits, regular or quick-cooking (Quaker Oats)	Farina (Pillsbury)	Corn Flakes (Kellogg's)	290
		Bran Chex (Ralston)	300
Cream of Wheat, regular or quick-cooking (Nabisco)	Oatmeal, regular or quick-cooking (Quaker Oats)	Corn Chex (Ralston)	310
		Product 19 (Kellogg's)	320
Cream of Rice (Nabisco)	Wheatena (Uhlmann)	*Hot Cereals*	
	Maypo (Uhlmann)	Cream of Wheat, instant, original flavor (Nabisco)	180
		Cream of Wheat, instant, various flavors (Nabisco)	180–240
		Oatmeal, instant, various flavors (Quaker Oats)	135–360
		Corn Grits, instant, regular flavor (Quaker Oats)	440
		Corn Grits, instant country bacon flavor (Quaker Oats)	590

TABLE 11.11
Guide to fat and sodium in cheese

SODIUM	FAT Low (less than 6 g/oz)	Medium (6–8 g/oz)	High (8–10 g/oz)
Low (less than 150 mg/oz)	Unsalted, dry-curd cottage cheese (½ cup) Part-skim mozzarella Part-skim ricotta (¼ cup)	Whole-milk mozzarella Neufchatel Swiss	Low-sodium cheddar Cream cheese Gruyere Whole-milk ricotta (¼ cup)
Medium (150–225 mg/oz)		Brie Tilsit	Brick Caraway Cheddar Chesire Colby Gjetost Monterey Jack Muenster Port-Salut
High (225–350 mg/oz)	Low-fat, processed cheese products Skim processed cheese	Camembert Edam Feta Gouda Limburger Provolone Romano Processed American cheese food	
Very high (350–550 mg/oz)	Low-fat or creamed cottage cheese (½ cup)	Parmesan (hard) Processed cheese spread Processed Swiss cheese Processed Swiss cheese food	Processed American cheese Blue Parmesan (grated) Roquefort

Data from HeartBriefs, American Heart Association, Alameda County Chapter, Oakland, CA. © 1980. Used with permission.

are quite high in sodium. Table 11.11 categorizes the different types of cheeses according to sodium and fat content. Part-skim mozzarella and ricotta are lower in both sodium and fat. Processed cheeses like American, Blue, Parmesan, and Roquefort have 350–500 mg of sodium per ounce and are also high in fat.

There are several choices one can make to reduce sodium intake, and they are summarized in Sidebar 11.1. In general, limiting foods known to be high in sodium, paying attention to food labels, reducing the amount of salt added during cooking or eating, and substituting low-sodium condiments for salt enable one to keep sodium intake at recommended levels. Also, emphasizing more fresh fruits and vegetables in the diet automatically cuts down the sodium intake while increasing potassium intake, thus improving the Na/K ratio.

Sidebar 11.2 outlines the many herb blends that can be used to enhance the flavors of food. Three blends are given as substitutes for salt. Americans love the taste of salt but may find that other tastes increase the enjoyment of eating. Herbs and spices can provide creative, tasteful alternatives to salt (20).

USDA Recommendations on How to Moderate Sodium Intake

What You Can Do

If you decide you want to moderate your sodium intake, there are choices you can make. If you want more details than this general listing provides, consult USDA's "The Sodium Content of Your Food."

First, When You Shop

- Read food labels. Labels that make specific claims such as "low in sodium" *must* show the sodium content on the label. Also, more and more manufacturers are voluntarily putting sodium information on labels. The amount of sodium is always stated in milligrams per serving and includes sodium in the raw ingredients as well as those added during processing.

    Even when the amount of sodium is not on the label, remember that the ingredients are listed according to their weight in the product's recipe — from most to least.

    Learn to recognize ingredients that contain sodium. Salt, soy sauce, salt brine, and any ingredient with sodium (such as monosodium glutamate) or soda (such as baking soda) as part of its name contain sodium.

- Finally, some companies don't list sodium information on their product labels, but do provide nutrition information to customers who write for it. Look for the firm's address on the label.

In the Kitchen

- Plan meals that contain less sodium.

    Consider the total amount of sodium in a meal, or in a day's meals. If you eat a high-sodium food, choose a low-sodium food to go with it.

    Take into consideration not only the sodium content of a food, but how much you will eat. Also consider the proportion of balance of calories and essential nutrients in the food.

    Remember that unprocessed foods usually contain less sodium than processed foods. When you start from scratch, you're in charge of the amount of salt you add.

- Reduce the salt you add to foods during cooking.

Start with moderate changes. That way you can cut back on your taste for salt gradually. You weren't born with a preference for salt, and it can be "unlearned."

Try gradually reducing the amount of salt in your favorite recipes until you've got it down to half or even less.

Look for recipes with a reduced sodium content.

Cut back or even cut out the salt used in cooking rice, noodles, pasta, or hot cereals.

Consider the sodium content of all the ingredients in a recipe. For instance, if you use cured meat, dehydrated or canned soup, cheese, or canned vegetables in a dish, you may not need to add any salt.

- Look for condiments and sauces with less sodium, or use lemon juice, spices, or herbs — such as onion or garlic powder (not onion or garlic salt), paprika, pepper, curry, or dill — for flavor. Make your own relishes and salad dressings, cutting back on the salt.

    Try adding new spices and herbs instead of salt to vegetables or the water you cook them in.

At the Table

- Taste food before you salt it. If you must add salt, try one shake instead of two.
- Watch the amount of prepared sauces or condiments you add.
- Try lemon juice, vinegar, or a homemade relish for zest.

At a Restaurant

- Choose foods without sauces. If you do prefer a sauce, ask for it "on the side" so you can control the amount.
- Ask to have your food served without added salt so you can add only as much as you want.
- Try to balance, as you do at home. If you have a high-sodium main dish, eat low-sodium side dishes with it; or if you eat a high-sodium dinner, eat a lower sodium breakfast and lunch.

From United States Department of Agriculture.

Herbs

Strengths of Herbs

Strong or Dominant Flavors: These should be used with care since their flavors stand out — approximately one teaspoon for six servings. They include bay, cardamon, curry, ginger, hot pepper, mustard, pepper (black), rosemary, and sage.

Medium Flavors: A moderate amount of these is recommended — one to two teaspoons for six servings. They are basil, celery seed and leaves, cumin, dill, fennel, French tarragon, garlic, marjoram, mint, oregano, savory (winter and summer), thyme, and turmeric.

Delicate Flavors: These may be used in large quantities and combine well with most other herbs and spices. This group includes burnet, chervil, chives, and parsley.

Herb Blends

Herbs can be combined for specific foods. Having the combinations on hand will speed cooking and enhance one's reputation as a gourmet. They can be added loose, or wrapped in cheesecloth and removed before serving. Following are some suggested herb blends:

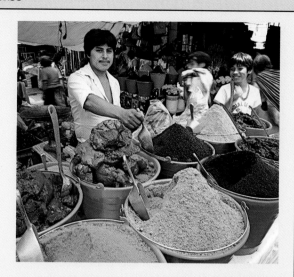

- Egg herbs: basil, dill weed (leaves), garlic, parsley.
- Fish herbs: basil, bay leaf (crumbled), French tarragon, lemon thyme, parsley (options: fennel, sage, savory).
- Poultry herbs: lovage, marjoram (two parts), sage (three parts).
- Salad herbs: basil, lovage, parsley, French tarragon.
- Tomato sauce herbs: basil (two parts), bay leaf, marjoram, oregano, parsley (options: celery leaves, cloves).
- Vegetable herbs: basil, parsley, savory.
- Italian blend: basil marjoram, oregano, rosemary, sage, savory, thyme.
- Barbecue blend: cumin, garlic, hot pepper, oregano.
- French herbal combinations: Fines herbes: parsley, chervil, chives, French tarragon (sometimes adding a small amount of basil, fennel, oregano, sage, or saffron).
- Bouquet garni mixtures: bay, parsley (two parts), thyme. The herbs may be wrapped in cheesecloth or the parsley wrapped around the thyme and bay leaf.
- Basic herb butter: one stick unsalted butter, one to three tablespoons dried herbs or two to six tablespoons fresh herbs, ½ teaspoon lemon juice, and white pepper. Combine ingredients and mix until fluffy. Pack in covered container and let set at least one hour. Any of the culinary herbs and spices may be used.

- Herb vinegars: Heat vinegar in an enamel pan and pour it into a vinegar bottle and add one or several culinary herbs (to taste). Do not let the vinegar boil. Let the mixture set for two weeks before using. Any type of vinegar may be used, depending on personal preference.

Herb Blends to Replace Salt

These can be placed in shakers and used instead of salt.

- Saltless surprise: 2 teaspoons garlic powder and 1 teaspoon each of basil, oregano, and powdered lemon rind (or dehydrated lemon juice). Put ingredients into a blender and mix well. Store in glass container, label well, and add rice to prevent caking.
- Pungent salt substitute: 3 teaspoons basil, 2 teaspoons each of savory (summer savory is best), celery seed, ground cumin seed, sage and marjoram, and 1 teaspoon lemon thyme. Mix well, then powder with a mortar and pestle.
- Spicy saltless seasoning: 1 teaspoon each of cloves, pepper, and coriander seed (crushed), 2 teaspoons paprika, and 1 tablespoon rosemary. Mix ingredients in a blender. Store in airtight container.

What Goes with What

- Soups: bay, chervil, French tarragon, marjoram, parsley, savory, rosemary.
- Poultry: garlic, oregano, rosemary, savory, sage.
- Beef: bay, chives, cloves, cumin, garlic, hot pepper, marjoram, rosemary, savory.
- Lamb: garlic, marjoram, oregano, rosemary, thyme (make little slits in lamb to be roasted and insert herbs).

continued

- Pork: coriander, cumin, garlic, ginger, hot pepper, pepper sage, savory, thyme.
- Cheese: basil, chervil, chives, curry, dill, fennel, garlic chives, marjoram, oregano, parsley, sage, thyme.
- Fish: chervil, dill, fennel, French tarragon, garlic, parsley, thyme.
- Fruit: anise, cinnamon, coriander, cloves, ginger, lemon verbena, mint, rose geranium, sweet cicely.

- Bread: caraway, marjoram, oregano, poppy seed, rosemary, thyme.
- Vegetables: basil, burnet, chervil, chives, dill, French tarragon, marjoram, mint, parsley, pepper, thyme.
- Salads: basil, borage, burnet, chives, French tarragon, garlic chives, parsley, rocket-salad, sorrel. (These are best used fresh or added to salad dressing. Otherwise, use herb vinegars for extra flavor.)

From H. H. Shimizu, "Herbs," *FDA Consumer* (April 1984): pp. 18–19.

*T*ABLE 11.12
Recommended seasonings

Salt Substitutes (no sodium, mainly KCl)*
   No-Salt (Norcliff Thayer, Inc.)
   Nu-Salt (Sweet 'n Low)
   Morton Salt Substitute
   Adolph Salt Substitute
   Featherweight "K" Salt Substitute

Seasoning Blends (no sodium, no KCl)
   Mrs. Dash
   Mrs. Dash-Low Pepper-No Garlic
   Slim Fixins
   Lawry's Pinch of Herbs
   Herbit-Herbal Seasoning
   New Vegit (Gayelord Hauser)
   Nature's Gourmet
   The "Blended Spices Salt-Free" Series: Italian, Oriental, French, Mexican, Curry

Salt Substitute (KCl) Seasoning Blends
   Lawry's Seasoned Salt-Free
   Instead of Salt
   Featherweight Seasoned Salt Substitute
   Morton Seasoned Salt Substitute

Other Seasonings with a Decreased Amount of Sodium
   Morton's Lite Salt (½ regular salt, ½ KCl)
   McCormick/Schillings Lite Seasoning Salt: Chicken, Onion, Garlic, Lemon Pepper, Season All—75% Less Salt

WATCH OUT for these!
Seasoning with a Fairly High Amount of Sodium
   Spike (Gayelord Hauser)
   Spike Dee-licious (Gayelord Hauser)
   Hain Vegetable Seasoned Salt
   Schilling Salad Supreme
   Schilling Salad Toppings
   Schilling Season All—Seasoned Salt
   Schilling Barbecue Spice
   Lawry's Seasoned Salt
   Cavender's All Purpose Greek Seasoning
   Vege-Sal (Gayelord Hauser)
   Jane's Krazy Mixed Up Salt
   Knorr Swiss Aromat All-Purpose Seasoning
   Konriko Creole Seasoning
   Morton's Nature's Seasoning
   Lawry's Lemon Pepper Seasoning
   Garlic Salt
   Onion Salt

*KCl=potassium chloride

In using salt substitutes or alternate seasonings, one needs to be careful that sodium levels are truly reduced. Table 11.12 categorizes seasonings according to their salt content. Notice that salt substitutes such as No-Salt or Nu-Salt use potassium chloride (KCl) instead of sodium chloride. The tastes of KCl and NaCl are very similar.

Chloride usually occurs in the diet as sodium chloride or salt. For this reason, an intake of chloride can be considered adequate as long as the sodium intake is in the recommended range.

Role in Body

Sodium and chloride ions tend to concentrate outside of body cell walls **(extracellular)**, whereas potassium tends to concentrate inside of body cell walls **(intracellular).** This arrangement is essential in maintaining the balance of tissue fluids inside and outside of cells, and it works like a tiny battery, with just enough electrical potential or difference to allow the movement of nutrients and waste products in and out of the cell.

Chloride also helps form **hydrochloric acid** from the stomach lining, which is required to help gastric juices digest protein and assists the blood in carrying large amounts of carbon dioxide to the lungs (3). Sodium, potassium, and chloride work with bicarbonate in regulating the acid-base balance of the body. Sodium has an important role in regulating normal muscle tone. Potassium helps influence both skeletal and heart muscle activity.

The kidney is the primary organ that controls sodium, chloride, and potassium levels in the body. Excess sodium, chloride, or potassium are readily excreted by the kidney and the skin (salty sweat) when extra amounts enter the body. This process appears to be under hormonal control. Some people are thought to retain electrolytes more easily than others, however, possibly contributing to high blood pressure (see Health-Promotion Insight at the end of this chapter).

Low Intake

The electrolytes are under precise regulation by the body. In rare instances, body electrolyte levels can fall, resulting in life-threatening complications. Prolonged fasting, cancer, liver disease, chronic infection, surgery, extensive trauma, excessive diarrhea or vomiting, kidney disease, or certain drugs may lower electrolyte levels. It is highly unusual for dietary electrolyte restriction to cause a drop in blood electrolyte levels.

High Intake

As discussed in this section, Americans tend to have a high diet Na/K ratio, which may be an important factor in high blood pressure in susceptible individuals. This is discussed in detail in the Health-Promotion Insight.

In certain disease states or medical situations, electrolyte levels can rise to very high levels in the body.

Minor Minerals

Iron

Iron was considered to be of heavenly origin in ancient Eastern Mediterranean civilizations. The "metal of heaven" was used in Egypt and Babylon for medical purposes (21). Although the total amount of iron in the human body is small (4–5 grams), it is one of the most important elements in nutrition and good health.

Recommended Intake/Low Intake

United States male adults consume 15.9 mg of iron per day and female adults only 10.0 mg/day (4), in comparison to the RDA of 10 mg and 15 mg/day, respectively. As figure 11.1 shows, U.S. women on the average are thus ingesting 30 percent less iron than is recommended.

TABLE 11.13
Iron in one-cup portions of food

Food	Iron per Cup of Food (mg)
Molasses (blackstrap)	51.2
Brewer's yeast (dry)	22.4
Sesame seeds	21
Cereal, Total	21
Cereal, Product 19	21
Pumpkin seeds	20.7
C. W. Post/Raisins cereal	16.4
Wheat germ	10.3
Sunflower seeds	9.8
Cashews	8.2
Wheat Chex cereal	7.3
Spinach	6.4
Dried apricots	6.1
Jerusalem artichokes (raw)	5.1
Navy beans, cooked	5.1
Mixed nuts, roasted	5.1
Grape Nuts	4.9
Great north beans (cooked)	4.9
Soybeans (cooked)	4.9
Almonds	4.8
Brazil nuts	4.8
Peanuts	4.7
Red kidney beans (cooked)	4.6
Lentils (cooked)	4.2
Prunes	4.0
Swiss chard	4.0
Dried pears	3.8
Blackeye cowpeas (cooked)	3.6
Lima beans (cooked)	3.5
Whole-wheat bread	3.4
Raisins	3.0
Fish, bass, broiled	2.9
Turkey	2.5
Ham, extra lean	2.1
Lobster	1.9
Tuna	1.5

The RDA for males is 10 mg/day, for females, 15 mg/day.

Table 11.13 shows that while lean meats, fish, and seafood are good sources of iron, many plant foods such as molasses, fortified breakfast cereals, seeds and nuts, dried fruits, and legumes are also high in iron. Figure 11.9 reveals that enriched grain products are the number-one source of iron in the U.S. diet, with various meat products also ranking high.

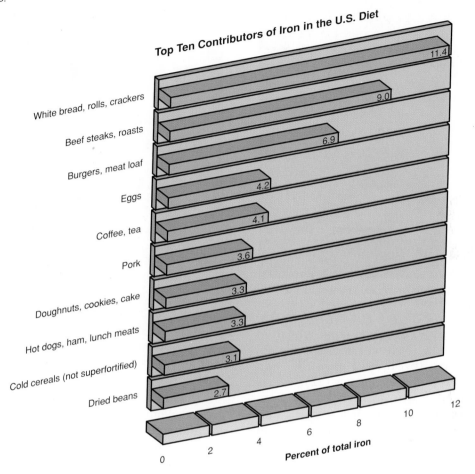

*F*IGURE 11.9

Most grain products in the U.S. are made with iron-enriched flour. This fact, plus the large use of grain products by Americans, makes grain products the number-one source of iron in the U.S.

Top Ten Contributors of Iron in the U.S. Diet

Food	Percent of total iron
White bread, rolls, crackers	11.4
Beef steaks, roasts	9.0
Burgers, meat loaf	6.9
Eggs	4.2
Coffee, tea	4.1
Pork	3.6
Doughnuts, cookies, cake	3.3
Hot dogs, ham, lunch meats	3.3
Cold cereals (not superfortified)	3.1
Dried beans	2.7

Percent of total iron: 0 2 4 6 8 10 12

The absorption of iron is a complex process that depends on many factors. In general, only about 10 percent of all dietary iron is absorbed through the small intestine into the blood (22). The rest passes out of the body with the feces. When an individual is iron-deficient, the body attempts to adjust by doubling or tripling the amount of iron absorbed.

The average loss of iron in the healthy adult man is approximately 1 mg/day. With women, there is an additional 0.5 mg/day average loss due to menstrual blood flow. This average loss of 1 to 1.5 mg/day for adults is balanced when 10 percent of dietary iron is absorbed. Pregnancy, lactation, and rapid growth increase iron requirements (see chapters 13 and 14).

Forty percent of the iron in animal products is called **"heme" iron.** The remaining 60 percent of the iron in animal products and all the iron in vegetable products is called **"non-heme" iron.** Heme iron is more easily absorbed by the body. Absorption of nonheme iron can be improved by including foods with vitamin C at mealtime, or by consuming some meat (22). Some foods and substances such as bran, nuts, soy protein, tannic acid in tea, and antacids can decrease absorption of nonheme iron.

In the U.S., iron intake is frequently inadequate during the following four periods in life: (1) from six months to four years of age (because of the low-iron content of milk and

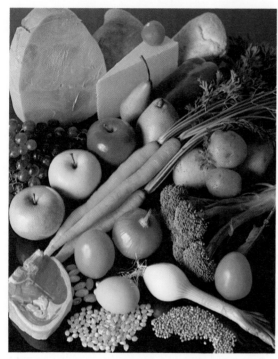
Meats, dairy products, fruits, grains, and vegetables are a source of vitamins and iron.

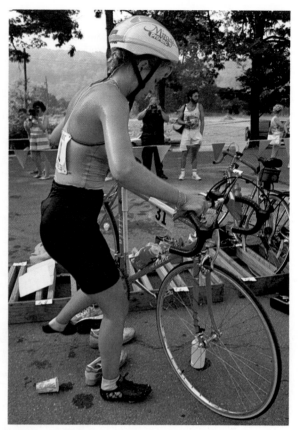
Highly trained female athletes tend to be at higher risk for iron deficiency.

rapid growth rate); (2) during rapid growth in early adolescence; (3) from puberty to menopause in women (because of menstrual iron losses); and (4) during pregnancy (22).

There are two basic types of iron-deficiency states. Mild iron deficiency or iron depletion is characterized by low iron stores in the body. Severe iron deficiency, or **anemia,** is characterized by low blood levels of **hemoglobin** (a protein molecule in red blood cells that contains iron). An extended deficiency of dietary iron will gradually deplete the body's iron stores in the bone marrow and liver. This first stage is known as iron depletion. Eventually anemia results because hemoglobin cannot be formed in adequate amounts (23). Anemia is diagnosed when hemoglobin levels in the blood fall below 13 g/dL for men, and below 12 g/dL in women.

Iron deficiency is the single most common nutritional deficiency in the world today, with more than 500 million people suffering from this problem (24). A total of 1–3.5 percent of U.S. males are iron-deficient, as are 3.4–5.4 percent of U.S. females. The percentage of Americans who are actually anemic is very small. Recent information shows that anemia is declining among low-income children in the U.S., a group that is at high risk for iron-defi-

ciency anemia (25). The prevalence of anemia in children between the ages of six months and five years has declined from eight percent in 1975 to three percent in 1985. It appears that this decrease is due to improvements in childhood iron nutrition.

Highly trained athletes appear to be at higher risk for iron deficiency than nonathletes (23). Various researchers have reported that runners may lose more than the normal amount of iron through their sweat or in their feces. Some female athletes have been found to have low dietary intakes of iron. Endurance athletes are urged to have their body iron stores evaluated periodically, and to consume iron-rich foods. In some cases, physicians may prescribe an iron supplement. When hemoglobin levels fall below normal, the ability to run, swim, cycle, or play sports decreases.

When a child is iron-deficient, the symptoms include fatigue, depressed growth, and decreased resistance to infection (21). Adults can become listless and tired and develop mouth sores.

Role in Body

Iron is an important component of hemoglobin, **myoglobin** (a muscle protein molecule that contains iron), and a number of enzymes (3). Hemoglobin is a special compound in red blood cells that carries oxygen to the body tissues. Myoglobin carries oxygen from the blood to the muscle cell. When oxygen is connected to hemoglobin, the blood is bright red.

Of the total amount of iron in the body, 70 percent is in hemoglobin, myoglobin, and enzymes. Thirty percent is stored in the body, primarily in the bone marrow, liver, and spleen. It is in the bone marrow that red blood cells are made.

High Intake

The minimum toxic dose of iron is approximately 100 mg, or 5.5 times the U.S. RDA (see table 11.5). There are approximately two thousand cases of iron poisoning each year in the United States, mainly in young children who ingest the iron supplements of their parents (22).

When iron intake is high from use of iron supplements, the absorption of zinc in the small intestine is reduced (26). Because zinc is important for tissue growth, iron supplements should be used only on the advice of a physician. Emphasizing high-iron foods in the diet is a much better practice than using iron supplements (see table 11.13).

Zinc

Early in this century, researchers discovered that the mineral **zinc** was important for normal growth in animals (21). Zinc deficiency in humans was first established during the 1960s, when adult patients in Iran who looked like ten-year-old boys were examined. Even though the patients were more than 20 years of age, they had the height and sexual organs of children. They were found to be consuming primarily unleavened bread made with coarse, whole-wheat flour. In addition, most of them were eating up to one pound of clay every day! This habit is called **geophagia** and is not uncommon in some rural Iranian villages. Researchers later speculated that because of the low zinc levels of their diets, subjects were ingesting the clay to obtain more zinc. When the subjects were treated with zinc for a few months, most of them grew rapidly and matured sexually.

Recommended Intake

In 1974, the Food and Nutrition Board established recommended dietary allowances for zinc for the first time. Metabolic studies indicated that 10 to 15 mg of zinc was adequate to maintain a positive balance of zinc in the body. The RDA for adult men and women is 15 mg/day and 12 mg/day, respectively. Presently, U.S. males 25–30 years of age average 16.2 mg of zinc per day, whereas women average only 9.6 mg per day (80 percent of the RDA) (see figure 11.1) (4). The Canadian RDA for zinc is 9 mg/day, a level that the majority of people are able to attain.

Table 11.14 shows that seeds and nuts, legumes, whole-grain cereals, dairy products, and lean meats are important sources of zinc. Zinc from whole-grain products may be harder for the body to absorb due to the presence of phytate, a chemical that can bind zinc (21).

Role in Body

Zinc plays an incredibly versatile and vital role in multiple functions of the body. The human body contains about 2 grams of zinc, found in all human tissues and fluids. Bone holds 50 percent of this zinc, with 30 percent found in the soft tissues and fluids, and 20 percent in the skin, hair, and nails. The retina of the eye and the male sex organs (prostate and gonads) contain about three times as much zinc as other soft tissues (11).

Zinc is a part of more than 70 major enzyme systems of the body. Zinc is important for synthesis of key tissue proteins and for the synthesis and repair of the basic genetic controllers of life, the nucleic acids DNA and RNA. These control growth, sexual maturation, wound healing, and the maintenance of skin, hair, nails, and the mucous membranes of the mouth, throat, stomach, and intestines.

Low Intake

The body pool of available zinc is rather small, and it has a rapid turnover. This means that if the diet is deficient in zinc, deficiency symptoms appear rapidly. The most prominent symptoms of zinc deficiency include loss of appetite, failure to grow, skin changes, impairment of wound healing and the immune system, delayed bone growth, behavioral problems, and decreased

Table 11.14
Zinc in one-cup portions of food

Food	Zinc Per Cup of Food (mg)
Wheat germ	18.8
Sesame seeds	11.2
Cereal, All Bran	11.2
Pumpkin seeds	10.3
Peanuts	9.6
Cashews	7.7
Peanut butter	7.5
Sunflower seeds	7.3
Brazil nuts	6.4
Cereal, Nutri-Grain	5.8
Mixed nuts, roasted	5.2
Peanuts, roasted	4.8
Turkey	4.3
Mozzarella, skim milk	4.2
Ham, lean, roasted	4.0
Soybean kernels, roasted	3.9
Almonds	3.8
Ricotta cheese, skim	3.3
Walnuts	2.7
Grape Nuts	2.5
Blackeye cowpeas (cooked)	2.4
Lentils (cooked)	2.0
Yogurt, plain, low-fat	2.0
Red kidney beans (cooked)	1.9
Great north beans (cooked)	1.8
Roman Meal cereal (cooked)	1.8
Coconut	1.7
Green peas (cooked)	1.5
Wheat Chex cereal	1.2
Rolled wheat cereal (cooked)	1.1
Oatmeal (rolled oats, cooked)	1.1

The RDA for males is 15 mg/day, and for females is 12 mg/day.

growth. When the children increased their zinc intake, they showed improved appetites and weight gain. Later, the same team of researchers tested children with poor growth rates from low-income families and found that two-thirds of them had lower-than-optimal zinc levels in their blood and hair (28).

Because of these studies, interest in zinc among the public has grown tremendously. People have been urged to send in their hair samples for analysis, to take zinc to restore or improve fertility, or to megadose with zinc to decrease acne. Advertisements which urge you to send a sample of your hair for zinc analysis should be ignored (11). Most experts agree that analysis of hair for determination of optimal body stores of important vitamins or minerals is close to worthless (29,30). Hair mineral content can be affected by many factors, including the type of shampoo used, the season of the year, the place on the body where the hair is obtained, and the age and sex of the person (29). The state of health of the body may be entirely unrelated to the chemical condition of the hair. Finally, insufficient research has been conducted to establish norms that indicate what concentration of minerals in the hair is optimal.

There is also no evidence that zinc supplementation will improve sexual function or clear up acne (11). It is a misconception that if a body organ is high in a certain nutrient, then excess intake of that nutrient will result in "super" function. Just because the prostate gland is high in zinc doesn't mean that zinc supplements will make the prostate function better. If this were true, then excess dietary cholesterol intake should improve brain function, because the brain is very high in cholesterol! When the body has sufficient zinc coming in from the diet, supplements will not produce miraculous results.

High Intake
A wide margin of safety exists between normal intakes of zinc from foods and the zinc intake likely to produce toxic effects in humans. The minimum toxic dose is 500 mg, or 33 times the RDA (14).

High doses, however, can be harmful. Zinc supplements can decrease the amount of high density lipoprotein circulating in the blood, increasing risk of heart disease (31). Excess zinc interacts with other minerals, such as copper and

ability to taste food flavors (3,27). Other deficiency symptoms include a weakening of the ability of the white blood cells to fight infection, diarrhea, loss of hair, and night blindness. Zinc deficiency in pregnant animals results in fetuses born with birth defects.

Mild zinc deficiency has been observed in U.S. children. In one survey of 150 apparently healthy children in Denver, 8 percent displayed deficiency symptoms, which included low levels of zinc in the hair, impaired ability to taste food flavors, poor appetite, and less-than-optimal iron, decreasing their absorption. In animals, zinc supplements decrease the absorption of iron so much that anemia is produced (32). When patients are given 150 mg of zinc per day, copper deficiency results. Intakes of zinc only 3.5 mg/day above the RDA decrease copper absorption (33). In animals, copper deficiency causes scarring of the heart muscle tissue and low levels of calcium in the bone (31). Excess zinc also decreases the functioning of the immune system.

One needs to be very careful about using heavy supplements of minerals. In the small intestine, minerals interact with one another, affecting the ability of some to be absorbed (26). There are many other examples in addition to those noted above. For example, excess calcium depresses the absorption of magnesium, iron, and zinc. Even vitamin supplements can interfere with mineral absorption. Folate supplements, for example, decrease absorption of zinc, increasing the amount of zinc lost in the stool (34). The best nutrition policy is to consume foods rich in nutrients and to avoid concentrated doses from supplemental pills unless their use is ordered by a physician.

Iodine

The ancient Greeks used burnt sponges (which are rich in **iodine**) in the treatment of human **goiter.** This knowledge helped the French physician Coindet to use iodine salts for the treatment of goiter. But it was not until the first quarter of this century that researchers in several countries were able to establish that goiters were due to deficiency of iodine in the food and water supplies of the affected regions of the world (21).

Recommended Intake

The RDA of iodine for adults is 0.15 mg/day. American males and females average 0.52 and 0.27 mg/day, respectively, well above the RDA (see figure 11.1).

Seafood is the only reliable food source of iodine, because ocean water contains consistent amounts of this mineral. In many sections of the world, including parts of the U.S. formerly known as "goiter belts," the amount of iodine in the water and earth is too low. Thus, the iodine content of dairy products and eggs depends on the composition of the animal feed, which depends on the region of the country where it was grown (3).

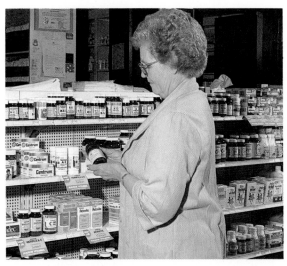

The best nutrition policy is to consume foods rich in nutrients and to avoid concentrated doses from supplemental pills unless their use is ordered by a physician.

Because of this problem, the U.S. federal government has encouraged the use of iodized table salt since 1924. One teaspoon of iodized salt provides 0.26 mg of iodine, nearly double the RDA. The Food and Nutrition Board has recommended that in all noncoastal regions of the U.S., iodized salt be used (3). In the coastal regions the need is less because of the higher amounts of iodine in the environment. Dietary iodine is also used as a supplement in some bread-dough conditioners.

Role in Body

The body of a healthy adult contains a total of 10–20 mg of iodine. Approximately three-fourths of this is concentrated in the thyroid gland. Iodine is an important component of thyroid hormones. Iodine deficiency decreases production of thyroid hormones, resulting in weight gain, lack of energy, low blood pressure, slow resting heart rate, and decreased muscle strength.

Low Intake

Iodine is obtained from food and water. Because some soils have little or no iodine, plant foods grown in these soils are low or lacking in iodine. Before the modern era when iodine was supplemented in table salt and other products, some people living in iodine-deficient areas developed simple goiter. Simple goiter is defined as an enlargement of the thyroid gland (10). The thyroid gland, which is located in the front of the neck, can grow as large as a person's head in severe cases.

High Intake

The Food and Nutrition Board warned in 1980 that although present iodine intake in the U.S. can be considered safe, any additional increases should be viewed with concern (3). The minimum toxic dose is 2 mg, or 13 times the RDA (14). In recent years, kelp (dried seaweed) has been promoted as an aid to dieting. Large amounts of kelp taken for long periods of time can cause thyroid problems, as has been described in the northern island of Japan and in China (10).

Fluoride

As early as 1901, the beneficial effect of **fluoride** on the incidence of dental caries was recognized. One researcher noted that dental caries (tooth decay) in children with brown stains on their tooth enamels were relatively rare (21). Later the mineral fluoride was identified as the substance causing both the mottling and the prevention of dental caries.

Recommended Intake/Role in Body

Fluoride is present in nearly all soils, water supplies, plants, and animals. However, the concentration of fluoride varies considerably. During the 1930s, various researchers reported that when the natural fluoride content of water was about 1 mg per liter, dental caries were reduced 50–60 percent if this water was consumed regularly before children grew permanent teeth (35). This level of fluoride did not cause brown stains to form on the teeth. As a result of this research, many communities during the 1940s adjusted the fluoride content of their water supplies to equal 1 mg per liter. Because some communities had to add fluoride to the water supply to reach this level, a vigorous public outcry resulted.

Dental caries are reduced 50–60 percent for the lifetime of the teeth if fluoride in water at a concentration of 1 mg per liter regularly washes over the teeth (35). If fluoride is withdrawn, dental caries increase.

Among people living for a lifetime in areas where the flouride content of the water is 3.5 mg per liter or higher, women experience reduced fractures of the spine. In other words, fluoride may also increase the hardness of bones (35).

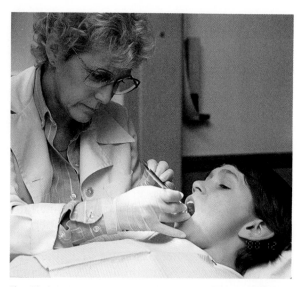

Fluoride in water at a concentration of one milligram per liter helps reduce dental caries.

The Food and Nutrition Board (3) in 1980 estimated that the safe and adequate intake for adults is 1.5–4.0 mg per day, a range easily obtained in communities whose water supplies contain 1 mg per liter. Table 11.15 shows that brewed tea, seafood, some fruits and vegetables, honey, wheat germ, and dairy products contain good amounts of fluoride. Drinking water, however, is the most reliable and consistent source for this mineral.

Fluoridation of the water supply is a popular target among quacks and food faddists. Opponents claim that fluoridation increases the risk of cancer, heart disease, Down's Syndrome (mongoloid births), birth defects, allergic responses, kidney disease, and warts (35). Thousands of scientific studies have shown all of these claims to be false. Fluoridation of the water supply has been found to be safe, effective, and beneficial.

High Intake

In areas with highly fluoridated water (both natural or added), severe mottling of the tooth enamel can appear (21). Mottled teeth are characterized by chalky white patches with yellow and brown staining. The enamel becomes weak, and in severe cases the enamel can become pitted.

Acute toxic doses are about 2.5–5 grams if consumed at one time.

TABLE 11.15
Fluoride in one-cup portions of food

Food	One-Cup Portion of Food (mg)
Tea, brewed	7.70
Fish, mackerel (canned)	2.52
Baked potato with skin	0.48
Honey	0.34
Crab, steamed	0.31
Wheat germ	0.28
Ricotta cheese, skim milk	0.22
Kale, cooked	0.21
Cottage cheese, low-fat	0.20
Mozzarella, skim milk	0.13
Almonds	0.12
Onions	0.10
Cheddar cheese	0.10
Grapefruit	0.07
Apples	0.07
Low-fat milk	0.07
Corn, cooked	0.06
Carrots	0.04

The RDA is 1.5–4.0 mg/day.

TABLE 11.16
Copper in one-cup portions of food

Food	One-Cup Portion of Food (mg)
Sesame seeds	5.88
Cashews	3.04
Oysters	2.88
Sunflower seeds	2.52
Peanuts, roasted	1.85
Crabmeat	1.71
Walnuts	1.28
Almonds	1.22
Cereal, All Bran	0.98
Tuna fish	0.93
Wheat germ	0.70
Prunes	0.69
Kidney beans	0.56
Dried apricots	0.56
Lentils, cooked	0.54
Sweet potato, cooked	0.53
Dates	0.51
Whole milk	0.50
Raisins	0.45
Cereal, C. W. Post, Raisins	0.40
Grape Nuts	0.38
Whole-wheat bread	0.34
Cooked cereal, Roman Meal	0.32

The estimated safe and adequate daily dietary intake is 1.5 to 3.0 mg.

Copper

In 1928, researchers discovered that **copper,** in addition to iron, was necessary for blood formation in animals (21). Only recently have researchers shown that it is required for humans.

Recommended Intake
Copper intake by American adults is low (4). U.S. males and females average 1.24 and 0.93 mg of copper per day, respectively, less than the estimated safe and adequate daily dietary intake of 1.5–3.0 mg. New research is showing that 1.3 mg per day is sufficient and that the safe and adequate daily range for copper may be too high (36). Table 11.16 shows that seeds and nuts, seafood, dried fruits, legumes, and whole-grain cereals are good sources of copper.

Role in Body
Copper is part of several important enzymes that are needed for proper utilization of iron and for the manufacture of hemoglobin and red blood cells in the bone marrow. The integrity of connective tissue, bones, nerves, the cardiovascular system, the immune system, and the blood-clotting system are all in part dependent on copper (36). A total of 100–150 mg of copper is found in adults. The liver, kidney, heart, hair, and brain contain the highest concentrations of copper (10).

Low Intake
Because copper is widely distributed in foods, copper deficiency in humans is very rare. In animals, copper-restricted diets lead to a decreased iron absorption from the small intestine, a reduction in red blood cells, defects in normal development of the bone, central nervous system, and connective tissue, abnormal hair texture and quality, and heart disease.

Excessive zinc, iron, molybdenum, or vitamin C supplements can reduce the absorption of copper (36,37). As discussed previously, in animals, zinc supplements can decrease copper absorption, leading to anemia and heart disease (36). Vitamin C supplements of 500 mg with each meal have been found to decrease copper status in young men (37). Whenever mega-doses of vitamins or minerals are taken, there are multiple interactions with other nutrients.

High Intake

The minimum toxic dose for copper is 100 mg, or 33 times the recommended range. Toxicity from dietary copper is rare and in humans is called **Wilson's disease,** a hereditary disorder in which copper accumulates in body tissues.

Selenium

Recent reports from the Chinese Academy of Medical Sciences have helped to affirm that **selenium** is essential for human life and health. Some children living in a wide area across China developed a fatal disease of the heart muscle. This disease, coined **Keshan disease** was reduced 80 percent by giving selenium to the children. Children with Keshan disease had racing heart rates, large hearts, abnormal heart electrical patterns, and low blood-selenium levels.

Recommended Intake

The recommended adult dietary intake for selenium is 70 μg for men and 55 μg for women. U.S. male and female adults consume 100 and 60 μg per day, respectively.

Table 11.17 shows that seafood, nuts, dairy products, and whole-wheat products contain good amounts of selenium.

Role in Body

The highest concentrations of selenium are found in the liver, kidney, heart, and spleen. Selenium is part of an important red blood cell enzyme that helps to destroy chemicals that damage cell membranes. For this reason, some researchers have shown that selenium may play a role in preventing cancer.

In the northeastern U.S., high rates of cancer have been associated with low selenium levels in the soil (38). Cancer patients have been found to have low selenium levels in their blood. More study is needed to better understand this association between selenium and cancer.

TABLE 11.17
Selenium in one-cup portions of food

Food	One-Cup Portion of Food (μg)
Tuna fish	180
Oysters	160
Brazil nuts	140
Cashew nuts	90
Brown rice	80
Pork, roasted	70
Cereal, whole wheat	60
Peanuts, roasted	60
Cottage cheese, low-fat	50
Chicken, roasted	40
Fish, sole/flounder, baked	40
Whole-wheat flour	40
Cereal, Grape Nuts	30
Macaroni, cooked	30
Mozzarella, skim milk	20
Walnuts	10
Cheddar cheese	10
Milk, low-fat	10

The RDA for males is 70 μg/day, and for females is 55 μg/day.

Low Intake

The selenium content of plants such as grains is determined by the selenium content of the soil (39). In certain parts of the world, such as New Zealand, selenium intake is very low because of the low amount of selenium in the soil. In the U.S., some areas have low selenium in the soil, but because the U.S. has a system whereby foods are transported over the entire nation, any local deficiencies are usually compensated for when people eat foods from other areas.

As previously mentioned, in certain parts of the world where selenium is low in the soil and foods from other areas are not transported in, a sickness called Keshan disease can occur (39). Selenium deficiency appears to be a major factor in this disease, which may also have a viral component. Kaschin-Beck disease is another disease occurring in eastern Asia that is related to selenium deficiency. Children develop joint stiffness at first, and then the disease progresses to growth retardation and severe joint problems.

Can Plants Grown on Mineral-Deficient Soils Be Low in Minerals?

Many food faddists claim that because mineral levels in American farmlands are low or out of balance, supplements are needed. There is no evidence that this is true. In fact, nutrient levels in the American food supply are now higher than ever before! (see chapter 2). And because of our nationwide distribution of food, our wonderful system of storing the foods under optimal conditions, and the wide variety of foodstuffs now available, the potential for consuming enough vitamins and minerals has never been better.

If soil lacks a mineral, then the plant limits its growth. For example, a plant may not produce as many tomatoes when the soil is weak in nutrients, but the tomatoes it does produce will have the essential nutrients they need. If the nutrients are not there, then the plant cannot grow.

Two minerals can be low in the soil, however, and not affect plant growth. These are iodine and selenium, as we have discussed previously. The plants can still grow fine with or without them. However, other minerals do not act this way.

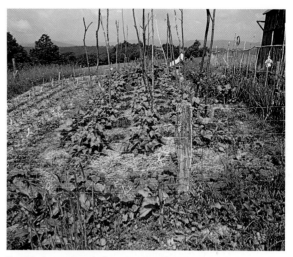

If soil lacks a mineral, then the plant limits its growth.

High Intake

In certain areas of the world where selenium levels are high in both soil and plant foods, defects in fingers, toenails, and hair can develop (39). Selenium toxicity has not been observed in humans but can develop in animals.

Some people feel that high intakes of selenium can prevent cancer. However, there is no evidence that intakes above recommended levels are beneficial.

Chromium

Chromium in tiny amounts has long been known to be essential for animals. In 1957, researchers observed that rats fed diets low in a certain factor that included chromium developed problems with their blood glucose levels (21). Now it is believed that trace amounts are also important for humans in maintaining normal blood glucose levels (40).

Recommended Intake

The Food and Nutrition Board has estimated that the safe and adequate dietary intake is 50–200 μg per day. Table 11.18 shows that peanuts, prunes, oils, various vegetables, whole-wheat bread, and chicken are good sources of chromium. Brewer's yeast is very high in chromium, and when given to diabetics or the elderly, blood glucose levels improve and insulin levels decrease. Intake of dietary chromium appears to have a wide range of safety.

Manganese

In 1931, **manganese** was found to be essential for the growth and reproduction in rats and mice. Later, manganese was discovered to prevent skeletal defects in chickens.

Recommended Intake

American males and females consume 2.72 and 2.05 mg of manganese per day, respectively, somewhat lower than the 2.0–5.0 mg/day estimated by the Food and Nutrition Board as the safe and adequate daily dietary intake (4).

Table 11.19 shows that nuts and seeds, whole grains, and various fruits and vegetables are good sources of manganese. Very little is present in animal products.

Role in Body

Manganese is a key part of a large number of enzyme systems. The total manganese content of an adult human is about 20 mg.

Table 11.18
Chromium in one-cup portions of food

Food	One-Cup Portion of Food (μg)
Peanuts, roasted	230
Prunes	160
Vegetable oil	100
Whole-wheat bread	60
Tomato, raw	60
Green peas, cooked	60
Corn, cooked	60
Chicken, roasted	40
Spinach, boiled	40
Macaroni, cooked	30
Pears, fresh	30
Potato, baked with skin	30
Onions, raw	30
Orange juice	30
Broccoli, cooked	30
Green beans, cooked	30
Cabbage, cooked	20
Mushrooms, raw	20
Cucumber, raw	20
Lentils, cooked	20
Apples	10
Celery	10
Lettuce	10

The estimated safe and adequate daily dietary intake is 50 to 200 μg.

Table 11.19
Manganese in one-cup portions of food

Food	One-Cup Portion of Food (mg)
Wheat germ	22.6
Walnuts	5.34
Pecans	4.87
Sesame seeds	3.54
Almonds	2.95
Sunflower seeds	2.91
Pineapple	2.56
Coconut	2.30
Blackberries	1.86
Peanuts	1.79
Rice	1.78
Lima beans	1.46
Whole-wheat cereal	1.41
Cooked oatmeal	1.37
Raspberries	1.25
Tea, brewed	1.19
Grape juice	0.91
Boysenberries	0.72
Mixed vegetables	0.69
Sprouted soybeans	0.67
Green peas	0.66
Grapes	0.66
Dried pears	0.59
Dates	0.53
Spinach, raw	0.50

The estimated safe and adequate daily dietary intake is 2.0 to 5.0 mg.

In animals, manganese deficiency is characterized by defective growth, bone abnormalities, reproductive deficiencies, central nervous system problems, and disturbances in the way the body handles fat (10). Although manganese deficiency has rarely been found in humans, it appears to be important for reproduction, skeletal development, and proper functioning of the brain and spinal cord.

Molybdenum

Recommended Intake
The Food and Nutrition Board has estimated that the safe and adequate daily dietary intake of **molybdenum** is 75–250 μg for adults. Table 11.20 shows that lean meats, legumes, whole grains, and various fruits and vegetables are good sources of molybdenum.

Role in Body
Molybdenum is a key part of the enzyme xanthine oxidase, which is needed by animals, humans, and many forms of plant life. Although deficiency can be produced in animals, molybdenum deficiency in humans has not been observed.

Cobalt

Although **cobalt** is essential, no recommended dietary allowance has been established. As discussed in chapter 10, cobalt is an essential component of vitamin B_{12} (cobalamin). When vitamin B_{12} from animal foods is consumed, cobalt is also ingested. Although no vitamin B_{12} is found in plant foods, cobalt by itself is found in green leafy vegetables.

Table 11.20
Molybdenum in one-cup portions of food

Food	One-Cup Portion of Food (μg)
Wheat germ	580
Pork, lean roasted	520
Cereal, All Bran	230
Lentils, cooked	140
Yams, baked	80
Green beans, cooked	80
Spinach, cooked	50
Cereal, Puffed Rice	30
Strawberries	20
Winter squash	20
Whole milk	20
Spinach, raw	10
Carrots, raw	10

The estimated safe and adequate daily dietary intake is 75 to 250 μg.

Other Minor Minerals That May Be Essential

There are several minerals that occur naturally in plants and animals, but their function is unknown (1). These include tin, nickel, silicon, and vanadium.

Human diets have been reported to contain 3.5–17 mg of tin per day. This dietary tin is poorly absorbed and is excreted in the feces. Nickel deficiency has been produced in chickens and rats. Traces of nickel are found in human tissues. Deficiencies of silicon have also been produced in laboratory animals. Silicon is ingested mainly from vegetable foods. Deficiencies of vanadium have been shown in chickens and rats, and it is present in human tissues.

Mineral Contaminants

As far as is known, the presence of lead, cadmium, mercury, arsenic, strontium, boron, aluminum, and lithium in the body is foreign to human and animal body function and health (1).

Twenty years ago, exposure to lead was much higher than it is today (41). At that time, close to one-third of Americans living in cities had blood levels of lead so high (greater than 0.03 mg/dL) that today they would be classified as toxic. Old lead water pipes, leaded gasoline, and lead in paint are all possible factors. Children can accumulate high levels of lead by eating old paint chips, drinking contaminated water, or inhaling too much car exhaust. Today, because of concertive action by many concerned citizens and lawmakers, only 2 percent of people nationwide have blood levels that are considered too high.

Lead toxicity is higher in children who are under six years of age, live in cities, and are from lower-income families. Signs and symptoms include constipation or diarrhea, irritability, weakness and fatigue, and a short attention span. If lead levels are too high, kidney damage, anemia, and gout can occur. Coma and death can then follow.

Aluminum is the third most abundant element in the earth's crust, and the human body contains 50–150 mg. The diets of Americans are believed to contain less than 150 mg per day, despite the use of aluminum cooking utensils (42). This amount of aluminum does not appear to impair the body's ability to absorb calcium, magnesium, zinc, iron, or copper. In addition, there is little evidence to support the theory that excessive exposure to aluminum causes Alzheimer's disease, a form of senility in elderly patients.

Exposure to high levels of mercury for long periods of time can damage the brain and nervous system (10). In the 1800s, makers of felt hats dipped the felt into mercury-nitrate solutions to make the felt easier to shape. The mercury was inhaled and absorbed through their skin. Tremors, incoherent speech, difficulty in walking, and feeble-mindedness resulted. The problem was immortalized in the phrase "mad as a hatter" and by the Mad Hatter in *Alice in Wonderland*. Recently, mercury poisoning has been reported in people eating fish from waters polluted with mercury compounds.

Exposure to smaller amounts of mercury vapor can cause less drastic symptoms, including insomnia, anxiety, and minor tremors.

Recently, some people have been claiming that dental fillings can lead to mercury poisoning. One hundred million Americans have "silver" dental fillings. The fillings are actually alloys of silver and other metals, including mercury. Some people claim that chewing can release minute amounts of mercury vapor from the old fillings, causing depression, fatigue, irritability, and other problems. The American Dental Association, however, states that "silver" fillings are safe. There is no need to have these old fillings replaced.

The Effects of Food Processing on Food Mineral Content

In this chapter we have noted that mineral supplementation is usually unnecessary if one consumes a wide variety of wholesome foods. However, the mineral quality of food can be diminished if improper processing and cooking procedures occur.

During the milling process of wheat, which involves the removal of the bran and wheat germ, many minerals are lost. Of the major minerals, 60–85 percent of calcium, phosphorus, magnesium, potassium, and sodium is removed. Sixteen percent of the selenium, and 40–89 percent of the minor minerals chromium, manganese, iron, cobalt, copper, zinc, and molybdenum is milled out. By law, only one of these minerals, iron, must be put back in before the white bread or refined grain product can be sold. Using whole-grain products, therefore, is one very helpful practice in ensuring that your intake of all minerals is optimal.

Cooking and canning can also affect the mineral quality of your food. For example, canned spinach has 82 percent less manganese, 71 percent less cobalt, and 40 percent less zinc than raw spinach. Canned beans have 60 percent less zinc, and canned tomatoes have 83 percent less zinc than the raw products.

Many of the minor minerals can be lost if cooking water or canning water is discarded. One study examining 16 different vegetables showed that boiling, as compared with steaming, more than doubled the loss of both iron and magnesium and tripled the loss of calcium. It is a good idea to steam your vegetables. If you boil them, save the water and use it as a base for homemade soup or other dishes.

HEALTH-PROMOTION INSIGHT
Minerals and High Blood Pressure

Blood pressure is the force of blood against the walls of the arteries and veins, created by the heart as it pumps the blood to every part of the body. When the heart pumps blood out of the heart, the pressure rises. This is called the **systolic blood pressure.** In between heartbeats, when the heart is resting, the pressure falls. This is called the *diastolic blood pressure.*

High blood pressure, or **hypertension,** is simply a condition in which the blood pressure is higher than is considered healthful. High blood pressure makes the heart and blood vessels work harder, and eventually it can contribute to failure of the heart or to heart disease. As discussed in chapter 6, one out of every two persons in the U.S. dies of heart disease. High blood pressure, along with smoking and too much cholesterol in the blood, is an important factor explaining this epidemic.

Table 11.21 shows that when the systolic blood pressure is higher than 140 mm Hg and/or the diastolic blood pressure is higher than 90 mm Hg, a person is classified as having high blood pressure. The blood pressure should be taken by a qualified health professional after you have been sitting for three to five minutes. It is a good idea to have your blood pressure taken on two separate days just in case you were a bit nervous the first time, which can raise your blood pressure.

Table 11.21
Blood pressure classification based on confirmed diastolic and systolic pressures in adults

Blood Pressure	Normal	Mild HX	Moderate HX	Severe HX
Systolic (mm Hg)	< 125	140–149	150–159	> 160
Diastolic (mm Hg)	< 85	90–104	105–114	> 115

Note: HX = hypertension; mm Hg = millimeter of mercury

Adapted from the 1988 Report of the Joint National Committee on Detection, Evaluation, and Treatment of High Blood Pressure. *Archives of Internal Medicine* 148:1023–1038, 1988.

*F*IGURE 11.10

Hypertension in U.S. adults is more common among blacks and the elderly. Nationwide, nearly one of three people has high blood pressure.

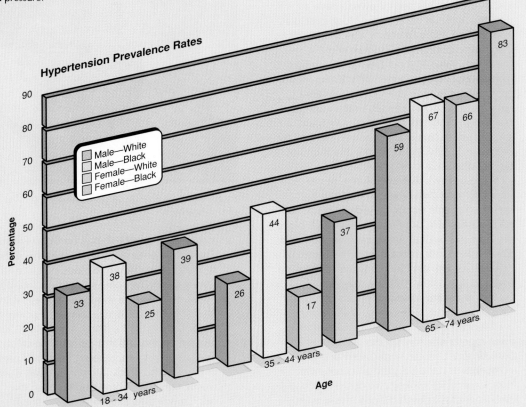

Hypertension Prevalence Rates

Legend:
- Male—White
- Male—Black
- Female—White
- Female—Black

Percentage axis: 0, 10, 20, 30, 40, 50, 60, 70, 80, 90

18 - 34 years: 33, 38, 25, 39
35 - 44 years: 26, 44, 17, 37
65 - 74 years: 59, 67, 66, 83

Age

More than 60 million American adults and children have high blood pressure, making this disease one of the most common in the United States. Figure 11.10 shows that nearly 40 percent of blacks are hypertensive, as compared to 33 percent of white males and 25 percent of white females. Researchers still have not yet figured out why blacks have more high blood pressure than whites. High blood pressure is more common among the elderly. In this country, 64 percent of people over age 65 have blood pressures greater than 140/90 (43).

Lowering Risk of High Blood Pressure

You may know someone who takes medication for high blood pressure. Many researchers are now advising that people with high blood pressure, in cooperation with their physician, should make some life-style improvements to see if their blood pressure can be controlled without the drugs. In the U.S.,

more than ten million hypertensive patients are using medications, at an annual estimated cost of $2.5 billion, a figure that exceeds that of any other disease.

Life-style improvements include weight loss to achieve ideal weight, reducing salt intake while increasing potassium consumption, restricting alcohol, and regular physical exercise. If these fail to lower the diastolic blood pressure below 95 mm Hg, then the physician may want to continue the same regimen but supplemented with drug therapy. So in other words, life-style first, and if this fails, continue the life-style improvements along with drug use (44).

Below is a description of life-style factors that can help you prevent high blood pressure. And if you know a friend or a family member who already has it, these methods can also help in treating the problem.

1. *Weight Loss.* The best way to lower high blood pressure is to reduce the body weight to optimal levels (45). In chapter 9 we discussed various ways in which this can be done. Losing just ten pounds has been shown to have a powerful effect in lowering the blood pressure.

2. *Less Sodium, More Potassium.* This chapter gives a complete description of sodium and potassium. Table 11.8 outlines the low-sodium, high-potassium foods, which include most fruits and their juices, vegetables, beans, unsalted nuts, and low-sodium cereals. When a person consumes 40 percent more potassium than sodium, risk of high blood pressure falls. And for people with high blood pressure, this is one of the best methods to help lower it.

    Some people's blood pressure is more sensitive to salt than others. These "salt-sensitive" people include the elderly, blacks, and people who have close relatives with high blood pressure. Although all Americans would do well to keep their sodium intake within the range of 1,100–3,300 mg/day, "salt-sensitive" people are urged to stay below 2,000 mg/day (44).

    Yes. According to several studies, the desire for salty food can be lessened. In one study, preference for salty food was lowered after three months of a low-salt diet (46).

3. *Less Alcohol.* Chapter 12 discussed alcohol consumption in the U.S., and all its potential risks. One risk of drinking two or three alcoholic drinks per day is elevated blood pressure. People with high blood pressure should restrict their alcohol intake or abstain entirely to see if the blood pressure will drop to more normal levels.

4. *More Physical Activity.* Regular physical activity like walking, cycling, swimming, jogging, or sports play has been found to both prevent high blood pressure and bring it down if it is too high (47). During exercise, the heart rate increases, and so does the systolic blood pressure. This is a normal response to the exercise. However, after the exercise is over, both the systolic and diastolic blood pressure fall lower than they were before the exercise session. If exercise is repeated day after day, the blood pressure stays lower.

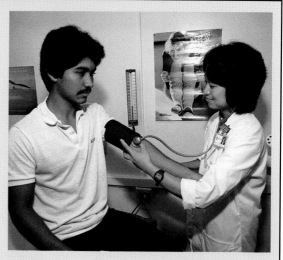

It's good to have your blood pressure taken regularly to remain healthy.

5. *Influence of Other Minerals on Blood Pressure.* There have been many studies regarding the relationship of calcium to blood pressure (48). During the 1970s, some researchers found that risk of heart disease was lower in areas with "hard" water. Calcium usually is the primary factor causing the hardness in the water. Some researchers thought that perhaps the calcium in the hard water was lowering the blood pressure of people who drank it, reducing heart disease. During the 1980s, some studies found that calcium was associated with lower blood pressure, and some did not (49). Much more research is needed to settle this issue. For now, consuming at least the RDA for calcium through use of low-fat dairy products, seeds and nuts, leafy green vegetables, and dried fruit is a good idea.

When rats are fed diets low in magnesium, they develop high blood pressure (49). Because research on humans is very scant, few recommendations can be offered at this time.

In conclusion, the strongest evidence points toward the importance of weight loss, a low sodium/potassium ratio, regular exercise, and alcohol restriction in preventing or treating high blood pressure. Other minerals may play a role, but more research is needed.

SUMMARY

1. The six major minerals are calcium, phosphorus, magnesium, and the three electrolytes — sodium, potassium, and chloride. The ten minor minerals are iron, zinc, iodine, fluoride, copper, selenium, chromium, manganese, molybdenum, and cobalt.

2. Average intake of most of the minerals is adequate for U.S. males and females. However, both males and females consume less than the recommended level of copper, and females consume less than the recommended amounts of manganese, selenium, potassium, magnesium, zinc, and iron. Part of the problem may be recommended dietary allowances that are too high for some of these minerals. For example, newer research has concluded that 1.3 mg of copper per day, instead of 2–3 mg, is sufficient.

3. Dairy products are rich sources of calcium. Nuts, legumes, seeds, and dried fruits are rich in calcium, magnesium, iron, zinc, copper, and manganese. Low-sodium, high-potassium foods include fruits and fruit juices, low-sodium cereals, unsalted nuts, vegetables, and legumes.

4. Calcium is the most abundant mineral in the human body and is important for strong bones, nerve and muscle function, blood clotting, and other important functions. Many experts recommend that calcium dietary intake exceed phosphorus to maintain proper levels of calcium in the bone.

5. Magnesium is required for more than 300 different enzyme systems of the body. Only 25 percent of Americans equal or exceed 100 percent RDA for magnesium.

6. No RDA for the three electrolytes (sodium, potassium, and chloride), has yet been established. Instead, the Food and Nutrition Board has established safe and adequate daily dietary intakes for each. For prevention of high blood pressure, a sodium/potassium ratio of 0.60 is recommended. In other words, 40 percent more potassium than sodium should be consumed.

7. Iron deficiency from inadequate intake is the most common single nutritional deficiency in the world today. This problem is more prevalent in developing countries. Iron is an important component of hemoglobin and a number of enzymes. When hemoglobin blood level falls below normal, this condition is called anemia. Iron from animal products (heme iron) is absorbed more easily by the human body than iron from plant products (nonheme iron).

8. Zinc is important for normal growth and is a part of more than 70 enzyme systems of the body. Mild zinc deficiency has been observed in U.S. children, resulting from lower-than-optimal dietary intakes. Hair sample analysis to determine zinc or mineral status is close to worthless.

9. Deficiency of iodine can lead to simple goiter. Fluoride is an important mineral in preventing dental caries.

10. If soil lacks a mineral (except for selenium and iodine), then a plant limits its growth. If the nutrients are not in the soil, then the plant cannot grow. Food supplements to counter low levels of minerals in foods because of alleged deficient U.S. farmland soils are not recommended or necessary. Food processing, however, such as occurs during the milling of wheat and other grains, does remove many important minerals. Use of whole-grain products is highly recommended.

11. The presence of lead, cadmium, mercury, arsenic, strontium, boron, aluminum, and lithium in the body is probably harmful to human health.

12. The most important way to prevent or treat high blood pressure is to keep body weight at optimal levels. A high-potassium, low-sodium diet is also helpful. More research on the relation of such minerals as calcium and magnesium to high blood pressure is needed before recommendations can be given.

REFERENCES

1. Anderson, C. E. 1983. Minerals. In *Nutritional Support of Medical Practice*, H. A. Schneider, C. E. Anderson, and D. B. Coursin, eds. Philadelphia: Harper & Row, Publishers.

2. Anderson, L., et al. 1982. *Nutrition in Health and Disease.* Philadelphia: J. B. Lippincott Company.

3. Food and Nutrition Board. Recommended Dietary Allowances. 10th rev. ed. 1989. Washington, D.C.: National Academy Press, 1989.

4. Pennington, J. A. T., et al. 1986. Mineral Content of Foods and Total Diets: The Selected Minerals in Foods Survey, 1982 to 1984. *Journal of the American Dietetic Association* 86:876–91.

5. Nordin, B. E. C., et al. 1987. The Problem of Calcium Requirement. *American Journal of Clinical Nutrition* 45:1295–1304.

6. Block, G., et al. 1985. Nutrient Sources in the American Diet: Quantitative Date from the NHANES II Survey. *American Journal of Epidemiology* 122:13–26.

7. National Institutes of Health, Consensus Conference. 1986. Osteoporosis. *Journal of the American Medical Association* 252:799–1685.

8. Riis, B., K. Thomsen, and C. Christiansen. 1987. Does Calcium Supplementation Prevent Postmenopausal Bone Loss? *New England Journal of Medicine* 316:173–77.

9. McDonough, F. E., et al. 1987. Modification of Sweet Acidophilus Milk to Improve Utilization by Lactose-Intolerant Persons. *American Journal of Clinical Nutrition* 45:570–74.

10. Shils, M. E. G., and V. R. Young. 1988. *Modern Nutrition in Health and Disease.* Philadelphia: Lea & Febiger.

11. Marshall, C. W. 1985. *Vitamins and Minerals: Help or Harm?* Philadelphia: George F. Stickley Company.

12. Nelson, R. L. 1987. Dietary Minerals and Colon Carcinogenesis. *Anticancer Research* (3 Pt A):259-69.

13. Gordon, G. S., and C. Vaugham. 1986. Calcium and Osteoporosis. *Journal of Nutrition* 116:319-22.

14. Hathcock, J. N. 1985. Quantitative Evaluation of Vitamin Safety. *Pharmacy Times* (May):104-13.

15. Wester, P. O. 1987. Magnesium. *American Journal of Clinical Nutrition* 45:1305-1312.

16. Consumer Nutrition Division, Human Nutrition Information Service, U.S. Department of Agriculture. Nationwide Food Consumption Survey, 1977-78. Nutrient Intakes: Individuals in 48 States. Report No. I-2. Hyattsville, Maryland: U.S. Department of Agriculture.

17. Seelig, M. S. 1980. *Magnesium Deficiency in the Pathogenesis of Disease.* New York: Plenum Press.

18. Jacobson, M. F. 1985. *The Complete Eater's Digest and Nutrition Scoreboard.* New York: Anchor Press/Doubleday.

19. Anonymous. Salt Heads Health Concerns. *FDA Consumer* (December 1984-January 1985):p. 3.

20. Shimizu, H. H. 1984. Herbs. *FDA Consumer* (April).

21. Prasad, A. S. 1978. *Trace Elements and Iron in Human Nutrition.* New York: Plenum Medical Book Company.

22. Herbert, V. 1987. Recommended Dietary Intakes (RDI) of Iron in Humans. *American Journal of Clinical Nutrition* 45:679-86.

23. Haymes, E. M. 1987. Nutritional Concerns: Need for Iron. *Medical Science and Sports Exercise.* 19:S197-S200.

24. Expert Scientific Working Group. 1985. Summary of a Report on Assessment of the Iron Nutritional Status of the United States Population. *American Journal of Clinical Nutrition* 42:1318-1330.

25. Yip, R., et al. 1987. Declining Prevalence of Anemia among Low-Income Children in the United States. *Journal of the American Medical Association* 258:1619-1623.

26. O'Dell, B. L. 1984. Bioavailability of Trace Elements. *Nutrition Review* 42:301-308.

27. Keen, C. L., et al., 1988. Studies of Marginal Zinc Deprivation of Rhesus Monkeys. III. Use of Liver Biopsy in the Assessment of Zinc Status. *American Journal of Clinical Nutrition* 47:1041-1045.

28. Hambidge, K. M., et al. 1976. Zinc Nutrition of Preschool Children in the Denver Head Start Program. *American Journal of Clinical Nutrition* 29:734-38.

29. Barrett, S. 1985. Commercial Hair Analysis: Science or Scam? *Journal of the American Medical Association* 254:1041-1045.

30. Klevay, I. M., et al. 1987. Hair Analysis in Clinical and Experimental Medicine. *American Journal of Clinical Nutrition* 46:233-36.

31. Anonymous. 1986. Adverse Effects of Zinc Megadoses. *Nutrition and the M.D.* (March).

32. Greger, J. L. 1987. Food, Supplements, and Fortified Foods: Scientific Evaluations in Regard to Toxicology and Nutrient Bioavailability. *Journal of the American Dietetic Association* 87:1369-1373.

33. Festa, M. D., et al. 1985. Effect of Zinc Intake on Copper Excretion and Retention in Men. *American Journal of Clinical Nutrition* 41:285-92.

34. Milne, D. B., et al. 1984. Effect of Oral Folic Acid Supplements on Zinc, Copper, and Iron Absorption and Excretion. *American Journal of Clinical Nutrition* 39:535-39.

35. Richmond, V. L. 1985. Thirty Years of Fluoridation: A Review. *American Journal of Clinical Nutrition* 41:129-38.

36. Turnlund, J. R. 1988. Copper Nutriture, Bioavailability, and the Influence of Dietary Factors. *Journal of the American Dietetic Association* 88:303-308.

37. Finley, E. B., and F. L. Cerklewski. 1983. Influence of Ascorbic Acid Supplementation on Copper Status in Young Adult Men. *American Journal of Clinical Nutrition* 37:553-56.

38. Greenwald, P., and E. Sondik. 1986. Diet and Chemoprevention in NCI's Research Strategy to Achieve National Cancer Control Objectives. *Annual Review of Public Health* 7:267-91.

39. Diplock, A. T. 1987. Trace Elements in Human Health with Special Reference to Selenium. *American Journal of Clinical Nutrition* 45:1313-1322.

40. Riales, R., and M. J. Albrink. 1981. Effect of Chromium Chloride Supplementation on Glucose Tolerance and Serum Lipids Including High-Density Lipoprotein of Adult Men. *American Journal of Clinical Nutrition* 34:2670-2678.

41. Rabinowitz, M. B. 1986. Lead and Nutrition. *Nutrition & the M.D.* 12(3):1.

42. Greger, J. L., and M. J. Baier. 1983. Effect of Dietary Aluminum on Mineral Metabolism of Adult Males. *American Journal of Clinical Nutrition* 38:411-19.

43. The Working Group on Hypertension in the Elderly. 1986. Statement on Hypertension in the Elderly. *Journal of the American Medical Association* 256:70-74.

44. Kaplan, N. M. 1986. Dietary Aspects of the Treatment of Hypertension. *Annual Review of Public Health* 7:503-19.

45. Langford, H. G., et al. 1985. Dietary Therapy Slows the Return of Hypertension after Stopping Prolonged Medication. *Journal of the American Medical Association* 253:657.

46. Blais, C. A., et al. 1986. Effect of Dietary Sodium Restriction on Taste Responses to Sodium Chloride: A Longitudinal Study. *American Journal of Clinical Nutrition* 44:232-43.

47. Kenney, W. L., and E. J. Zambraski. 1984. Physical Activity in Human Hypertension. *Sports Medicine* 1:459.

48. Kaanja, N., and D. A. McCarron. 1986. Calcium and Hypertension. *Annual Review of Nutrition* 6:475-94.

49. Council for Agricultural Science and Technology. 1987. Diet and Health, Report No. 111. Ames, IA: Council for Agricultural Science and Technology.

HEALTH-PROMOTION ACTIVITY 11.1
Do You Know Your Blood Pressure?

Have your blood pressure taken by a trained health professional (perhaps at your school's health center). Answer the following questions.

1. What is your blood pressure _____ / _____ mm Hg.
   systolic   diastolic
   NOTE: your blood pressure should be rechecked on a separate day if outside normal levels.
2. According to table 11.21, what classification would you give yourself?
   a. normal
   b. mild hypertension
   c. moderate hypertension
   d. severe hypertension

3. According to information given in the Health-Promotion Insight, what are three important life-style habits to prevent or treat high blood pressure?

a. _____

b. _____

c. _____

HEALTH-PROMOTION ACTIVITY 11.2
Foods High in Minerals

Study tables 11.3, 11.4, 11.6, 11.7, and 11.13 through 11.20. Rank foods in each table, and see which ten foods have the highest average ranking. List below the ten foods that rank highest on all of the lists.

Top Ten Foods for Overall Mineral Status (Highest Average Ranking)

Food	Average Ranking	Food	Average Ranking
1.		6.	
2.		7.	
3.		8.	
4.		9.	
5.		10.	

*H*EALTH-PROMOTION ACTIVITY 11.3
Lowering Sodium in Your Diet

Study the section in this chapter on sodium. Think through your personal salt and sodium intake, and then list below *five* ways that you individually can lower your sodium intake.

Ways to Lower Your Sodium Intake

1.

2.

3.

4.

5.

12

Water and Other Beverages

INTRODUCTION

S oft drinks, coffee, and beer are three of America's favorite beverages. This chapter will emphasize the importance of drinking more water and moderating intake of coffee and beer. Evidence is mounting that the human body does not tolerate high intakes of caffeine or alcohol very well. Many of the most common diseases in Western culture are now being associated with the regular abuse of these substances.

People who exercise heavily need liberal amounts of water to help restore that which is lost in the sweat. Dehydration can decrease one's ability to exercise and can make the difference between victory and defeat. The Health-Promotion Insight at the end of this chapter will explore the fascinating topic of sports nutrition.

Water

Water is vital for life and optimal health. All humans need water: from the hot and thirsty desert traveler to the secretary working at a desk.

Where Water Is Found

Within the Body

Our bodies contain more water than any other substance or chemical. Approximately 60 percent of adult human body weight is water. The muscles are about 75 percent water, and the bones are a mere 20 percent water. Blood is 90 percent water, and teeth are only 5 percent water.

Infants have an even higher percentage of water weight, and the elderly have a lower percentage. Because body fat tissue contains very little water, obese individuals have a lower percentage of water weight than do lean muscular people.

Most of the body's water is found inside the cells of the body. This is known as intracellular water. Extracellular water is located in the blood, lymph, and fluid surrounding each body cell (see figure 12.1). Electrolytes (sodium, potassium, and other minerals) regulate the balance of intracellular and extracellular water (1). Potassium is found primarily inside the cells, and sodium is on the outside. Water flows back and forth across the cell wall according to the mineral concentration on either side. Water moves toward the area of higher concentration and di-

lutes it to the same concentration as the other side. This process is called **osmosis.** Thus the body's total fluid balance occurs at the cellular level and is regulated by electrolyte concentrations (2).

Within Beverages and Foods

All beverages contain more water than any other ingredient. Club soda is 100 percent water. Tea, coffee, and diet drinks are 99 percent water. Other drinks, such as lemonade, milk, and alcoholic beverages, contain higher amounts of dissolved solids that displace the water (see table 12.1).

Many foods also contain a significant amount of water. As outlined in table 12.1, fruits and vegetables and certain dairy products have a relatively high water content, whereas nuts, dried fruit, and cereals, for example, have a low water content.

Role of Water in the Body

A regular supply of water is even more essential to the body than food. One can exist for weeks without food, but only for several days without water. Every body function depends on an ample water supply (3). And we use water for many other daily activities as well, with the average person in the U.S. using 110 gallons of water per day.

The Digestive System and Nutrient Transport

Water is needed to form the two gallons of digestive enzymes and juices produced every 24 hours. After the food is softened and broken into

*F*IGURE 12.1

Water moves back and forth across the cell wall according to the concentration of salt.

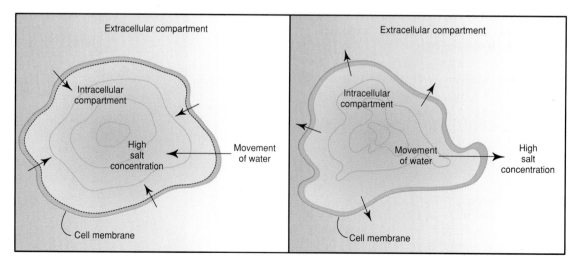

small particles, water is the solvent that carries nutrients to the absorption sites on the wall of the small intestine. As nutrients are absorbed, water in the blood and lymph provides further transport throughout the body (4).

The Filtering System
The high water content of blood provides more than just a solution for nutrient transport. Additionally, metabolic waste products such as urea, uric acids, electrolytes, glucose, sulfates, phosphates, nitrates and creatinine are dissolved in the blood and carried to the kidneys (2). About 48 gallons of water pass through the kidneys' filtering system daily; most of it is reabsorbed. The amount of actual urine produced depends on the concentration of cell waste products and the body's water intake. On the average, urine is 97 percent water.

Lubrication
Water is the primary constituent of the various lubricants the body produces for the joints and muscles. These substances lower the friction between the moving parts of the body. Fluid substances also help cushion and protect the internal organs, and mucous and saline solutions protect the sensitive linings of the nose and eyes.

Maintenance of Body Temperature
The water contained within the body also helps to regulate body temperature (2). Slight perspiration occurs continuously, as anyone who has ever worn plastic gloves can testify. Normally this perspiration quickly evaporates from the skin. Gloves, heavy clothing, and high humidity diminish the rate of evaporation, leaving the skin damp and clammy.

During heat waves and intense physical exertion, the sweat glands in the skin secrete increased amounts of fluid. As the sweat evaporates from the surface of the skin, the body temperature is lowered (see the Health-Promotion Insight at the end of this chapter). To prevent dehydration and an elevated body temperature, the fluid lost from sweating must be replaced by increased water consumption.

Preventing Dehydration

Daily Water Loss
Optimal health is dependent on the right balance of fluid intake and output. Abnormalities in this delicate balance can be life threatening. Fluid intake and output are closely monitored

TABLE 12.1
Percent water in foods (by weight)

Category	Food	Percent Water
Dairy Products	Whole milk	87
	Cheese	40
	Cottage cheese	78
	Yogurt	89
Meat	Eggs	74
	Beef	53
	Chicken	58
	Pork	42
	Sardines	62
Nuts	Almonds	5
	Peanut butter	2
Vegetables	Broccoli	91
	Carrots	88
	Corn	74
	Lettuce	95
	Peas	82
Fruit	Tomato	94
	Apples	85
	Oranges	86
	Bananas	76
	Watermelon	93
Dried Fruit	Dates	22
	Prunes	28
Cereals	White bread	36
	Whole-wheat bread	36
	Corn flakes	4
	Oats	3
	Rice	12
	Shredded Wheat	7
Fats	Margarine	16
	Corn oil	0
Favorite American Beverages	Club soda	100
	Iced tea	99+
	Coffee	99+
	Cola (diet)	99
	Kool-aid (presweetened)	99
	Beer	92
	Ginger ale	92
	Milk (skim, butter)	90.5
	Cola (regular)	90
	Root beer	90
	Soda (fruit flavor)	88
	Kool-aid (sugar added)	88
	Lemonade	88
	Milk (whole)	87
	Martini	80
	Wine	76.7

Data from U.S. Department of Agriculture Food Composition Tables (Handbook No. 8 series).

FIGURE 12.2

Optimal health depends on the right balance of fluid intake and output. Most sedentary people lose nearly three quarts of water per day from the body—this must be replaced.

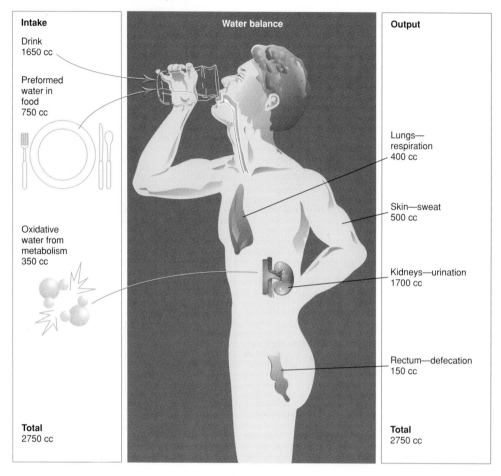

Intake	Water balance	Output
Drink 1650 cc		Lungs—respiration 400 cc
Preformed water in food 750 cc		Skin—sweat 500 cc
Oxidative water from metabolism 350 cc		Kidneys—urination 1700 cc
		Rectum—defecation 150 cc
Total 2750 cc		**Total** 2750 cc

in hospital patients to detect or prevent serious complications. It is a good idea for people out of the hospital to also pay close attention to their body's water balance.

During a 24-hour period, water loss averages just under three quarts a day (3,4) (see figure 12.2). This varies greatly among individuals, depending on body size, the amount of water consumed beyond body needs, medical complications, and environmental conditions.

The four routes of water loss are shown in figure 12.2. The majority of water leaving the body each day is routed through the kidneys, and the rest through the skin, lungs, and rectum.

Water Conservation within the Body

Although human adults average nearly three quarts of water loss per day, this amount would be much greater if the body did not recycle its

water over and over. The actual daily water need is 2,500 gallons a day! This is why any defect in the fluid balance system can have a major effect.

Dehydration causes a change in the **electrolyte** (sodium, potassium, chloride) balance. The extracellular water becomes concentrated and pulls water out of the cells. As the cells become dehydrated and shrink in size, the thirst response is triggered by the **hypothalamus,** a small but important command post in the brain (see figure 12.3). The pituitary gland then secretes the **antidiuretic hormone,** which signals the kidney to preserve water. When the person drinks more water, cell volume is finally restored, turning off the thirst desire. The function of the thirst mechanism is to make sure that body water will be promptly replenished when a deficit occurs (2).

*F*IGURE 12.3

The function of the thirst mechanism is to make sure that body water will be replenished when a deficit occurs.

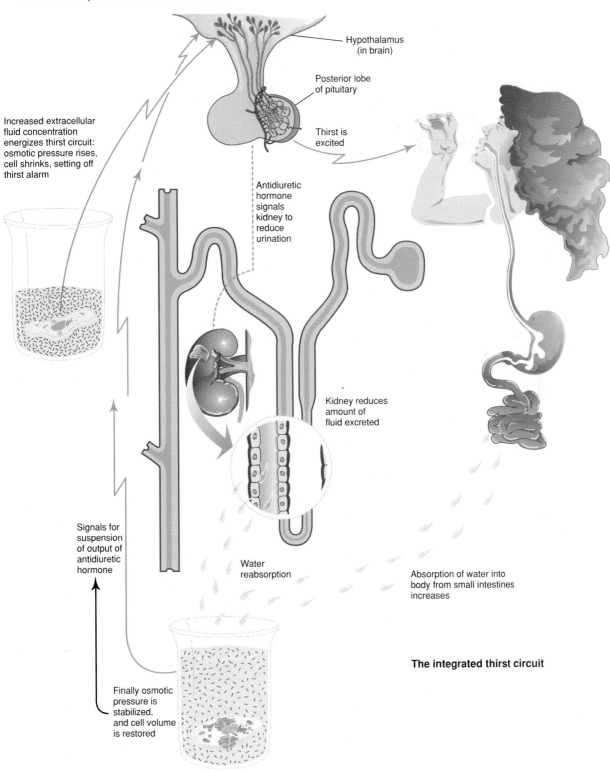

Hypothalamus
(in brain)

Posterior lobe
of pituitary

Thirst is
excited

Increased extracellular
fluid concentration
energizes thirst circuit:
osmotic pressure rises,
cell shrinks, setting off
thirst alarm

Antidiuretic
hormone
signals
kidney to
reduce
urination

Kidney reduces
amount of
fluid excreted

Signals for
suspension
of output of
antidiuretic
hormone

Water
reabsorption

Absorption of water into
body from small intestines
increases

Finally osmotic
pressure is
stabilized,
and cell volume
is restored

The integrated thirst circuit

Among persons doing hard running in hot, humid weather, sweat rates as high as three quarts per hour have been recorded! Such excessive sweating for prolonged periods of time can result in depletion of both water and electrolyte levels in the body (see the Health-Promotion Insight at the end of this chapter).

Three groups are at risk for dehydration—infants, the elderly, and athletes engaging in long endurance events like marathons or triathalons. Infants given concentrated milk formulas without adequate water cannot handle the high solute level. The infant must draw on its own water stores to dilute the concentrated milk, leading to dehydration. If a baby has very few wet diapers, insufficient water intake is likely.

The elderly sometimes neglect to maintain adequate fluid intake. Many elderly people admitted to hospitals have a range of complications related to dehydration, including mental confusion and extreme fatigue.

To prevent dehydration, fluid intake must equal the output (see figure 12.2). The majority of fluid intake must come from consumption of water and beverages. Water contained within the food eaten is another important source of water intake. A small amount of water is obtained during the final stages of fat, protein, and carbohydrate metabolism.

The Significance of Dehydration

A loss of 30–40 percent of a person's muscle and fat stores is serious but not life threatening. In contrast, a ten percent loss of body water is a very serious matter, and a 20 percent loss is fatal. If a person loses six percent of body water per day, death results within three to four days.

The most common cause of mild dehydration is the failure to consume sufficient amounts of water each day. Additionally, various factors may accelerate fluid loss. High-protein diets require extra water for kidney filtration. This results in increased urine and temporary weight loss from dehydration. Infections with high fever, vomiting, and diarrhea can quickly deplete body water stores. Various medications used for controlling high blood pressure, such as **diuretics,** can increase urination, thereby decreasing body water stores. Vigorous exercise in high altitudes or humid, hot environments also can lead to serious dehydration. See the Health-Promotion Insight for a description of the signs and symptoms of dehydration.

TABLE 12.2
Drinking water drunk per individual per day

Sex and Age (years)	Individuals Reporting No Water (%)	Cups (average)
Males and females		
Under 1	51.6	1.4
1–2	10.5	2.1
3–5	7.1	2.5
6–8	6.3	2.6
Males		
9–11	8.2	2.8
12–14	4.9	3.4
15–18	6.1	3.8
19–22	7.5	3.9
23–34	13.4	3.8
35–50	12.5	3.9
51–64	9.1	3.9
65–74	7.3	4.1
75 and over	5.9	3.9
Females		
9–11	5.7	2.8
12–14	6.6	3.1
15–18	10.0	3.0
19–22	13.8	3.2
23–34	15.8	3.1
35–50	11.7	3.2
51–64	8.6	3.6
65–74	6.3	3.6
75 and over	8.5	3.2
All individuals	10.1	3.3

Data from Nationwide Food Consumption Survey, 1977–78, Report No. I-2, May 1984. U.S. Department of Agriculture.

Daily Habits to Prevent Dehydration

The average person drinks only 3.3 cups of water per day (see table 12.2) (6). This is far below the recommended six to ten cups of water. Many Americans avoid "plain water" and use flavored, sweetened, carbonated, caffeinated, dyed, chilled, and bottled beverages. Total fluid intake from all sources for the average American varies widely, ranging from one to six quarts per day (7). The Food and Nutrition Board of the National Academy of Sciences recommends one quart of water per 1,000 calories consumed per day. This means that the average woman in this country should consume about 1.5 quarts of water a day and the average man should consume 2.5 quarts a day.

Because both coffee and alcohol tend to act as diuretics, these are poor sources for meeting body fluid needs. In other words, because coffee and alcohol increase the loss of body water through the urine, other beverages are considered better sources.

Following is a simple plan (for a non-athlete) to ensure that sufficient fluid is consumed:

Upon arising: drink two cups of water.
Mid-morning or 30–45 minutes prior to lunch: drink two cups of water.
Mid-afternoon or 30–45 minutes prior to supper: drink two cups of water.
Evening: drink one to two cups of water, 90 minutes prior to bedtime.

Drinking the water 30–45 minutes prior to mealtimes helps to make the blood more fluid, allowing digestive glands to more easily form their digestive juices. It also helps prevent the feeling of thirst that can often follow meals, and it may reduce feelings of fatigue as well.

Athletes need much more water than nonathletes to replace the large amounts of water lost through sweat. Also, during illnesses that result in fluid loss from vomiting, diarrhea, or fever, one should consume extra fluids in the form of water, juice, or soup.

Safety and Purity of the Water Supply

Purity of water is essential for prevention of infectious disease. Undeveloped countries continue to have problems in providing unpolluted sources of drinking water for their citizens, resulting in thousands of needless deaths every year.

In the United States, the quality of our drinking-water supply, although considered excellent, still continues to be a cause for concern among some segments of the population. Some people believe that tap water cannot be trusted as a safe and pure source for their drinking and cooking water. However, there is little evidence to support this concern.

The U.S. Environmental Protection Agency (EPA) has set new drinking-water standards for eight pollutants (8). The EPA reports that for each pollutant, under the new standards, if a million people drink two quarts of polluted water every day for 70 years, only one will develop cancer as a direct result of one of the chemicals. Only 2.3 percent of the nation's 79,000 public water systems do not meet these very strict standards. Even for these, the risk of disease is considered very remote.

Of all the water used in the United States, about 6 percent is for residential, 14 percent is for industrial, and 80 percent is for agricultural purposes. On the average, it takes 1,000 gallons of water to produce each pound of food we eat (9). To feed one person in the U.S. for a year requires about five acre-feet, or 1,630,000 gallons, of water.

Nationwide, we are drawing on groundwater reserve resources at a rate of over 30 trillion gallons every year. Not only are some of these groundwater reserves steadily dropping; many are vulnerable to contamination from chemical dumping and industrial waste. Our water supply is precious, and concerted action is needed to safeguard its future.

Many people have turned to bottled water for safety and taste (10). During the early 1980s, Americans were consuming over 600 million gallons of bottled water a year, not including imported mineral water or carbonated products. As concerns about the quality of tap water continue to grow, Americans will probably continue to be willing to spend money for bottled water.

Caffeinated Beverages

Definition of Caffeine

Caffeine is a naturally occurring substance found in over 60 different plants (11). Coffee beans, cocoa beans, cola nuts, and tea leaves are the most common sources of caffeine. Chemically, its structure is a methylxanthine (see figure 12.4).

Caffeine Consumption

Most adults consume caffeine daily in one form or another. Not only is caffeine present in coffee, tea, soft drinks, and chocolate products, but it is also found in many drugs. The average American adult who uses caffeine consumes 227 mg per day (12). A dose of just 200 mg caffeine causes many druglike effects (stimulation of the brain, elevation of blood hormones and glucose).

Beverages

Caffeine content varies considerably in coffee and tea. The type of coffee bean or tea leaf, the quantity used, and the length of time brewed or steeped affect the caffeine level (13). Brewed coffee, in general, has more caffeine than does instant coffee (see table 12.3). One cup (5 oz) of coffee, in general, has about 100 milligrams of caffeine, whereas the same amount of tea has

FIGURE 12.4

Caffeine is a naturally occurring substance found in more than 60 different plants, including coffee beans and cola nuts.

Caffeine
(1, 3, 7-trimethyl-
xanthine)

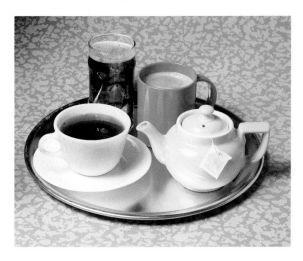

TABLE 12.3

Caffeine content of popular beverages and foods

Item	Caffeine Content (mg)
Coffee (5-oz cup)	
Drip method	110–150
Percolated	64–124
Instant	40–108
Decaffeinated	2–5
Instant decaffeinated	2
Tea, loose or bags (5-oz cup)	
1-min brew	9–33
3-min brew	20–46
5-min brew	20–50
Tea products	
Instant (5-oz cup)	12–28
Iced tea (12-oz can)	22–36
Chocolate products	
Hot cocoa (6 oz)	2–8
Dry cocoa (1 oz)	6
Milk chocolate (1 oz)	1–15
Baking chocolate (1 oz)	35
Sweet dark chocolate (1 oz)	5–35
Chocolate milk (8 oz)	2–7
Chocolate-flavored syrup (2 tbsp)	4

Data from Consumers Union, Food and Drug Administration, National Coffee Association of the U.S.A., and National Confectioners Association of the United States.

TABLE 12.4

Coffee drinkers in different age groups (percentage of Americans of various age groups who are coffee drinkers)

	1962	1987
	(%)	(%)
10–19 years	25.1	5.3
20–29	81.0	33.1
30–59	90.8	67.2
60+	88.4	77.8
All ages	74.7	52.0

Data from International Coffee Organization, London, England.

about 50 mg. Many restaurants serve 5-oz portions of coffee, but coffee mugs used at home or work may hold more than double this amount.

Coffee consumption has decreased dramatically during the past 25 years. Both the number of coffee drinkers and the quantity they drink have diminished (13). Table 12.4 shows that in 1962, approximately 75 percent of Americans ten years and older drank coffee. By 1987, this had dropped to 52 percent. Three cups of coffee per day is now the average quantity consumed by Americans, down from the four-cup average in 1962. Many people have switched to decaffeinated coffee, while others prefer soft drinks instead.

Table 12.5 shows that cola-type and other soft drinks contain caffeine. Some of this caffeine comes from the cola nut, but the majority is derived from coffee beans. Unlike coffee and tea, each brand of soft drink has a regulated, consistent amount of caffeine. There is wide variation, however, among brands.

Soft-drink consumption has risen sharply since 1970. Between 1970 and 1985, per capita consumption of soft drinks rose 92 percent (see chapter 2). Table 12.6 shows that soft drinks are now America's favorite beverage, with 58 percent using them. Use of coffee is second, at 52 percent of the U.S. population, and milk is third, at 47 percent. Studies show that the primary caffeine-containing food for children in this country is carbonated beverages (12). Half of the total caffeine intake of young adults comes from soft drinks.

Although coffee consumption is declining, coffee still remains the greatest source of caffeine in this country. Ounce per ounce, coffee contains more caffeine than any other beverage.

TABLE 12.5
Caffeine content of various soft drinks

Soft Drinks Containing Caffeine[a]	Caffeine Content (mg/ 12-oz serving)
Jolt	72.0
Sugar-Free Mr. PIBB	58.8
Mountain Dew	54.0
Mello Yello	52.8
TAB	46.8
Coca-Cola	45.6
Diet Coke	45.6
Shasta Cola	44.4
Shasta Cherry Cola	44.4
Shasta Diet Cola	44.4
Shasta Diet Cherry Cola	44.4
Mr. PIBB	40.8
Dr. Pepper	39.6
Sugar-Free Dr. Pepper	39.6
Big Red	38.4
Sugar-Free Big Red	38.4
Pepsi-Cola	38.4
Aspen	36.0
Diet Pepsi	36.0
Pepsi Light	36.0
RC Cola	36.0
Diet Rite	36.0
Kick	31.2
Canada Dry Jamaica Cola	30.0
Canada Dry Diet Cola	1.2

[a]There are at least 200 flavors, varieties, and types of soft drinks, manufactured by the leading bottlers, that contain no caffeine.

Data from National Soft Drink Association.

Chocolate
Table 12.3 shows that chocolate milk and cocoa also contain caffeine. Concentrated chocolate products, such as baking chocolate, have relatively high amounts of caffeine but are usually diluted when eating in their final form.

Drugs
For many years, caffeine has been added to certain drugs, such as pain relievers, cold tablets, diuretics, and diet pills (11) (see table 12.7). Its addition to headache remedies helps to constrict the swollen blood vessels that cause pain.

TABLE 12.6
Consumption of coffee and other beverages (percentage of U.S. population who drink various beverages)

	1962	1987
	(%)	(%)
Coffee	74.7	52.0
Tea	24.7	29.3
Milk	53.6	47.3
Soft drinks	32.6	58.1
Juices	41.4	42.8

Data from International Coffee Organization, London, England.

TABLE 12.7
Caffeine content of drug preparations[a]

Classification	Caffeine Content	
	mg/tablet or capsule	mg/day[b]
Over-the-Counter Stimulants		
NoDoz Tablets	100	200
Vivarin Tablets	200	200
Pain Relievers		
Anacin	32	64
Excedrin	65	130
Excedrin P.M.	0	0
Midol (for cramps)	32	64
Midol (P.M.S.)	0	0
Plain aspirin, any brand	0	0
Vanquish	33	66
Diuretics		
Aqua-Ban	100	200
Cold Remedies		
Coryban-D	30	30
Dristan	0	0
Weight-Control Aids		
Dexatrim	200	200
Dexatrim, caffeine-free	0	0
Dietac	200	200
Dietac, caffeine-free	0	0
Prescription		
Amaphen	40	—[c]
Cafergot	100	100
Darvon compound	32.4	64.8
Darvon compound-65	32.4	64.8
Fioricet	40	40 or 80
Fiorinol	40	40 or 80
Migralam	100	800 to 1,000
Percaps	40	—[c]
Synalgos-DC	30	360
Triad	40	—[c]
Two-Dyne	40	—[c]
Wigraine	100	—[c]

[a]Information on caffeine content and standard dosages obtained from Physician's Desk Reference (1986) and Physician's Desk Reference for Nonprescription Drugs (1986).
[b]Depending on the type drug, a single dose is recommended once a day or as often as once every 4 hours.
[c]Recommended daily dosage not listed in Physician's Desk Reference (1986).

Caffeine tablets (NoDoz, Vivarin) are used by some individuals to stay awake while working, driving, or studying. Habitual use can lead to caffeine addiction and "rebound" fatigue.

The Effects of Caffeine

For years, people have questioned the safety of consuming varied amounts of caffeine (see chapter 2). Confusing and conflicting results from numerous studies have failed to provide clear answers. However, there is a growing consensus that regular use of such caffeinated beverages such as coffee is associated with various health problems.

Metabolic Effects

Caffeine is a stimulant to the central nervous system. It can increase the heart rate, increase the basal metabolic rate, cause stomach acid secretion, increase urine production, dilate and constrict blood vessels, and function as a bronchodilator in asthma patients (11).

Caffeine reaches its peak level in the blood thirty minutes after consumption. It saturates other body tissues at a level proportional to their water content. Unborn infants can receive caffeine through the placenta, and breast-fed infants can obtain caffeine through human breast milk.

It takes time for caffeine to be eliminated from the body. Age, sex, hormone levels, medications, smoking status, and pregnancy affect the elimination process. Newborns, pregnant women, and women taking birth control pills have slower rates of caffeine removal. Only 50 percent of caffeine is removed (**half-life**) three to four days after consumption by newborns because they lack enzymes to metabolize caffeine. The half-life of caffeine in nonsmoking adults is five to seven hours, but in pregnant women it is 18–20 hours.

Caffeinism

Five to six cups of coffee per day may lead to **caffeinism** in some individuals. It is a behavioral, psychophysiological affliction with the following characteristics: restlessness, anxiety, irritability, agitation, muscle tremor, insomnia, headache, lightheadedness, heart palpitations, diarrhea, and increased urination. Individuals

with caffeinism are advised to gradually taper down their consumption. Sudden withdrawal can intensify the symptoms. However, the best treatment is to progress to abstinence of all caffeinated products.

Health Problems

Heart Disease

Recent studies have linked heavy coffee consumption to elevations in serum cholesterol levels. Several studies have now also shown that coffee drinking is associated with increased risk of heart disease. In one of the best-designed studies, at Johns Hopkins University, researchers studied the effect of coffee consumption on coronary heart disease in 1,130 male medical students. The length of the follow-up varied from 19 to 35 years (14). Men who drank five or more cups of coffee per day, as compared with nondrinkers, increased their risk of heart disease by 250 percent. Similar results were found in a 19-year study of 1,910 white males aged 40–56 from the Chicago Western Electric Company Study (15).

Breast Disease

Early reports suggested that a woman might increase her risk of breast cancer by drinking coffee. Many women have read articles in lay publications that suggest that risk of breast lumps and cysts, perhaps early markers for breast cancer, is increased with caffeine consumption. However, recent studies provide little evidence to support the association between caffeine consumption and fibrocystic breast disease (16).

Birth Defects

In some animal studies, birth defects are increased when the mother uses caffeine. At this time there is no human evidence to suggest that moderate caffeine consumption by pregnant women causes birth defects. However, in one study of 3,891 pregnant women, maternal caffeine intake was associated with decreases in the birth weight of their infants, probably through growth retardation (17). More research is needed to verify these results.

Cancer

Some animal studies have suggested that caffeine may enhance the risk of cancer, while others have not (18). Various studies with

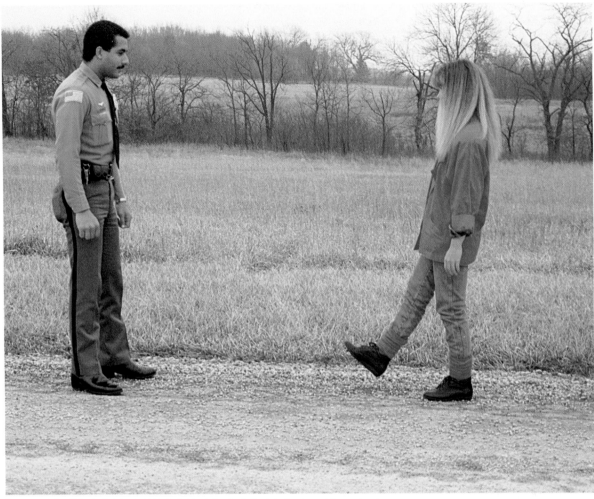

States vary in giving sobriety tests to individuals in alcohol-related automobile accidents.

humans are also mixed, but there is some data to suggest that heavy use of coffee may be associated with colon cancer, bladder cancer, and ovarian cancer. More study is needed before definitive conclusions can be made.

Decaffeination

There are two basic coffee decaffeination processes used in the U.S.: water extraction, and direct solvent extraction with methylene chloride. Some people have been concerned that methylene chloride may end up in decaffeinated coffee, causing health problems (13). However, the FDA has determined that methylene chloride concentrations in decaffeinated coffee are very low and pose no danger to humans. Nonetheless, most companies have switched to the water extraction technique to allay public fears. Drinking decaffeinated coffee is a better choice than drinking regular coffee.

Alcoholic Beverages

Alcohol Consumption in the U.S.

Most standard portions of beverages containing alcohol have one-half ounce of ethanol. This amount of ethanol is found in

12 oz, or one can, of beer
4 oz, or one glass, of wine
1.25 oz of 80-proof gin, rum, vodka, whiskey.

As a rule of thumb, one standard drink (.5 oz ethanol) consumed within one hour will produce a blood-alcohol level (BAL) of .02 in a 150-pound male. Five beers consumed within one hour will cause the BAL to rise to .10, which violates the drinking and driving laws of most states (see figure 12.5).

*F*IGURE 12.5

Of all fatal traffic accidents, 50–55 percent involve a drinking driver or pedestrian. The Department of Motor Vehicles distributes this information to increase awareness among drivers.

IF YOU DRINK, DON'T DRIVE!
But if you do drink and drive...KNOW YOUR LIMIT!!

There is no safe way to drive after drinking. These charts show that a few drinks can make you an unsafe driver. They show that drinking affects your **BLOOD ALCOHOL CONCENTRATION (BAC)**. The **BAC** zones for various numbers of drinks and time periods are printed in white, grey, and black. **HOW TO USE THESE CHARTS;** First, find the chart that includes your weight. For example, if you weigh 160 lbs., use the "150-169" chart. Then look under "Total Drinks" at the "2" on this "150 to 169" chart. Now look below the "2" drinks, in the row for 1 hour. You'll see your **BAC** is in the grey shaded zone. This means that if you drive after 2 drinks in 1 hour, you could be arrested. In the grey zone, your chances of having an accident are 5 times higher than if you had no drinks. But, if you had 4 drinks in 1 hour, your **BAC** would be in the black shaded area...and your chances of having an accident 25 times higher. What's more, it is **ILLEGAL** to drive at this **BAC** (.10% of greater). Before reaching the white **BAC** zone again, the chart shows you would need 4 more hours...with no more drinks.

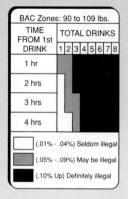
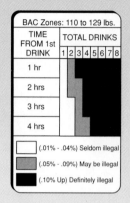
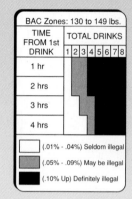
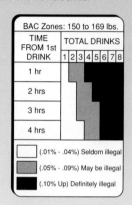

REMEMBER: "One drink" is a 12-ounce beer, or a 4-ounce glass of wine, or 1 1/4-ounce shot of 80-proof liquor (even if it's mixed with non-alcoholic drinks). If you have larger or stronger drinks, or drink on an empty stomach, or if you are tired, sick, upset, or have taken medicines or drugs, you can be **UNSAFE WITH FEWER DRINKS.**

TIPS TO HELP AVOID
*"Driving under the influence of alcohol and/or drugs" (DUI)**

- Set a safe limit in advance and don't go above it.
- Space your drinks...try not to have more than one drink per hour.
- Taper off and STOP DRINKING at least one hour before you drive.
- Eat before and during drinking.
- Don't drink alcohol if you're taking medicine or drugs.

> Distributed by the Department of Motor Vehicles and prepared in cooperation with the California Highway Patrol, The Office of Traffic Safety, the Department of Alcohol and Drug Programs, and the Department of Justice.

By strictly following these tips, you can greatly lower your chances of being arrested or having an accident.

Remember, coffee can't help, **ONLY TIME CAN LOWER YOUR BLOOD ALCOHOL CONCENTRATION (BAC)**...Some drivers can be under the influence at .03% **BAC.**

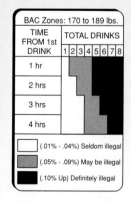
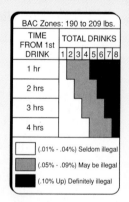
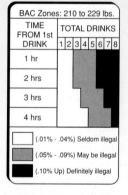
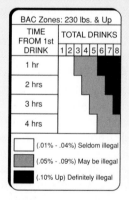

TECHNICAL NOTE: These charts are intended to be guides and are not legal evidence. Although it is possible for anyone to exceed the designated limits, the charts have been constructed so that fewer than 5 persons in 100 will exceed these limits when drinking the stated amounts on an empty stomach. Actual values can vary by body - type, sex, health status, and other factors.

*Violation of Vehicle Code Section 23152 or 23153 – driving under the influence of alcohol and/or drugs.

FIGURE 12.6

Between the years 1971 and 1985, the percentage of people drinking varying levels of alcohol has changed little.

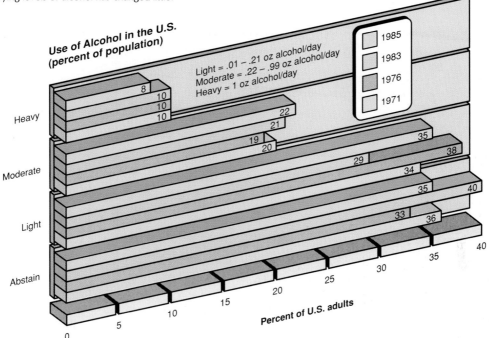

Use of Alcohol in the U.S.
(percent of population)

Light = .01 – .21 oz alcohol/day
Moderate = .22 – .99 oz alcohol/day
Heavy = 1 oz alcohol/day

1985
1983
1976
1971

Heavy: 8, 10, 10, 10

Moderate: 22, 21, 19, 20

Light: 35, 38, 29, 34

Abstain: 35, 40, 33, 36, 40, 35

Percent of U.S. adults

0, 5, 10, 15, 20, 25, 30, 35, 40

Figure 12.6 shows that between the years 1971 and 1985, the percentage of people drinking varying amounts of alcohol has changed very little. While 35 percent of Americans abstain totally from alcohol, 35 percent drink lightly (less than three drinks per week), 22 percent drink moderately (between three drinks per week and two drinks per day), and 8 percent drink heavily (two or more drinks per day) (19).

An estimated 18 million adults 18 years and older in the U.S. currently experience problems as a result of alcohol use. Of these, 10.6 million suffer from the disease of **alcoholism.** Alcohol-related problems may include symptoms of alcohol dependence such as memory loss, inability to stop drinking until intoxicated, inability to cut down on drinking, binge drinking, and withdrawal symptoms. Nearly 25 percent of adults experience acute monthly binge drinking, which is defined as consuming five drinks or more per occasion (20). Nearly five percent of high school seniors drink every day, and 37 percent drink heavily at least once every two weeks. Seventy percent of those 12–17 years old in the U.S. have used alcohol.

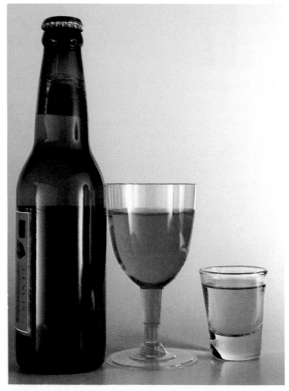

The same quantity of absolute alcohol is present in a bottle of beer, a glass of wine, and a shot of whiskey.

*F*IGURE 12.7

Increasing use of beer during the last 20–30 years has finally leveled off. Total ethanol consumption has also plateaued.

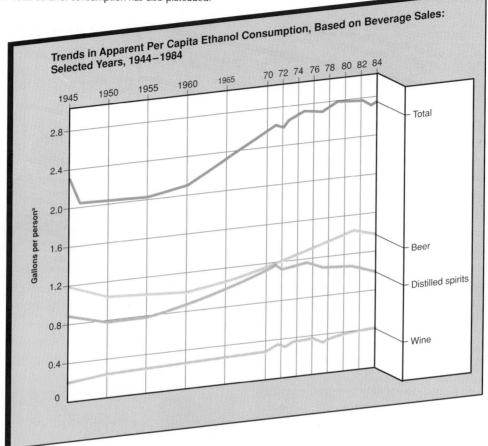

Trends in Apparent Per Capita Ethanol Consumption, Based on Beverage Sales: Selected Years, 1944–1984

[a]In U.S. gallons

Two-thirds of the adult U.S. population drink alcoholic beverages; however, the ten percent of these who drink most heavily drink half of the total amount of alcohol consumed. Alcohol abuse and alcoholism costs the U.S. nearly $120 billion per year in reduced productivity, premature death, and medical treatment.

Figure 12.7 shows that per capita rates of alcohol consumption rose approximately 21 percent during the 1960s, 10.3 percent during the 1970s, and 8.3 percent during the period from 1970 through 1982 (21).

Figure 12.8 shows that the estimated per capita consumption of alcohol in the U.S. was 2.65 gallons in 1984, the lowest since 1977 and the third consecutive annual decrease. The period 1981–1984 marked the first three-year decline since Prohibition. One of the 1990 Health Objectives for the Nation is that per capita consumption of alcohol not exceed 1978 rates. Although this objective has been achieved, producers of alcoholic beverages are increasing their promotional budgets and are expanding their product lines to appeal to both changing tastes and special-market segments in order to retain profitability (wine coolers, for example) (22).

Many individuals and organizations are very active in their efforts to reduce problem drinking, and this may be helping in reducing per capita consumption. The national effort to raise the minimum purchase age to 21 has been effective in an increasing number of states. Some states have enacted "dramshop" legislation, which makes the server responsible if a patron is involved in an accident after having consumed too much alcohol. There is also a move

*F*IGURE 12.8

One of the 1990 objectives for the nation is that per capita consumption of alcohol not exceed 1978 rates. This objective has been achieved, but producers are increasing their promotional budgets.

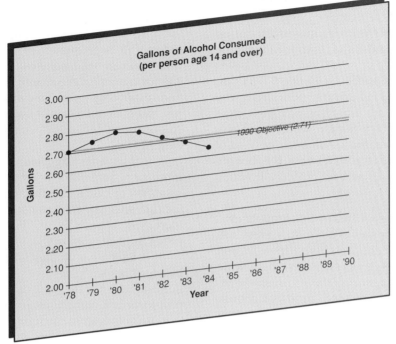

in some states to ban special low prices on drinks, such as for "happy hours" and "two-for-one" specials. Congress recently enacted legislation that modestly raises the excise tax on distilled spirits. Further, the increasing health consciousness of adults has led to a shift toward consumption of beverages with lower alcohol content and less drinking overall. In the 26 states that have raised their minimum drinking age between 1975 and 1984, nighttime fatal automobile crashes among 18- and 19-year-old drivers decreased 13 percent.

What Is Alcohol?

Ethyl alcohol (ethanol) is a social drug that is called a "sedative-hypnotic" because of its dramatic effects on the brain. Ethanol (CH_3CH_2OH) is a small, water-soluble molecule that is absorbed rapidly and completely from the stomach and small intestine. In the fasting state, after ingestion of ethanol, peak blood levels occur within 40 minutes. The presence of food in the stomach will delay absorption (23).

More than 90 percent of the ethanol ingested is broken down or oxidized in the liver, with the rest excreted through the lungs and urine. The amount of ethanol oxidized per unit of time is proportionate to body weight or liver weight. However, the amount of time that the liver takes to get rid of the alcohol varies widely among individuals. People accustomed to alcohol have an accelerated ethanol oxidation.

Ethanol increases urination (depresses secretion of the body's antidiuretic hormone). It also causes the blood vessels to dilate, so when the skin blood vessels are dilated after one drinks alcohol, body heat is released. Thus, when a person drinks high levels of alcoholic beverages in cold weather, hypothermia (loss of body heat which can lead to death) can result. The last drink you want that Saint Bernard (the famous rescue dog of the Swiss Alps) to bring you is an alcoholic beverage!

Alcohol-Related Disease and Mortality

Alcohol-Related Deaths

Alcoholics die earlier, with death rates from various causes being 2.5 times greater than that of nonalcoholics (24). Nearly 20,000 Americans die each year from cirrhosis of the liver and other alcohol-related diseases, and almost 8,000 more die from alcohol-related cancers, especially cancers of the mouth and throat areas. Deaths due to alcohol-related accidents, suicides, homicides, and other causes add nearly 140,000 more deaths to these figures.

Cirrhosis of the liver is most often caused by alcohol abuse and is the ninth leading cause of death in the U.S.

Of all fatal traffic accidents, 50–55 percent involve a drinking driver or pedestrian. The major cause of death among young persons is alcohol-related motor-vehicle accidents. Teenaged drivers account for less than six percent of motor-vehicle miles traveled in the U.S. but are involved in almost 15 percent of alcohol-related fatal crashes.

The Burden of Illness — Health Consequences

Even moderate amounts of alcohol can result in significant impairment in ability to drive, fly, and other activities requiring complex skills. A wide variety of psychomotor skills is adversely affected, such as reaction time, hand-eye coordination, accuracy, and balance. A consistent finding is the impairment of information processing. Blood alcohol levels as low as .04–.06 (two or three beers, for example) have been found to be sufficient to impair driving skills in the majority of subjects, leading to decreased peripheral vision, slower eye reaction, reduction of visual acuity by 30 percent, slower recovery from headlight glare, reduction in reaction time by 25 percent, impaired ability to concentrate on driving, impaired judgment of speed and distance of objects, increased self-confidence and risk-taking, and increased irresponsible driving. For these reasons, the American Medical Association is urging that all states adopt the 0.05 percent blood alcohol concentration levels as the legal limit, and that 21 years of age be designated as the legal drinking age (25).

The brain is markedly affected by ethanol more than any other organ. Effects include sedation, relief of anxiety, slurred speech, difficulty in walking, impaired judgment, and uninhibited behavior. There is some evidence that in alcoholics there is irreversible damage of brain cells (26). More research is needed to determine what effect, if any, social drinking has on brain cells.

Alcoholics experience more cancers of the mouth, tongue, throat, and esophagus than nonalcoholics. In some studies, excessive beer drinking has been associated with increased risk of colorectal cancer. There is some evidence of increased liver cancer following liver injury and cirrhosis from excessive ethanol consumption. Ethanol in large quantities acts in concert with inhaled cigarette smoke to further increase the risk for cancers of the mouth, larynx, esophagus, and respiratory tract. New evidence shows that just three alcohol drinks per week increase the risk of breast cancer in women by 40 to 50 percent (27).

Alcohol ingestion suppresses the immune system of the body, seriously impairing its ability to battle invading microbes (28). Risk for tuberculosis, infections, and cancer is thus increased, especially in people who drink alcohol in high amounts.

Excessive alcohol use is a major factor in liver diseases (fatty liver, cirrhosis, and alcoholic infection of the liver, or hepatitis). Stomach problems and chronic infection of the pancreas that are common in alcoholics are probably the result of heavy, long-term drinking.

Ethanol can lead to low blood glucose levels by reducing liver glucose output. Ethanol is also an irritant to the lining of the stomach and small intestine. In the stomach, this can lead to increased acid secretion, decreased mobility, decreased gastric emptying time, and acute infection of the stomach lining. In the small intestine, ethanol can lead to a decrease in nutrient absorption, a disruption of the normal gastrointestinal waves, and an alteration of the enzymes. Pancreatic function can be disturbed, and liver bile salts altered. Nutrient deficiencies can thus arise. Table 12.8 outlines the many nutritional consequences caused by chronic alcohol consumption. Recommendations center around a high nutrient-dense diet to counter some of these alcohol-related problems. For individuals suffering from these physical problems, the best policy is to stop alcohol consumption entirely.

Reduced sexual drive and/or impotence and infertility have been reported in 70–80 percent of alcoholics. Some 50 percent of alcoholic males develop feminine pubic hair patterns, and 20 percent experience breast enlargement.

TABLE 12.8
Effects of alcohol

Physical Problems	Nutrition Consequences	Recommendations
Mouth Poor hygiene, neglect. Decreased sense of taste. Sores, infection, sensitivity.	Avoiding foods that may irritate sores means less variety, loss of appetite. Dentures no longer fit.	Increase nutrient-rich foods; limit spicy, salty and acidic foods to promote healing; limit sugar to prevent decay.
Throat Pyloric valve malfunctioning. Swallowing difficulties. Problems from vomiting. Enlarged and twisted veins.	Heartburn, increased sensitivity leading to avoidance of many foods.	Take fluids between meals; eat slowly and chew thoroughly; try soft texture foods to aid in swallowing.
Stomach 20% of alcohol is absorbed directly in the stomach—this causes ulcers and cramps. Alcohol increases acid secretion and delays stomach emptying.	Alcohol absorption interferes with nutrient absorption; more nutrients are needed to compensate for those lost.	Increase nutrient-rich foods; eat slowly and chew food thoroughly.
Intestines 80% of alcohol is absorbed in the intestines—this causes ulcers and indigestion. Digestive enzymes impaired by alcohol. Food nutrients can't be absorbed—diarrhea results.	Malabsorption of nutrients caused by injured intestinal wall; many foods not tolerated; fat can't be digested; thiamin, folate, vitamin B_{12}, vitamin C, and vitamin K deficiency.	Increase nutrient-rich foods; low-fat diet; therapeutic vitamin supplement.
Liver Decreased ability to detoxify leads to increased level of fatty acids and uric acid—also decreased energy (glucose) and protein production. Fatty liver, hepatitis, cirrhosis.	Increased fat and cholesterol in the blood; gout; up-and-down blood sugar levels; indigestion; malabsorption; weight loss; malnutrition; anemia.	Increase nutrient-rich foods; low-fat diet; increase complex carbohydrate; therapeutic vitamin supplement.
Pancreas Decreased release of digestive enzymes.	Malabsorption of fat and protein; constipation or diarrhea; intense pain and weakness.	Low-fat diet.
Central Nervous System Decreased ability to think logically. "Fuzzy" perception. Poor memory. Vision problems. Hand and foot numbness and weakness (polyneuropathy). Increased temperature and blood pressure. Severe coordination problems and psychosis (Wernicke-Korsakoff Syndrome).	Impulsive and poor food selection; fatigue; malnutrition—especially B-vitamin deficiency; false perception of hunger.	Increase nutrient-rich foods; therapeutic vitamin supplementation; hospitalization during acute stage.
Heart Increased risk for heart disease. Fluid build up around heart.	Increased fat and cholesterol in blood; increased blood pressure; thiamin deficiency.	Low-fat diet; sodium restriction; exercise program; therapeutic vitamin supplement.
Kidneys Decreased hormone production which results in fluid loss. Kidney infection.	Mineral (magnesium, zinc, calcium) and vitamin (B,K) loss from increased excretion; cycle of dehydration and fluid retention; decreased vitamin D levels.	Increase nutrient-rich foods; increase high-potassium foods; decrease caffeine (it causes fluid loss); therapeutic vitamin supplement.
Hormones and Sexual Reproduction Increased estrogen level. Testicular atrophy, impotence.	Fat tissue buildup; food cravings; fluid retention.	Low-fat diet; moderate weight loss; extra vitamin E and zinc supplements are not helpful.
Bones and Body Tissue Decreased calcium in bones which may lead to osteoporosis. Increased % of body fat. Muscle loss and weakness.	Inactive vitamin D; low calcium intake; diet too low in Calories to preserve the muscle.	Increase calcium; low-fat dairy foods and green leafy vegetables are good sources; high complex carbohydrate, low-fat diet; decrease fat pounds; exercise program.

TABLE 12.9
Alcohol-related violence

	Victimization[1] Levels	Approximate Percentage[2] Alcohol-Related
Rape	39,000	19,500–50% of rape offenders
Completed		12,090–31% of rape victims
Attempted	134,000	67,000–50% of rape offenders
		41,540–31% of rape victims
Assault	1,707,000	
Aggravated		1,229,040–72% of offenders
Simple	3,041,000	1,348,530–79% were victims
Robbery	1,209,000	84,630–265,890–7–22% of offenders had been drinking
Fire — total fatalities	6,357	5,276–83% of fatalities
		2,796–53% of fatalities were alcoholics
Child abuse fatalities	210	84–40% of the parents have a history of problem drinking
Family violence	–	6% to 50% of marital violence is alcohol-related
Fetal alcohol syndrome[3]	–	1 per 2,000 live births . . . estimated at 1,650 cases per 3.3 million live births in 1977

[1]Bureau of Justice Statistics, Technical Report, March 1983.
[2]Fact Sheets, NCALI, October 1981.
[3]Facts About Alcohol and Alcoholism, NIAAA, 1980.

Data from NIAAA *Quick Facts*, August 1984.

Heavy use of alcohol by pregnant women may result in **fetal alcohol syndrome** (FAS) in their offspring. The effects of FAS may include growth retardation with decreased weight, height, and head circumference, and impairment of intellectual and motor functions and head abnormalities. Studies indicate that pregnant women should abstain completely from alcohol because no safe level of alcohol consumption has been established.

Having two to three drinks a day has now been closely related to elevated blood pressure. In moderate to heavy drinkers, the prevalence of systolic blood pressures over 140 mm Hg is four times greater than in people who abstain completely from alcohol.

Recent evidence has demonstrated that people who drink more than three drinks per day have four times the risk of stroke than light drinkers (29).

With an ethanol blood concentration of 100 mg/dL (BAC = .10, the legal limit when driving an automobile) the heart muscle cannot contract properly. Actual damage to the heart muscle can occur when alcohol consumption continues for ten or more years. This can lead to an increased risk of sudden death from abnormal heart electrical patterns.

Some research suggests that persons having ten drinks per week versus only one per week have increased death rates from various causes. Other studies have shown that death from coronary artery disease is less frequent in those who drink moderately versus those who totally abstain. Some researchers claim that alcohol increases the levels of high density lipoprotein cholesterol (HDL-C), which helps protect one from coronary heart disease. The Institute of Medicine, however, has reviewed the data and states that there are inconsistencies and conflicts among the studies, and that more study is needed to resolve the matter (30).

Even if moderate alcohol consumption is found to be associated with less coronary heart disease, advocating the use of alcohol for this reason would be unwise and simplistic. Ten percent of the population who use alcohol become problem drinkers. Table 12.9 shows that much of the violence in this country is alcohol-related.

A U.S. Department of Justice survey showed that nearly one-third of the nation's 523,000 state prison inmates drank heavily before committing rapes, burglaries, and assaults. Alcohol is involved in 40 percent of family court cases and one-third of child-abuse incidents. As many as 45 percent of the country's more than 250,000 homeless are alcoholics. Alcohol was involved in up to 70 percent of the 4,000 drowning deaths in 1986 and in 30 percent of the nearly 30,000 suicides. In addition, cancer rates are higher in those who drink alcoholic beverages regularly. Alcohol is considered the second leading cause of death in America, after cigarette smoking. There are too many problems associated with drinking to even think of recommending this approach for heart disease reduction. The "cure" would be far worse than the disease.

The Disease of Alcoholism

Alcoholism is a chronic, progressive, and potentially fatal disease. "Chronic and progressive" means that the physical, emotional, and social changes that develop are cumulative and become worse as the drinking continues. In time, the brain adapts to the presence of high concentrations of alcohol, and one feels "bad" when alcohol levels are low. Withdrawal symptoms occur from decreasing or ceasing consumption of alcohol. The alcoholic cannot consistently predict on any drinking occasion how much alcohol he or she will consume or how long the drinking will continue. In other words, there is little control. In time, the liver, brain, nerves, stomach, and small intestine develop life-threatening changes.

A person who is experiencing problems as a result of alcohol consumption needs professional help. Problems include the following:

Health problems: person reports that drinking has been harmful to health or that a physician has advised cutting down on alcohol intake.

Belligerence: gets into heated arguments after drinking.

Problems with friends: friends are advising that drinking needs to be cut back.

Symptomatic drinking: loss of control is experienced (drinking is secretive, drinks are gulped, memory lapses occur (blackouts), meals are skipped to allow more drinking, or drinking is engaged in to relieve a hangover).

Job problems: fellow workers are advising that drinking should be cut back because of decreased job performance.

Problems with the law, police, or traffic accidents: arrested while driving because of intoxication, or accident occurred because of drinking.

Binge drinking: intoxication has occured for several days in a row during past 12 months.

Psychological dependence: drinking is regularly engaged in to change a mood, e.g., to cheer up or calm down.

Problems with spouse: spouse has threatened to leave during the past two to three years because of drinking.

More than 500,000 Americans were reported to be in treatment for alcohol abuse and alcoholism in late September 1984. Studies show that about two-thirds of the treated alcoholics improve, helping to contain costs throughout the health-care system (24).

There are now more than 7,000 treatment programs for alcoholism, a 65 percent increase during the first six years of the 1980s. Alcoholics Anonymous is the single biggest source of support for chronic drinkers.

Alcoholics Anonymous (AA) is an organization composed of alcoholics who are trying to help themselves and others abstain from alcohol by offering encouragement and discussing experiences, problems, feelings, techniques, and issues. AA also sponsors similar groups for the spouses of alcoholics (Al-Anon) and for the children of alcoholics (Al-Teen). AA has groups in most cities in the U.S. and is listed in telephone books.

Researchers are finding more evidence that alcoholism can result from the interaction of both heredity and environment (31). Seventy percent of alcoholics have a family history of alcoholism. Children of alcoholics that are adopted have four times the risk for alcoholism than children of nonalcoholics. Thus, a genetic factor appears to explain why some people become alcoholics and others don't.

Two types of genetic predisposition to alcoholism have been identified: male-limited, which occurs early in males and with severe consequences; and environment-limited, which occurs later in life, is milder, and involves environmental influence (24).

Water and Electrolytes in Exercise

During heavy exercise like marathon running, the amount of heat produced by the body is so great that if it were not released from the body, lethal heat injury (hyperthermia) would occur within 20 minutes.

Obviously, the body must get rid of the heat quickly or one may end up exercising no more. The body's chief avenue of heat loss is evaporation of sweat. For every liter of sweat evaporated, close to 600 kcal are eliminated from the body (32).

It is not uncommon for humans to sweat 1.5 liters (about one quart) every hour during endurance sports like running, cycling, or soccer. In extremely hot conditions, sweat rates exceeding 2.5 liters per hour have been measured in fit individuals. Dr. Lawrence Armstrong of the U.S. Army Research Institute of Environmental Medicine reported that Alberto Salazar lost 12 pounds during the Olympic marathon. This means Salazar lost one pound of water (approximately one-half quart) every 11 minutes, or just over 2.5 quarts per hour.

When the body sweats profusely so that two percent or more of body weight is lost, the ability to perform is decreased because of high body temperatures and decreased blood flow from the heart. In other words, if a 150-pound person loses three pounds during exercise, the loss of water from the body is so great that performance is impaired.

One study has shown the dramatic effects of fluid replacement during exercise. A physically active, middle-aged male performed treadmill simulations of ten-mile races on two separate days in a heated chamber (95 degrees F). In the first trial, cold fluids were force-fed in 400-ml volumes at 20-minute intervals before and during the run. In the second trial, the exercise was repeated in the same fashion but without fluids. Results from the study showed that the water improved the ability to exercise, and heart rates and body temperatures were lower. In the no-fluid trial, premature exhaustion occurred at 6.8 miles because of high body temperatures (32). This experiment and others show the importance of drinking fluids beyond the thirst desire during exercise to enhance performance. In fact, most exercise physiologists say that runners, cyclers, and other athletes should drink more than they desire (at least one-third more) because during exercise, thirst falls behind actual body needs.

Table 12.10
Adverse effects of dehydration

Percent Weight	Symptoms
.5	Thirst
2.0	Stronger thirst, vague discomfort, loss of appetite
3.0	Increasing hemoconcentration, dry mouth, reduction in urine
4.0	Increased effort for exercise, flushed skin, impatience, apathy
5.0	Difficulty in concentrating
6.0	Impairment in exercise temperature regulation, increased heart rate
8.0	Dizziness, labored breathing in exercise, mental confusion
10.0	Spastic muscles, inability to balance with eyes closed, general incapacity, delirium and wakefulness, swollen tongue
11.0	Circulatory insufficiency, marked hemoconcentration and decreased blood volume, failing renal function

From J. E. Greenleaf and W. J. Fink. "Fluid Intake and Athletic Performance." In *Nutrition and Athletic Performance* (W. Haskell, ed.). © 1982. Palo Alto: Bull Publishing Co. Used with permission.

How much water should you drink during hard exercise? Forcing down 200–400 ml of water (at least one cup) every 20 minutes is advised. Fifteen minutes after drinking 400 ml of water 60–70 percent of the water is out of the stomach, being absorbed in the small intestine. Pure water is the best fluid to drink. Drinks that contain sugar can cause nausea and interfere with the body's ability to absorb the water.

The water should be cold (40–50 degrees F or "refrigerator cold") when drunk during exercise. The coldness increases gastric motility, allowing the stomach to empty the fluid more quickly into the small intestine, where it can be absorbed. The cold fluid will also help stabilize the core temperature of the body.

If water intake during exercise is low, dehydration can result. Table 12.10 outlines the adverse effects of dehydration.

Those most vulnerable to these adverse effects are the obese, unfit, dehydrated, unacclimatized (those not accustomed to the heat), or ill individuals who exercise on hot, humid, sunny days. Early warning signals include clumsiness, stumbling, excessive sweat, cessation of sweating, headache, nausea, or dizziness.

Should electrolytes be added to the exercise drink? The electrolyte content of sweat is very low compared to the body fluids. Although sodium, chloride, potassium, magnesium, calcium, zinc, and some vitamins are excreted with the sweat, most studies have shown that such losses in properly nourished individuals very rarely result in significant deficiencies of any essential nutrients (32).

Should people who exercise in the heat use salt tablets? No! People who have become used to exercising in the heat are very unlikely to develop sodium chloride deficiency despite high sweat rates, because with training they acquire adaptative mechanisms that lead to less salt loss in the urine and sweat. The salt content of a trained athlete's sweat is one-third that of the untrained. It usually only takes four to eight days of gradually increasing amounts of exercise in the heat to become adapted to it.

So in summary, one of the most important measures an athlete can take is to develop the habit of drinking plenty of water just before, during, and after exercise. The water should be cold, and drunk in 200–400 ml quantities every 20 minutes. This amount of water will be more than the athlete desires. There is no need for mixing sugar with the drink. There is no evidence that electrolytes need be included in the fluid drink. Most individuals will easily obtain all needed electrolytes in the food they eat following the exercise.

The Importance of Carbohydrate for Endurance Exercise

In addition to water, people who exercise heavily need carbohydrate. As we shall see, the harder and longer the exercise (such as marathon running), the greater the need for carbohydrate by the working muscles. During heavy exercise, the primary fuel for the muscle is *glycogen,* or stored carbohydrate, and the source for this glycogen is the carbohydrate you eat during your meals — pasta, potatoes, grains, and dried fruit, for example.

Outlined below are some of the reasons why carbohydrate is so important for endurance athletes (32).

1. *Body glycogen (carbohydrate) stores play an important role* in hard exercise that is both prolonged and continuous, such as in running, swimming, and cycling. Other sports that are of an aerobic nature, like soccer and basketball, also require large amounts of glycogen. Table 12.11 shows that the harder the intensity, the greater the demand for carbohydrate (CHO).

Table 12.11
How intensity affects what fuel the muscle uses

Exercise Intensity	Fuel Used by Muscle
Slow walking	Mainly muscle fat stores
Very brisk walking or slow jogging	Fat and CHO used evenly
Hard running — marathon	Mainly CHO
Very hard — near sprinting	Nearly 100% CHO

From D. C. Nieman, *The Sports Medicine Fitness Course.* © 1986. Palo Alto: Bull Publishing. Used with permission.

2. *Exhaustion during prolonged, hard exercise is tied to low muscle glycogen levels.* Glycogen is stored in the body from the carbohydrate you eat in your diet. During hard exercise, the primary fuel of the muscle is glycogen. Carbohydrate stores are thus the *limiting* factor in ability to perform such exercise. This has been repeatedly confimed in both cycling and treadmill-running experiments.

3. *During strenuous training, muscle glycogen stores undergo rapid day-to-day fluctuation.* Athletes, because of their hard training, have up to double the glycogen stores that sedentary people do. However, as figure 12.9 shows, these high levels in athletes can be quickly depleted during repeated, daily two-hour workouts. However, a high-carbohydrate diet can help counter this glycogen depletion.

In general, the greater the amount of carbohydrate eaten, the greater the amount of glycogen stored. On the basis of many experiments, it is recommended that athletes in heavy training consume a diet of 70 percent carbohydrate. This type of diet can help the body glycogen stores to keep at a high level, allowing the athlete to continue heavy training. Researchers have found, however, that this amount of carbohydrate is more than most athletes desire. Therefore, they need to be educated to arrange their diets to take in this large amount of carbohydrate. Athletes commonly underestimate their carbohydrate needs, and thus become energetically "stale" from glycogen depletion.

*F*IGURE 12.9

A low-carbohydrate diet results in a progressive reduction in muscle glycogen, whereas the high-carbohydrate diet helps to keep muscle glycogen stores near normal.

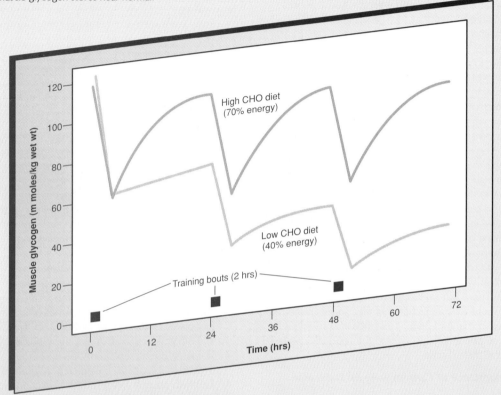

Table 12.12 outlines a sample menu for a high-carbohydrate diet. Notice that all of the minerals and vitamins and protein are adequately supplied by a high-carbohydrate diet. There is no need to use nutrient or protein supplements during heavy exercise training because a varied and healthy diet more than matches body demands. Several studies have shown that food supplements do not enhance performance (32).

People who exercise heavily need to emphasize two major changes in their diet — more water and more carbohydrate. With these changes, all other body nutrient needs will be supplied.

4. *Carbohydrate loading before the endurance event can improve performance.* When an athlete exercises longer than 75 minutes, body glycogen stores can drop very low, decreasing the ability to perform. However, it is possible to store more than the normal amount of glycogen by **"carbohydrate loading."** The old classical method had two stages.

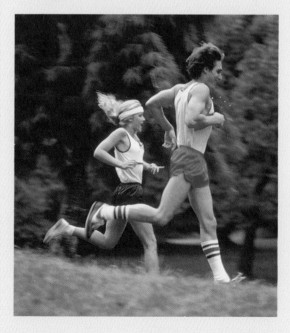

Table 12.12

Sample Menu of 3,500 kcal, high-carbohydrate (79% total kcal) diet

The foods listed below represent a one-day sample of the type of diet recommended for endurance training. This sample diet meets the RDA for all nutrients and follows the guidelines of the "prudent diet." Simple carbohydrates are avoided, and most of the Calories come during breakfast and lunch, with a lighter supper.

	Portion	Food	Kilocalories
Breakfast	1 cup	Grape Nuts	404
	2 cups	2% Low-fat milk	242
	1 whole	Banana	105
	.5 cup	Seedless raisins	247
	2 cups	Orange juice	224
	1 piece	Whole-wheat bread	84
	2 tsp	Honey	43
Lunch	2 pieces	Whole-wheat bread	168
	1 tbsp	Peanut butter	96
	2 whole	Apple	162
	2 cups	Cooked brown rice	464
	2 cups	Mixed vegetables	105
	1 tsp	Seasonings	5
	1 cup	Low-fat yogurt	231
	2 whole	Bagels (cinnamon)	330
Supper	.5 whole	Fresh tomato	12
	.5 cup	Loose leaf lettuce	5
	2 oz	Cooked chicken	108
	2 pieces	Whole-wheat bread	168
	1 tbsp	Low-cal dressing	35
	2 cups	Canned pineapple juice	278

Meal	Kilocalories	Total CHO	%CHO
Breakfast	1,349	290	86%
Lunch	1,561	292	75%
Supper	606	108	71%
Totals	3,516	690	79%

Nutrients	Protein	Iron	Zinc	Calcium	Vit C	Vit A	Vit B₁
Day Totals	116 g	25 mg	18 mg	1,579 mg	425 mg	15,009 I.U.	4.2 mg

Stage 1: Starve muscles of glycogen by eating a low-carbohydrate diet for three days while engaging in two intense, prolonged exercise sessions.

Stage 2: Supercompensate muscle glycogen by resting for three days before competition while eating a 90-percent carbohydrate diet.

This regimen has been found to create very high muscle glycogen levels. Unfortunately, several undesirable side effects occur during the depletion phase, including marked physical and mental fatigue, depression, and irritability. During replenishment, the athlete often feels heavy and stiff in the legs.

Because of these side effects, researchers have sought to modify the depletion phase. Instead of three days of low-carbohydrate and hard exercise, the modified scheme utilizes a slow tapering of exercise over a six-day period. During the first three days of this tapering, the diet is a normal mixed diet of 50 percent CHO Calories. During the last three days, a diet that is 70 percent CHO is consumed. This modified regimen has been found to create muscle glycogen levels nearly as high as the old classical method, without all undesirable depletion side effects.

Table 12.13
Alcoholic beverages (percent USRDA)

Type of Alcoholic Beverage (% Calories alcohol)	Quantity	Calories	Vit A	Thiamin	Riboflavin	Vit C	Calcium	Iron	Magnesium
80-proof gin, rum, vodka, whiskey (100%)	1.25 oz	80	0%	0%	0%	0%	0%	0%	0%
Wine — red (89%)	4 fl oz	85	0%	0%	2%	0%	1%	3%	4%
Wine — white (96%)	4 fl oz	79	0%	0%	0%	0%	1%	2%	3%
Beer — regular (61%)	12 fl oz	146	0%	1%	5%	0%	2%	1%	5%
Beer — light (79%)	12 fl oz	100	0%	2%	6%	0%	2%	1%	4%
Bloody Mary (80%)	5 fl oz	116	5%	3%	2%	34%	1%	3%	3%
Daiquiri (85%)	2 fl oz	111	0%	1%	0%	2%	0%	0%	0%
Manhattan (94%)	2 fl oz	128	0%	0%	0%	0%	0%	0%	0%
Martini (99%)	2.5 fl oz	156	0%	0%	0%	0%	0%	0%	0%
Screwdriver (54%)	7 fl oz	174	1%	9%	2%	111%	2%	1%	4%

Note: Notice that the Bloody Mary and Screwdriver are high in vitamin C because they contain tomato juice and orange juice, respectively.

Data from U.S. Department of Agriculture Food Composition Tables (Handbook No. 8 series).

Do Alcoholic Beverages Aid in Athletic Performance?

Long endurance athletes are being advised by various magazines to drink alcoholic beverages to gain certain benefits. Beer has been presented as a "soup to replace lost electrolytes." The alcohol of beer or wine will "relax muscles and improve emotional state." Runners are urged to "have a beer with your pasta" to carbohydrate load before a race. To recover from a race, athletes are advised they would do well to drink wine or beer to remove aches and pains.

Some athletes believe that drinking wine or beer during long endurance events will enhance performance. For example, during the 1979 Great Hawaiian Footrace, a 500-km road run held over 20 days, athletes averaged seven cans of beer per day.

The combination of alcohol and exercise is not new. The ancient Greek games were accompanied by great revelry and the drinking of prodigious amounts of wine. Spiridon Loues, winner of the first Olympic marathon in 1896 drank several cups of white-resin wine during the race, supposedly to power him to victory. At the turn of the century, it was standard practice for runners to quaff champagne or brandy immediately before a race.

The claims that wine and beer provide good amounts of carbohydrate and electrolytes for the athlete cannot be substantiated. According to the Nutrient Data Research Group of the USDA, one 12 fl oz portion of beer provides only about 50 Calories of carbohydrate, enough to run about one-half mile. Red or white wine contain less than ten Calories of carbohydrate per serving. Since these servings of beer or wine also contain one-half ounce of ethanol, which raises the blood alcohol to .02 (in a 150-pound man), to obtain enough carbohydrate to run just 2.5 miles would mean the blood alcohol level would rise to 0.10, which violates the drinking and driving laws of most states. In other words, to get enough carbohydrate from beer or wine to get anywhere, one would be too drunk to be a legal driver.

The amounts of minerals and vitamins in beer and wine are too low to be of health value. (See table 12.13.) All the electrolytes are very low, by the RDA standards.

The ethanol in alcoholic beverages is unavailable to the working muscle for energy. Researchers have documented that alcohol elimination is increased during exercise but that the alcohol is not being used in any form by the muscle (32). The enhanced alcohol elimination during exercise is probably due to increased liver enzyme activity induced by an increase in body temperature.

Alcohol has various side effects that are detrimental to exercise performance. Lactate levels are increased, urine output increases, the central nervous system is sedated, heart muscle contraction is depressed, the blood vessels dilate, and blood glucose levels decrease (159). Small to moderate doses for alcohol have a deleterious effect on a wide variety of psychomotor skills. In cold environments, alcohol leads to impairment of the body's blood glucose levels and ability to keep body temperature levels normal.

For all these reasons, the American College of Sports Medicine and the American Dietetic Association have both concluded that alcohol has no real benefits during exercise and, in most instances, appears to be detrimental to optimal performance (32).

SUMMARY

1. Approximately 60 percent of adult human body weight is water, with most of this water found inside the cells of the body (intracellular water). Sodium, potassium, and other minerals regulate the flow of water in and out of body cells.
2. Every body function depends on an ample supply of water. Digestion, nutrient transport, kidney function, joint lubrication, and maintenance of body temperature are important examples.
3. The body loses at least three quarts of fluid a day, depending on sweat losses. The majority of water leaving the body is routed through the kidneys, followed by the skin, lungs, and rectum.
4. Dehydration causes a change in the electrolyte balance. Cells become dehydrated, and the thirst alarm is set off in the hypothalamus. The antidiuretic hormone is then secreted to signal the kidney to preserve water. Infants, the elderly, and athletes are at risk for dehydration.
5. The average American drinks only 3.3 cups of water per day, far below the recommended six to ten cups. Total fluid intake from all sources varies widely, ranging from one to six quarts a day.
6. In the U.S., the quality of the drinking water supply is considered by most public health experts to be excellent.
7. Caffeine consumption is quite high, averaging 227 mg per day for U.S. adults. Coffee consumption, however, has decreased dramatically during the past 25 years. Soft drinks, however, are now the primary source of caffeine for children. Chocolate and many drugs also contain caffeine.
8. High levels of caffeine intake are associated with various health problems, including caffeinism, heart disease, and cancer.
9. An estimated 18 million U.S. adults experience problems with alcohol. Per capita consumption of alcohol is at its lowest level since 1977.
10. Alcohol is a social drug that has dramatic effects on the brain. More than 90 percent of the ethanol ingested is broken down in the liver.
11. Abuse of alcohol is associated with many health problems, including cirrhosis of the liver, impairment of psychomotor skills, cancer, impairment of the immune system, disruption of normal stomach and intestine function, reduced sexual drive, fetal alcohol syndrome, elevated blood pressure, and violence-related deaths.
12. Alcoholism is a chronic, progressive, and potentially fatal disease that needs professional treatment.
13. Sports nutrition is based on two factors—increasing intakes of both water and carbohydrate. Alcohol, vitamin and mineral supplements, and other substances do not improve performance.

REFERENCES

1. Anderson, B., L. G. Leksell, and M. Rundgren. 1982. Regulation of Water Intake. *Annual Review of Nutrition* 2:73-89.
2. Vokes, T. 1987. Water Homeostasis. *Annual Review of Nutrition* 7:383-406.
3. Robinson, J. R. 1970. Water, the Indispensible Nutrient. *Nutrition Today* (Spring):pp. 16-29.
4. Shils, M. E., and V. R. Young. 1988. *Modern Nutrition in Health and Disease*. Philadelphia: Lea & Febiger.
5. National Research Council. 1980. Recommended Dietary Allowances. 9th ed. Washington, D.C.: National Academy of Sciences.
6. Consumer Nutrition Division, Human Nutrition Information Service, U.S. Department of Agriculture. 1984. Nutrient Intakes: Individuals in 48 States, Year 1977-78. Nationwide Food Consumption Survey 1977-78, Report No. I-2 (May).

7. Stumbo, P. J., et al. 1985. Water Intakes of Lactating Women. *American Journal of Clinical Nutrition* 42:870–76.
8. EPA Sets Drinking Water Standards for Eight Pollutants. 1987. *The Nation's Health.* (August):p. 16.
9. Coelho, T. 1982. Water and Food Supply. *Journal of the American Dietetic Association* 80:311.
10. Ballentine, C. L., and M. L. Herndon. 1983. The Water That Goes into Bottles. *FDA Consumer* (May):pp. 5–7.
11. Institute of Food Technologists Expert Panel on Food Safety and Nutrition. 1987. Evaluation of Caffeine Safety — A Scientific Status Summary. *Food Technology* (June):pp. 105–13.
12. Arbeit, M. L., et al. 1988. Caffeine Intakes of Children from a Biracial Population: The Bogalusa Heart Study. *Journal of the American Dietetic Association* 88:466.
13. Lecos, C. W. 1987–88. Caffeine Jitters: Some Safety Questions Remain. *FDA Consumer* (December 1987-January 1988):pp. 22–27.
14. LaCroix, A. Z., et al. 1986. Coffee Consumption and the Incidence of Coronary Heart Disease. *New England Journal of Medicine* 315:977–82.
15. LeGrady, D., et al. 1987. Coffee Consumption and Mortality in the Chicago Western Electric Company Study. *American Journal of Epidemiology* 126:803–12.
16. Levinson, W., and P. M. Dunn. 1986. Nonassociation of Caffeine and Fibrocystic Breast Disease. *Archives of Internal Medicine* 146:1773–1775.
17. Martin, T. R., and M. B. Bracken. 1987. The Association between Low Birth Weight and Caffeine Consumption during Pregnancy. *American Journal of Epidemiology* 126:813–21.
18. Pozniak, P. C. 1985. The Carcinogencity of Caffeine and Coffee: A Review. *Journal of the American Dietetic Association* 85:1127–1133.
19. National Center for Health Statistics: Health, United States, 1986. DHHS Pub. No. (PHS) 87–1232. Public Health Service. Washington, D.C.: U.S. Government Printing Office.
20. Office of Disease Prevention and Health Promotion, U.S. Public Health Service, U.S. Department of Health and Human Services. 1988. *Disease Prevention/Health Promotion: The Facts.* Palo Alto: Bull Publishing.
21. U.S. Department of Health and Human Services. Prevention '86/'87: Federal Programs and Progress. Washington, D.C.: U.S. Government Printing Office.
22. Public Health Service, U.S. Department of Health and Human Services. Office of Disease Prevention and Health Promotion. 1986. The 1990 Health Objectives for the Nation: A Midcourse Review. Washington, D.C.: U.S. Government Printing Office.
23. Katzung, B. G. 1982. *Basic and Clinical Pharmacology.* Los Altos: Lange Medical Publications.
24. Sixth Special Report to Congress on Alcohol and Health. National Clearinghouse on Alcohol and Drug Information.
25. AMA Council on Scientific Affairs. 1986. Alcohol and the Driver. *Journal of the American Medical Association* 255:522–27.
26. Harper, C., J. Kril, and J. Daly. 1987. Are We Drinking Our Neurones Away? *British Medical Journal* 294:534–36.
27. Schatzkin, A., et al. 1987. Alcohol Consumption and Breast Cancer in the Epidemiologic Follow-Up Study of the First National Health and Nutrition Examination Survey. *New England Journal of Medicine* 316:1169–1173.
28. MacGregor, R. R. 1986. Alcohol and Immune Defense. *Journal of the American Medical Association* 256:1474–1478.
29. Gill, J. S., et al. 1987. Stroke and Alcohol Consumption, *New England Journal of Medicine* 315:1041–1046.
30. Hamburg, D. A. 1982. *Health and Behavior.* Washington, D.C.: National Academy Press.
31. Schuckit, M. A. 1985. Genetics and the Risk for Alcoholism. *Journal of the American Medical Association* 254:2614–2617.
32. Nieman, D. C. 1986. *The Sports Medicine Fitness Course.* Palo Alto: Bull Publishing.

*H*EALTH-PROMOTION ACTIVITY 12.1
How Much Water Do You Drink Each Day?

As discussed in this chapter and as outlined in table 12.2, males 19 to 22 years of age drink just under four cups of water a day, and females of the same age drink 3.2 cups per day. At least six to eight cups of water should be ingested every day, and much more than this if sweating from exercise occurs.

In this Health-Promotion Activity, you will keep a record of how much water (*not* flavored beverages, just plain water) you drink for one 24-hour period. Try to follow your normal habits, and fill in the worksheet below. Compare your results with table 12.2. How close did you adhere to the recommended pattern of water consumption outlined in this chapter?

Worksheet to Measure Water Consumption for One 24-Hour Period

Time of Day	Amount of Water Consumed (in cups) (1 cup = 8 fl oz)	Place

Total cups of water/24-hour period = _____

HEALTH-PROMOTION ACTIVITY 12.2
How Much Caffeine Did You Consume Today?

As outlined in tables 12.3, 12.5, and 12.7, caffeine is found in many beverages, foods, and drugs. Because caffeine has been related to a host of health problems, it is wise to keep total caffeine intake below 100 mg a day. In this Health-Promotion Activity, you will record in the worksheet below all the caffeine-containing foods, drugs, and beverages you ingest during one 24-hour period, and then use tables 12.3, 12.5, and 12.7 to calculate how many milligrams of caffeine you consumed. Be sure to note portion sizes carefully.

Worksheet to Calculate Total Caffeine Intake for One 24-Hour Period

Time of Day	Food, Beverage, or Drug	Portion Size	Caffeine Content

Total caffeine intake _____ mg

HEALTH-PROMOTION ACTIVITY 12.3
Do You Have a Problem with Alcohol?

This questionnaire is designed to help you determine whether you have a problem with alcohol. Record your answer to each question in the right-hand column. Follow the scoring instructions at the end of the questionnaire.

Health Problems   *Yes*   *No*

Have your drinking habits been harmful to your health, or has a physician advised you to cut down on alcohol intake? _____ _____

Belligerence

Do you get into heated arguments after drinking? _____ _____

Problems with friends

Are friends advising you that your drinking needs to be cut back? _____ _____

Symptomatic drinking

Do you drink secretly? _____ _____

Do you gulp your drinks? _____ _____

Do you suffer memory lapses? _____ _____

Do you skip meals to allow more drinking? _____ _____

Do you drink to relieve a hangover? _____ _____

Job problems

Are fellow workers advising you that your drinking should be cut back because of decreased job performance? _____ _____

Problems with the law

Has your drinking gotten you into trouble with the police? _____ _____

Has your drinking led to a traffic accident? _____ _____

Have you been arrested while driving because of intoxication? _____ _____

Binge drinking

Have you been drunk for several days in a row during the past 12 months? _____ _____

Psychological dependence

Do you drink to change your mood (e.g., to cheer up or calm down)? _____ _____

Problems with family

Have you been fighting with your family over your drinking habits? _____ _____

Scoring:

Number of "yes" responses:

None	No apparent problem with alcohol.
1–2	Early warning signals that drinking is becoming a problem.
3 or more	You are a problem drinker and should seek professional help.

UNIT

IV

Nutrition throughout the Life Cycle

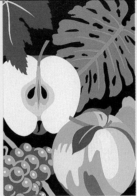

Nutrition is important throughout the life cycle, but there are certain time periods when nutrition is critical. Pregnancy makes many nutritional demands on the prospective mother, the most important need being that of the unborn infant. Other critical time periods include the first year of life, when the infant is growing quickly and the mother may be breast-feeding; the turbulent adolescent years; and the "twilight" years, when humans draw near the close of life. Chapters 13 through 15 review the influence of nutrition throughout the life span.

Special topics of interest will also be discussed, including the importance of breast-feeding, the relationship between diet and behavior, the role of nutrition in the prevention and treatment of osteoporosis (low mineral mass in the bone), and the significance of a healthy diet for the optimal functioning of the immune system.

FIGURE 13.2
Development of a fetus.

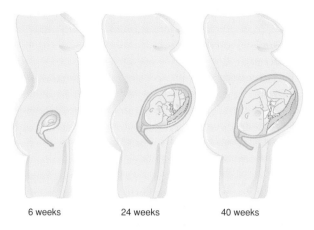

6 weeks   24 weeks   40 weeks

At the close of the first trimester of pregnancy, all the major structures, internal and external, have begun to form. Therefore, this period is the most critical phase of human development (see figure 13.3). Anything that disrupts development at this time will most likely result in a major birth defect or in the death of the embryo. Drugs, alcohol, viruses, chemicals, and radiation are some of the agents that can lead to birth defects during this period.

Second Trimester
During the second three-month period the mother becomes keenly aware of the movements within her growing abdomen. All organs are fairly well formed, and the fetus weighs about two pounds by the end of this stage. However,

FIGURE 13.3
Critical periods of development. Teratogens can cause anatomical and physiological defects during fetal development.

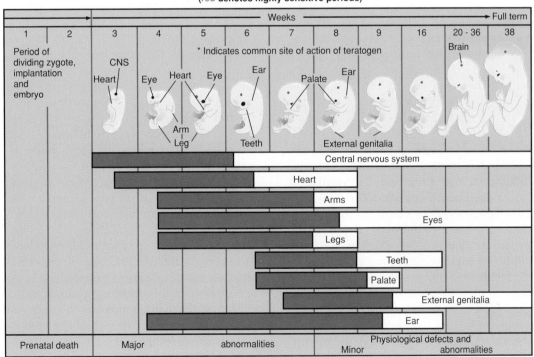

if the fetus is born during the second trimester, chances of survival are only fair to poor because the respiratory system is too immature to sustain life outside the womb.

Third Trimester

The fetus gains more than two-thirds of its birth weight during these last three months of pregnancy. A full-term baby weighs, on the average, 7.5 pounds and measures 20 inches in length. Chances for survival of a fetus born during the last trimester are excellent because the fetus is just acquiring the "finishing touches," and the vulnerable lungs are fairly well developed.

Nutritional Concerns during Pregnancy

Weight Gain during Pregnancy

The idea of gaining weight during pregnancy often creates mixed emotions. Some women fear the weight gain. Others see pregnancy as an opportunity to eat anything they want since they are "eating for two," and any extra weight will be due to the baby, not fat. Clearly, there is a distinction between being fat and being pregnant. A pregnant woman needs to focus on producing a healthy baby and on consuming the amount and type of nutrients that will accomplish this.

From the 1950s until the 1970s, physicians often advised limiting weight gain during pregnancy to between 10 and 15 pounds. This resulted in smaller babies that were easier to deliver, thus reducing the need for a cesarean-section delivery, a very dangerous procedure at that time. A limited weight gain was also thought to decrease the chances of another serious complication of late pregnancy: **toxemia,** or **pregnancy-induced hypertension.** This condition is characterized by edema (the accumulation of excess water in the body tissues), high blood pressure, and kidney damage. As pregnancy-induced hypertension progresses, it may lead to convulsions, coma, and even death of the mother and fetus. The sudden, rapid weight gain that occurs with pregnancy-induced hypertension is not caused by the overconsumption of Calories, as was once thought, but to the edema. Research studies have now confirmed that the restriction of weight gain during pregnancy does not prevent pregnancy-induced hypertension.

Current medical opinion on the topic of weight gain differs greatly from that of 20 to 30 years ago. The American College of Obstetrics

Component	Pounds Gained
Fetus	7.3
Placenta	1.4
Amniotic fluid	1.8
Uterus	2.0
Breast tissue	0.9
Blood supply	2.7
Total accounted for	16.1
Increase in maternal fat reserves and other weight gain	7.9–18.9
Total body-weight gained	24.0–35.0

TABLE 13.1
Components of weight gain during pregnancy

From Committee on Maternal Nutrition. Food and Nutrition Board, National Academy of Sciences. *Maternal Nutrition and the Course of Pregnancy,* 1977.

and Gynecology now recommends a weight gain of 22 to 28 pounds (2). Women who are more than 20 percent underweight may be advised by their physicians to gain more, while those who are 20 percent or more overweight may be advised to gain slightly less. Adequate weight gain for the mother is one of the best predictors of pregnancy outcome (3). Within the recommended limits, the more weight a women gains during pregnancy, the more the baby will weigh, and vice versa. One of the biggest problems with gaining more than 30 pounds is getting rid of the weight afterwards.

Low-birth-weight infants (under 5.5 pounds) are 40 times more likely to be ill and/or die during the first year of life (4). In a national study on the effect of weight gain on pregnancy outcome, women who gained between 26 and 35 pounds were the least likely to have low-birth-weight infants, and those who gained less than 21 pounds were twice as likely to have low-birth-weight infants (5). Therefore, dietary restriction for weight gains of less than 21 pounds is not recommended during pregnancy.

If the average newborn weighs only 7.5 pounds, what does the rest of the weight gain consist of? (See table 13.1.) The fetus is supported by a placenta, **amniotic fluid** (fluid that surrounds the fetus in utero), a uterus, and an increase in the maternal blood supply. The breast tissue also develops in preparation for nursing after delivery, and fat is accumulated to store energy to produce milk. All of these are essential in producing a healthy baby.

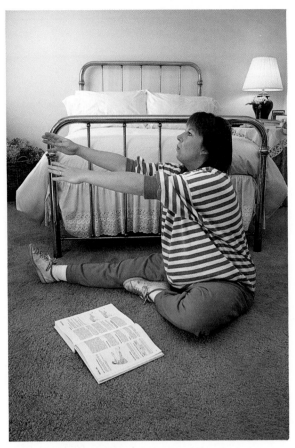
Two-thirds of the weight gained during pregnancy is accumulated in the last trimester.

certainly expected; however, the tissues need a constant supply of nutrients available for growth. It is therefore helpful if the addition of Calories is fairly uniform over the last six months.

Suppose that a pregnant woman has already gained twenty pounds by the beginning of her eighth month. This is not the time to diet. Perhaps a diet record would be beneficial in discovering the source of extra Calories. This record may reveal overconsumption of sweets, soft drinks, and high-Calorie snack foods. The object is not to stop weight gain but to slow it, to no more than one pound per week.

Nutritional Needs during Pregnancy

Calories In order to have a gradual but steady weight gain, the body will need to take in more Calories. The Food and Nutrition Board currently recommends that no additional Calories are needed during the first trimester. However, 300 extra Calories per day are required during the last two trimesters.

Obviously, with this small increase in Calories, the pregnant woman is not "eating for two." In addition, pregnancy often causes a woman to decrease her activity level due to morning sickness, fatigue, excess weight, or aches and discomforts. If this occurs, energy is being saved, and less than 300 extra Calories per day will need to be added. Keeping weekly records of the pregnant woman's weight gain will help to assess how much to adjust her intake of food (6).

Protein Calories alone are not sufficient to support the growth of a baby. Approximately two pounds of protein are deposited in the fetus and accessory tissues of the woman. The additional daily requirement is 10 g of protein, or one additional serving of milk daily. A total of two protein servings and three to four milk servings per day is required during pregnancy.

Although protein is generally regarded as extremely important for the pregnant woman, it is seldom a problem. Most women in the United States get enough protein to support a pregnancy.

Knowing where the weight goes makes it easier to understand how to distribute the weight gain during the nine months.

In the first trimester, qualitative nutritional needs are of primary importance. A two- to four-pound weight gain is sufficient for this initial period. The last two trimesters demand not only quality but quantity.

Most of the accumulation of weight in the second trimester is due to maternal tissue growth. In particular, the breasts, uterus, and blood volume are all increasing in size. The fetus, the placenta, and the amniotic fluid are responsible for the majority of the weight gain needed in the last three months. In the last two trimesters almost one pound per week should be gained. Fluctuations in this weight gain are certainly expected; however, the tissues need a constant supply of nutrients available for growth. It is therefore helpful if the addition of Calories is fairly uniform over the last six months.

TABLE 13.2
Recommended daily dietary allowances for girls and women at various ages, and for pregnancy

	Recommended Daily Allowances for Nonpregnant Women				Recommended Daily Allowances for Pregnancy
	11–14* Years Old	15–18† Years Old	19–24‡ Years Old	25–50§ Years Old	
Energy (kcal)	2,200	2,200	2,200	2,200	2500 2nd & 3rd trimester
Protein (g)	46	44	46	50	60
Vitamin A (μg RE)//	800	800	800	800	800
Vitamin D (μg)#	10	10	10	5	10
Vitamin E (mg α-TE)**	8	8	8	8	10
Ascorbic acid (mg)	50	60	60	60	70
Folacin (μg)	150	180	180	180	400
Niacin (mg NE)††	15	15	15	15	17
Riboflavin (mg)	1.3	1.3	1.3	1.3	1.6
Thiamin (mg)	1.1	1.1	1.1	1.1	1.5
Vitamin B_6 (mg)	1.4	1.5	1.6	1.6	2.2
Vitamin B_{12} (μg)	2.0	2.0	2.0	2.0	2.2
Calcium (mg)	1,200	1,200	1.200	800	1,200
Phosphorus (mg)	1,200	1,200	1,200	800	1,200
Iodine (μg)	150	150	150	150	175
Iron (mg)	15	15	15	15	30
Magnesium (mg)	280	300	280	280	320
Zinc (mg)	12	12	12	12	15

*Weight, 46 kg height, 157 cm.
†Weight, 55 kg height, 163 cm.
‡Weight, 58 kg height, 164 cm.
§Weight, 63 kg height, 163 cm.
//Retinol equivalents. 1 retinol equivalent = 1 mcg retinol or 6 mcg beta-carotene.
#As cholecalciferol. 10 mcg = 400 IU of vitamin D.
**Alpha-tocopherol equivalents. 1 mg d-alpha-tocopherol = 1 α-TE.
††1 NE (niacin equivalent) is equal to 1 mg niacin or 60 mg of dietary tryptophan.

Reprinted with permission from: Food and Nutrition Board. Recommended Dietary Allowances. 10th rev. ed. 1989. Washington, DC: National Academy Press, 1989.

Vitamins In order to utilize extra energy and build fetal and maternal tissues, additional vitamins are needed. Table 13.2 lists the 1989 RDA for the pregnant woman. If the extra Calories are chosen wisely, the vitamins will be present in the pregnant woman's food.

One serious vitamin deficiency that is common during pregnancy is that of folacin. Folacin functions as an essential coenzyme in cell division, so there is a substantial increase in demand for this nutrient. The RDA is 400 micrograms per day, double that of the nonpregnant female. Folacin deficiency is associated with low birth weight, miscarriages, birth defects, and toxemia in some studies (7). Folacin deficiency may also be a factor in morning sickness.

Good food sources of folacin include grain products, legumes, green vegetables, oranges, strawberries, bananas, and cantaloupe. Supplementation may be neccesary for those manifesting symptoms of morning sickness or for those who have an inadequate intake as revealed by diet history. Consultation with a health-care provider is recommended before taking folacin supplements because of possible deleterious interaction with other nutrients.

Minerals The requirements for all minerals are increased during pregnancy, as shown in table 13.2. Most of these requirements will be met by good choices of whole grains, legumes, dairy products, fruits, and vegetables. Usually, if a mother does not ingest adequate nutrients, the fetus is deprived. However, the fetus will drain the mother's stores of the minerals calcium and iron. The greatest need for these minerals is during the last trimester of pregnancy.

Adequate supplies of calcium and phosphorus are required to supply the needs of the mother and the growing fetus. Approximately 30 g of calcium are found in the full-term infant, most of which (300 mg daily) is deposited during the last three months of pregnancy (8). The mother also appears to store extra calcium in anticipation of the greatly increased requirements of lactation.

The current RDA for calcium in pregnancy is 1,200 mg, or 400 mg more than that recommended for the nonpregnant female. It is virtually impossible to meet these requirements with natural foods other than dairy products. The 1,200 mg per day allowance is contained in one quart, or four cups, of milk. Pregnant women who develop the habit of drinking milk will not only supply the fetus with needed calcium but can set a valuable example for her family. Other good sources of calcium include green leafy vegetables and some canned fish (sardines and salmon).

Inadequate calcium intake increases the chance of developing osteoporosis. Pregnancy, because of its high demands for calcium, may place a woman at serious risk for this bone-crippling disease. Therefore, if a woman is not able to get four servings of milk per day, a calcium supplement should be considered.

Women of childbearing age must also be concerned about getting enough iron. Women normally lose iron when they menstruate, but during pregnancy this iron is conserved. Despite this, the RDA for pregnant women is 15 mg per day more than that recommended for nonpregnant women. There are several reasons for this increase. The pregnant woman's blood volume increases by about 33 percent, a small portion of which is additional red blood cells. Iron is needed for their manufacture. Also, the placenta and uterus require iron as they grow. Iron is particularly important during the last trimester because it is transferred from the mother to the infant for storage. This is necessary to sustain the infant for the first four to six months after birth, when milk, a poor source of iron, makes up the diet.

The best food sources of iron are meats, dried legumes, whole grains, dried fruits, and some dark green leafy vegetables. The absorption of iron from plant sources is enhanced by vitamin C. Therefore, pregnant women try to consume citrus fruits and juices, melons, strawberries, broccoli, green pepper, and other good sources of vitamin C, along with foods high in iron.

The majority of physicians in the United States favor routine supplementation of iron during pregnancy. Levels of supplementation of 30 mg per day result in normal hemoglobin and hematocrit values (screening measures of iron status) for the mother and child at delivery (9). Iron supplements should be continued for two to three months after delivery, if necessary, to replenish the mother's stores.

Supplementation   The need for nutritive supplements other than iron for pregnant women is not fully supported in the literature. Nonetheless, the standard practice of most physicians is to prescribe prenatal vitamins and minerals. There are several points to remember about this recommendation. Although vitamins play a very essential role in making energy available, they do not replace food. Once again, after making sure that one consumes the recommended increases of milk and protein, complex carbohydrates are an excellent source of fuel, vitamins, and minerals.

The pregnant woman should take a prenatal vitamin and mineral supplement if one is prescribed for her. These are based on the RDA and contain safe levels of the nutrients needed by mother and baby. It can be dangerous to self-medicate on supplements that are not prescribed. High doses of vitamins are known to cause defects in the developing fetus. For example, excess vitamin C can cause a rebound scurvy after the birth of the infant, even if the infant is receiving adequate vitamin C. Likewise, large doses of vitamin A can lead to deformities in the urinary system of the infant, and megadoses of vitamin D can deform the head, face, and heart valves (10). Since vitamins and minerals interact with each other, high doses of one may decrease the bioavailability of another. Large doses of iron, for instance, can decrease the absorption of zinc.

Guidelines for Nutritious Eating While Pregnant

The daily food guides can provide some valuable insight into a pregnant woman's current eating habits. They can also be used to make a daily eating plan to help her meet her nutritional needs. (See Health-Promotion Activity 13.1.)

Food-Related Discomforts of Pregnancy

Pregnancy has many ups and downs, and some of these can be eased by additions or deletions of certain foods.

Nausea and/or Vomiting

The term "morning sickness" can be quite misleading. Although this feeling of nausea often occurs when the stomach is empty, as it is in the morning, some women have it all day. Symptoms may range from slight sickness to vomiting several times per day. The cause of morning sickness is not fully understood, but it is most certainly related to the rising levels of various hormones during the first trimester of pregnancy.

There are several dietary strategies for avoiding or alleviating morning sickness. Sipping warm water and eating a few dry crackers or toast upon waking may ease the discomfort. Eating six small meals per day, or several small snacks, may be beneficial since morning sickness worsens when the stomach is empty. As a general rule the pregnant woman should avoid greasy fried foods, tobacco, and the smells of foods or perfumes that may make her queasy.

If vomiting is a problem, the pregnant woman should make sure to drink plenty of fluids to replace the lost water. It is wise to report any symptoms to a physician. The pregnant woman should beware of antinausea medication because some are related to birth defects. Most women do stop feeling sick by the fourth month of pregnancy, although a few may remain ill for longer.

Constipation

Another common complaint during pregnancy is constipation. **Progesterone,** a hormone present in high levels during pregnancy, slows peristalsis, the wavelike contraction of the digestive tract. This often leads to a hardening of the stool and irritates the veins in the anal region, a painful condition known as hemorrhoids. The enlarging uterus also puts added pressure on these veins. The preventive measures for both constipation and hemorrhoids is the same. Drink a lot of fluids and eat natural laxatives, such as dried fruits, prune juice, whole grains, and raw fruits and vegetables.

Heartburn

As the uterus continues to enlarge in the last trimester, it presses against the stomach and causes a reflux of acidic stomach contents into the esophagus. This irritation, commonly called **heartburn,** produces a feeling of pressure and burning. To ease heartburn, the pregnant woman should eat slowly, in a relaxed environment, and eat five or six smaller meals per day rather than three large ones. Some foods (spicy dishes, for example) seem to create more problems than others, so they should be avoided. Also, assuming an upright posture after a meal will help prevent heartburn. Taking a walk would be ideal.

Edema

Some edema in the last trimester of pregnancy is normal. As the blood volume expands, some cells, particularly in the extremities, become water-filled. In the past, salt restriction was recommended to prevent pregnancy-induced hypertension. Thus, it is not surprising that low-sodium diets would be encouraged. However, current research suggests that sodium restriction may actually be risky (11). Authorities now believe that there is an increased need for sodium in plasma, muscle, bone, and brain due to the large prenatal fluid-volume expansion. A physician should be consulted when edema occurs.

If edema is diagnosed as the only problem, salt consumption should not be restricted or increased, and water consumption should not be limited. Elevation of the feet at every opportunity may keep the swelling down. The pregnant woman should wear comfortable, low-heeled shoes. Although a nuisance, the edema should disappear within one week after delivery.

Cravings

Some women report cravings for certain foods like ice cream and pickles, watermelon, or chocolate. Such cravings are harmless and do not reflect any deep-seated need for a nutrient, as folk lore suggests (12). Having an occasional chocolate shake or piece of watermelon certainly will not cause any problems, but substituting a large

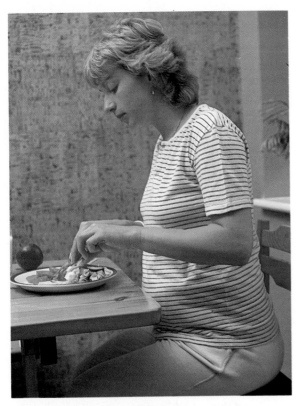

An occasional treat may be harmless, but the diet of a pregnant woman must be chosen wisely.

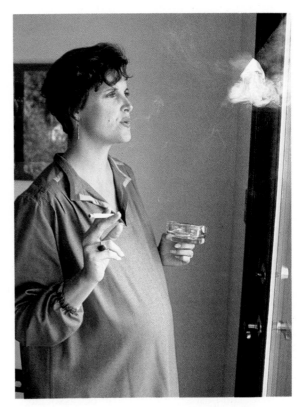

Life-style has a dramatic impact on the developing fetus.

portion of your Calories for any one particular food choice, or for an array of low-nutrient foods, may. Occasionally, cravings are for nonnutritive substances such as clay or starch. The craving for nonnutritive materials like these is known as **pica.** Cravings that are uncontrollable or nonnutritive should be reported to your health-care provider. Under no circumstances should cravings be allowed to crowd a balanced diet, either with too many Calories or too few nutrients.

Hazards for the Developing Fetus

Pregnancy brings a desire to know how to provide the best environment for a fetus to develop. Obtaining adequate nutrients is just one way. But there are some habits that need special attention during this time because of their potentially harmful effects on the baby.

Smoking

Smoking has several adverse effects on the fetus. Research has consistently shown that women who smoke are twice as likely to give birth to a low-birth-weight infant (less than 5.5 pounds) than women who don't smoke. This may not seem important, but it places the infant at higher risk of death in the first year of life. Other risks associated with maternal smoking during pregnancy include miscarriage, stillbirth, premature birth, sudden infant death syndrome (formerly called crib death), and respiratory distress syndrome (13).

Research indicates that low birth weight is dose-responsive, meaning that the more the mother smokes, the less the baby will weigh. Therefore, the sooner she quits, the better it will be for her baby. Pregnancy is a stressful time, which makes it even more difficult to quit, but the motivation is great. Stop-smoking programs are available from health agencies such as the American Cancer Society or the American Lung Association.

Alcohol

The consumption of alcoholic beverages during pregnancy is another factor that can have profound negative consequences for the fetus. Possible birth defects related to alcohol may include fetal growth or mental retardation, minor or major malformations, and a variety of behavioral problems, such as poor sleep habits, decreased alertness, or feeding difficulties.

FIGURE 13.4

The third leading cause of birth defects is alcohol consumption. This child has fetal alcohol syndrome.

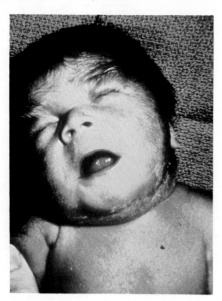

The best-known birth defect associated with alcohol is fetal alcohol syndrome (FAS). Infants born to mothers who are heavy drinkers have an increased risk of this syndrome. It is characterized by central nervous system disorders, growth deficiencies, a specific cluster of facial abnormalities (the eyes are narrow and round, the nose is short and upturned, the upper lip is thin, and the face is flatter than normal), and other malformations (see figure 13.4). The child is often mentally retarded, too. According to the National Institute on Alcohol Abuse and Alcoholism, alcohol-related birth defects are the third leading disorder associated with mental impairment, ranking after Down's syndrome and spina bifida (a defect in which vertebrae fail to fuse, exposing the spinal cord). The difference in the three, however, is that alcohol-related birth defects are preventable.

How much alcohol, then, can be considered a safe amount? As little as two drinks per day can retard growth. Fetal alcohol syndrome occurs in babies whose mothers drink only one or two ounces (30–60 ml) of alcohol a day about ten percent of the time. Heavy drinkers have a 30 to 45 percent risk (14,15). Alcohol readily crosses the placenta to the fetus. Unfortunately, the fetus is not capable of metabolizing alcohol because the specific enzyme necessary for breakdown is still lacking. The question of safety still remains unanswered, but the severity of defect does seem to increase with increased consumption of alcohol. Since no safe level has been established, pregnant women should be urged to abstain from alcohol throughout pregnancy. If a woman has been drinking during the early part of her pregnancy, she may still be at low risk if she stops as soon as possible.

Caffeine

The consequences of consuming caffeinated products during pregnancy are not as clear as those associated with alcohol. Caffeine stimulates the nervous system, increases the heartbeats per minute, and crosses the placenta. Concerns about the detriment of caffeine to the fetus have arisen mainly from animal studies. Defects that have been reported include low birth weight, premature births, and malformations. In a recent human study of 3,800 pregnant women, maternal caffeine consumption was associated with decreased birth weight (16).

Despite conflicting studies, in 1980 the Food and Drug Administration advised pregnant women to avoid caffeinated products or use them sparingly. In order to do this, the pregnant woman should consider what products she currently consumes that contain caffeine. The nation's primary source of caffeine is coffee, followed by soft drinks. Other important sources include tea, chocolate, cocoa, and many over-the-counter medications. Chapter 12 provides further insight into ways to reduce caffeine consumption.

Returning to Prepregnancy Weight

During delivery a woman loses the combined weight of the fetus, amniotic fluid, and placenta—perhaps ten or more pounds. The abdominal region, however, is still soft and unfirm. No new mother leaves the hospital with a prepregnancy figure.

In the week after delivery, much of the accumulated water in the mother's body will be excreted via the skin or kidneys, an additional weight loss of about five pounds. Typically, another four to six pounds will be lost by six weeks after delivery, and any additional weight can usually be lost within three months (see table 13.3). Chapter 9 offers some tips on losing weight that can be applied to the new mother.

TABLE 13.3
Returning to prepregnancy weight

Time	Pounds Lost
Delivery	10
Week 1	5
Weeks 2-6	5
Weeks 7-16	10
Total	30

A breast-feeding mother will use some "maternal reserve" pounds for the production of milk. As will be discussed in the next section, breast-feeding requires an extra 500 to 1,000 Calories per day. Of these Calories, approximately 200 to 500 can remain a deficit, leading to a loss of one-half to one pound per week. A word of caution is needed here. Excessive restriction of Calories (1,000 Calories or more per day) to lose weight while breast-feeding can decrease milk production and is not necessary.

Exercise is another method of regaining the prepregnancy figure. Toning exercises for the abdomen and thighs are a must. Aerobic exercise such as walking will also increase the fat loss. The whole family may enjoy doing this together.

Lactation

It should not be too surprising that after providing for the needs of the developing fetus for nine months, the new mother can continue to meet the baby's nutritional demands. Breast-feeding was the main way to nourish babies until this century. In the 1920s food manufacturers marketed evaporated milk, which could be used to make baby formula. This was soon followed by commercially modified formulas. By the 1950s, only 20 percent of women in the U.S. chose to breast-feed. The renewed interest in breast-feeding in the last 20 years was due at first to greater interest by mothers themselves, and later to pediatric recommendations. With the renewed recognition of the nutritional, bacteriological, and psychological benefits of breast-feeding, more than 60 percent of women in some segments of the population, especially the upper social and educational strata, now elect to breast-feed at the time they leave the hospital (17).

Physiology

The female breast is a delicate organ consisting of glandular, connective, and fatty tissues. The milk-producing glands in the breasts are called alveoli. Milk ducts lead from the alveoli to reservoirs near the nipples (see figure 13.5). The nipples contain 15 to 25 openings from which milk flows. Surrounding the nipples is an area of darker-colored skin known as the areola. Small pimplelike glands on the surface of the areola are called Montgomery's glands. They enlarge during lactation and secrete a lubricating substance that helps protect the nipples.

Early in pregnancy the breasts begin to increase in size in preparation for lactation. As pregnancy progresses, estrogens and progesterones (hormones produced by the placenta), stimulate development of the breast tissue. (All mature breasts contain about the same amount of glandular tissue; therefore, breast size has nothing to do with the ability to produce milk or to succeed at nursing.) Progesterone stimulates the mammary gland so that it is capable of producing milk, and estrogen causes the ducts to grow and become branched.

After childbirth, the breasts begin to change again due to the expulsion of the placenta and the consequent reduction in the hormones it produced. The hormone prolactin then stimulates the production of milk in the alveoli. Finally, the "let-down" reflex is triggered by the baby's sucking. It is controlled by the hormone oxytocin, which causes tiny muscles in the cells surrounding the ducts to contract, moving milk from the alveoli toward the nipple. Sucking causes additional prolactin to be released; therefore, the baby not only gets the immediate gratification of milk but also "places an order" for a future meal.

Nutritional Concerns during Lactation

Breast milk is the perfect food for a baby. It is uniquely formulated and can meet changing demands. The composition and amount of breast milk will vary with the infant's age, from a premature infant to a toddler. Breast milk is made up of lactose, protein, lipids, and other constituents. Although the basic composition is not affected by the mother's diet, she is wise to continue a well-balanced food plan for herself and her family.

FIGURE 13.5
Functional structures in the human breast.

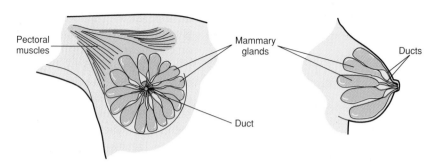

The Food and Nutrition Board recommends that a breast-feeding mother eat about 500 extra Calories per day. Breast milk contains 20 Calories per ounce (20 kcal/30 ml), and a baby consumes, on the average, 30 ounces (900 ml) per day for the first few months. Of course as the infant grows, the demand for milk increases. Also note that adjustments to decrease Calories must be made when breast-feeding is supplemented by solid food, formula, or weaning.

Along with the need for increased Calories, the lactating woman needs 15 g more of protein per day. Once again, this is not a problem in the United States, where women often eat more than double the RDA for nonpregnant women. Table 13.4 shows the increase in RDA for lactating women. All other nutrients are increased to some extent, except for iron. Iron is not secreted significantly in breast milk, so the mother can return to the nonpregnant RDA of 15 mg.

Supplements for the Lactating Mother
If the breast-feeding mother consumes a diet that represents the servings recommended in the daily food guide and chooses a variety of foods, she does not need to take supplements. A physician, however, may want the new mother to continue on the prenatal nutritive capsules until solid foods are introduced to her baby. One reason for this is that breast milk can lack some vitamins, such as vitamin D, if the mother is not consuming adequate amounts. Also, the mother may need to build up depleted iron stores. Of course, if a good diet history shows any nutrients consistently lower than the RDA, and dietary improvements are not possible, supplements become necessary.

TABLE 13.4
Recommended dietary allowances for the lactating woman 25 to 50 years, 63 kg, 163 cm

Nutrient	Amount 1st Six Months	Amount 2nd Six Months
Energy (kcal)	2,700	2,700
Protein (g)	65	62
Vitamin A (IU)	6,500 (1,300 RE)	6,000 (1,200 RE)
Vitamin D (μg)	10	10 μg (400 IU)
Vitamin E mg α-TE	12	11
Ascorbic acid (mg)	95	90
Folacin (μg)	280	260
Niacin (mg)	20	20
Riboflavin (mg)	1.8	1.7
Thiamin (mg)	1.6	1.6
Vitamin B_6 (mg)	2.1	2.1
Vitamin B_{12} (μg)	2.6	2.6
Calcium (mg)	1,200 mg	1,200
Phosphorus (mg)	1,200 mg	1,200
Iodine (μg)	200	200
Iron (mg)	15	15
Magnesium (mg)	355	340
Zinc (mg)	19	16

Reprinted with permission from: Food and Nutrition Board. Recommended Dietary Allowances. 10th rev. ed. 1989. Washington, DC: National Academy Press, 1989.

Practical Eating for the Lactating Woman
The beginning of lactation provides an excellent opportunity to review eating patterns. A diet record of what the lactating woman eats can help identify any nutritional inadequacies (see Health-Promotion Activity 13.1).

There is a considerable increase in the need for water while lactating. Breast milk contains water that must be replaced; therefore, the lactating woman should drink about three quarts of water or more per day. Insufficient fluid may actually decrease the amount of breast milk produced (17). Drinking a glass of water or low-fat milk at each breast-feeding will help with hydration.

The Breast versus Bottle Decision

Among the many decisions parents-to-be make is, How will we feed the baby? The previous discussion on physiology should assure the new mother that she is equipped to breast-feed her infant. But both bottle-feeding and breast-feeding have advantages, and neither is trouble free (see table 13.5). Feeding a baby involves much more than just nutrition, so this section and the Insight on breast-feeding have been designed to help the new parents make a comfortable and well-informed choice (see Health-Promotion Activity 13.2).

Composition

Surprisingly, each species' milk is unique in composition. Cow's milk is most often substituted for human milk in the United States, although they do differ. Table 13.6 compares the composition of human milk to cow's milk (18).

Human milk is higher in polyunsaturated fats, lactose, and cholesterol. In human milk, lactose increases the absorption of calcium. Cholesterol and galactose (from lactose) are used in the formation of myelin, which surrounds nerve fibers and is essential in the normal functioning of the brain. Deficits in linoleic acid (from polyunsaturated fatty acids) could result in dermatitis and growth retardation.

On the other hand, cow's milk has high levels of calcium and phosphorus that are not in the best ratio to one another for a human infant. The protein level in cow's milk is also higher, which produces a strain on the still-maturing kidney of a newborn. Although cow's milk serves the calf very well, the American Academy of Pediatrics recommends that it should not be given to an infant until six months to one year of age (19).

Formula

Commercially prepared formulas use protein from either cow's milk or soybeans. The fat in cow's milk is replaced with vegetable oil to increase the polyunsaturated fatty acids. Corn syrup may be added to increase the carbohydrate content of the formula. The formulas are then fortified with vitamins and minerals. A variety of formulas are now available.

Breast Milk

Human milk varies in composition. If an infant is delivered prematurely, the "preterm" milk of the mother is richer in protein and lipids than if the baby is full term. "Preterm milk" also contains taurine and cysteine, which may be essential amino acids for the premature infant. Controversy surrounds the issue of formula versus breast milk for the premature infant, but it does appear that preterm breast milk may meet the needs of a larger premature infant (greater than 1,800 g in weight) (20).

During the first few days after birth, a watery liquid called colostrum is produced by the mother's breasts. Colostrum is actually a concentrated "super food;" it is rich in disease-protective factors and meets the unique nutritional needs of the newborn. The laxative properties of colostrum assist in the elimination of meconium, which is the first stool. Encouraging the baby to drink as much colostrum as possible is beneficial in producing mother's mature milk.

Even after the mature milk is well established, the composition changes during a feeding. At the beginning of any breast-feeding, a very dilute milk, foremilk, is released, which tends to quench the baby's thirst. As the feeding continues, the fat content of the breast milk increases, satisfying the baby's hunger more quickly. This is referred to as the hindmilk.

Nutrition for the First Year

Recommended Calories and Nutrients

Calories

Infants require much greater energy per unit of body weight than older children or adults. The RDA for energy is set at 108 Calories per kilogram of weight at birth and 98 Calories per kilogram of weight after six months of age (see table 13.7). This is 2.5 to 3.0 times that of an adult.

TABLE 13.5
Breast- versus bottle-feeding

Consideration	Breast-Feeding	Bottle-Feeding
Nutrients	Nutrients are provided in amounts and proportions needed.	If prepared properly, all known nutrients are present.
Safety	Safe, properly mixed, and the right temperature.	Depends on sanitation and sterilization practices used.
Allergies	Rare.	Possible allergies to protein or other substances.
Protection from illness	Provides antibodies that protect against viruses, bacteria, and other microbes. Contains bifidus factor that promotes helpful bacteria and decreases the chance of diarrhea.	Provides no particular protection.
Tooth, gum, and jaw development	Promotes good development.	Need orthodontic nipple. Babies should not take formula or juice to bed because it promotes cavities and may be related to middle-ear infections.
Presence of hazardous substances	Possibly unacceptable levels of PCB's, DDT, or other pesticides. Many drugs, and alcohol, can pass into the breast milk.	Not likely.
Cost	Depends on cost of extra 500 Calories, but is not "free."	Commercial formulas are usually more expensive than breast milk. Cost increases with convenience.
Convenience	Mother or pumped milk must be available.	Proper mixing and sterilizing take time, but a day's supply can be mixed. Disposable bottles are time savers but more expensive.
Frequency	Every two to three hours at first, since breast milk is more digestible.	Usually a four-hour schedule.
Infant's eating habits	Eats what he needs, no way to "force feed." Breast-fed babies usually weigh less at one year of age.	Requires less work and is easier to overeat. Tendency to finish bottle.
Supplements	Not necesary until four to six months.	Most are fortified.
Emotional satisfaction	Close body contact required. Encourages bonding.	Similar to breast-feeding if bottle is not propped up for baby. Other people besides mother can experience satisfaction. Mother is not tied down as much.
Eating out	May be discreet with practice. Ready anytime, anywhere.	Bottle acceptable anywhere. Formula should be kept cold to decrease microbial growth, and warmed for drinking.
Physical benefits to the mother	Sucking stimulates uterus to contract back to normal size faster, and also provides a pleasant sensation. Aids mother in losing fat.	An option for woman who have debilitating or chronic disease or are malnourished.
Father	Sometimes feels left out and must be encouraged to cuddle baby at other times. Needed for support.	Father can have an active role.
Work	Must pump or feed at least every three to four hours to maintain supply.	Anyone can feed.
Premature Infant	"Preterm milk" is richer in protein and lipids. Contains amino acids that premature infants cannot make. Immunity advantages.	Can mimic "preterm" milk except for immunity.

TABLE 13.6
Composition of human milk, cow's milk, and cow's-milk formula (per one fluid ounce)

Nutrient	Human Milk	Cow's Milk	Cow's-Milk Formula
Water (oz)	0.89	0.85	0.88
Calories	21	27	20
Protein (g)	0.3	1	0.5
Fat (g)	1.4	1	1.1
Saturated	0.6	0.6	0.5
Polyunsaturated	0.2	0.03	0.34
Cholesterol (mg)	4	4.3	0.5
Carbohydrate (g)	1.4	1.4	2.1
Sodium (mg)	5	15	6
Calcium (mg)	10	36	14
Phosphorus (mg)	4	28	9
Iron (mg)	0.7	tr	0.03
Vitamin C	1	0.6	2

From J. A. T. Pennington and H. N. Church. *Food Values of Portions Commonly Used.* © 1985. J. B. Lippincott Co., Philadelphia.

TABLE 13.7
Recommended dietary allowances for infants during the first year

	0–6 Months, 6 kg-60 cm	6–12 Months, 9 kg-71 cm
Energy (kcal)	108 kcal/kg	98 kcal/kg
Protein (g)	2.2 g/kg (13)	1.6 g/kg (14)
Vitamin A (RE)	375 (1,875 I.U.)	375 (1,875 I.U.)
Vitamin D (μg)	7.5 (300 I.U.)	10 (400 I.U.)
Vitamin E (mg α-TE)	3	4
Ascorbic acid (mg)	30	35
Folacin (μg)	25	35
Niacin (mg NE)	5	6
Riboflavin (mg)	0.4	0.5
Thiamin (mg)	0.3	0.4
Vitamin B_6 (mg)	0.3	0.6
Vitamin B_{12} (μg)	0.3	0.5
Calcium (mg)	400	600
Phosphorus (mg)	300	500
Iodine (μg)	40	50
Iron (mg)	6	10
Magnesium (mg)	40	60
Zinc (mg)	5	5

Reprinted with permission from: Food and Nutrition Board. Recommended Dietary Allowances. 10th rev. ed. 1989. Washington, DC: National Academy Press, 1989.

Protein
Protein requirements gradually decrease, from a very high 2.2 g per kilogram of weight during the first six months to 1.6 g per kilogram of weight for the second six months of life. Although the requirements are high, breast milk or formula supply all that is needed for most of the first year.

Vitamins and Minerals
Table 13.7 lists the RDA for the first year. Breast milk or formula is sufficient to meet these needs during the first four to six months of life. A few vitamins and minerals, however, may need special attention. Most infants are given an injection of vitamin K at birth because the intestinal bacteria are not yet present to manufacture it. Unless the infant receives sufficient sun, which is hard to judge, many pediatricians recommend vitamin D supplements as well (21). In addition, fluoride is usually supplemented for breast-feeding infants and for those on formula if the preparation water has less than 0.3 parts per million of fluoride (22).

There is still debate over supplementation of iron for the infant. Most experts feel that the newborn has enough iron in storage to last for the first six months of life (23). However, some believe that if iron is supplemented, the infant won't deplete its stores and risk anemia. Iron seems to have several negative effects on the infant younger than four months. Some infants have experienced gastrointestinal distress and poor absorption of zinc. High intakes of iron may also worsen infections, as has been seen in babies from developing countries. By the sixth month, the baby needs additional iron, and iron-fortified cereals should be introduced.

Water

Of course infants need water, and breast milk or formula usually supplies it. A good indicator of adequate hydration is six to eight wet diapers per day. If this does not occur, or if the baby has diarrhea or is vomiting, a physician should be consulted. Only boiled water from a sterile bottle should be given to an infant.

Introduction of Solid Foods

In the 1920s, easily prepared and pureed foods were marketed (24). These could readily be introduced to the infant at a very early age. By the 1950s some mothers were starting babies on solid foods as early as the first month. Many hoped this would help the baby sleep through the night sooner, although there was never any evidence that it did. Early eating of solids also implied advanced intellectual and physical development, at least in the minds of the parents. Conversely, the manipulations needed to get a newborn to swallow food led to serious investigation of the physical readiness of an infant to accept solid food.

Physical Readiness

The decision of when to add solid foods to an infant's diet should be based on the physical readiness of an infant. In the first few months of life, the baby is only able to suck and swallow. The swallowing is part of an involuntary reflex. At this same time an "extrusion reflex" pushes out of the mouth any solid matter that is placed on the tongue.

Several developments occur between four to six months that allow babies to eat food without having to be forced. The extrusion reflex disappears, and the baby learns to swallow voluntarily. The baby is also able to hold in the upper lip, thus keeping food in the mouth. Other signs of readiness in the infant include opening the mouth to show desire for table foods, and the ability to lean forward to reach them. The

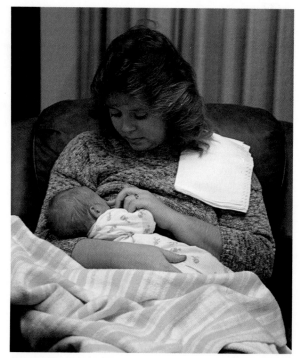

Breast milk can meet all the nutritional needs of an infant for the first six months of life.

baby is now able to sit in a highchair and can signal that he or she does not want any more food by turning his or her head away. All of these developments are necessary in creating an enjoyable eating experience for the infant, and one that avoids force feeding.

When and What to Introduce

In the first year, it is important to remember that breast milk or formula provides the basis for an infant's diet and that solid foods are only supplemental. Solid foods are added after the fourth month to give a baby the few extra Calories needed for its increasing activity level and size. Inappropriate or early introduction of solid foods may lead to poor eating habits, obesity, or allergies. Solid foods may also exceed the functional capacity of the infant's kidneys. Foods can be introduced slowly and in a preferred order to avoid these problems.

The sequence of solid foods added to an infant's diet traditionally starts with an iron-fortified infant cereal when the baby is four to six months old. Rice is usually the first choice because it causes less allergies than wheat cereals. Mixed with breast milk or formula, cereals give the baby an opportunity to get used to eating from a spoon and manipulating the semisolid food down the throat. It is important to introduce single-ingredient foods one at a time and to allow a week before adding the next. This allows the parents to spot any allergic reaction the baby may have. Gradually, strained vegetables and fruits can be added, progressing to more challenging textures as the months continue. Protein foods and finger foods are introduced after the ninth month. A suggested timetable for the addition of infant foods is shown in table 13.8.

By about six months, babies are interested in anything that is placed in front of them. Feeding is a perfect opportunity to capitalize on an infant's developing hand skills. Oven-dried toast can be given to help in teething. Later, as fruits are added to the diet, mashed banana, peeled peach halves, or other soft fruits can be placed on the highchair tray, and the baby can self-feed. A list of favorites at this time includes bananas, applesauce, peaches, pears, carrots, green beans, squash, sweet potatoes, avocados, cereal, rice cakes, and dried toast.

At about nine months of age, a baby is able to use the thumb and forefinger as pinchers, adding a new dimension to self-feeding. Finger foods certainly become more appealing because the baby can now easily pick them up. Some favorite foods at this time are dried cereal, rice cakes, bite-sized cooked carrots, and cooked spaghetti. Cold peach slices and frozen bananas or strawberries may soothe the sore gums of teething infants. Drinking from a cup may be messy, but it helps the child develop hand and eye coordination.

The goal during this first year is to create a healthy eating attitude. It is best accomplished by watching for cues from the baby, adding foods gradually, and encouraging self-feeding—all in a positive environment (see Health-Promotion Activity 13.3).

Allergies

If time is taken to introduce foods slowly and one at a time, there is more opportunity to isolate any food that is causing an allergy. An **allergic reaction** results from contact with a substance (antigen) to which the body has become sensitized (formed antibodies against). Cow's-milk protein, wheat protein, orange juice, and chocolate contain common allergenic substances (25). The most frequent allergy symptoms reported among babies are bloating and

TABLE 13.8
Introduction of solid foods

Age in (months)	Food	Feeding Behavior
1-6	Human milk or formula only 14 to 50 oz	Look for signs of physical readiness for solid foods.
6-12	Human milk or formula plus solid foods	
6	Cereal*: 3-5 tbsp Rice, then barley Feedings: 2	Mouth opens to receive food. Infant helps with spoon.
7	Cereal: 3-5 tbsp Fruit: 2-5 tbsp strained or junior Feedings: 2 to 3	Teeth erupt and chewing begins as tongue moves food.
8	Cereal: 5-9 tbsp Fruit: 9-18 tbsp strained or junior Vegetables: 9-18 tbsp strained or junior Feedings: scheduled by infant	Infant uses hands in feeding. Holds handle on cup. Shows desire or dislike for food. Shows satiety.
9	Cereal: 6-12 tbsp Protein: ½ oz ground meat, cheese, or ¼ c mashed beans Fruit: 9-18 tbsp Vegetables: 9-19 tbsp Finger foods: assorted from above Feedings: scheduled by infant	Chews easily. Bites correct amount. Picks up food well.
10-12	Cereal: ½-¾ Protein: ½-1 oz Starch: ¼-¾ c mashed potato or pasta Fruits: ½-¾ c mashed or chunks Vegetables: ¼-½ c mashed or finger foods Juice: 2-6 oz c vitamin-C fortified Finger foods: oven-dried toast, crackers, pasta, etc. Calcium rich: yogurt, cottage cheese, pudding, ice cream	Follows family eating schedule plus snacks. Pincer grasp apparent. Picks up bite-sized pieces. Mimics adult behavior. Begins self-feeding with utensils at about 11 months.

*All cereal should be iron-fortified.

gassiness, a sandpaperlike rash on the face, runny nose and watery eyes, and chronic cranky behavior (25). Other symptoms to be aware of are sneezing, coughing, asthma, hives, eczema, vomiting, colic, abdominal pain, and shock. Allergies tend to run in families, so close observation of an infant may help to identify similar allergies.

Commercial versus Homemade Baby Foods

Some parents prefer to use commercial baby foods, whereas others make their own from the family's food. Either choice requires safety and nutritional considerations.

Commercially prepared baby foods are convenient and safe, although more expensive than homemade. Single-ingredient baby foods are cheaper and more concentrated in nutrients than are dinners. In the past, commercial baby foods were high in sugar, salt, and preservatives, but this is generally not true today. Baby foods now are available in a wider range of textures, from pureed to chunks, offering more challenge to the maturing infant.

Once a baby food jar has been opened, the portion needed should be removed and the rest stored in the refrigerator for up to three days. The food jar should not be heated if only part of the contents will be used. Some nutrients will be destroyed by reheating. For safety, leftover portions should never be saved because they may be contaminated with saliva or microorganisms.

Several rules should also be followed if baby food is to be home-prepared. Honey or corn syrup should not be used to sweeten foods for an infant under one year of age (26). These products may contain spores that will produce a lethal toxin in the immature gastrointestinal tract of the infant, resulting in the disease called infant botulism.

When preparing baby foods, the food handler should be meticulous about washing hands and equipment, always using hot soapy water. Wooden cutting boards should be avoided because they are notorious for causing contamination. Utensils that have been used to taste-test should not be used to prepare food.

Vitamins and minerals may be preserved in foods by using appropriate heating and storage procedures. Once the food is ready, it should be served immediately. If food sits at

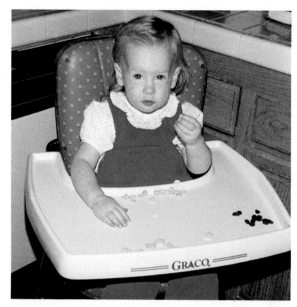

Allow children to discover food with all of their senses.

room temperature for a half hour, it serves as a perfect medium for bacterial growth. No salt, sugar, or excessive spices should be used for baby food. Allow the child to enjoy the wonderful flavor of the natural food.

Whether individuals decide to use mainly commercially prepared or homemade baby foods, the goal is to provide safe, nutritious, and challenging food for the infant. Homemade foods should eventually be introduced and can provide more variety in texture and selection.

How Much to Feed?

Unlike adults, babies do not look around at other babies and wish they were thinner or rounder. For the most part, wait for the inner distress signal of hunger to trigger their desire for food. Parents' influence on eating behavior is thought to begin in infancy. Some researchers believe that overfeeding during infancy can lead to a continual struggle with obesity into the adult years.

Breast Milk or Formula

When deciding if an infant is eating enough during the first four to six months of life, refer to the RDA guide of 108 Calories per kilogram of body weight. Generally, breast milk or formula provides 20 Calories per ounce, so all that is needed is the infant's weight to estimate the

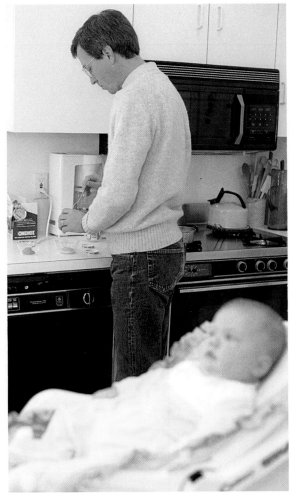

Serve food soon after preparation to assure the best quality.

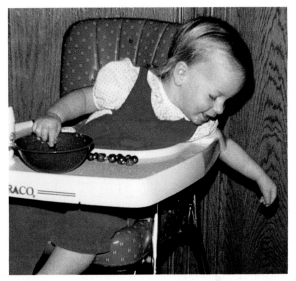

Toddlers can signal their parents when they are full.

ounces he will need each day. An infant may begin by eating 20 ounces of milk in the first week and increase to double that by six months. Once solid foods are introduced, milk consumption will drop to about one quart per day for the remainder of the first year.

The baby is the best judge of how much he needs to eat. A sleepy baby may not eat as much as one who has been napping for a few hours.

Solid Foods
Even after the baby has started eating solid foods, the risks of overfeeding will be small if parents listen and watch for her to signal fullness. Often the baby is quite direct and spits the food out, but there are other subtle messages. Playing with food, turning the head, not opening the mouth, and reaching to get down from the table may mean that the baby feels full and is not just distracted.

Sometimes adults compare what an infant eats to the amount they themselves eat. This further convinces the parents that the child is eating too little. At six months an infant will consume only a few teaspoons of cereal, and that will be enough. When introducing new foods, start with one-fourth teaspoon. Initially, the objective is to introduce new tastes, textures, temperatures, and colors—not to fill the baby up. Breast milk or formula still provides the majority of the needed Calories. Each child needs quite different amounts of food and is often the best judge. Indications that a baby is still hungry include crying, reaching for food on the table, or opening the mouth (see Health-Promotion Activity 13.3).

Growth Charts
Height and weight charts are a good indicator of whether a baby is eating enough. Although comparing individual children may lead to frustration at times, growth charts represent large numbers of children throughout the U.S. and provide a better comparison. Figure 13.6 is one such growth chart for the first two years of life. The dashed lines on the graph show the high and low ranges in weight gains for girls, and the solid lines for boys. The growth figures and the stages of development are only averages; growth of individual babies may differ.

A pediatrician usually plots an infant's growth from birth. Using similar charts, the doctor can advise parents on any abnormalities in growth that are observed.

FIGURE 13.6

Growth and development chart.

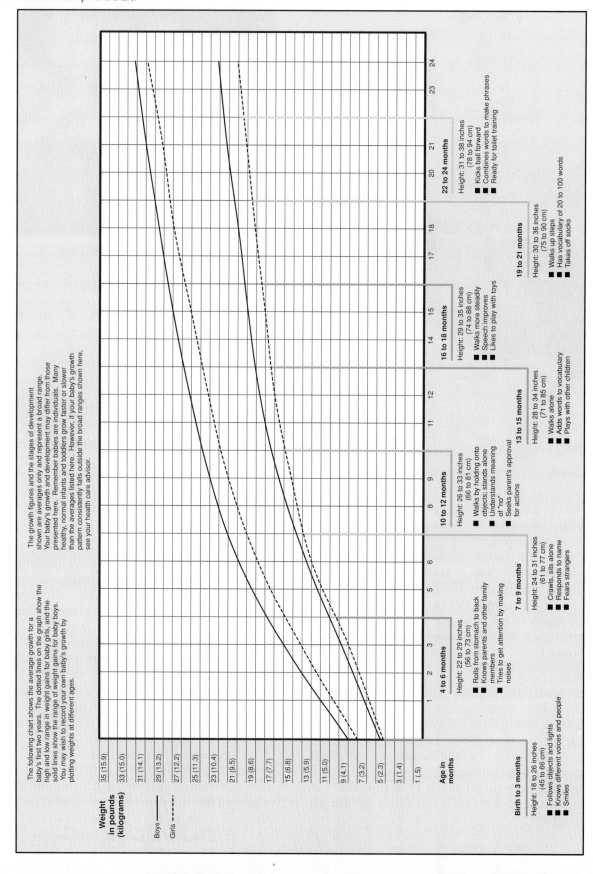

The following chart shows the average growth for a baby's first two years. The dotted lines on the graph show the high and low range in weight gains for baby girls, and the solid lines show the range of weight gains for baby boys. You may wish to record your own baby's growth by plotting weights at different ages.

The growth figures and the stages of development shown are averages only and represent a broad range. Your baby's growth and development may differ from those presented here. Remember babies are individuals. Many healthy, normal infants and toddlers grow faster or slower than the averages listed here. However, if your baby's growth pattern consistently falls outside the broad ranges shown here, see your health care advisor.

Weight in pounds (kilograms)

35 (15.9)
33 (15.0)
31 (14.1)
29 (13.2) Boys ——
27 (12.2) Girls - - - - -
25 (11.3)
23 (10.4)
21 (9.5)
19 (8.6)
17 (7.7)
15 (6.8)
13 (5.9)
11 (5.0)
9 (4.1)
7 (3.2)
5 (2.3)
3 (1.4)
1 (.5)

Age in months

1 2 3 4 5 6 7 8 9 10 11 12 13 14 15 17 18 20 21 23 24

Birth to 3 months

Height: 18 to 26 inches (45 to 66 cm)
■ Follows objects and lights
■ Knows different voices and people
■ Smiles

4 to 6 months

Height: 22 to 29 inches (56 to 73 cm)
■ Rolls from stomach to back
■ Knows parents and other family members
■ Tries to get attention by making noises

7 to 9 months

Height: 24 to 31 inches (61 to 77 cm)
■ Crawls, sits alone
■ Responds to name
■ Fears strangers

10 to 12 months

Height: 26 to 33 inches (66 to 81 cm)
■ Walks by holding onto objects; stands alone
■ Understands meaning of "no"
■ Seeks parent's approval for actions

13 to 15 months

Height: 28 to 34 inches (71 to 85 cm)
■ Walks alone
■ Adds words to vocabulary
■ Plays with other children

16 to 18 months

Height: 29 to 35 inches (74 to 88 cm)
■ Walks more steadily
■ Speech improves
■ Likes to play with toys

19 to 21 months

Height: 30 to 36 inches (75 to 90 cm)
■ Walks up steps
■ Has vocabulary of 20 to 100 words
■ Takes off socks

22 to 24 months

Height: 31 to 38 inches (78 to 94 cm)
■ Kicks ball forward
■ Combines words to make phrases
■ Ready for toilet training

HEALTH-PROMOTION INSIGHT
Breast-Feeding

Today, 60 percent of American women start to breast-feed their babies while still in the hospital (17). After two months, however, only 45 percent of these women are still breast-feeding. At four months it drops to 35 percent, and by six months to 25 percent. There are several explanations for this dramatic decline.

The two most common causes of unsuccessful feeding are an insufficient knowledge of the process and technique, and a nonsupportive environment. The mothers and possibly the grandmothers of pregnant women today probably were bottle-fed. Thus, the traditional passage of knowledge is blocked and the family support weakened. For the new parents who chose to breast-feed, and for those who will help to support them, advice is offered to increase the chances of succeeding.

Getting Started

The pregnant woman should arrange to nurse her baby as soon as possible after delivery. Ideally, the baby will not suck a rubber nipple until at least three to four weeks after birth, when lactation is firmly established. Although a new mother may have preconceived notions about her baby immediately taking to the breast, this may not happen; the baby must learn to breast-feed. Even if the mother has breast-fed before, each child is different. It will take from one month to four months to feel comfortable with breast-feeding. Breast-feeding, like any other feeding method, has both positive and negative aspects, and at times the mother may not feel adequate. This is not necessarily due to the feeding method; the newborn can be very unpredictable, and the mother may be a novice. Confidence will come with time and practice.

Supportive Environment

A pregnant woman needs to build her support team before delivering her baby. This should include friends, relatives, significant others, other breast-feeding mothers, and, most important, the father. These people should be included in classes and share literature on the topic. This support group should support the mother's decision to breast-feed and be able to offer encouragement to a mother who feels inadequate.

Positioning the Baby

Getting the baby to take the nipple correctly is a key to avoiding numerous difficulties with breast-feeding. Tips to ensure a proper nursing position follow.

1. Position the baby so that the head is facing the nipple. The baby should lie on its side, with the stomach and knees directed toward the mother's abdomen. The lower arm should be tucked behind the mother's arm that is holding the baby in a cradle hold.
2. Grasp the breast behind the areola with thumb and forefinger.
3. Tickle the cheek of the baby to stimulate it to turn toward the breast. Then brush the nipple against the lower lip, and wait for the baby to open its mouth wide, as in yawning.
4. Position the baby's mouth so that it surrounds the areola. If the baby takes only the nipple, it will hurt, and soreness may develop. Proper positioning may take several tries.
5. To release the baby's mouth, use a finger to break the suction at the corner of the baby's mouth.

Milk Supply

A frequent concern of breast-feeding mothers is that they do not have enough milk to feed their baby. The breast tissue does respond to the infant's need for milk. Mothers should not give supplemental feedings to newborn infants during the first four months of life, because this will only decrease the mother's milk supply. Following are some tips for a mother to keep her milk supply adequate.

1. Feed the baby on demand. During the first few months a baby may wish to eat every one and one-half to two hours.
2. Drink at least six to eight glasses of liquid each day. Water, juice, or milk is best.
3. Eat a balanced diet, and don't reduce Calories.
4. Limit visitors and major chores for a month after delivery.
5. Get plenty of rest, and nap when the baby is sleeping.

Preventing Sore Nipples

Sore nipples are a common reason why women stop breast-feeding during the first few months. To prevent sore nipples,

1. do no use soap to wash nipples; use only plain water;
2. keep nipples dry between feedings. At first leaky nipples will be a problem. Let nipples air dry when possible, and change nursing pads frequently;
3. position the infant correctly on the breast;
4. break the suction before removing the infant from the breast; and
5. do not let the infant sleep while nursing.

Length of Time for Breast-Feeding

The American Academy of Pediatrics recommends that breast-feeding be continued for one year. However, even six months of breast-feeding can be beneficial to the infant. Once milk is well established (by about the third month) nursing mothers can leave their infant for short periods and miss an occasional feeding. Breast milk can also be expressed by hand or with a pump, and it can be left for the infant. Expressed milk will be safe for 24 hours in the refrigerator, and it can also be frozen.

SUMMARY

1. Pregnancy is divided into three trimesters lasting about three months each. During the first trimester all the major structures of the fetus are formed. Therefore, the first trimester is the most critical phase of human development. During the last two trimesters the fetus gains the majority of its total delivery weight.

2. The pregnant woman should gain between 22 and 28 pounds. Weight gains of less than 21 pounds are associated with low-birth-weight infants, who have an increased risk of death in the first year of life.

3. The Food and Nutrition Board adds 300 extra Calories and 10 extra grams of protein to the diet of a pregnant woman.

4. A pregnant woman should consume a minimum of four servings of dairy products, three servings of protein, four servings of fruits and vegetables, and four servings of grains per day. A vitamin and mineral supplement is not necessary unless a diet history or laboratory values indicate a deficiency. Folacin, calcium, and iron may be deficient in the diet of a pregnant woman.

5. Pregnancy may bring food-related discomforts that can be relieved by adjusting intake of particular foods and beverages. Common discomforts include nausea and vomiting, constipation, heartburn, and edema.

6. Smoking, alcohol, and caffeine pose hazards to the developing fetus that may result in growth or mental retardation, and even death.

7. A lactating mother needs 500 extra Calories and 15 extra grams of protein. The need for most other nutrients, except iron, are also increased during lactation. Although these can be obtained through the diet, a physician may recommend that prenatal nutritive capsules be continued for three to six months after delivery.

8. Both breast- and bottle-feeding have advantages and disadvantages. A table of these is contained in the chapter.

9. Infants require more energy per unit of body weight than adults. Protein requirements are also high, at 2.2 grams per kilogram during the first six months of life and 1.6 grams per kilogram for the rest of the first year.

10. An infant may require supplements of three nutrients: vitamin D, iron, and fluoride. Vitamin K is administered at birth because the bacterial flora of the gut, which usually manufacture it, are not yet present.

11. Infants may require additional water during periods of diarrhea or vomiting. This water must be sterile.

12. The introduction of solid foods to an infant should be based on the physical readiness of the infant to accept them. Several physical developments occur between four to six months that allow the infant to hold food and swallow it.

13. By six months, an infant needs an iron-fortified cereal. Other single-ingredient foods may then be added. Encouraging the infant to self-feed can make eating a more enjoyable experience for the infant.

14. Either commercial or home-prepared baby foods are acceptable. The goal is to provide the infant with foods that are nutritious, safe, and challenging.

15. Although it is difficult to know how much to feed an infant, each infant gives cues or signals that he or she is either hungry or full. Growth charts can also indicate whether the infant is changing weight dramatically enough to adjust eating habits.

16. Breast-feeding definitely offers nutritional, immunological, psychological, and bacteriological benefits to the infant. However, many women lack the knowledge needed to succeed at using the procedure, and many lack support from family members. Measures to increase the chances for successful breast-feeding are offered.

REFERENCES

1. Worthington-Roberts, B. 1987. Nutritional Support of Successful Reproduction: An Update. *Journal of Nutrition Education* 19:1.
2. McCarthy, E. Report of a Montreal Diet Dispensary Experience. 1983. *Journal of the Canadian Dietetic Association* 44:71-75.
3. Mitchell, M. C., and E. Lerner. 1989. Weight Gain and Pregnancy Outcome in Underweight and Normal Weight Women. *Journal of the American Dietetic Association* 89:5:634-41.
4. Correlations Underscored: Maternal Weight Gain, Infant Birth Weight. 1986. *The Nation's Health* (September):p. 1.
5. Drife, J. O. 1986. Weight Gain in Pregnancy: Eating for Two or Just Getting Fat? *British Medical Journal* 293:903.
6. Lawrence, M., et al. 1984. Maintenance Energy. Costs of Pregnancy in Rural Gambian Women and Influence of Dietary Status. *Lancet* (August 18): Vol. II, pp. 363-65.
7. Huber, A. M., L. L. Wallins, and P. DeRusso. 1988. Folate Nutriture in Pregnancy. *Journal of the American Dietetic Association* 88:7:791-95.
8. Mitchell, H. W., et al. 1982. *Nutrition in Health and Disease.* Philadelphia: J. B. Lippincott Co.
9. Schneider, H. A. 1983. *Nutritional Support of Medical Practice.* Philadelphia: Harper and Row.
10. Leader, A., et al. 1985. Maternal Nutrition in Pregnancy, Part I: A Review. *Canadian Medical Journal* 125:545.
11. Ott, D. B. 1984. Nutrition during Pregnancy. *Journal of the American Dietetic Association* 84:5:572.
12. Worthington-Roberts, B., et al. 1989. Dietary Cravings and Aversions in the Postpartum Period. *Journal of the American Dietetic Association* 89:5:647-51.
13. Hoff, C. W., et al. 1986. Trend Associations of Smoking with Maternal, Fetal and Neonatal Morbidity. *Obstetrics and Gynecology* 68:317-21.
14. Beagle, W. S. 1981. Fetal Alcohol Syndrome: A Review. *Journal of the American Dietetic Association* 79:274.
15. Sulaiman, N. D., et al. 1988. Alcohol Consumption in Dundee Primigravidas and Its Effects on Outcome of Pregnancy. *British Medical Journal* 296:1500.
16. Martin, T. R., and M. B. Bracken. 1987. The Association between Low Birth Weight and Caffeine Consumption during Pregnancy. *American Journal of Epidemiology* 126:813-21.
17. Greecher, C., et al. 1986. Position of the American Dietetic Association: Promotion of Breast Feeding. *Journal of the American Dietetic Association* 86:11:1580-1585.
18. Pennington, J. A. T., and H. N. Church. 1985. *Food Values of Portions Commonly Used.* Philadelphia: J. B. Lippincott Co.
19. American Academy of Pediatrics Committee on Nutrition. 1983. Use of Whole Cow's Milk in Infancy. *Pediatrics* 72:253.
20. Brady, M. S., et al. 1982. Formulas and Human Milk for Premature Infants: A Review and Update. *Journal of the American Dietetic Association* 81:547.
21. Finberg, L. 1981. Human Milk Feeding and Vitamin D Supplementation. *Journal of Pediatrics* 99:228.
22. American Academy of Pediatrics Committee on Nutrition. 1979. Fluoride Supplementation: Revised Dosage Schedule. *Pediatrics* 63:150.
23. Siimes, M. A., L. Salmenpera, and J. Perheentupa. 1984. Exclusive Breast Feeding for Nine Months: Risk of Iron Deficiency. *Journal of Pediatrics* 104:196.
24. Weigley, E. S. 1988. Infant Feeding Practices. A Century of Transitions. *Nutrition Today* (March/April):20-24.
25. Butkus, S. N., and L. K. Mahan. 1986. Food Allergies: Immunological Reactions to Food. *Journal of the American Dietetic Association* 86:5:601-608.
26. Arnon, S. S., et al. 1979. Honey and Other Environmental Risk Factors for Infant Botulism. *Journal of Pediatrics* 94:331.

HEALTH-PROMOTION ACTIVITY 13.1
Just Eating for Two, or, Choosing Foods for a Well-Nourished Mother and Baby

1. On the Food Group Chart on page 366, circle the items in column I that you tend to include in your normal diet. If there are foods that you commonly eat that are not listed in column I, write them in column I.
2. Total the number of servings (use the appropriate food-group serving sizes) for each food group in column II.
3. On the bottom of the Food Group Chart, circle the extra foods that you regularly eat, and write in others as appropriate.
4. Compare column II to the recommended daily servings table in the left-hand corner of the Food Group Chart. What improvements could you make?
5. For each of the four food groups in column I, the healthier choices are listed first. Where do most of your circled foods appear?
6. What would you be willing to eat to improve your choices in the four food groups? Make a plan in column III.
7. Circle the extra food category that you now feel would be a detriment to a pregnant woman or her developing fetus.

Source: Dairy Council of California. © 1983, 1984. Reprinted by permission.

Food Group Chart

Recommended Daily Servings					
	Adult	Child	Teen	Pregnant/ Nursing Woman	Pregnant/ Nursing Teen
Milk	2	3	4	4	5
Meat	2	2	2	3	3
V-F	4	4	4	4	4
B-C	4	4	4	4	4

	Column I List of foods from the Four Food Groups which provide the major nutrients we need.	Column II Recommended number of servings needed daily	Column III Your Daily Food Pattern Use this column for preparing your personal food plan.

Milk ~ Milk Products

Major Source of: calcium, riboflavin, protien, Vitamin B$_{12}$, magnesium

- Nonfat milk, buttermilk, low-fat milk, plain yogurt
- Whole milk, cheese, fruit-flavored yogurt, cottage cheese
- Custard, milkshake, pudding, ice cream

4

1. _____
2. _____
3. _____
4. _____
_____

Meat ~ Meat Alternates

Major Source of: protein, iron, niacin, thiamin, Vitamins B$_6$ and B$_{12}$, folic acid, magnesium, zinc

- Poultry, fish, lean meat (beef, lamb, pork), dried peas and beans, eggs
- Beef, lamb, pork, luncheon meats, refried beans
- Hot dogs, peanut butter, nuts

3

1. _____
2. _____
3. _____
_____
_____
_____
_____

Vegetable ~ Fruit

Major Source of: vitamins A and C, folic acid

- Apricots, bean sprouts, broccoli, Brussels sprouts, cabbage, cantaloupe, carrots, cauliflower, cucumber, grapefruit, green beans, green peas, leafy greens (spinach, mustard, and collard greens), lettuce, mushrooms, orange, orange juice, peach, strawberries, tomato, winter squash
- Apple, banana, canned fruit, corn, pear, potato
- Avocado, dried fruit, sweet potato

4

1. _____
2. _____
3. _____
4. _____
_____
_____
_____

Bread ~ Cereal

Major Source of: thiamin, niacin, iron, zinc

- Whole-grain and enriched breads, rolls, tortillas
- Rice, cereals, pastas (macaroni and spaghetti), bagel
- Pancake, muffin, cornbread, biscuit, pre-sweetened cereals

4

1. _____
2. _____
3. _____
4. _____
_____
_____

Extra Foods

Extra Foods tend to be high in sugar, fat, salt, or alcohol and in most cases, Calories

Sugar

Cake, pie, cookies, donuts, sweet rolls, candy
Soft drinks, fruit drinks, jelly, syrup, gelatin desserts
Sugar, honey

Fat

Margarine, salad dressing, oils, mayonnaise
Cream, cream cheese, butter
Gravy, sauces

Salt (sodium)

Potato chips, corn chips, pretzels
Pickles, olives, bouillon
Mustard, soy sauce, steak sauce
Salt, seasoned salt

Alcohol
Wine, beer, liquor

Other

Spices, herbs, coffee, tea, diet soft drinks

Refer to Table 13.6 and list two important considerations in making a decision to support either breast- or bottle-feeding.

Is there a significant other that holds the opposite view to your decision? What evidence from table 13.6 and from the Health-Promotion Insight could you share to support your position?

What are two possible drawbacks to the method you would support?

List two people that you could call on for support of your decision.

*H*EALTH-PROMOTION ACTIVITY 13.3
Planning Meals for Infants

Jason is a ten-month-old infant who is excited about eating solid foods. However, he seems to get full in the middle of his meals, and it's a constant battle to keep him focused on food. Often Jason twitches in his highchair, wanting to get down, and shakes his head. Oddly, at snack times he gulps his juice and requests more. After studying a typical daily menu for Jason, perhaps you can offer some suggestions.

10:00 A.M.	½ cup rice cereal
	½ oz ground beef
	½ tortilla in small pieces
	¼ cup carrots
2:00 P.M.	1 6-oz bottle of apple juice
4:00 P.M.	¼ cup mashed beans
	½ cup rice
	¼ cup strained pears
8:00 P.M.	1 6-oz bottle of apple juice taken to bed

Is the quantity of food adequate for a ten-month-old infant? If not, what needs to be added? (See table 13.8.)

Evaluate this typical meal for quality, based on the chapter discussion and on table 13.8. For example, look for calcium, vitamin C, and iron sources. What could be changed or added?

Is the timing of the meals throughout the day appropriate? A better meal pattern for an infant who wakes at 7:00 A.M. and goes to bed at 8:00 P.M. would be three meals and two snacks.

Picture the texture, color, and variety of this meal plan. How can these factors be improved? What would encourage self-feeding?

Compile all your thoughts and ideas from the previous question into a day's menu for Jason, improving his nutrition and creating a healthy feeding attitude.

14

Nutrition in Childhood and Adolescence

OUTLINE

INTRODUCTION

To experience firsthand the growth of a child is one of life's greatest pleasures. In this chapter, the relationship of nutrition to three phases of growth and development will be reviewed: the preschool years, or ages 1–5; childhood, or ages 6–12; and adolescence, or ages 13–19. Growth characteristics and developmental traits of each phase will be explored. In addition, the nutritional needs of each time period will be discussed.

Special attention will be given to several popular topics, including food advertising directed to children, the influence of television viewing on health and eating behaviors, the school lunch program, and factors that may affect nutritional habits among adolescents, such as tobacco, alcohol, and drug use. The Health-Promotion Insight will review the relationship of diet and brain function, with special attention given to public misconceptions concerning sugar and learning problems in children.

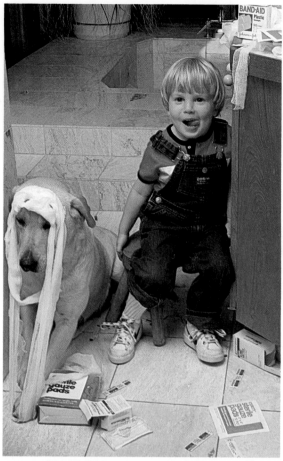

By eighteen months of age, babies can move rapidly and confidently, exploring their environments with high levels of curiosity and energy.

The Preschool Years: Ages 1–5

Physical Growth

A child's rate of growth and development is influenced by the level of nutrition received and by environmental stimulation. The preschool years are therefore a critical period in the total life span.

Developmental Traits

After the First Year: Brain growth is rapid before birth and for the first two years. Proper nourishment during this time helps to ensure optimal motor development and intellectual abilities.

By 12 months, a child should be able to grasp and manipulate objects, including a cup, fairly well. The variety and number of intriguing objects increase steadily, along with new ways to bang, throw, roll, and, of course, taste them. By 18 months, little ones become more adept at stacking blocks and making marks with a crayon.

Babies learn to walk at about 12 months of age. By 18 months, they are able to move quite rapidly and confidently. The range of scenery awaiting exploration provides constant opportunities. Children rarely remain still at this age, and they often tax every bit of the caretaker's energy. Between climbing stairs and furniture, running from room to room, checking out bathroom fixtures, and opening anything with a door or lid, a child's desire to learn about the surrounding environment never ceases.

Tender and loving attention, stimulating surroundings, safety precautions, and a basic routine enhance a child's development and positive self-image.

Two and Three Year Olds: Healthy two and three year olds are intensely curious and active. Their motor skills progressively become more developed and capable. They are able to scribble, name parts of the body, walk up steps, walk in a straight line, perform simple tasks independently, and express the word "no" without a moment's hesitation. Their vocabulary and the length of their phrases expand, and their attention span increases gradually. Left-or right-hand dominance begins to emerge.

Four, Five, and Six Year Olds: Children this age are less likely to scurry rapidly from one activity to another. Their increased concentration level and attention to detail allow a new type of learning to take place. Looking at books, watching television programs like Sesame Street, role playing with other children, running, jumping, hopping, and drawing various shapes are popular activities. Their problem-solving ability and memory become more sophisticated.

The following anecdote helps to illustrate the distinction between ages. An active four-year-old boy loved playing outside with the water hose far better than any toy or activity. Consequently, his parents had removed all the water faucet handles to prevent large, muddy messes. One morning, upon spying a water faucet handle inadvertently left in place, the four-year-old very calmly told his father to go inside, thus hoping (unsuccessfully, as it turned out) to remove the obstacle to unihibited play. In a similar situation, the two or three year old would have simply made a beeline to the cherished object.

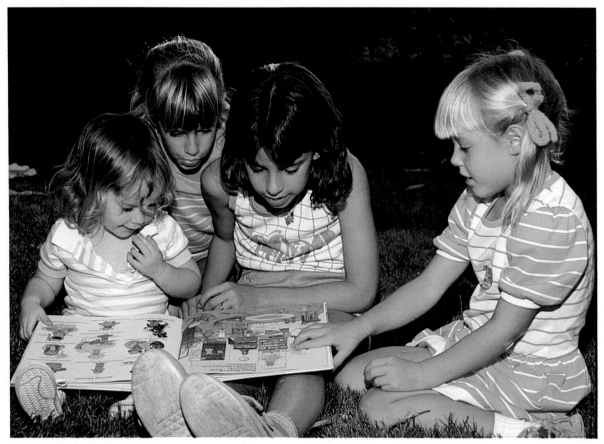

Children from four to six years of age enjoy looking at books because their problem-solving abilities are increasing.

Physical Growth Rate

After the First Year: The first year is without parallel in a child's growth. Most infants triple their birth weight during this time. As the first birthday passes, the rate of growth slows, with yearly increases approximating the birth weight. For example, if a child weighs seven pounds at birth, by age one the weight averages close to 21 pounds, and by age two, 28 pounds.

An infant's length at birth usually increases 50 percent by age one. Height doubles by age four and triples by age 13. For example, an infant 20 inches long at birth would be about three feet, four inches tall (40 inches total) at age four, and approximately five feet tall (60 inches) at age 13.

Two to Six Year Olds: After the second birthday, a child's weight gain usually slows down to about five pounds per year for the next seven or eight years. As mentioned, the birth length should double by age four. Slowly the roly-poly look of infancy disappears as height increases at a faster rate than weight. Body proportions also change. By age two, the head has reached a disproportionate two-thirds of its adult size. During the rest of growth, the trunk of the body slowly catches up to the head proportions. Meanwhile, the leg length increases. In summary, young children cannot be considered to be "miniature adults" in body shape.

Figure 14.1 shows growth charts that are used to determine the percentile track into which a child's rate of growth falls when compared to other children the same age. Plotting a child's height and weight every few months clearly illustrates the overall pattern. Growth far below or greatly in excess of the middle range warrants a closer look. Also, sudden changes in a child's growth percentile track should be investigated. For example, a child with average growth (50th percentile) who drops down to the 10th percentile one year later may very well have medical or nutritional problems.

FIGURE 14.1

These growth charts are used to compare the rate of growth of one child with other children of the same age. Plot the child's height and weight every three months. Growth far below or above the 50th percentile, or growth that deviates from a given percentile tract, needs to be checked with a physician.

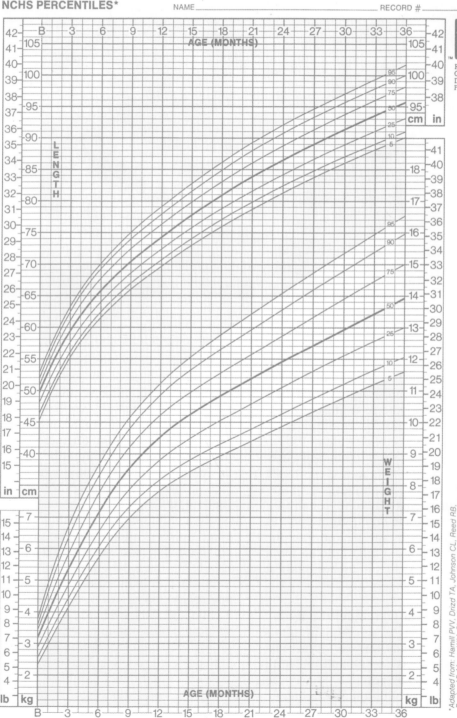

GIRLS: BIRTH TO 36 MONTHS
PHYSICAL GROWTH
NCHS PERCENTILES*

NAME _____ RECORD # _____

*Adapted from: Hamill PVV, Drizd TA, Johnson CL, Reed RB, Roche AF, Moore WM: Physical growth: National Center for Health Statistics percentiles. AM J CLIN NUTR 32:607-629, 1979. Data from the Fels Research Institute, Wright State University School of Medicine, Yellow Springs, Ohio.

© 1980 ROSS LABORATORIES

Ross
Growth &
Development
Program

NAME_____ RECORD #_____

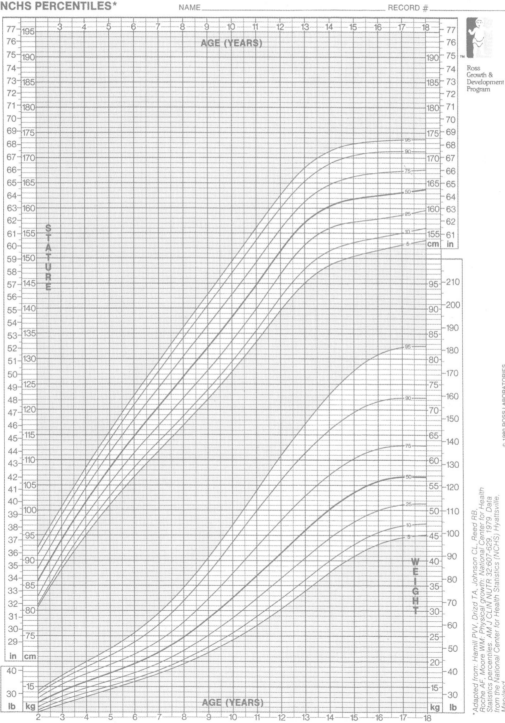

Ross
Growth &
Development
Program

© 1980 ROSS LABORATORIES

*Adapted from: Hamill PVV, Drizd TA, Johnson CL, Reed RB,
Roche AF, Moore WM. Physical growth: National Center for Health
Statistics percentiles. AM J CLIN NUTR 32:607-629, 1979. Data
from the National Center for Health Statistics (NCHS) Hyattsville,
Maryland.

*F*IGURE 14.1
continued

BOYS: BIRTH TO 36 MONTHS
PHYSICAL GROWTH
NCHS PERCENTILES*   NAME_____   RECORD #_____

*Adapted from: Hamill PVV, Drizd TA, Johnson CL, Reed RB, Roche AF, Moore WM. Physical growth: National Center for Health Statistics percentiles. AM J CLIN NUTR 32:607-629, 1979. Data from the Fels Research Institute, Wright State University School of Medicine, Yellow Springs, Ohio.

© 1980 ROSS LABORATORIES

NAME _____ RECORD # _____

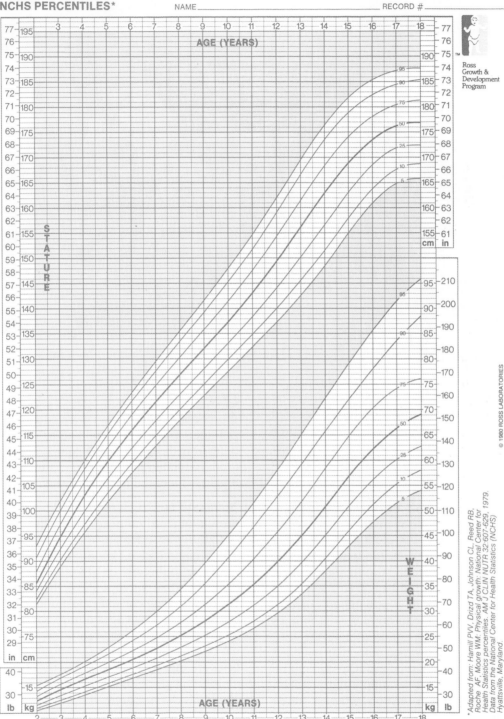

Ross
Growth &
Development
Program

© 1980 ROSS LABORATORIES

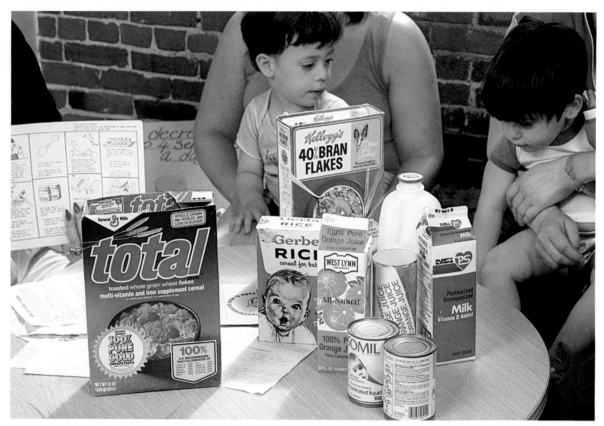

Nutrition seminars provide supplemental food and nutrition information for many families.

Delayed Growth: Children receiving inadequate Calories and protein will suffer stunted growth and development. Studies with children from low-income families reveal marginal, lower Caloric intakes in contrast to children from higher-income families.

Government programs such as the **Women, Infants, and Children (WIC)** provide supplemental food and nutrition classes for low-income families. WIC provides vouchers, or coupons, for high-nutrient foods such as dairy products, infant formulas, baby cereals, juice, peanut butter, and dried beans. In addition to receiving these food supplements, parents attend brief nutrition education classes. Studies show that infants and children receiving WIC support are taller and weigh more than matched groups not involved with the WIC program (1). For every dollar spent on supporting pregnant women in the WIC nutrition program, three dollars are saved in future medical costs, such as for treatment of low-birth-weight or anemic infants (2).

Diet

Preschool children need a varied and nutrient-rich diet. Their nutritional and health concerns differ from those of an adult. Simply serving adult foods in smaller portions to children will not adequately meet their special needs.

Nutritional Needs

Preschool children need almost the same level of Calories as sedentary adults (see table 14.1). The recommended Caloric intake for children from one to three years of age is 1,300 Calories daily. National surveys show that the average child of this age consumes just under 1,200 Calories per day. From ages four to six, the recommended intake is 1,800 Calories per day, with national surveys showing that close to 1,500 Calories are ingested. Considering the small size of children at these ages, this represents quite a challenge: to consume all the Calories needed, it is often necessary for children to eat foods higher in Calories than those eaten by adults. Generally, diet recommendations for adults emphasize foods that are low to moderate in Ca-

TABLE 14.1
Recommended dietary allowances for children (males and females)

Age (Years)	1–3 (13 kg)	4–6 (20 kg)
Energy (kcal)	1300	1800
Protein (g)	16	24
Vitamin A (μg – RE)	400	500
Vitamin D (μg)	10	10
Vitamin E (mg – αTE)	6	7
Ascorbic acid (mg)	40	45
Folacin (μg)	50	75
Niacin (mg – NE)	9	12
Riboflavin (mg)	0.8	1.1
Thiamin (mg)	0.7	0.9
Vitamin B_6 (mg)	1.0	1.1
Vitamin B_{12} (μg)	0.7	1.0
Calcium (mg)	800	800
Phosphorus (mg)	800	800
Iodine (μg)	70	90
Iron (mg)	10	10
Magnesium (mg)	80	120
Zinc (mg)	10	10

Reprinted with permission from: Food and Nutrition Board. Recommended Dietary Allowances. 10th rev. ed. 1989. Washington, DC: National Academy Press, 1989.

loric content, or foods that are high in dietary fiber and low in fat content. Such a diet is advised to help prevent heart disease, cancer, and obesity in adults. Although these principles also apply to children, such foods as nuts, dried fruits, cheese, and plant oils are needed to help provide sufficient Calories for active, growing children.

The Caloric ranges given for children are designed so that about half the Calories will maintain bodily functions and the other half will be used for activity and growth. As previously mentioned, there are three sources of Calories in the diet. Calories from protein are needed primarily for growth. Calories from carbohydrate provide the body's preferred source of energy, especially during physical activity. Calories from fat are a form of concentrated energy for storage and special body demands. For optimal growth and development, an appropriate balance of these three Calorie sources is needed.

Protein: The protein recommendation for children ages one to three is 16 grams per day, and for children four to six, 24 grams per day (see table 14.1). National surveys show that children of these ages consume nearly 50 grams of protein per day, far above the recommended level. The actual amount of protein a child needs may be somewhat higher or lower, depending on the child's weight and rate of growth. Also, if there is an overall Calorie shortage, some of the protein in the diet must be used to supply energy, decreasing the supply available for growth. Ideally, 10 to 15 percent of the total daily Caloric intake should come from protein.

Carbohydrate: For most U.S. children, carbohydrate supplies almost half of the Calories. As discussed in chapter 5, there are two types of carbohydrate—the simple sugars (as found in candy and fruit), and the complex carbohydrate (including starches). Sugar has been blamed for countless evils in children, from hyperactivity to allergies. As will be reviewed in this chapter's Health-Promotion Insight, scientific evidence fails to support these claims but does show that sugar causes cavities and often displaces more nutritious foods in the diet (3). With a growing child's need for Calories and nutrients, there's little room for high-sugar foods that supply Calories with few nutrients.

Complex-carbohydrate foods such as whole-grain breads and cereals, rice, pasta, and beans supply an excellent quantity of energy, B vitamins, and dietary fiber. Although a very-high-fiber diet is not recommended for children because of their need to consume high levels of Calories despite their small size (and stomachs), a moderate amount of fiber is important. For example, bran supplements or high-bran breakfast cereals are not recommended. Learning to eat a balanced diet that includes food sources of fiber lays the foundation for a healthy diet in later years. As reviewed in chapter 5, research shows that adults consuming a complex-carbohyrdrate, fiber-rich diet reduce their risk of acquiring such diseases as colon cancer, diabetes, diverticulosis, and heart disease.

Fat: The third source of Calories is fat. Fat, by definition, is the most concentrated form of Calories (see chapter 6). One gram of fat has nine Calories, which is more than twice the four Calories found in a gram of protein or carbohydrate (see chapter 8). Since dietary fats, especially saturated, animal fats, are related to heart disease, cancer, and obesity, some parents have thought it important to strictly reduce the fat content of their children's diets. Stunted growth in children can result from an overzealous attempt to eliminate fat Calories. The National Institute of Health and the American Heart Association both recommend a moderate decrease in fatty foods beginning at age two (4,5). However, total Calories from fat should be in the range of 30 to 40 percent. This is higher than what is recommended for adults (see chapter 6).

Vitamins and Minerals: In addition to an imbalance in the three Calorie sources, several key nutrients may be lacking in young children's diets. The USDA Nationwide Food Consumption Survey (NFCS) (6) and the National Health and Nutrition Examination Surveys (7,8) show low iron, calcium, vitamin B_6, and vitamin C intakes among young children. The Selected Minerals in Foods Survey conducted by the Food and Drug Administration (9) also reported low iron intakes among young children, as well as low zinc intakes. Other studies (10) point to low vitamin-A intakes. Place of residence, ethnic background, family income, the nutrition knowledge of the parents, and seasonal changes are factors influencing the vitamin and mineral levels of children's diets.

As reviewed in chapter 11, iron is vital for blood transport of oxygen throughout the body and is involved in many enzyme systems of the body. During periods of growth, demands for iron are especially high. Table 14.1 shows that the RDA for one to three year olds and for four to six year olds is 10 mg per day. Including foods such as fortified cereals, dried fruits, lean meats, seeds, nuts, and dried beans helps to meet these high requirements. Iron supplements are not recommended unless a physician advises them for medical reasons. Including vitamin-C-rich foods with each meal increases the absorption of iron from plant foods (see chapter 11).

Another important nutrient is calcium, which is recommended in quantities equal to that of adults (800 mg per day) (see Sidebar 14.1). As reviewed in chapter 11, calcium is needed for building bones and teeth, in addition to regulating nerve and muscle function. Dairy products are the major source of calcium, but whole grains, dried beans, dark green leafy vegetables, seeds, and nuts also supply good

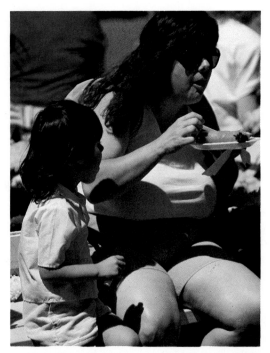

Children need the structure of regular mealtimes that offer a variety of wholesome foods and appropriate portion sizes.

amounts. Using milk in soups, sauces, pancakes, and baked goods can help children obtain the high amounts of recommended calcium. Children who are allergic to milk can be given soy milk or other milk substitutes fortified with calcium.

Food Patterns and Choices

Two principles govern the food patterns and choices of healthy diets for children: variety and portion size. When a child consumes a wide variety of healthful foods in adequate amounts, the potential for health and proper growth is excellent. However, if a three year old, for example, consumes only cottage cheese and applesauce, the chance of health problems rises.

Children's portions are much smaller than adults'. One guideline is to serve one tablespoon for each year of life. For example, the three year old can be given a portion of fruit equal to three tablespoons. When larger servings are given, several problems may occur. The child may be discouraged and leave the food untouched, or may eat it all, leaving less room for other nutritious foods needed to balance the diet.

How Much Do You Need?

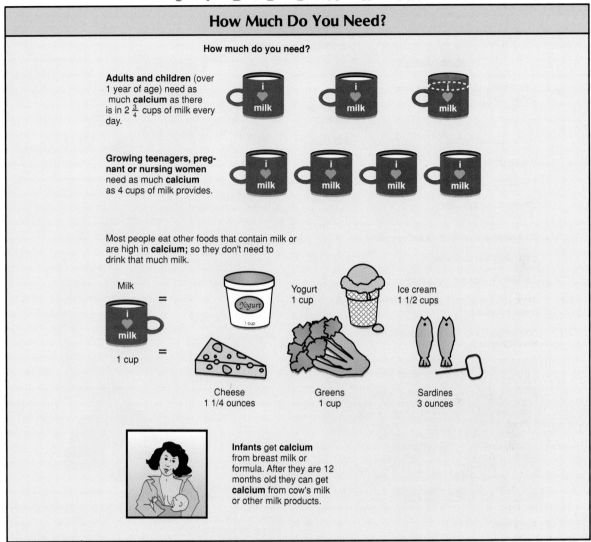

How much do you need?

Adults and children (over 1 year of age) need as much **calcium** as there is in 2 ¾ cups of milk every day.

Growing teenagers, pregnant or nursing women need as much **calcium** as 4 cups of milk provides.

Most people eat other foods that contain milk or are high in **calcium**; so they don't need to drink that much milk.

Milk

= Yogurt 1 cup

= Ice cream 1 1/2 cups

1 cup = Cheese 1 1/4 ounces

= Greens 1 cup

= Sardines 3 ounces

Infants get **calcium** from breast milk or formula. After they are 12 months old they can get **calcium** from cow's milk or other milk products.

From *Women, Infants, Children* (Supplemental Food Section). California Department of Health Services, Sacramento. Used with permission.

Obesity is another concern with some young children. As discussed in chapter 9, close to one out of four children and youth in this country is considered obese. Because a significant portion of overweight adults were also overweight as children, avoidance of overeating by children is an important goal. Figure 14.2 describes various methods that can be used to help children avoid becoming obese.

Study figure 14.3, which outlines the recommended food patterns for three preschool groups: one year olds, two and three year olds, and four to six year olds. The number of servings is the same for each food group; only the portion sizes vary. Children need four servings from the milk group, three servings from protein sources, four servings from the bread and cereal group, and four servings from the fruit and vegetable group, including one vitamin-C-rich food and one vitamin-A-rich food (from dark green and yellow sources).

**Helping Your Child to Avoid
Becoming Overweight**

1. FOOD CHOICES

Offer foods from each of these food
groups daily

	Number* of Servings
Milk and milk products	2 -3 Cups
Protein group	3
Breads, cereals, grains	4
Vitamin-C-rich fruits and vegetables	1
Dark green and yellow fruits and vegetables	1
Other fruits and vegetables	2

*Smaller servings for young children.

Think about what you feed your child and how you
prepare the food

Choose foods with less fat and sugar, therefore
low in Calories.

Higher Calories	Lower Calories
French fries	Baked potato
Ice cream	Frozen juice popsicles
Whole milk	Low/nonfat milk
Chips	Soda crackers
Cookies, cake, pie	Piece of fruit
Doughnuts	Toast
Sour cream	Plain yogurt
Fried hamburger	Broiled hamburger
Hi - C, Kool - aid, or soda	Water

Remember:

1. Food high in sugar and fat is also high in Calories.
2. Choose lower - Calorie foods.
3. Bake or broil instead of fry.
4. One cookie is better than six cookies.
5. Avoid buying high-Calorie foods.

2. OVEREATING

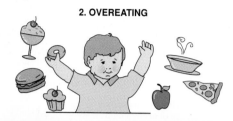

DO YOU...	TRY...
• Use food as a reward or bribe?	Hugs and kisses instead of food.
• Let your child drink all he wants from a bottle?	Use a cup or put water in bottle.
• Push your child to "clean the plate"?	Serve smaller portions on small plates.
• Let your child eat **whenever** he wants?	Set regular meal and snack times.
• Let your child eat **whatever** he wants?	Say "no" to junk-food requests. Give a choice of low-Calorie foods.
• Quiet your child with food?	Comfort your child.

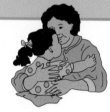

Things to Do !

1. Encourage eating slowly.
2. Keep portions small; let your child ask for seconds.
3. Store food out of sight and reach.
4. Set a good example.

3. ACTIVITY

Take your child's mind off food.
Encourage active play every day.

Take a walk with your child
Play in the park
Ride tricycles
Swim
Play ball
Running, jumping, skipping
Dance to music
Set aside "family exercise time"

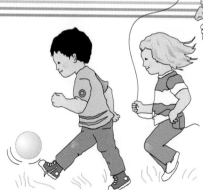

Remember...

• Make activities fun
• Limit TV watching
• Active play uses Calories
• Active children sleep better

FIGURE 14.3

Foods for your child—every day

	Milk and Milk Products	Protein Foods	Breads, Cereals and Grain	Vitamin-C-Rich Fruits / Vegetables	Dark Green and Yellow Fruits / Vegetables	Other Fruits/ Vegetables
Number of Servings	4	3	4	1	1	2
Servings Eaten						
Serving Size **1** year old	1/2 c milk, yogurt 3/4 oz cheese	1 oz meat, poultry, fish 1 egg 1/2 c cooked beans 2 tbsp peanut butter	1/2 slice bread, tortilla 1/4 c rice, pasta 1/4 c cooked cereal 1/3 c dry cereal	1/4 c fruit juice 1 small fruit 2 tbsp cooked vegetables	1 small fruit 2 tbsp cooked vegetables	1/4 c fruit juice 1 small fruit 2 tbsp cooked vegetables
2 - 3 year old	1/2 - 3/4 c milk, yogurt 3/4 - 1 oz cheese	1 oz meat, poultry, fish 1 egg 1/2 c cooked beans 2 tbsp peanut butter	1 slice bread, tortilla 1/3 c rice, pasta 1/3 c cooked cereal 1/2 c dry cereal	1/2 c fruit juice 1 small fruit 1/4 c cooked vegetables 1/2 c raw vegetables	1 small fruit 1/4 c cooked vegetables 1/2 c raw vegetables	1/2 c fruit juice 1 small fruit 1/4 c cooked vegetables 1/2 c raw vegetables
4 - 5 year old	3/4 c milk, yogurt 3/4 oz cheese	1 - 2 oz meat, poultry, fish 1 egg 1/2 - 3/4 c cooked beans 2 - 4 tbsp peanut butter	1 slice bread, tortilla 1/2 c rice, pasta 1/2 c cooked cereal 3/4 c dry cereal	1/2 c fruit juice 1 small fruit 1/4 c cooked vegetables 1/2 c raw vegetables	1 small fruit 1/4 c cooked vegetables 1/2 c raw vegetables	1/2 c fruit juice 1 small fruit 1/4 c cooked vegetables 1/2 c raw vegetables

FIGURE 14.4

Age	Breakfast	Snack	Lunch	Snack	Dinner
1 year old	1/2 c milk 1/4 c hot cereal 1/2 small banana	1/4 c orange juice 1 hard-boiled egg 1 graham cracker	1/2 c milk 1/2 peanut butter sandwich 2 tbsp. peas 1/2 peach	1/2 c milk 1/4 c dry cereal	1/2 c milk 1 chicken leg 1/4 c rice 2 T. carrots 1/4 c applesauce
2–3 year old	1/2 c milk 1/2 c orange juice 1/2 c dry cereal	1/2 c apple juice cheese cubes	1/2 c milk 1/2 c ham and split pea soup 1 slice bread apple slices	1/2 c yogurt 3–4 crackers	1/2 c milk 2 oz hamburger patty 1/3 c noodles 1/4 c broccoli 1/2 c lettuce salad
4–5 year old	3/4 c milk 1 scrambled egg 1 slice toast 1/2 c orange juice	1/2 c pineapple juice 3–4 crackers	3/4 c milk 1 tuna sandwich 3–4 carrot sticks	3/4 c milk peanut butter & celery	3/4 c milk 3/4 c chili con carne 1/2 c tossed spinach salad 1 piece cornbread

Sample menu

Snacks are needed by the very young child and should be offered as part of their daily diet. Include such foods as: fruits and fruit juices, vegetables, cheese, crackers, peanut butter, hard-cooked eggs, yogurt, custards, dry cereal.

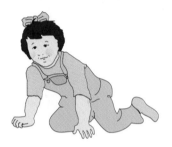

Many small children are not able to eat enough at each meal to last four to five hours. It is also difficult for them to eat all the recommended foods in just three meals. For these reasons small, nutritious snacks are recommended. When snacks are a part of the meal plan described in figure 14.3, they serve a positive function. There is no place in a growing child's diet for regular snacks high in sugar, fats, and salt. This practice sets a bad precedent for future health habits. Children who are brought up eating healthfully may find it easier during adulthood to follow recommended dietary practices. Problems arise if snacking occurs all day and interferes with more structured meals. Mealtimes provide children an opportunity to learn about balanced food choices and also to become skilled in social relations.

Figure 14.4 illustrates a sample menu for the preschool age groups. The food choices include a variety of foods rich in such key nutrients as protein, vitamin A, vitamin C, iron, and calcium.

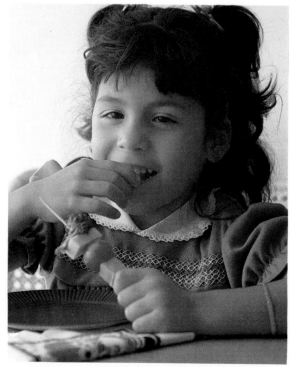

When new foods are introduced, children are often attracted to bite-sized portions that they can eat with their hands.

382 Chapter 14

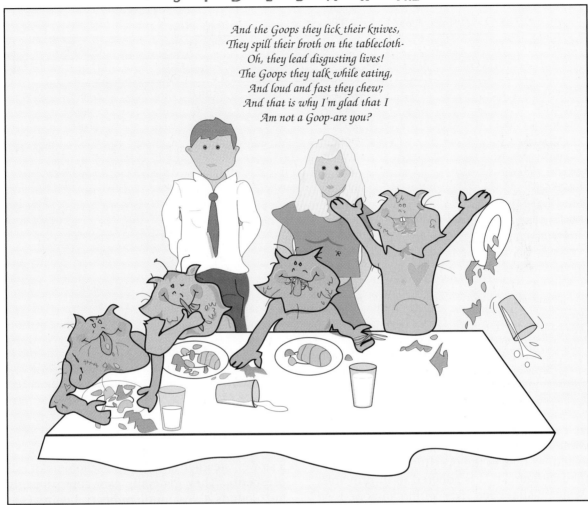

And the Goops they lick their knives,
They spill their broth on the tablecloth-
Oh, they lead disgusting lives!
The Goops they talk while eating,
And loud and fast they chew;
And that is why I'm glad that I
Am not a Goop-are you?

Promoting a Healthy Life-Style

The foundation for lifelong eating habits and food choices is laid in early childhood. Forced feeding, using food as a reward, eating when bored or upset, irregular and unbalanced meals, and tension-filled mealtimes leave lasting impressions. Children need the structure of regular mealtimes at which a variety of wholesome foods and appropriate-size portions are offered.

When new foods are introduced, children are often attracted to bite-sized portions that can be eaten with their hands. These "finger foods" can include cut up pieces of raw "broccoli trees" or a slice of fresh "papaya suns". The attitude of those nearby is meaningful when a child is deciding whether to try something new. Also, repeated exposure to new foods can make each additional experience a bit easier, especially if it occurs without fanfare.

When parents nag and coerce a child to eat, the child quickly realizes that his behavior can be used to control his parents. Food becomes a power issue. Generally, a more relaxed approach works best, while at the same time limiting access to unhealthy foods. A child who is unwilling to touch dinner should not be allowed to run to the cookie jar instead. It is normal for young children to experience periods of rejecting various types of food or eating a few special foods. As the child's unique personality develops and unfolds, so too does his or her special style of eating behavior (see Sidebar 14.2). Wails of protest such as "but I only

TABLE 14.2
Recommended dietary allowances for children and youth

Age (Years)	Males and Females 7–10	Males 11–14	Females 11–14
Energy (kcal)	2000	2500	2200
Protein (g)	28	45	46
Vitamin A (μg—RE)	700	1000	800
Vitamin D (μg)	10	10	10
Vitamin E (mg—αTE)	7	10	8
Ascorbic acid (mg)	45	50	50
Folacin (μg)	100	150	150
Niacin (mg—NE)	13	17	15
Riboflavin (mg)	1.2	1.5	1.3
Thiamin (mg)	1.0	1.3	1.1
Vitamin B_6 (mg)	1.4	1.7	1.4
Vitamin B_{12} (μg)	1.4	2.0	2.0
Calcium (mg)	800	1200	1200
Phosphorus (mg)	800	1200	1200
Iodine (μg)	120	150	150
Iron (mg)	10	12	15
Magnesium (mg)	170	270	280
Zinc (mg)	10	15	12

Reprinted with permission from: Food and Nutrition Board. Recommended Dietary Allowances. 10th rev. ed. 1989. Washington, DC: National Academy Press, 1989.

eat half sandwiches and whole bananas, not whole sandwiches and half bananas" can be expected. As long as the overall food plan as outlined in figure 14.3 is adhered to in principle, specific dislikes and likes within any one food group are fine. However, if a child completely avoids all foods in a particular food group (for example, no dark green or yellow vegetables and fruit), this is a more serious problem, and if necessary, counseling with a dietitian may be indicated.

Children Ages 6–12

Physical Growth

Developmental Traits
As children enter school, they become increasingly independent. The parenting role gradually changes from primarily physical caretaking to providing and guiding. The influence of other children and adults grows as activities outside the home increase.

Physical Growth Rate
School-age children from six to twelve grow at a slower, steadier rate than preschoolers or **adolescents.** They generally gain approximately five pounds a year until **puberty** begins (see figure 14.1).

Diet

Nutritional Needs
The Caloric demands for children aged six to twelve range from 1,800–2,500 (see table 14.2 for average recommended levels). Younger and less active children should consume Calories at the lower end of this range, whereas older, physically active children typically consume more. Beginning at age eleven, the caloric RDA for boys (2,500 Calories) exceeds that of girls (2,200 Calories). From this age on, caloric, vitamin, and mineral recommendations differ between the sexes.

The years between ages six and twelve are sometimes known as the "lull before the storm." A good diet helps provide adequate stores of nutrients, such as calcium, that will be needed during the adolescent growth spurt.

TABLE 14.3

Food substitutions to improve the quality of the diet in elementary school children

Substitute good foods for undesirable ones — don't merely take them away.

Instead of:	Try:
Soft drinks or punch	Fruit juice
Ice cream	Frozen yogurt or juice popsicle
Cookies	Whole-wheat crackers with cheese
Potato chips	Popcorn
Candy	Dried fruit
Cake, pie, doughnuts	Cut up fresh fruit or vegetables

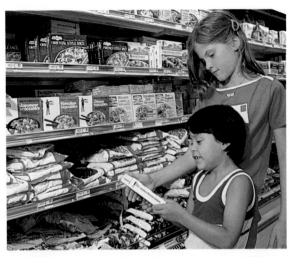

The grocery store can be an excellent place to review nutrition principles that have been discussed at home.

Likewise, the development of a strong, healthy body through proper dietary and exercise habits during these years helps to ensure optimal growth and development during adolescence.

As with preschool children, diet surveys of elementary school children also indicate that several nutrients may be low in the diet. Iron deficiency is most common. During childhood, the body's demand for iron is much higher per pound of body weight than for an adult, and it equals the total (15 mg) recommended for an adult woman. Special care should be taken to include iron-rich and fortified foods in the daily diet.

Elementary school children may also have low intakes of some of the B vitamins, vitamin A, vitamin C, and calcium. Generally, nutrient deficiencies at this age are simply the result of not eating enough food. However, the quality of the food choices becomes critical when children refuse to eat the amounts of food recommended. Table 14.3 outlines some of the foods that can be substituted for less nutrient-dense foods to improve the quality of the diet for elementary school children.

Food Patterns and Choices

Variety and portion size are still key elements in the diets of elementary school children. The number of servings from each food group remains basically the same as in the preschooler meal plan, but the portion sizes are larger. Faster growing and more active children are encouraged to select more food from each of the food groups, but in particular the bread and cereal group (see table 14.4 for the daily food pattern recommended for elementary school age children).

Other Factors Affecting Nutritional Status

As children grow older, an increasing number of factors influence their nutritional status. Peer preferences, school lunch programs, television viewing, snacking habits, potential food allergies, activity levels, growth rate, family attitudes, and a wider variety of food offerings all contribute to the nutritional status of the elementary school child.

Food Marketing: Children are a popular target among food advertisers. Well-known television and movie stars who promote various types of foods make lasting impressions on susceptible children (and adults). Nutrition misinformation is widespread, and unfortunately, advertising media generally make little effort to screen the accuracy of information presented.

Grocery-store displays and vending machines are also enticing to children. When children see products in the store that have been advertised on television, "grocery-store tantrums" can occur, especially if the parent attempts to seek alternate products. To avoid such problems, parents need to spend time educating the child about the motives of food companies and advertising agencies. In addition, the grocery store can actually be an excellent site to review nutrition principles that have been discussed at home. If children and parents plan meals together at home, grocery shopping becomes more focused on selecting menu ingredients.

Daily food pattern for children ages 6–12

Milk/Milk Products (Four Servings)	Protein Foods (Three Servings)	Breads and Cereals (Four or More Servings)	Vitamin-C-Rich Fruit/Vegetables (One or More Servings)	Dark Green or Yellow Fruit/ Vegetables (One or More Servings)	Other Fruit/ Vegetable (Two or More Servings)
For Ages 6–9					
¾ c low-fat Milk/ yogurt or ¾ oz cheese	2 oz lean meat or one egg or ½ to ¾ c cooked beans or 3 tbsp peanut butter	1 slice or ½ c rice, pasta, cooked cereal or ¾ c dry cereal	½ c juice or 1 fruit or ⅓ c cooked veg or ½ c raw veg	1 small or ⅓ c cooked veg or ½ c raw veg	½ c juice or 1 fruit or ⅓ c cooked veg or ½ c raw veg
For Ages 10–12					
1 c low-fat Milk/ yogurt or 1 oz cheese	2 oz lean meat or one egg or ½ to ¾ c cooked beans or 3 tbsp peanut butter	1 slice or ½ c rice, pasta, cooked cereal or ¾ c dry cereal	½ c juice or 1 fruit or ½ c cooked veg or ¾ c raw veg	1 small or ½ c cooked veg or ¾ c raw veg	½ c juice or 1 fruit or ½ c cooked veg or ¾ c raw veg

Television Viewing: In addition to the marketing influence of television, there are other associated concerns. Time spent watching television is time away from playing outdoors, interacting with friends and family, or reading and doing homework. Additionally, television viewing is frequently associated with snacking. Several studies have confirmed these concerns. One study showed that children who were rated as light television viewers scored significantly better than moderate and heavy television viewers on a comprehensive physical fitness test (11). The researchers concluded that "for purposes of good physical fitness, television viewing should be limited to one hour or less per day." In another study, results showed that television can have a major impact on children's knowledge, attitudes, and behavior (12). For example, aggressive behavior can be increased, racial and sex-role stereotypes can be strengthened, interest in reading and school activities can be decreased, and poorer health habits and attitudes can be developed. Another study showed that the prevalence of obesity among children watching television for five or more hours per day was twice as high when compared to children watching less than one hour per day (13). Obviously, parents need to help children manage their television viewing habits.

School Lunches: Most children participate in the nationwide school lunch program. Federal guidelines regulate the balance of food groups and portion sizes for each age group served. One-third of the RDA for children must be supplied by school lunches. Compliance is essential before school districts can receive monetary support and supplemental foods at reduced costs. Provisions are made for lower-income children to receive free or reduced-price lunches.

Food-service personnel responsible for planning and preparing school lunches face a challenging task. At issue is selecting a variety of nutritious foods that children like (or can at least tolerate) while attempting to stay within a very lean budget. Recent trends have included student, teacher, and parental involvement with menu planning, more options for children to choose from, the serving of lower-fat milk, better lunchtime scheduling, and greater attention to preparation methods.

Some factors continue to interfere with the nutritional balance provided by school lunches. As young children first begin eating away from home, they are often reluctant to try any food that looks or tastes different. Generally, elementary school children eat a lower percentage of their food than high schoolers (14). Vegetables are the most frequently rejected item.

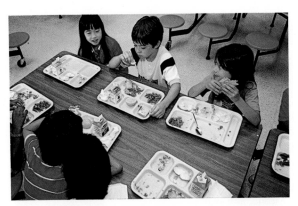

Federal guidelines regulate the balance of food groups and portion sizes in the nationwide school lunch program.

Another problem is the availability of vending machines. Many school districts have debated this issue, balancing revenue income with nutritional concerns. Some schools have successfully limited vending machines to healthier food choices such as milk, juice, fruit, and nuts.

Some children choose not to participate in the school lunch program, bringing a lunch from home instead. Although not true in all cases, one study showed that school lunches tend to be nutritionally superior when compared to lunches brought from home (15).

Early Changes in the Diet of Young Girls: Research indicates that girls begin to adopt adult eating habits at an earlier age (nine to eleven) than boys. Unfortunately, this means a decrease in consumption of milk, breads, and cereals, with an increase in use of coffee, tea, and soft drinks (16). Evidently, girls see milk as a young child's beverage and begin cutting back to look "adultlike" at the very time when calcium needs begin increasing. Many girls also subscribe to the popular misconception that starches are fattening and should therefore be limited. As explained in chapter 5, foods high in starches are usually very low in fat but high in dietary fiber, a combination that bodes well for health and prevention of obesity and chronic disease.

Promoting a Healthy Life-Style

The ages six to twelve are an ideal time to teach good nutrition and life-style habits. As children become more independent in their decisions, they have more control over their own eating and activity choices. As mentioned, adult eating behavior has an influence, generally first observed in girls. To help prevent the formation of health-endangering habits, parents can provide their children with both accurate nutrition information and good role models. As children enter adolescence, peer pressure introduces a whole new set of problems to cope with, such as substance abuse, binge-eating, avoidance of entire food groups, reliance on fast foods, and meal skipping. Good nutrition habits, when taught during the receptive elementary school years, may help the adolescent "weather the storm."

The Adolescent Years: Ages 13–19

Physical Growth

Individual variation is the single most important trait of adolescent growth. Some adolescents shoot up to towering heights even before they become teenagers. Others amble through high school with junior high school bodies. Sooner or later, however, adolescents do undergo growth spurts almost as dramatic as the changes that occur during infancy.

Males

Generally, males start their puberty growth two years after females, with the peak velocity at approximately 14 years of age. The beginning of this growth period is signaled by the secondary sex characteristics of voice change, pubic hair growth, and genital development. Muscular and skeletal development continues, often with body fat decreasing. Bone density increases during the adolescent growth spurt, which requires an adequate supply of calcium.

Although full height is usually attained by age 19, it is possible for slight increases to occur during the early twenties (17). Figure 14.1 demonstrates normal growth rates, and as stated before, the best comparison is the adolescent's present growth rate versus individual past growth rate. The overall trend is what is important.

Females

Females usually begin puberty growth around ten to eleven years of age, and reach peak velocity between 12 and 13. During these years, girls are often taller and heavier than boys. Physical development includes pubic hair growth, breast development, and the onset of menstruation. The percentage of body fat increases to a level almost double that of boys. By age 15 or 16, girls have generally completed their growth spurt.

Recent Growth and Development Trends

Evidence shows that children now mature at younger ages compared to 50 to 100 years ago. Girls begin their periods earlier, reach taller heights at earlier ages, and have an accelerated sexual maturation (18). Environmental factors including improved quality and quantity of food, decreased physical hardship, and improved medical care and sanitation are thought to be primarily responsible.

Diet

Nutritional Needs

The Caloric needs of adolescents are higher than at any other time of life. For females the recommendation is 2,200 Calories per day, and for males it is 3,000. National surveys show that teenage girls average 1,800 Calories a day, and teenage boys average 2,600 Calories per day. Although pound for pound the Caloric demands of preschoolers are actually higher than for adolescents, the total Caloric requirement for adolescents is greater. After the slower-growing middle years, another critical growth period begins, with demands for high levels of Calories and nutrients (see table 14.5).

According to national surveys, the diets of adolescent boys are fairly adequate due to their high Caloric intakes (6,7,8). Most of the required nutrients are found among the large quantities of food they ingest.

The diets of adolescent girls, however, are often lacking in essential nutrients. Vitamin B_6, iron, calcium, magnesium, and copper are the key nutrients lacking. Low Caloric consumption and poor food choices make it somewhat difficult for girls to ingest the level of nutrients needed during their high growth period and

Age (Years)	Males	Females
	15–18	15–18
Energy (kcal)	3000	2200
Protein (g)	59	44
Vitamin A (μg—RE)	1000	800
Vitamin D (μg)	10	10
Vitamin E (mg—αTE)	10	8
Ascorbic acid (mg)	60	60
Folacin (μg)	200	180
Niacin (mg—NE)	20	15
Riboflavin (mg)	1.8	1.3
Thiamin (mg)	1.5	1.1
Vitamin B_6 (mg)	2.0	1.5
Vitamin B_{12} (μg)	2.0	2.0
Calcium (mg)	1200	1200
Phosphorus (mg)	1200	1200
Iodine (μg)	150	150
Iron (mg)	12	15
Magnesium (mg)	400	300
Zinc (mg)	15	12

TABLE 14.5
Recommended dietary allowances for children and youth

Reprinted with permission from: Food and Nutrition Board. Recommended Dietary Allowances. 10th rev. ed. 1989. Washington, DC: National Academy Press, 1989

time of sexual maturation. Other factors, such as dieting, activity levels, eating disorders, substance abuse, and meal skipping, may impair their nutritional status.

Adolescents have protein needs comparable to adults (see table 14.4). Like adults, teenaged boys and girls have been found to consume far more protein than is required (100 and 66 grams per day, respectively). Fat intake for teenaged boys and girls averages 37 percent and 43 percent of total Calories, respectively, which is higher than recommended. Carbohydrate intake is on the low side, as a result.

As with the earlier years, iron deficiency continues to be of concern for some teenagers. Adolescent girls are at higher risk of anemia because of three factors: iron losses during menstruation, rapid growth rate, and lower than recommended Caloric intakes. An emphasis on foods rich in iron is important (see chapter 11).

Calcium is another vital nutrient especially needed during high growth periods. The RDA for calcium during adolescence is very high—1,200 mg per day, or 50 percent higher

TABLE 14.6
Daily food pattern for teenagers, ages 13–19

Milk/Milk Products	Protein Foods	Breads and Cereals	Vitamin-C-Rich Fruit/Vegetables	Dark Green Yellow Fruit/ Vegetables	Other Fruit/ Vegetables
		Males			
Four Servings	*Three Servings*	*Eight or More Servings*	*One or More Servings*	*One or More Servings*	*Three or More Servings*
1 c low-fat milk/ yogurt or 1 oz cheese	2–3 oz lean meat or one egg or ¾ c cooked beans or 4 tbsp peanut butter	1 slice or ½ c rice, pasta, cooked cereal or ¾ c dry cereal	½ c juice or 1 fruit or ½ c cooked veg or ¾ c raw veg	1 small or ½ c cooked veg or ¾ c raw veg	½ c juice or 1 fruit or ½ c cooked veg or ¾ c raw veg
		Females			
Four Servings	*Three Servings*	*Six or More Servings*	*One or More Servings*	*One or More Servings*	*Two or More Servings*
1 c low-fat milk/ yogurt or 1 oz cheese	2 oz lean meat or one egg or ½ to ¾ c cooked beans or 3 tbsp peanut butter	1 slice or ½ c rice, pasta, cooked cereal or ¾ c dry cereal	½ c juice or 1 fruit or ½ c cooked veg or ¾ c raw veg	1 small or ½ c cooked veg or ¾ c raw veg	½ c juice or 1 fruit or ½ c cooled veg or ¾ c raw veg

than during adulthood. Adolescent girls who think milk is only for babies and young children would do well to reconsider. Without milk (preferably low-fat) and other dairy products, obtaining 1,200 mg of calcium daily is very difficult unless large amounts of dark green vegetables, whole grains, and seeds and nuts are consumed, or a calcium supplement is taken.

Food Patterns and Choices

The best strategy for acquiring all the Calories, protein, fiber, vitamins, calcium, iron, and other nutrients recommended for adolescents is by eating a well-balanced diet. There is no shortcut, no magical substance or food.

Many similarities exist between the ideal diet recommended for adults and the one recommended for adolescents. Both need adequate protein, moderate to low levels of dietary fat, and need to obtain most of their Calories from complex carbohydrate. Teenagers do require more Calories than adults, however. Often the extra Calories come from high-fat foods such as cheeseburgers, french fries, milkshakes, and other fast foods. Ideally, high complex-carbohydrate foods such as pasta, rice, potatoes, breads and cereals, and fruits should be substituted.

Evidence indicates that the "typical teenager diet" may be associated with very adultlike diseases. Autopsies of young men in their early twenties who were killed in Vietnam have revealed extensive atherosclerosis (19). As explained in chapter 6, this means that fatty streaks and deposits (plaque material) had already begun to narrow the major arteries of the heart muscle in many of these young men, laying the foundation for premature death from heart attack. Such studies show that heart disease starts early in life and that teenagers (even children) should adopt an optimal diet with their future health in mind.

Table 14.6 outlines the daily food pattern recommendations for teenagers. The present weight and activity levels of the teenager must always be taken into consideration. Caloric recommendations and food choices for a sedentary, underweight, teenaged girl would vary considerably from the recommendations given to an active, muscular teenaged boy.

Table 14.7
Comparison of fast-food dinner vs home-cooked dinner

Fast-Food Dinner	Home-Cooked Dinner
Cheeseburger	Baked chicken (no skin)
French fries (1 serving)	(3 oz)
Cola-type soda (12 fl oz)	Brown rice (½ cup)
	Broccoli (½ cup)
	Whole-wheat dinner roll (1)
	Peanut butter (low sodium)
	(1 tsp)
	Tossed salad (lettuce,
	tomato, carrot, cucumber)
	(1 cup)
	Salad dressing, sweet &
	sour (2 tsp)
	Low-fat milk (12 fl oz)

Nutrient Analysis	Fast-Food Dinner	Home-Cooked Dinner
Calories	745	613
Protein (gm)	19	50
Fat (gm)	25	15
Sodium	817	485
Potassium (mg)	733	1305
Vitamin A (I.U.)	345	6722
Vitamin C (mg)	16	66
Iron (mg)	4.2	3.9
Calcium (mg)	153	620
Dietary fiber (gm)	4	9
Sugar (gm)	45	23
Caffeine (mg)	37	0

Note: the fast food meal is higher in calories, fat, sodium, sugar and caffeine, but lower in protein, potassium, vitamin A, vitamin C, calcium, and dietary fiber.

Table 14.7 demonstrates that a diet based on fast foods provides less nutrients, but more dietary fat, caffeine, sugar, and sodium than a diet based on wholesome home cooking. Ethnic restaurants (for example, Mexican, Chinese, or Italian) generally provide healthier food choices than most fast-food restaurants. However, several fast-food restaurant chains are now offering healthier alternatives, such as salads, baked potatoes, whole-grain buns, and baked fish, making it easier to follow health and diet recommendations.

Other Factors Affecting Nutritional Status

Fast foods are by no means the only obstacle to good nutrition during adolescence. Fatigue, stress, peer pressure, eating disorders, substance abuse, physical activity levels, and pregnancy are also important issues. Adolescents are literally bombarded with thousands of choices, each demanding decision and action. Unfortunately, many of the decisions made do not consider the potential impact on health status. During the past 30 years, adolescents have been the only population group in the U.S. not experiencing an improvement in their health status (20). Violence is now the primary cause of death among teenagers. More than 77 percent of adolescent deaths are caused by accidents, homicide, and suicide. Self-destructive life-styles, substance abuse, and other risk-taking behaviors make an enormous impact on health. The presence or lack of health habits can make a critical difference.

Tobacco Use: Of adults who smoke regularly, 95 percent began their habit before the age of 20 (21). The choice to smoke is often based on a false perception of the number of peers smoking and on inaccurate information regarding health consequences (22). Adolescents frequently believe they won't become addicted to nicotine or susceptible to smoking-related diseases. When asked why they smoke, many adolescents reply that "everyone else does it." The truth is that the last ten years have witnessed an overall decline in smoking, from 25 percent of 12 to 17 year olds in 1974 to 16 percent in 1985 (23) (see table 14.8 for more information).

A study comparing young adults that began smoking during adolescence with non-smokers showed that the smokers had higher blood cholesterol levels (24). As explained in chapter 6, increased cholesterol in the blood corresponds with an increase in risk of heart disease. In addition, smokers are also at higher risk for certain types of cancer. Eighty-five percent of all lung cancer, our nation's number-one cancer killer, is caused by cigarette smoking. Every year, close to 400,000 deaths are directly attributable to cigarettes.

TABLE 14.8

Use of selected substances in the past month by youths 12-17 years of age, according to age and sex: United States, selected years 1972–85

Substance, age, and sex	1972	1974	1976	1977	1979	1982	1985
Cigarettes				*Percent of population*			
All ages, both sexes	(¹)	25	23	22	(¹)	15	16
12–13 years	(¹)	13	11	10	(¹)	*3	6
14–15 years	(¹)	25	20	22	(¹)	10	15
16–17 years	(¹)	38	39	35	(¹)	30	26
Male	(¹)	27	21	23	(¹)	16	16
Female	(¹)	24	26	22	(¹)	13	15
Alcohol²							
All ages, both sexes	(¹)	34	32	31	37	27	31
12–13 years	(¹)	19	19	13	20	10	12
14–15 years	(¹)	32	31	28	36	23	35
16–17 years	(¹)	51	47	52	55	45	48
Male	(¹)	39	36	37	39	27	34
Female	(¹)	29	29	25	36	27	29
Marijuana							
All ages, both sexes	7	12	12	17	17	12	12
12–13 years	*1	*2	*3	*4	4	*2	4
14–15 years	6	12	13	16	17	8	12
16–17 years	16	20	21	30	28	23	22
Male	9	12	14	20	19	13	13
Female	6	11	11	13	14	10	11

Data are based on household interviews of a sample of the population 12 years of age and over in the coterminous United States.
[1]Data not comparable because definitions differ.
[2]In 1979, 1982, and 1985, private answer sheets were used for alcohol questions; in earlier years, respondents answered questions aloud.
*Relative standard error greater than 30 percent.

Data from *National Household Survey on Drug Abuse: Main Findings, 1979,* by P. M. Fishburne, H. I. Abelson, and I. Cisin; *National Household Survey on Drug Abuse: Main Findings, 1982,* by J. D. Miller et al.; and *National Household Survey on Drug Abuse: Population Estimates, 1985.* National Institute on Drug Abuse, U.S. Department of Health and Human Services publications.

Use of **smokeless tobacco** is also associated with health risks, especially oral cancers. And unfortunately, its use is increasing among adolescents. Chewing tobacco and snuff were used by approximately four percent of adolescents in 1975. In the 1980s, usage reached ten percent (25, 26). Despite myths to the contrary, smokeless tobacco does cause a higher risk of mouth and throat cancer. It is by no means a safe alternative to cigarette smoking.

Use of Alcohol: Nearly all adolescents have tried alcohol at one time or another. Along with experimentation comes the decision of whether to abstain from alcohol or increase consumption. Certainly not all teenagers who drink have a problem, but those developing regular and binge-drinking patterns may lose control.

The profile of teens more frequently abusing alcohol has the following characteristics: generally male, less religious, indifferent to school performance, greater family tolerance for alcohol, and other substance abuse (20).

Table 14.8 indicates that as of 1985, 31 percent of teenagers reported drinking alcohol within the past month (see figure 14.5). Some sections of the country report even higher teenager drinking rates (27).

As with smoking, the reason most often given by adolescents for drinking alcohol is that "everyone else does it." An unspoken desire to participate in an "adult-level practice" to prove "maturity" may also influence the decision to drink.

*F*IGURE 14.5

The National Institute on Drug Abuse's 12th annual survey of high school seniors shows that despite a stop in the declining use of some drugs in 1985, the general downward trend in illicit drug use among high school seniors continued in 1986. This figure shows a 30-day prevalence (i.e., the percentage of high school seniors who used marijuana/hashish, cocaine, or alcohol in the last 30 days) and 30-day prevalence of daily use (i.e., the percentage who used these types of drugs daily in the last 30 days). The survey results show that the percent of high school seniors who ever used marijuana/hashish has been on the decline since 1979; cocaine "ever used" trends show peaks in 1981 and 1985 but a slight decline in 1986; and alcohol use has shown a small downward trend since 1980. Some of the declines may be attributed to the fact that many high school seniors are aware of the potential harmfulness of drugs, alcohol abuse, and cigarette smoking.

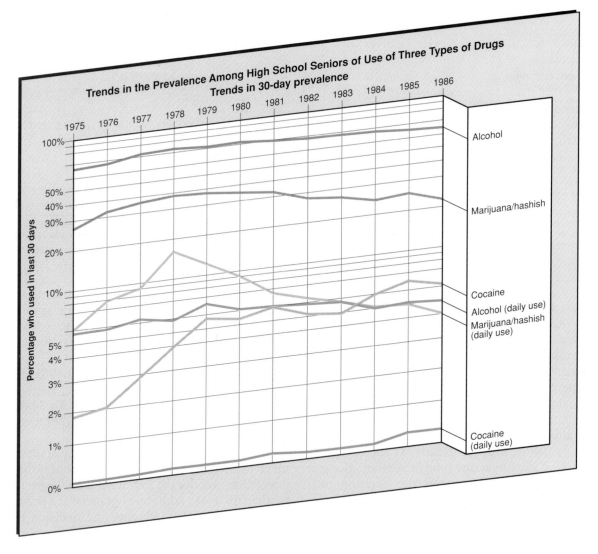

Some people seem to be born with a susceptibility to alcohol abuse. There is evidence that a strong family history of alcoholism can predispose offspring to becoming alcoholics. When teenagers with such a background strive to be accepted among peers, they may be swept into an escalating spiral of alcohol abuse that is beyond their control.

Alcohol use is defined as alcohol abuse when it leads to driving under the influence, trouble with the law, school problems, psychological turmoil, and physical abuse to self and others. Interpersonal relationships begin to suffer. Often drinkers blame everything and everyone else for their problems, angrily denying that alcohol is the underlying cause. Frequently, the excuse of "I drink to escape from all the problems in my life" is given. Myths such as "teenagers are too young to be alcoholics" and "you can't be an alcoholic just by drinking beer" are promoted; however, these are very false.

Nutritionally, alcohol abuse has multiple effects. First, alcohol Calories take the place of nutritious food Calories. Alcohol contains a high amount of Calories (7 Calories per gram), but insignificant amounts of vitamins and minerals. Also, the more people drink, the less they tend to eat. This combination may lead to disruptions with the growth spurt of adolescents.

Additionally, the toxic effect of alcohol is responsible for much harm to body organs and interferes with vitamin and mineral absorption in the small intestine, and metabolism by the liver. The liver works hard to detoxify the alcohol in the body, but when the intake is too high, the liver can't keep up. Liver and pancreas damage can result, further hindering the nutrient state of the body. Ultimately, almost every part of the body is harmed by alcohol abuse. If this disease is left untreated, it is fatal (see chapter 12 for more information).

When alcohol abuse is evident, professional help is needed. Calling a local treatment center or nearby chapter of Alcoholics Anonymous (AA) can provide guidance on the steps for overcoming this disease. Most counselors are very willing to answer questions and provide referrals.

Drugs: Experimenting with various chemical substances, including marijuana, is common during adolescence. By itself, experimentation does not constitute substance abuse.

Abuse results when a regular or binge pattern sets in, with multiple consequences in the physical, social, familial, educational, and psychological areas.

Surveys suggest that **marijuana** smoking has increased during the past decade. Table 14.8 indicates that seven percent of youth ages 12 to 17 reported marijuana usage during the past month in 1972, versus 12 percent in 1985. Figure 14.5 shows the trends in use of drugs in high school seniors. Less than 25 percent now use marijuana, a decline from nearly 40 percent in 1978 (28, 29).

Heavy use of marijuana can cause multiple side effects. In addition to legal problems, the ability to think logically can be affected, and perceptions of time, space, and social relationships may be altered. Decreased motivation and interest in school matters also develop, and lung damage can occur. Nutritionally, marijuana smoking alters the appetite control center, often leading to intense cravings for all types of snack foods—"the munchies." Needless to say, in this state, teenagers are not striving to choose wisely from the basic four food groups.

Other drugs such as **cocaine, crack, amphetamines, LSD, PCP,** and **heroin** are used by some adolescents with varying frequencies. Figure 14.5 shows that use of cocaine by high school seniors is finally starting to drop after rising strongly during the mid-1980s. Currently, LSD, PCP, and heroin use is less prevalent, while cocaine and amphetamine use is more common (27).

Table 14.9 describes some of the physical problems and nutritional consequences that arise from cocaine, crack, and amphetamine abuse. Mouth, nose, and throat inflammation, indigestion, diarrhea, decreased appetite, and heartbeat irregularities are among the most common side effects. These medical problems then lead to nutritional disturbances. Loss of appetite, poor food choices, inability to absorb nutrients properly, and weight loss are common symptoms of heavy drug usage. The end result is malnutrition and loss of health.

Many drug treatment programs include education on good nutritional practices. The importance of regularly scheduled, well-balanced meals is emphasized. Diet recommendations are generally for a low-fat, moderate

TABLE 14.9
Effects of cocaine, crack, and amphetamines

Physical Problems	Nutrition Consequences

Mouth and Nose
    Inflammation
    Gum disease
	Avoiding foods that may irritate; less variety.

Throat
    Inflammation
    Damage to vocal cords
    Difficulty breathing and
    swallowing
	Loss of appetite.

Stomach
    Decreased digestive
    enzymes
    Indigestion
	Stomach cramps; loss of appetite.

Intestines
    Food rushes through
    causing diarrhea
    Increased urination
	Nutrients not absorbed, B-vitamins, zinc and calcium deficiency; constipation upon withdrawal.

Central Nervous System
    Suppressed appetite
    Increased temperature
    and blood pressure
    Vision problems
    Insomnia
    Seizures
	Weight loss; malnutrition; may experience "rebound appetite" after period of not eating; fatigue.

Heart
    Rapid heartbeat,
    skipped beats
    Chest pain, chest
    congestion
    Heart enlargement
    Heart attack
	High sodium intake is harmful.

Kidneys Kidney infection	Decreased immune system function; malnutrition.

protein, high complex-carbohydrate diet. Initially patients are usually given large amounts of juice and water during the detoxification period. Underweight patients may need to include more of the Calorically dense foods, such as dried fruits and nuts. Often drug rehabilitation results in a "rebound appetite" in the patient. Some patients end up consuming large quantities of food as the body attempts to adjust for the long periods of erratic eating habits.

Teenage Pregnancy: By age 19, one-fourth of all females have had one pregnancy (30). Therefore, it is important that young women know of the extra nutritional demands of a pregnancy during the adolescent growth spurt.

Evidence reveals that pregnant teenagers and their unborn babies are at very high risk for nutritional deficiencies. The younger the teen mother, the higher the risk for anemia, hypertension, low-birth-weight infants, and birth complications. When a young mother-to-be is still going through her own growth spurt, there may be competition with the fetus over nutrients in the diet. In other words, if both have a strong need for calcium, and a glass of milk is consumed, how much calcium will they each get? Answers to these types of questions are not fully known yet, but it is obvious that either the mother or the fetus, or both, might be deprived.

There are other problems as well. Studies have shown that many pregnant adolescents skip meals, rely heavily on fast foods and/or snack foods, avoid certain food groups (such as milk), diet to hide weight gain, and smoke and/or take drugs. With each of these practices, there is a risk to the unborn child. An indicator that the pregnancy is not progressing healthfully is poor weight gain.

Consuming an inadequate diet can lead to vitamin, mineral, and Calorie deficiencies in the fetus. Fetuses that are not properly nourished may be born underweight, which is associated with a multitude of complications as well as birth defects. Smoking during pregnancy also lowers birth weight (see chapter 13). Alcohol consumption can cause fetal alcohol syndrome, with associated physical and mental abnormalities. There is no safe level of alcohol use during pregnancy; total abstinence is recommended. Marijuana use is also associated with low birth weight, birth defects, and extra long labor (31). Cocaine use can lead to miscarriages and decreased nourishment to the fetus (32).

For a better chance of a successful pregnancy and a healthy infant, the avoidance of all chemical substances and cigarettes is highly recommended. Eating regularly from all the food groups and taking a prenatal vitamin and iron supplement, if prescribed, are encouraged for pregnant adolescents. Often this entails a change in the life-style and habits of the pregnant teen. This is never easy, and is especially difficult when friends are leading a different life-style. The unselfish changes made for a healthier way of life during pregnancy are well worth the sacrifice, however.

Johnny, a new fourth grader at Wilson Elementary School, simply cannot sit still at school. He squirms, throws spitballs, has an extremely limited attention span, and impulsively blurts out whatever first comes to mind during class discussions. In other words, he drives his teachers nuts. During one lunch break, as the teachers reviewed Johnny's progress, a consensus was reached that his diet must contain high amounts of food additives and sugar. The teachers decided to call his parents to see if they would cooperate with the school nurse and nutritionist in remedying the situation.

Is it true that "hyperactive" children can trace their problem to diet? Is there a relationship between diet and behavior?

Before answering this question, let's review the human brain for a moment (see figure 14.6). The developed human brain is composed of approximately 100 billion nerve cells (neurons) and an equivalent number of supporting cells (glial) (33). Even though the brain comprises only two percent of adult body weight, it receives 15 percent of the blood pumped out of the heart and accounts for 20 to 30 percent of the oxygen used by the body at rest (34). The constant electrical activity of the brain probably accounts for most of the brain's energy requirements.

Unlike other organs of the body, the brain does not store carbohydrate or fat for energy. Therefore, it is heavily dependent upon a constant supply of oxygen and glucose from the blood. As a result, it is not surprising to learn that brain function is relatively sensitive to the quality of diet.

Brain cells or neurons use many chemicals to communicate with each other and to send messages to the rest of the body. Between 30 and 40 of these chemicals, known as neurotransmitters, have been identified. Figure 14.7 shows that these neurotransmitters help brain messages to jump the small space (called the synapse) between brain cells. Amazingly, the synthesis of these neurotransmitters depends on enzyme systems that use vitamins and minerals from the diet. Also, many amino acids from

FIGURE 14.6
The human brain is composed of approximately 100 billion nerve cells (neurons) and receives fifteen percent of the blood pumped out of the heart.

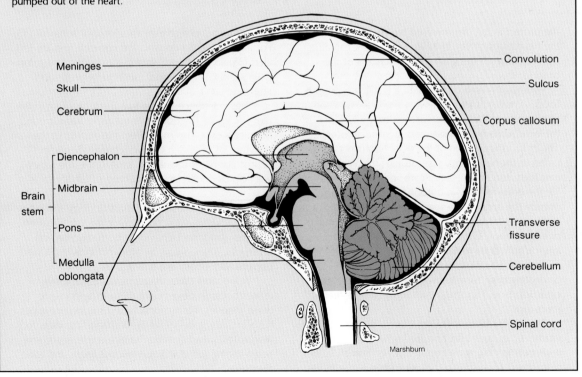

Meninges
Skull
Cerebrum
Diencephalon
Midbrain
Brain stem
Pons
Medulla oblongata

Convolution
Sulcus
Corpus callosum
Transverse fissure
Cerebellum
Spinal cord

Marshburn

FIGURE 14.7

Chemicals known as neurotransmitters help brain messages jump the small synapse, or space, between brain cells.

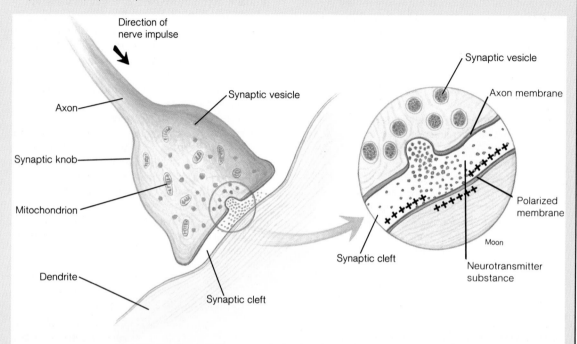

the protein in the diet are used by the brain to make the neurotransmitters. In other words, diet can affect the formation of the chemical messengers of the brain (33)!

Although research in this area is still very limited, food is known to affect the way the brain functions. Here is one of the best researched examples. One of the brain's chemical messengers is called serotonin. The brain cells use one of the essential amino acids, called **trytophan,** to make serotonin (35). When one eats high amounts of sugar (carbohydrate), it is easier for the brain to draw in trytophan from the blood outside the brain. More than the normal amount of serotonin is formed by the brain cells, and this makes one feel sleepy. On the other hand, high-protein, low-carbohydrate meals tend to increase the amount of the amino acid tyrosine going into the brain, promoting brain formation of the neurotransmitter catecholamine. This may make some people feel more alert.

Many nutrients, including vitamin B_6, iron, vitamin C, copper, and zinc are known to aid the brain cells in making neurotransmitters. Some researchers have shown that when iron is low in the diet, some people change their normal behavior (33). For example, children who are iron deficient are less alert (35). In addition, if infants survive protein-calorie malnutrition, lasting impairments in behavior and cognition can result (36).

New evidence shows that the type of fat in the diet influences the quality of the membrane around brain cells (33). This may affect the activity of the enzymes of the brain cell, which may then affect neurotransmitter formation. Research in the future will help us understand what type of dietary fat is best.

Because of these preliminary findings, there has been much discussion concerning the link between diet and abnormal behavior in both children and adults (33, 37). Could it be true that individuals who behave abnormally are eating poorly?

Advocates claim that criminals commit their crimes because of deficient diets. In response to these theories, correctional facilities in several states have actually gone so far as to change the diets fed to inmates, provide megavitamin supplements, and begin testing for low blood glucose levels and food allergies.

The belief that diet has a major influence on criminal behavior has already made its way into the courtroom. The most famous example of this was the "Twinkie defense" in the Dan White murder trial. Dan White was a former San Francisco supervisor who went to the city hall with a loaded gun, climbed through a window to avoid a metal detector, and then killed both Mayor George Moscone and Supervisor Harvey Milk. On the surface, this appeared to be a clear case of premeditated murder, but White's attorney used a "diminished capacity" defense to argue that White's ability to "maturely and meaningfully" reflect on the evil nature of his intended action was impaired as a result of depression. White's "penchant for wolfing down junk food — Twinkies, Cokes, doughnuts, and candy bars — exacerbated his depression and indicated a chemical imbalance of the brain (38)". As a result, White was given a reduced sentence for manslaughter, creating a tremendous public controversy.

The belief that sugar causes behavior and learning problems in children is widely held by the general public (39). Popular interest in this position has been heightened by media reports of the "Halloween effect" and the writings of the late Dr. Ben Feingold. In 1973, Dr. Feingold, a California allergist, proposed that artificial flavors and food colors were a cause of hyperactivity in children (40). Dr. Feingold recommended a diet free of these substances as both treatment and prevention of the condition. He published two popular books on the subject, *Why Your Child is Hyperactive* (1974), and *The Feingold Cookbook for Hyperactive Children*

(1979). Others later urged that sugar was also a factor explaining hyperactivity and aggression in children. Many parents adopted the diet for their "hyperactive" children, and beliefs persist to this day that Feingold's writings are the truth of the matter.

However, well-controlled, double-blind studies have not been able to show that children thought to be hyperactive are actually affected when sugar, artificial food dyes, or other food additives are added to meals (33). In one study (39), children who were believed by their parents to have adverse responses to sugar were brought to a clinic for seven sessions. During each session, varying levels of either aspartame (Nutra-Sweet) or sugar in water were fed to the children. However, neither the researchers or the children knew which sweetener they were consuming. A complex series of physical and psychological tests showed no effect of sugar on behavior. Other similar tests with food dyes and food additives have also shown no negative effects on behavior.

Studies on changes in the diets of inmates are also unsupportive. It appears that the diet will have to be abnormally extreme to produce any meaningful change in behavior. In other words, although there is plenty of evidence showing that substances from the diet can have subtle effects on human behaviors, and that brain chemicals are derived from the diet, there is no support for the theory that abnormal behavior (criminality or hyperactivity) can be traced to the diet. Johnny is probably throwing spitballs and squirming for other reasons.

*S*UMMARY

1. Brain growth is rapid before birth and for the first two years. Proper nourishment during this time helps to ensure optimal motor development and intellectual abilities.
2. The physical growth rate is dramatic during the first year of life, with most infants tripling their birth weight. After the second birthday, a child's weight gain usually slows down to about five pounds per year for the next seven or eight years.
3. Preschool children need a varied and nutrient-rich diet, having almost the same energy needs as sedentary adults. When a child consumes a wide variety of healthful foods in adequate amounts, the potential for health and proper growth is excellent.
4. Obesity is a concern for some young children, with nearly 25 percent considered overweight. Various methods for avoiding obesity in young children were reviewed.
5. The foundation for lifelong eating habits and food choices is laid down in early childhood. Regular mealtimes, wholesome food choices, and the introduction of new foods in a pleasant manner are important.
6. School-age children from six to twelve years old grow at a slower, steadier rate than preschoolers or adolescents. A good diet helps provide adequate stores of nutrients, such as calcium, that will be needed during the adolescent growth spurt.

7. Variety and portion size are key elements in the diets of elementary school children. As children grow older, an increasing number of factors influence their nutritional status, such as peer preferences, school lunch programs, television viewing, snacking habits, activity levels, family attitudes, and food advertising.

8. Individual variation is the single most important trait of adolescent growth. Males generally start their puberty growth two years after females. The beginning of this period is signaled by many secondary sex changes.

9. The Caloric needs of adolescents are higher than at any other time of life. The diets of adolescent girls are often lacking in essential nutrients. Many similarities exist between the ideal diet recommended for adults and the one recommended for adolescents.

10. Several factors can effect the nutritional status of teenagers, including regular consumption of some fast foods, peer pressure, eating disorders, substance abuse, tobacco and alcohol use, and early pregnancy.

11. Although research is still very limited, food is known to affect the way the brain functions. However, the belief that diet has a major influence on criminal behavior or that sugar and food additive consumption can cause hyperactivity in children is not supported by data from high-quality research projects.

REFERENCES

1. Mora, J. O., et al. 1981. The Effects of Nutritional Supplementation on Physical Growth of Children at Risk of Malnutrition. *American Journal of Clinical Nutrition* 34:1885.

2. Kennedy, E. T. 1979. Evaluation of the Effectiveness of the WIC Supplemental Feeding Program on Prenatal Patients in Massachusetts, Doctoral Thesis. Boston: Harvard School of Public Health.

3. Glinsmann, W. H., H. Irausquin, and Y. K. Park. 1986. Executive Summary: Evaluation of Health Aspects of Sugars Contained in Carbohydrate Sweeteners. Report of Sugars Task Force, 1986. *Journal of Nutrition* 116:(11 suppl):S1-S216.

4. National Institutes of Health, Office of Medical Applications Research. 1985. Lowering Blood Cholesterol to Prevent Heart Disease. Consensus Development Conference Statement. December 10-12, 1984. *Journal of the American Medical Association* 253:2080.

5. American Heart Association. Nutrition Committee. 1986. *Circulation* 74:1465A.

6. U.S. Department of Agriculture. 1985. Nutrient Intakes: Individuals in 48 States, Year 1977-78, Nationwide Food Consumption Survey, 1977-78, Report No. 1-2. Human Nutrition Information Service. Washington, D.C.: U.S. Government Printing Office.

7. Preliminary Findings of the First Health and Nutrition Examination Survey: Dietary Intake and Biochemical Findings. DHEW Publ. No. (HRA) 74-1219-1, 1974.

8. National Center for Health Statistics, Dietary Intake Source Data: United States, 1976-1980. 1983 (March). DHHS Publication (PHS) 83-1681, Public Health Service (Vital and Health Statistics; Series 11; No. 231). Washington, D.C.: U.S. Government Printing Office.

9. Pennington, J. A. T., et al. 1984. Selected Minerals in Food Surveys, 1974 to 1981/82. *Journal of the American Dietetic Association* 84:771.

10. Pipes, P. L. 1985. *Nutrition in Infancy and Childhood.* 3d. ed. St. Louis: Times Mirror/Mosby Publishing.

11. Tucker, L. A. 1986. The Relationship of Television Viewing to Physical Fitness and Obesity. *Adolescence* 21(84):797-806.

12. Zuckerman, D. M., and B. S. Zuckerman. 1985. Television's Impact on Children. *Pediatrics* 75(2):233-40.

13. Patterson, R. E., et al, 1986. Factors Related to Obesity in Preschool Children. *Journal of the American Dietetic Association* 86:1376-1381.

14. Jansen, G. R., and J. M. Harper. 1978. Consumption and Plate Waste of Menu Items Served in the National School Lunch Program. *Journal of the American Dietetic Association* 73:395.

15. Emmons, L., M. Hayes, and D. L. Call. 1972. A Study of School Funding Programs, II. Effects on Children with Different Economic and Nutritional Needs. *Journal of the American Dietetic Association* 61:268.

16. Crockett, A. F., and H. A. Guthrie. 1986. Alternative Eating Patterns and the Role of Age, Sex, Selection, and Snacking in Nutritional Quality. *Clinical Nutrition* 5:34-42.

17. Garn, S. M., and B. Wagner. 1969. The Adolescent Growth of the Skeletal Mass and Its Implications to Mineral Requirements. In *Adolescent Nutrition and Growth.* F. P. Heald, ed. New York: Meredith Corp.

18. Wyshak, G., and R. E. Frisch. 1982. Evidence for a Secular Trend in Age of Menarche. *New England Journal of Medicine* 306:1033.

19. McNamara, J. J., et al. 1971. Coronary Artery Disease in Combat Casualities in Vietnam. *Journal of the American Medical Association* 216:1185.

20. Blum, R. 1987. Contemporary Threats to Adolescent Health in the U.S. *Journal of the American Medical Association* 257:3390-3395.

21. National Center for Health Statistics: Health, United States, 1986. DHHS Pub. No. (PHS) 87-1232. Public Health Service. Washington, D.C.: U.S. Government Printing Office.

22. Leventhal, H., K. Glynn, and R. Fleming. 1987. Is the Smoking Decision an Informed Choice? *Journal of the American Medical Association* 275:3373-3376.

23. National Institute on Drug Abuse: National Survey on Drug Abuse: Main Findings 1979, by P. M. Fishburne, M. I. Abelson, and I. Cisin. DHHS Pub. No. (ADM) 80-976. Alcohol, Drug Abuse, and Mental Health Administration. Washington, D.C.: U.S. Government Printing Office; National Survey on Drug Abuse: Main Findings 1982, by J. D. Miller, et al. DHHS Pub. No. (ADM) 83-1263. Alcohol, Drug Abuse, and Mental Health Administration. Washington, D.C.: U.S. Government Printing Office; Unpublished data from the Division of Epidemiology and Statistical Analysis.

24. Freedman, D. S., et al. 1986. Cigarette Smoking Initiation and Longitudinal Changes in Serum Lipids and Lipoproteins in Early Adulthood: The Bogalusa Heart Study. *American Journal of Epidemiology* 124:207-19.

25. U.S. Department of Health, Education, and Welfare. 1979. Smoking and Health. Publication (PHS) 79-50066. Washington, D.C.: U.S. Government Printing Office.

26. Guggenheimer, J., et al. 1986. Changing Trends of Tobacco Use in a Teenage Population in Western Pennsylvania. *American Journal of Public Health* 76:196-97.

27. Robinson, T. N., et al. 1987. Perspective on Adolescent Substance Use: A Defined Population Study. *Journal of the American Medical Association* 258:2072-2076.

28. Johnston, L., et al. 1975. Use of Illicit Drugs by American High School Students, 1975-1984. U.S. Dept of Health and Human Services.

29. Johnston, L., J. Bachman, and P. O'Malley. 1985. Highlights from Drugs and the Class of '84. Behaviors, Attitudes, and Recent National Trends. Rockville, Md.: National Institute on Drug Abuse.

30. Miller, C. A. 1986. Monitoring Children's Health: Key Indicators. Washington, D.C.: *American Journal of Public Health Association.*

31. Tennes, K. 1984. National Institute on Drug Abuse Research. Monograph Series 44:115.

32. Chasnoff, I., et al. 1985. Cocaine Use in Pregnancy. *New England Journal of Medicine* 313:666.

33. Council for Agricultural Science and Technology. 1987 (March). Diet and Health. Report No. 111. Ames, Iowa: Council for Agricultural Sciences and Technology.

34. Krassner, M. B. 1986. Diet and Brain Function. *Nutrition Review* (suppl) 44:12-15.

35. Wurtman, R. J. 1986. Ways the Foods Can Affect the Brain. *Nutrition Review* 44:2-6.

36. Sandstead, H. H. 1986. Nutrition and Brain Function: Trace Elements. *Nutrition Review* 44:37-41.

37. Spring, B. J., et al. 1986. Effects of Carbohydrates on Mood and Behavior. *Nutrition Review* (suppl) 44:51-60.

38. Gray, G. E. 1986. Diet, Crime, and Delinquency: A Critique. *Nutrition Review* (suppl) 44:89-94.

39. Ferguson, H. B., C. Stoddart, and J. G. Simeon. 1986. Double-Blind Challenge Studies of Behavioral and Cognitive Effects of Sucrose-Aspartame Ingestion in Normal Children. *Nutrition Review* (suppl) 44:144-50.

40. Stare, F. J., E. M. Whelan, and M. Sheridan. 1980. Diet and Hyperactivity: Is There A Relationship? *Pediatrics* 66:521-25.

*H*EALTH PROMOTION ACTIVITY 14.1
Food Patterns and Choices of Preschoolers (Ages 1-5)

Interview the parent of a preschooler and answer the following questions:

1. What are the usual foods eaten by the preschooler during a regular 24-hour period? Report the types of foods, number of servings per day, and the serving sizes by the food groups listed below. See Figure 14.3.

Milk/Milk Products	Protein Foods	Breads, Cereals, Grains	Vitamin-C-Rich Fruit, Vegetables	Dark Green, Yellow Fruits, Vegetables	Other Fruit, Vegetables

2. How does the food list above compare with the recommendations given in figure 14.3? Compare number of servings in each food group and serving sizes.

3. What food problems or quirks does the child currently have?

4. How are the parents handling these problems? Give some additional strategies that you learned from this chapter.

5. What recommendations do you have for helping this preschooler to improve the diet?

In this Health Promotion Activity, the procedures of the previous activity will be followed, but for children aged 6–12.

Interview the parent of a child aged six to twelve and answer the following questions:

1. What are the usual foods eaten by the child during a regular 24 hour period? Report the types of foods, number of servings per day, and the serving sizes by the food groups listed below. See table 14.4.

Milk/Milk Products	Protein Foods	Breads, Cereals, Grains	Vitamin-C-Rich Fruit, Vegetables	Dark Green Yellow Fruits, Vegetables	Other Fruit, Vegetables

2. How does the food list above compare with the recommendations given in table 14.4? Compare number of servings in each food group and serving sizes.

3. What food problems or quirks does the child currently have?

4. How are the parents handling these problems? Give some additional strategies that you learned from this chapter.

5. What recommendations do you have for helping this child to improve the diet?

Sam is 17 years old, a senior in high school. He works part-time several afternoons a week and on the weekend at a fast-food restaurant. On Friday and Saturday nights Sam goes out drinking with his friends and usually has four or five beers. During the week he gets up late, skips breakfast, and rushes to school. Lunch is eaten in the school cafeteria, and generally his dinner is consumed at the fast-food restaurant. He usually has a cheeseburger, fries, chocolate milkshake, and a cola drink. Sam has put on 15 pounds of extra weight during the past year, feels tired most of the time, and has started smoking cigarettes on a regular basis (ten per day).

If you could talk with Sam privately about his lifestyle and eating habits, what counsel would you give him? Review the section in this chapter on the adolescent years.

15

Nutrition and Aging

INTRODUCTION

You may have heard of the baby boom. Well, get ready for the senior citizen explosion. By the year 2030, every fifth person you pass on the sidewalk will be 65 years old or older. For the first time in U.S. history, older people are living longer, increasing in number, and representing a growing proportion of the total population.

This chapter will explore the aging process, obstacles to adequate intake of nutrients in the elderly, results from national surveys showing that many elderly individuals have inadequate diets, drug use by the elderly, and nutritional requirements of the elderly. The topic of "life extension" and the role of nutrition in improving life expectancy will be discussed. The relationship of diet and osteoporosis, an age-related disorder characterized by decreased bone mass, will be elaborated. The examples of two remarkable elderly women, Hulda Crooks and Mavis Lindgren, will be highlighted. Finally, the immune system and its relationship to diet will be reviewed.

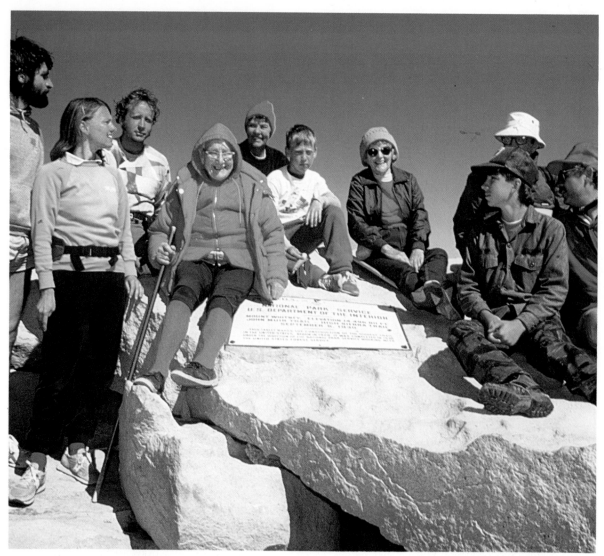

Hulda Crooks, at the age of 91, became the oldest person in history to make it to the top of Mt. Whitney (14,495 feet).

Grandma Whitney

During the summer of 1987 Hulda Crooks, at the age of 91, climbed unaided to the top of both Mt. Fuji, in Japan, and Mt. Whitney, in California. Dubbed "Grandma Whitney" by the press, Hulda has climbed to the top of 14,495-foot Mt. Whitney 23 times, all since turning 66 years of age.

Tests on Hulda in the Loma Linda University Human Performance Laboratory prior to her 1987 achievements revealed a woman in remarkable shape. Her heart and lung fitness were found to be that of a woman 30 years her junior.

Hulda's blood pressure and blood lipid profile were equal to those of a college-age woman. When asked to explain this amazing vitality and fitness despite her old age, Hulda listed several factors, including her vegetarian diet; her daily three-mile walks; avoidance of alcohol, tobacco, and other drugs; and her abiding faith in God.

In this chapter, the relationship between diet and the aging process will be reviewed. Do the elderly suffer from inadequate diets? Could improved nutrition delay the aging process, or at least increase vitality in old age? Is there a relationship between diet and osteoporosis, the age-related bone disorder?

FIGURE 15.1

The fastest growing minority in the United States today is the elderly — those who are 65 years of age and older. *Note:* Increments in years on horizontal scale are uneven.

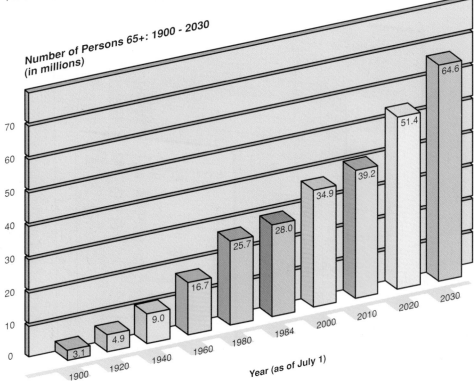

Number of Persons 65+: 1900 - 2030 (in millions)

Year (as of July 1)

Statistics and Trends

The fastest-growing minority in the United States today is the **elderly**—those who reach or pass the age of 65 (1). Figure 15.1 shows that there are now nearly 30 million elderly persons in the U.S., which will climb to 64.6 million, or 21 percent of the total population, by the year 2030. The 65-and-over population is growing twice as fast as the rest of the population (2). The baby boom is being replaced by the senior citizen explosion. Consider these statistics (1,2):

It is difficult to comprehend that in 1900, only 25 percent of individuals in the U.S. lived beyond age 65, whereas by 1985 approximately 70 percent survived age 65, and 30 percent lived to be 80 or more. If present trends continue, within the next 10 or 20 years almost half of deaths will occur after age 80.

Cardiovascular diseases (diseases of the heart and stroke combined) and cancers account for 72 percent of all deaths among the

elderly (see figure 15.2). The number-one cause of death among the elderly population is heart disease, accounting for 42.5 percent of all deaths among the elderly. Cancer ranks second to heart disease, comprising 20 percent of deaths among persons 65 and older. Cancer deaths are increasing in the elderly at a rate of nearly one percent per year.

In recent years, the death rate for the elderly population has declined considerably, particularly since 1968, due to reductions in death from cardiovascular disease. Heart disease death rates are declining 1.4 percent per year for the elderly. People who are 65 years of age can now expect to live 16.8 more years, to the ripe old age of nearly 82, higher than ever before (see figure 15.3).

Diseases of the heart are declining among the elderly but are still the number-one cause of death.

Leading Causes of Older Adult[a] Deaths: 1950, 1979, and 1985
Rate per 100,000 population

Rank		Year	Rate
e	Diseases of heart	1985*	2,187.8
1		1979	2,255.6
1		1950	2,861.9
e	Cancer[b]	1985*	1,038.4
2		1979	986.4
3		1950	856.5
e	Stroke[c]	1985*	461.2
3		1979	576.5
2		1950	923.9
e	COPD[d]	1985*	210.6
4		1979	152.2
4		1950	23.4
f	Pneumonia and influenza	1985*	203
5		1979	145.6
5		1950	191.3
e			

Percent distribution of older adult deaths by cause: 1950, 1979, and 1985

	1985*	1979	1950
Diseases of heart	42.5	44.6	45.6
Cancer[b]	20.2	19.5	13.7
Stroke[c]	9.0	11.4	14.7
COPD[d]	4.1	3.0	0.4
Pneumonia and influenza	4.0	2.9	3.1

Total older adult mortality rate

1985*	5,145.2
1979	5,059.5
1950	6,270.5

*Provisional data
[a]Older adult = 65 years and older
[b]Cancer = malignant neoplasms, including neoplasms of the lymphatic and hematopoietic tissues
[c]Stroke = cerebrovascular diseases
[d]COPD = chronic obstructive pulmonary diseases and allied conditions
[e]Rank not available for 1985 provisional data
[f]Not ranked in first 10 leading causes of death

Length of life has increased remarkably during the twentieth century (see figure 15.4).

Life expectancy at birth (the number of years a newborn baby can expect to live) reached a new high of 74.7 years in 1985 (3). Much of the increase in life expectancy is due to the dramatic drop in heart disease and stroke death rates in the U.S. (see chapter 6, Health-Promotion Insight). Nonetheless, the U.S. still ranks behind 11 other nations in male life expectancy at birth (see figure 15.5).

Although approximately two-thirds of the elderly perceive their health as "good" or "excellent," 50 percent have arthritis, 39 percent are hypertensive, 30 percent have a hearing impairment, 26 percent have heart disease, 17 percent have a deformity or orthopedic impairment, 15 percent have chronic problems with their sinuses, 10 percent have vision problems, and 9 percent have diabetes.

Osteoporosis, defined as the decrease in the amount of bone, leading to fractures, is present in a large number of the elderly. One-third of women over 65 develop fractures of their spinal bones, and by extreme old age, one of every three women and one of every six men will have had a hip fracture. Osteoporosis costs Americans $6.1 billion annually (4).

In 1980 the number of cases of **senile dementia** was estimated at two million,

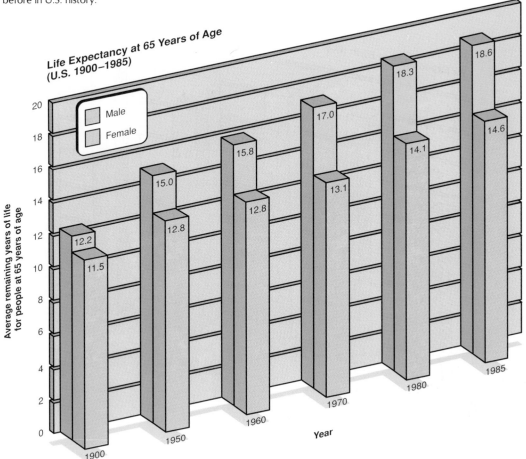

*F*IGURE 15.3
The elderly can now expect to live more years beyond age 65
than ever before in U.S. history.

Life Expectancy at 65 Years of Age
(U.S. 1900–1985)

☐ Male
☐ Female

Average remaining years of life
for people at 65 years of age

Year

with a mean age of 80. Projections for the year 2000 estimate the number to rise to 3.8 million, and by 2050, 8.5 million (see figure 15.6).

The forecasted increase in the number of people 85 years of age and older may lead to a large increase in use of nursing homes in the future. One study showed that by the year 2012, state Medicaid nursing home payments will increase 280 percent, to $6.3 billion annually (5,6). Financing the health care of the elderly for the future is now considered to be a serious dilemma.

There are several major principles to keep in mind when reviewing these statistics. For the first time in human history, older

people are living longer, increasing in number, and representing a steadily increasing proportion of the total population. The central issue in all this is quality of life. Unfortunately, most studies reveal that despite improved life expectancy, the number of years that elderly individuals live with disease and disability is increasing even more rapidly (1). However, as demonstrated by Hulda Crooks, this does not need to be the case. Although many elderly people have long years of disability and disease, needing extensive care, others live fully, actively, and independently into their ninth and tenth decades.

FIGURE 15.4

Length of life increased remarkably during the twentieth century.

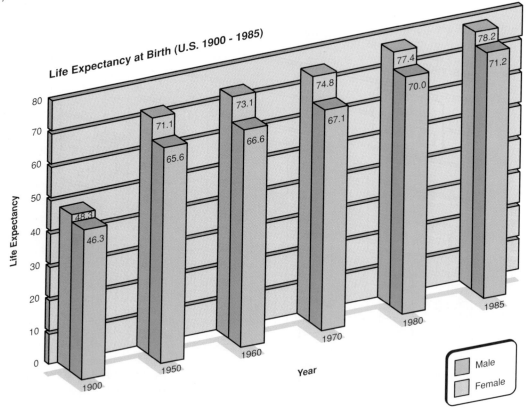

Life Expectancy at Birth (U.S. 1900 - 1985)

Male
Female

FIGURE 15.5

The U.S. ranks behind 11 other nations in male life expectancy at birth.

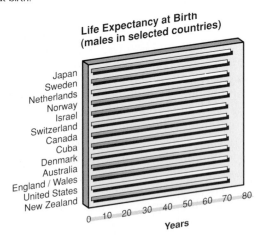

Life Expectancy at Birth
(males in selected countries)

Japan
Sweden
Netherlands
Norway
Israel
Switzerland
Canada
Cuba
Denmark
Australia
England / Wales
United States
New Zealand

Years

FIGURE 15.6

Projected number (in millions) of demented persons in the United States, by age: 1980–2050. With the increase in the number of elderly people is projected an alarming increase in the number of demented or senile persons.

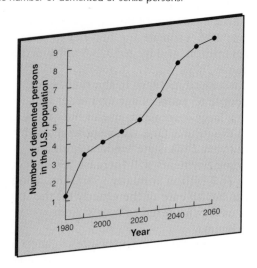

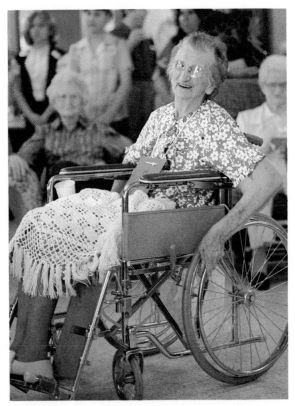

As a person ages, many changes take place in the body.

The Aging Process

Aging refers to the normal yet irreversible biological changes that occur during the total years that a person lives (7). The aging process occurs in all people, but for those over 65 years of age, it often results in significant changes in quality of life.

There are several theories of aging (8). Some researchers feel that human body cells can only divide a certain number of times before stopping, leading to death. Various biochemical and hormone theories suggest that there are important changes in body chemicals that finally lead to death. Finally, it is well known that the immune system is less effective in the elderly (see Health-Promotion Insight). The body may be less able to combat infection or destroy abnormal body cells. Two things are certain—there is no single cause of death, and death is inevitable.

As a person ages, many changes take place in the body that are important from a nutritional point of view (9,10,11,12).

Decrease in lean body weight. As a person ages, body fat increases while the muscle and bone weight (or lean body weight) decreases. This leads to a decrease in energy expended during rest, partially explaining why elderly individuals consume less Calories than younger people. National data show that elderly men and women weigh more than is recommended for optimal health.

Loss of taste and smell. The elderly often complain of a decreased ability to taste and enjoy food. Taste buds decrease in number and size, affecting sweet and salty tastes in particular. About 40 percent of people 80 years or older appear to have difficulty identifying common substances by smell.

Periodontal (bone area around the teeth) bone loss. The majority of the elderly suffer bone loss and disease in the tissues around the teeth as they grow older. As a result, 50 percent of the population over 60 have lost all of their teeth, and about 65 percent have lost all teeth in at least one arch. Older people therefore tend to choose foods that are easy to chew, leading to a reduced consumption of fresh fruit and vegetables high in dietary fiber (13).

Decrease in gastrointestinal function. With increase in age, the stomach cells are less able to secrete digestive juices. There is also a decrease in the secretion of gastric acid (hydrochloric acid) with aging. This may interfere with protein digestion. The stomach may also decrease its secretion of intrinsic factor, which is needed to help absorb vitamin B_{12}. Ulcers in the stomach wall, leading to bleeding, are present in large numbers of elderly persons. The small intestine becomes less capable of absorbing some nutrients, including protein, carbohydrate, fat, some vitamins, and minerals. Some older people may suffer from cramps and diarrhea after eating dairy foods containing lactose because they lack the enzyme lactase.

There may also be a reduced ability of the intestine to move its contents through the digestive tract, resulting in constipation.

Loss in visual and auditory function. Visual function starts to decline around the age of 45 and worsens gradually throughout life. After age 80, less than 15 percent of the population has 20/20 vision. Among the most common problems are presbyopia (loss of the ability of the lens to change its shape), cataracts (lenses become cloudy), and glaucoma (pressure inside the eyeball increases). Gradual hearing loss generally begins at about age 20 and has been estimated to occur in as many as 66 percent of people reaching the age of 80 years. Hearing loss is associated with depression and social embarrassment, which can affect normal eating behavior.

Loss of bone mineral mass. Loss of bone (osteoporosis) is an almost universal phenomenon with increasing age among white men and women. About 1.3 million fractures attributable to osteoporosis occur annually in people 45 years and older. These fractures are often difficult to mend, resulting in long periods of decreased physical activity and social interaction, both of which affect eating behavior.

Mental impairment. Senility, also called senile dementia or organic brain syndrome, affects about 60 percent of the elderly to varying degrees. Some of the problems associated with senile dementia include impairment of memory, judgment, feelings, personality, and ability to speak. Senile dementia of the Alzheimer's type accounts for at least half of all dementia in old age. Clinical depression can occur in 5–25 percent of the elderly. Men aged 65 and older are four times more likely to commit suicide than men younger than 25. Estimates have been made that two to ten percent of individuals over the age of 60, and up to 20 percent of some nursing home populations, suffer from alcoholism.

Decrease in heart and lung fitness. With aging, there is a decrease of about eight to ten percent per decade in the ability of the heart and lungs to supply oxygen to the muscles. Most of this is due to decreasing physical activity by the elderly. Several studies have shown that the elderly are capable of high degrees of heart and lung fitness if they exercise regularly (see Sidebar 15.1).

Decreased ability to metabolize drugs. The elderly have a decreased ability to absorb, distribute, metabolize, and excrete both prescription and nonprescription drugs. The majority of the elderly take more than one prescription drug, and these can interact with each other, affecting the nutritional status of the individual.

High prevalence of chronic disease. Up to 85 percent of the elderly suffer from at least one chronic disease (e.g., heart disease, cancer, and other life-style diseases), with one-third requiring special diets because of them. A variety of diseases are more common among the elderly, including diabetes, cancer, heart disease, high blood pressure, stroke, and arthritis.

Neuromuscular changes. Reaction time, ability to balance, and strength of muscles, tendons, and ligaments decrease with aging, limiting normal activity in some of the elderly. Accidents may increase, and ability to shop and prepare food may be hampered.

Urinary incontinence. Up to 20 percent of the elderly living in the community, and 75 percent of those in long-term care facilities, cannot control the muscle that controls urination. This can lead to social isolation, embarrassment, and the decision to live in a nursing home environment.

Decrease in liver and kidney function. The size and function of the liver decreases steadily with aging. The content of glycogen and vitamin C in the liver decreases, and its ability to synthesize protein is diminished. Alcohol becomes more toxic to the liver as its ability to detoxify ethanol decreases. The kidneys also decrease in size and function. The number of kidney nephrons decreases, and the membrane thickens, decreasing the ability of various substances to pass through. Thus the aged kidney may be inefficient in the removal of metabolic waste products. The older individual may also be susceptible to dehydration, resulting from a diminished thirst mechanism.

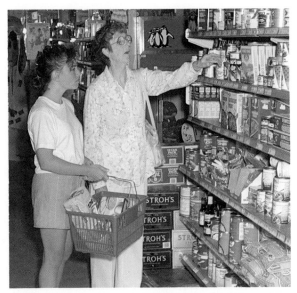

As people become more frail, limited access to food shopping and inability to carry groceries may influence whether they eat properly.

Other Obstacles to Adequate Intake of Nutrients in the Aged

In addition to limitations imposed by normal physiological decline and chronic disease conditions, many psychological, social, and economic factors influence food selection, dietary habits, and nutritional status of the elderly (14,15,16,17) (see table 15.1). It has been estimated that taken together, these factors are responsible for inadequate diets and malnutrition in 13 million of the elderly in the United States.

For example, as people become more frail, limited access to food shopping or inability to carry groceries may become a major factor in obtaining enough food. Individuals who live in inner city areas may not be able to take the bus to get to food stores that have a wide selection of fresh foods at a reasonable cost. They then become dependent on small grocery stores with high prices and limited selection. Individuals in rural areas may no longer be able to maintain gardens that previously provided fresh fruits and vegetables. Because vision, hearing, taste, and smell are important factors associated with the enjoyment of eating, some of the elderly experience loss of appetite. Depression from loss of loved ones may remove the desire and energy to shop for and prepare healthy foods.

Improving the Nutrition of the Elderly

Community feeding programs can greatly assist in providing the elderly with an adequate diet (11,12,17). Meals on Wheels is an example of a home-delivered meal service in which at least one meal a day (containing at least one-third of the RDA) is provided for five to seven days each week. These programs may be managed, run, and financially supported by community groups or be federally funded under Title VII of the Older Americans Act of 1965.

The Food Stamps program allows eligible individuals living on a limited income to buy food stamps whose purchasing power is greater than the amount that is paid for them. The stamps must be used for food purchases in cooperating retail stores.

A nutrition program for older Americans, Title VII of the Older Americans Act, was reorganized under Title III-C in 1978. This program was developed to meet both nutritional and social needs of persons 60 years of age and over. The program is designed to provide both group and home-delivered meals, as well as nutrition services and education, for the elderly. This federally funded program was a major turning point

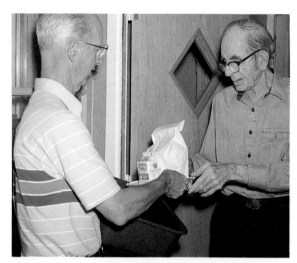

Meals on Wheels delivers meals to elderly persons in their homes.

TABLE 15.2
Practical suggestions for improving the nutrition of the elderly

1. Serve meals attractively, using a variety of foods with different flavors, colors, shapes, temperatures, textures, and smells.
2. Use a variety of herbs and spices to enhance the flavor of the food (but be moderate in the use of salt).
3. Serve a meal as if the person were in a nice restaurant. Use appetizers, salads, soups, and other attractive features. Eat out when possible at a variety of restaurants that offer unique and tasteful foods.
4. Try a variety of new foods, explaining their background.
5. Bring in friends and family members as often as possible to improve the social setting of the meal.
6. Stimulate the appetite with a walk (if possible) before the meal.
7. Use nutrient-dense foods as the basis of the menu.
8. At the dinner table, improve the setting with flowers and plants, attractive dishware and utensils, tablecloths and napkins.
9. If the elderly person has a physical handicap that limits normal eating movements, simplify the tasks and eliminate wasted motions. For example, cut the food ahead of time for easy self-feeding, use utensils with deep sides or handles that can be easily grasped, and purchase special utensils made for the elderly if needed.
10. If poor dentition limits normal food intake, chop, grind, or blend foods that are hard to chew. Mash or strain cooked vegetables or fruit, shred raw vegetables, remove tough skins or seeds, substitute softer, protein-rich foods such as peanut butter, cheese, baked beans, or yogurt for regular meat. Prepare soups, stews, cooked whole-grain cereals, and casseroles.

for the elderly at risk of developing not only nutritional problems but also further physical and mental deterioration because of adverse circumstances in their environment (11).

Some community agencies provide home health or neighborhood aides to assist elderly persons with meal management in their own homes. These aides provide advice, nutrition counseling, education, and support in food preparation, handling, budgeting, and shopping. This help may enable an elderly person to continue to stay at home longer than would otherwise be possible.

Not all aged individuals can or will participate in feeding programs offered by the government or community. Nutrition education through the mass media, senior citizen centers, and local community organizations is one way in which the elderly can get the information they need to improve their diets.

Table 15.2 outlines practical suggestions for improving the nutrition of the elderly. By being creative and attentive to the needs of the elderly, much can be done to improve their nutritional status and overall health (12).

Nutrient Intake of the Elderly

Several national surveys of the dietary habits of our aged population have now been conducted. Measurements of the quantity and quality of food consumed, physiological markers in the blood, and physical evaluation of the subjects have been made (11).

Taken as a whole, evidence indicates that the elderly as compared to other groups in our society suffer a relatively high incidence of malnutrition and suboptimal nutritional status (15). In general, the intake of most vitamins and minerals has been found to decrease with age in this country. The nutrients most often found to be consumed in amounts significantly below the RDA include folate, vitamin B_{12}, thiamin, riboflavin, vitamin B_6, and calcium. Intakes of vitamins A and C are low in certain groups of elderly people.

Table 15.3 outlines the average vitamin and mineral intakes of the elderly as measured by the USDA Nationwide Food Consumption Survey (18), and the FDA's Total Diet Study (19). This table shows that total Caloric consumption is nearly 20 percent below the recommended level. Nutrients below 100 percent RDA include calcium, magnesium, zinc, copper, and vitamin

TABLE 15.3

Food energy, protein, carbohydrate, fat, vitamin and mineral intakes by elderly individuals in the United States

Nutrient	Intake		Percent Recommended Dietary Allowance	
	Male	Female	Male	Female
Kilocalories	1,932	1,453	84%	76%
Protein (g)	80	62	127	130
Fat (g)	89	65		
Carbohydrate (g)	204	157		
Calcium (mg)	653	494	82	62
Iron (mg)	14	10	140	100
Magnesium (mg)	246	184	70	66
Phosphorus (mg)	1,248	880	156	110
Sodium (mg)	2,656	1,917	Ok	Ok
Potassium (mg)	2,527	1,954	Ok	Ok
Zinc (mg)	13	9	84	75
Copper (mg)	1.2	0.9	low	low
Manganese (mg)	2.6	2.1	Ok	Ok
Selenium (μg)	80	60	114	109
Iodine (μg)	0.34	0.25	227	167
Vitamin A (I.U.)	6,728	6,534	135	163
Thiamin (mg)	1.4	1.1	118	110
Riboflavin (mg)	1.8	1.5	131	122
Niacin (mg)	21	16	140	125
Vitamin B_6 (mg)	1.6	1.3	80	81
Vitamin C (mg)	100	96	167	160

Note: values are compared with the Recommended Dietary Allowances for the 51+ age group. Whether percent RDA is not given, either the RDA does not exist or estimated safe and adequate daily dietary intake ranges are given (if the nutrient average is within the range, "ok" is given, if below the range, "low" is given).

Adapted from E. M. Pao, S. J. Mickle, and M. C. Burke. "One-day and 3-day Nutrient Intakes by Individuals—Nationwide Food Consumption Survey Findings, Spring 1977." *Journal of the American Dietetic Association* 85:313–324, 1985. J. A. T. Pennington, et al. "Mineral Content of Foods and Total Diets: The Selected Minerals in Foods Survey, 1982 to 1984." *Journal of the American Dietetic Association* 86:876–891, 1986.

B_6. These figures represent the *average* intake of elderly people in the U.S. (ages 65–74 for the vitamins, ages 60–65 for the minerals). In addition, nutrient intake from vitamin and mineral supplements was not included in these figures. It is obvious that a wide range is found among the elderly, and that these averages could be misleading for the very old and frail. This is why most authorities recommend that the nutrient intakes of elderly people be measured singly, with individualized attention given to each.

Although intake of certain nutrients is low among the elderly, the prevalence of clinical signs of malnutrition is low (20). Clinical signs of malnutrition are found, however, in some elderly people, especially those in nursing homes. In one study, for example, between 22 percent and 33 percent of elderly patients in a nursing home were found to have varying degrees of malnutrition (21).

Should the elderly consume vitamin and mineral supplements to improve their nutrient status? Recent estimates indicate that approximately 50 percent of the elderly use vitamin and mineral supplements, with many users consuming supplement doses several times in excess of the recommended dietary allowances (22). Among ill-informed consumers, regular use of excessively high supplement doses can lead to potential toxicity and disturbances in nutrient absorption. The use of multiple vitamin and mineral supplements with nutrient levels kept below 100 percent RDA can be useful for some elderly people.

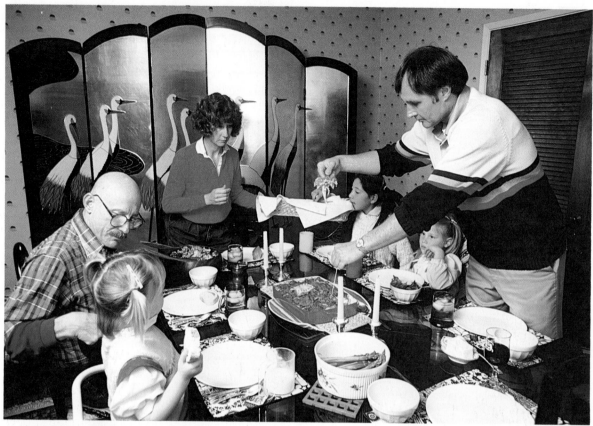

Little is known regarding optimal nutritional requirements for the elderly or how they differ from those of younger adults.

Improvement in the quality of the diet is needed by many. One nationwide study showed that elderly people have the lowest variety of foods consumed when compared to other age groups (23). Increasing the variety of fruits and vegetables, whole grains, low-fat dairy and meat products, and legumes, seeds, and nuts is a goal that all elderly people should aim for.

Nutritional Requirements of the Elderly

The great challenge for medical research over the next 50 years is to find a means of reducing the diseases and disabilities that occur with aging so that older people may continue healthy and productive lives (24,25,26,27,28,29). Nutrition has a role in the prevention of many of the diseases associated with aging; however, little is known regarding optimal nutritional requirements for the elderly and how they differ from those for younger adults.

Total Caloric Intake

The present RDA takes into account the declining need for Calories that is associated with aging (largely as a result of decreased physical activity). For example, the recommended daily energy intake for males between the ages of 25 and 50 is 2,900 Calories, whereas the recommendation for males 51 years of age and older is 2,300 Calories. For females, the recommendations are 2,200 and 1,900 Calories, respectively. However, for practically all other nutrients, the present RDA for the elderly is the same as the RDA for younger adults (see chapter 3 and table 15.4). Age factors have not been adjusted for, primarily because little is known about actual decreases or increases in nutrient needs that may accompany aging (25).

As a person ages, studies show that total daily intake of Calories decreases (24,25). A study by the National Institutes of Health showed that between the ages of 30 and 80, there is a 22 percent decline in total Caloric intake (25). Most

Table 15.4
National Research Council, recommended dietary allowances for individuals 51 years of age or older

	Men	Women
Calories[a]		
Ages 51+	2,300	1,900
Protein[a] (g)	63	50
Vitamin A (μg-RE)	1,000	800
Vitamin D (μg)	5	5
Vitamin E (mg α-RE)	10	8
Vitamin C (mg)	60	60
Thiamin (mg)	1.2	1.0
Riboflavin (mg)	1.4	1.2
Niacin (mg NE)	15	13
Vitamin B$_6$ (mg)	2.0	1.6
Folacin (μg)	200	180
Vitamin B$_{12}$ (μg)	2.0	2.0
Calcium (mg)	800	800
Phosphorus (mg)	800	800
Magnesium (mg)	350	280
Iron (mg)	10	10
Zinc (mg)	15	12
Iodine (μg)	150	150
Minimum Requirements of Healthy Persons		
Sodium (mg)	500	
Potassium (mg)	2000	
Chloride (mg)	750	

[a]Both Caloric and protein guidelines are for standard-size males and females. Caloric intake may vary according to physical activity and body size, while the protein allowance is based on a requirement of 0.8 grams per kilogram of body weight per day. In addition to the nutrients listed in the RDA, fiber is an important factor to consider.

Reprinted with permission from: Food and Nutrition Board. Recommended Dietary Allowances. 10th rev. ed. 1989. Washington, DC: National Academy Press, 1989.

of this decline in Calories can be accounted for by declining physical activity. With this decline in Caloric intake comes a decrease in vitamin and mineral intake.

The basal metabolic rate (BMR), or the energy expended during rest to keep one alive, has been determined to decrease by 15–20 percent with increasing age. This is primarily because the elderly decrease their activity and exercise less. This leads to a loss of muscle tissue, and as a consequence, BMR is lowered. A number of studies have shown that regular exercise can help maintain muscle tissue in the elderly.

As noted earlier in this chapter, a large number of elderly people have more body fat than they should. For elderly individuals trying to lose weight, the primary method should be decreasing intake of dietary fat (oils, margarine, butter, high-fat meats, and high-fat dairy products). Fat Calories are the most concentrated (9 kcal/g) and should be replaced with complex-carbohydrate foods, which have fewer Calories and more vitamins and minerals.

Protein
Several studies have concluded that the elderly require more dietary protein than younger adults (11,24). Others, however, suggest that a lower intake is required, and also results in less strain on the kidneys. Researchers from the USDA Human Nutrition Research Center on Aging at Tufts University have concluded that elderly people in the U.S. consume more than enough protein and that there is no need to emphasize increased usage (30).

Several research groups are recommending that the intake of protein for the elderly should average 12–14 percent of total Calories. The majority of the elderly are consuming more than this amount of protein. However, those living on limited incomes or who have limited transportation are of concern. In addition, protein requirements increase drastically for a number of health problems, including infection, broken bones, surgery, and burns. The amount of protein needed is directly proportional to the severity of the health problem.

Carbohydrate
Complex carbohydrate (carbohydrate foods high in dietary fiber, such as fruits, vegetables, and whole grains) is very important for the elderly. An increase in complex carbohydrate improves the intake of many vitamins and minerals. When less food is eaten, foods rich in nutrients are especially needed to ensure adequate intake.

The number of diabetics in the U.S. has been estimated at 11 million, and 40 percent of them are over the age of 65 (11). One-fourth of those over the age of 85 have diabetes. The American Diabetic Association is recommending that weight loss and a diet high in complex carbohydrate are helpful in treating diabetes (see chapter 5, Health-Promotion Insight). Because heart disease is the number-one cause of death among diabetics, a diet low in saturated fatty acids is also recommended.

Fat

Fat intake among the elderly in the U.S. averages 40 percent of total Calories, an amount considered higher than optimal for health (18). Although fat contributes to making foods taste better, provides essential fatty acids, and aids in the absorption of fat-soluble vitamins, it is also a high-energy source. In addition, hard-saturated animal fats contribute to the development of both heart disease and cancer (see chapter 6), diseases that are responsible for the deaths of many elderly people in this country. For these reasons, most health professionals advise that the elderly decrease their fat consumption to less than 30 percent of total Calories.

Vitamins

As already discussed, intake of some vitamins, in particular folate, vitamin B_{12}, thiamin, riboflavin, and vitamin B_6 have been found to be low in the elderly. In general, low dietary intakes (as a result of the low total Caloric intake due to decreasing physical activity levels and BMR) can account for much of this reported low vitamin intake (26). The first line of therapy should be to improve the variety and quality of the diet and to exercise more to stimulate the appetite.

A review of the literature shows that present RDA for thiamin, riboflavin, and vitamin C seem appropriate for the elderly (26). However, RDA for vitamin A may be too high, whereas RDA for vitamin D, vitamin B_6, and vitamin B_{12} may be too low, due to age-related changes in the metabolism of these vitamins. For vitamin E, vitamin K, niacin, biotin, and pantothenic acid, there is not yet enough evidence to make a judgment about the appropriateness of the present RDA for the elderly (26).

The reason vitamin A requirements are believed to be too high for the elderly is that national surveys show that despite the fact that large numbers of the elderly consume less than the RDA for this vitamin, serum levels are normal for the vast majority. For example, although up to 65 percent of the elderly have been reported to have vitamin intakes below two-thirds of the RDA, only 0.3 percent were found to have low serum levels of vitamin A.

Vitamin D is absolutely essential for the maintenance of a healthy skeleton throughout life (29). There is increasing evidence that the elderly are prone to develop vitamin-D deficiency and the associated bone disease osteomalacia. This is due to a decrease in milk consumption (the major dietary source of vitamin D), decrease in outdoor activities (sunshine on the skin results in vitamin D production), and age-related decreases in the capacity of the skin to produce vitamin D. The elderly would do well to spend at least 30 minutes a day exposed to sunshine, and perhaps use a low-dose vitamin-D supplement (10 mcg/day).

The majority of the elderly do not consume sufficient vitamin B_6, despite its wide distribution in food. With increasing age, there is a decline in blood levels of vitamin B_6. This may be due to specific age-related changes' in the body's ability to metabolize vitamin B_6. More research is needed before a specific RDA recommendation for the elderly can be given.

With increasing age, there is a tendency for blood levels of vitamin B_{12} to fall (26). Most elderly, however, are able to maintain normal serum vitamin B_{12} levels despite intakes below the RDA. Some of the elderly, however, who do not secrete sufficient gastric digestive juices or intrinsic factor, may require more dietary vitamin B_{12} than is presently recommended.

Minerals

Currently, the two major health concerns for the elderly are related to low intakes of iron and calcium, which are associated with anemia and osteoporosis, respectively (11). Iron absorption is reduced in the elderly. Several factors are related, including reduced hydrochloric acid secretion in the stomach (which is needed to help change iron into the form it can be absorbed from), and use of antacids, which can bind the iron. Nonetheless, national surveys have shown that relatively few elderly people develop iron deficiency (4.2 percent of elderly men and 6.8 percent of elderly women). Little evidence supports increasing the RDA for iron above 10 mg in the elderly.

Calcium absorption also decreases with increase in age (24). Several studies have shown that adequate intake of calcium throughout life is associated with decreased risk of osteoporosis in old age (see section on osteoporosis). However, the RDA of 800 mg per day appears to be adequate for the majority of elderly people, with estrogen replacement in elderly women being a more important therapy.

Although intake of some other minerals is below 100 percent RDA (magnesium, zinc, copper, and manganese for women) there is little evidence to suggest that the elderly are suffering ill health as a consequence. More research is needed regarding these issues.

Can Diet Alter the Life Span?

The topic of "life extension," or "maximum life span," has been receiving a lot of attention recently. Americans appear more eager than ever to seek out ways to ensure a longer life.

What is the potential for human longevity? What sort of vitality is possible in later life? Is it possible, as the Bible says, to "come to the grave in full vigor, like sheaves gathered in season"? (Job 5:26).

Before discussing this, the difference between life expectancy and life span needs to be explained (31). Life expectancy is the average number of years of life expected in a population at a specific age, usually at birth. **Life span** is the maximal obtainable age by a particular member of the species.

Since 1900, life expectancy at birth has jumped 27.6 years (from 47 to 74.7). But life expectancy for those at age 75 has only climbed 3 years since 1903, indicating perhaps a genetic limit for humans. Infectious diseases have been conquered, dramatically reducing infant mortality. But it appears that once a person reaches old age, the most that can be expected is a reduction in the duration of disabling morbidity and disability from chronic disease (32).

So the emphasis by many researchers today is not so much "life extension," or adding years to the life span of the human species, as it is a search for methods that will allow us to approach our true biogenetic potential for longevity. Medicated survival is a destiny to be avoided—and many health professionals now say it can be avoided, that it is possible for one to go to the grave "in full vigor" if various health habits are adopted.

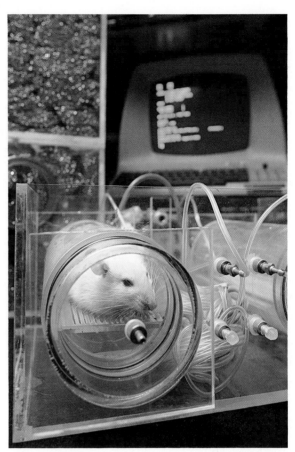

When rats eat 40 percent fewer Calories than normal, they live 50 percent longer.

Health habits are clearly identified as a strong factor in how quickly we age. Breslow of UCLA, for example, in his famous study of more than six thousand people in the San Francisco Bay area (33), showed a 520 percent difference in death rate between those who followed seven simple health habits (never smoked, moderate alcohol consumption, daily breakfast, no snacking, 7–8 hours of sleep per night, regular exercise, ideal weight) and those who did not.

Seventh-day Adventists (SDA), who tend to live longer than the average U.S. citizen (SDA males live an average of six years longer), have unusually low mortality rates from heart disease and cancer, due to virtually no cigarette smoking or alcohol consumption, low meat intake, and higher intake of fruits, vegetables, and whole grains (34).

If we keep winning the fight against heart disease and other chronic diseases, the possibility exists that a higher percentage of people will live to old age, reaching the theoretical limits of biological longevity.

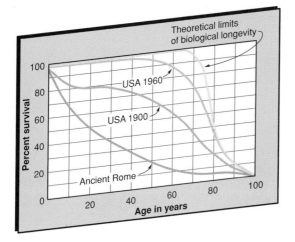

Some researchers, however, claim that diet can do more than reduce the obstacles of heart disease and cancer that lead to an improvement in life expectancy. They claim that by decreasing Caloric intake, the biological aging clock can actually be slowed down, thus increasing the life span.

Nearly 50 years ago, researchers first demonstrated that restricting the amount of food consumed increased the length of life in laboratory rats. Many other studies since then have shown that when rats are fed a low-fat, high-carbohydrate diet, with Calories reduced to 60 percent of normal intake, rats can live nearly 50 percent longer (35). Whether or not these studies will be found to be true in humans is questionable. Long-lived individuals in Vilcabamba, in rural Ecuador, have been found to consume only 1,200 Calories per day. However, verifying their actual ages has proven to be a difficult task.

Figure 15.7 summarizes this discussion. The primary factor explaining the increase in longevity of humans from early in this century to the present is the success in fighting infectious diseases. If we keep winning the fight against heart disease and other chronic diseases, the possibility exists that a high percentage of people will live into old age, reaching the theoretical limits of biological longevity. Whether or not we extend the biological limit remains to be seen.

Osteoporosis and Diet

Primary osteoporosis is an age-related disorder characterized by decreased bone mass and increased susceptibility to fractures in the absence of other recognizable causes of bone loss (36) (see figure 15.8).

Osteoporosis is a common condition affecting as many as 15–20 million people in the U.S. Loss of bone is an almost universal phenomenon with increasing age among white men and women in the U.S. About 1.3 million fractures attributable to osteoporosis occur annually in people aged 45 years and older. Among those who live to be 90, 32 percent of women and 17 percent of men will suffer a hip fracture, most related to osteoporosis. The cost of osteoporosis in the U.S. has been estimated at $6.1 billion annually (4). The number of hip fractures is projected to rise sharply over the next 50 years (see figure 15.9).

Peak bone mass is achieved at about 35 years of age for cortical bone (compact bone) and earlier for trabecular bone (spongy, internal bone) (see figure 15.10). Bone mass is approximately 30 percent higher in men than in women and approximately 10 percent higher in blacks than in whites.

After reaching its peak, bone mass declines throughout life. Over their lifetimes, women lose about 35 percent of their cortical bone and 50 percent of their trabecular bone, whereas men lose about two-thirds of these amounts. The following is a list of those who are at risk for osteoporosis (4):

White or Asian women
Underweight women, or those with short
    stature and small bones
Women who have an early menopause
Women who have never given birth
Women who have mothers that have
    experienced osteoporosis
Cigarette smokers
Those who use alcohol heavily
The physically inactive
Those who have low calcium intakes over a
    lifetime

The mainstays of prevention and management of osteoporosis are **estrogen replacement,** adequate calcium intake, and appropriate exercise. Estrogen replacement is highly effective for preventing osteoporosis in women (37).

FIGURE 15.8

Osteoporosis is characterized by decreased bone mass and increased susceptibility to fractures.

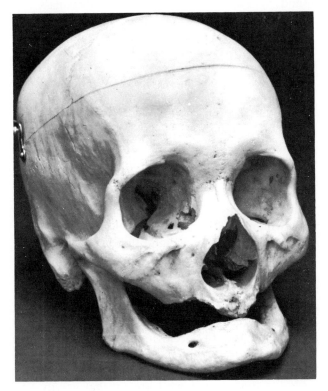

FIGURE 15.9

Projected number of hip fractures annually in the United States, by age: 1980–2050. The number of hip fractures is projected to rise sharply over the next 50 years.

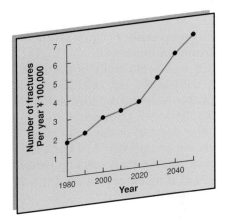

FIGURE 15.10

Some facts about bone. Osteoporosis affects as many as 15 to 20 million individuals in the United States. Thirty-two percent of women who live to be age 90 will suffer a hip fracture. The cost of osteoporosis in the United States has been estimated at $6.1 billion annually. There are two major forms of bone: cortical and trabecular. Cortical bone forms the external "envelope" of the skeleton, while trabecular, or spongy, bone forms a network that traverses the internal cavities of bone. The axial skeleton, especially the vertebral bodies, is primarily trabecular bone, while the appendicular skeleton is primarily cortical bone. Bone undergoes continuous remodeling, or turnover, throughout life. Osteoclasts resorb bone; osteoblasts then reform the bone. This bone resorption and formation are closely linked until about the fourth or fifth decade, when bone resorption begins to exceed bone formation, leading to decreased bone mass.

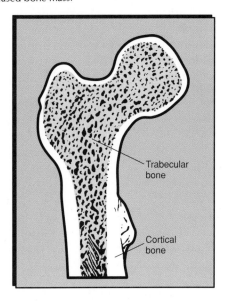

At menopause, women normally have an accelerated loss of bone mineral mass (2.5–5 percent per year) for several years. The result is that by 65 years of age, 50 percent of all women have a bone-mineral density below the normal fracture threshold of a 20-year-old woman. Estrogen helps to retard this process.

Estrogen therapy has risks, however, including possible endometrial cancer, gallbladder disease, hypertension, deep venous disease, and thromboembolic disease. The evidence for these risks, however, is weak and conflicting, and until more data are in, physicians may prescribe estrogen therapy for high-risk patients.

The usual intake of dietary calcium in the U.S. is 450–550 mg/day, well below the RDA of 800 mg/day (see chapter 11). Some calcium metabolic balance studies suggest that premenopausal and estrogen-treated women may need up to 1,000 mg/day to help retard osteoporosis; postmenopausal women may need 1,500 mg/day for calcium balance.

However, recent studies are showing that women most likely to benefit from increase in calcium intake are those with low intakes to begin with (4,38,39). For example, people with a lifelong low intake of dairy products because of lactase deficiency have an increased incidence of osteoporosis. Calcium supplements for these people are beneficial.

In a two-year study of postmenopausal women, daily 2,000 mg calcium supplements were not able to retard the loss of bone mineral loss (38). Estrogen treatments, however, prevented the loss of bone minerals. The researchers concluded that in large parts of the Western world, the daily calcium intake is 500 mg/day, and supplements beyond this may not be necessary or beneficial.

It is recommended that women at high risk for osteoporosis increase their calcium intake by consuming calcium-rich foods such as low-fat dairy products, leafy green vegetables, nuts, and seeds. The bones of elderly women who are lacto-ovo-vegetarians (eat no meat, poultry, or fish, but consume dairy products and eggs with the plant foods) have been found to have more mineral mass than those who are omnivores (no restrictions on animal flesh). There is some speculation that the high-protein diets of omnivores may increase the urinary excretion of calcium from the body, but more research is needed to verify this hypothesis.

Vitamin D is required for calcium to be absorbed from the small intestine. Elderly women are at risk for vitamin-D deficiency due to reduced intake, reduced exposure to sunlight, or impaired kidney and liver conversion of vitamin D. In one study, vitamin-D supplements reduced the rate of bone loss (40), suggesting that low vitamin-D levels in elderly women may increase the rate of bone loss.

Physical activity is a strong factor in maintaining bone density (41,42). In general, most studies show that for every week one spends in bed, one percent of bone mineral mass will be lost. Humans lose bone mass rapidly when gravitational or muscle forces on the legs are decreased or absent, as in weightlessness, bed rest, or spinal cord injury. Studies on astronauts have shown that weightlessness leads to rapid and significant loss of calcium from their bones.

Athletes have a greater bone density than people who do not exercise. Weight-bearing activities such as walking, running, and racket sports are more effective in maintaining the mineral density of leg and spinal bones than nonweight-bearing activities such as bicycling and swimming. The athletes with the greatest bone mineral mass are weightlifters, followed by athletes throwing the shotput and discus, then runners, soccer players, and finally swimmers. One study showed that the bone density in the arm with which tennis players serve and rally is 35 percent greater than that of the bones in their nonplaying arm (42). Obviously, physical activity is very important in keeping calcium in your bones.

Although it is well known that gravity and longitudinal force exerted on the bone will increase bone size and density, and that inactivity due to weightlessness and bed rest will lead to bone loss, whether or not exercise can delay bone aging and loss of calcium in elderly women has been a very controversial topic. In one study, researchers conducted a long-term study on 30 elderly women (mean age 81), who were divided into an exercise group and a control group. During the three years of the study, the exercise group participated in a 40-minute program three times a week. The sedentary control group had a bone mineral content loss of 3.28 percent during the 36 months, whereas the physical activity group had a 2.29 percent gain (41).

The evidence is mounting that women have much to gain by being physically active. Activity does appear to reduce osteoporosis, but more research is needed to define the kinds of whole-body activity needed and to determine just to what extent such exercise can counter the effects of aging on the skeleton.

One note of caution for younger women: excessive exercise that leads to loss of menstrual periods has been associated with increased risk of bone mineral loss (43). In Seattle, researchers showed that spinal bone mineral density in 14 amenorrheic athletes, whose average age was 25 and who ran 42 miles per week, was equivalent to that of women 51 years of age. Two of the athletes had a vertebral mineral density below the fracture threshold.

Drugs and the Elderly

The elderly are prescribed more drugs than any other segment of the U.S. population (44,45). A very large proportion of older people use drugs. About 84 percent of Medicare patients take prescription drugs, and 95 percent of elderly people in nursing homes use them. Surveys show that nursing home patients average 3.33 different drugs, or 6.34 pills, per day. Elderly people living independently average 2.9 prescription drugs per day.

The use of multiple drugs by the elderly poses many problems. As discussed previously, the elderly cannot metabolize and excrete the drugs as well as younger adults. Therefore, the action of the drug may last longer in the elderly person. In addition, drugs can interact, resulting in exaggeration of toxic or undesired effects.

Drugs also affect nutrient absorption and utilization by the body. Table 15.5 outlines some of the major effects of drugs on nutrients. Aspirin, for example, can increase loss of iron through bleeding. Laxatives can inhibit the absorption of fat-soluble vitamins, and diuretics taken for high blood pressure can increase the urinary loss of potassium and calcium. Alcohol use can decrease the absorption of folate and thiamin. The elderly should consult with a physician, pharmacist, and dietitian to discuss alterations in the diet to adjust for these effects.

TABLE 15.5
Commonly used drugs that affect nutrients

Drug	Nutrient	Mechanism
Cholestyramine (cholesterol-lowering agent)	Fats and fat-soluble vitamins	Inhibit absorption
Aspirin	Iron Folic acid	Increasing bleeding Compete for transport
Laxatives	Fat-soluble vitamins (A,D,K) Phosphorus	Inhibit absorption Depletion from bones
Antacids	Phosphorus	Inhibit absorption
Diuretics	Potassium Calcium	Increase excretion Increase excretion
Anticoagulants	Vitamin K	Inhibit utilization
Anticonvulsants	Vitamin D Folic acid	Inhibit utilization
Corticosteroids	Vitamin D Vitamin B_6 Zinc	Increase utilization Increase requirements Increase excretion
Alcohol	Folic acid Thiamin Vitamin B_6	Decreased absorption Increased requirement and decreased absorption Impaired conversion to active form
Nicotine (cigarettes)	Zinc and magnesium Vitamin C Vitamin B_6 Vitamin B_{12}	Increased excretion Uncertain Uncertain Uncertain

Exercise and Aging—Activated Longevity

Amazing Mavis!

She stands only five-foot-two and weighs just 102 pounds, but this 81-year-old nurse is big on achievement. Called "Amazing Mavis" by *Sports Illustrated* and many of her admirers, Mavis Lindgren is the hard-working owner of many national and world age-group records for various running events, from the 10K to the 26.2 mile marathon.

Mavis is a true "late-bloomer," having endured and overcome an unhealthy past. As a child in Canada, she suffered through whooping cough and pneumonia. Her lungs weakened, Mavis experienced annual bouts of severe bronchitis throughout her adulthood.

In her early 60s, while at a summer meeting in Canada, Mavis was inspired to take responsibility for her own health after listening to a lecture by Dr. Charles Thomas, a professor from Loma Linda University. Hoping and praying that exercise might help cure her worsening lung ailment, Mavis began walking faithfully every day.

At first she couldn't walk very far. Decades of inactivity had added 20 extra pounds of body fat and weakened her heart and skeletal muscles as well. Slowly she increased her walking distance, and after several weeks she began adding more and more jogging steps to her exercise routine.

As the months passed, Mavis experienced renewed health. She lost those 20 extra pounds of weight and was both gratified and overjoyed to discover that her lung problem had been cured. Those first few faltering steps marked the end of a lifetime illness.

Mavis also discovered that she loved to run. After a long period of adaptation, she found herself running five miles, six days per week, and enjoying it. She maintained this regimen for several years.

The running world discovered Mavis when she was 70 years old. At the strong urging of her son, a medical doctor who realized her unusual potential, she increased her training, entered her first marathon, and set an age-group world record for the 26.2 mile event. And from the ages of 70 to 81, Mavis has raced in 48 total marathons, resetting her own world record four different times (her world record is now 4 hours and 34 minutes). In the fall of 1984, Mavis also established a world best time for women over the age of 70 in the 10 kilometer (6.2 mile) event, racing to a 57 minute, 34 second finish.

Mavis has been the object of much attention from the press, and has a busy traveling schedule, flying to all parts of the United States, Canada, and the Carribean. Nonetheless, she keeps up with her demanding training schedule, which averages 50 miles of running per week. Mavis maximizes her training by eating a high-carbohydrate, vegetarian diet, which helps restore her muscle glycogen levels for the next training bout.

Recently, extensive physiological tests were conducted on Mavis at the Loma Linda University Human Performance Laboratory. It was discovered that Mavis has the oxygen intake capabilities of a college-age woman. The best measure of heart, lung, and blood vessel fitness is the $VO_{2\,max}$, which is the maximum amount of oxygen that the body can utilize during extremely heavy exercise. This can be measured directly, with a computerized metabolic cart, while the subject runs on a treadmill. Mavis tested out with a $VO_{2\,max}$ of 39 ml O2/kg per minute, which is equivalent to that of a college-age woman. In other words, Mavis has the heart and lungs of a woman 58 years younger than herself!

Body composition testing showed that Mavis is only 12 percent body fat. To put this in perspective, the average college-age woman is 25 percent body fat, and the average middle-aged woman is 32 percent body fat.

Other results showed that Mavis is able to ventilate 82 liters of air per minute during very heavy exercise, while breathing 52 times per minute. This is 40 percent above what is predicted for other women her age, an amazing statistic in light of her former lung problems.

Mavis is still training hard, seeking to break her own marathon world record. She enjoys the tough challenge of running through the wooded hills surrounding her northern California home. Mavis, a Seventh-day Adventist Christian, plans to continue as long as God gives her strength, for she looks upon her running as a means to help others improve their own life-styles and better glorify God.

The story of Mavis is particularly compelling because she appears to be defeating "Old Man Time." An elderly, overweight woman with lung problems, she seemed to throw off the shackles of age, and run her way to the "fountain of youth." The story of Mavis gives hope to the millions who today seek a more vibrant life.

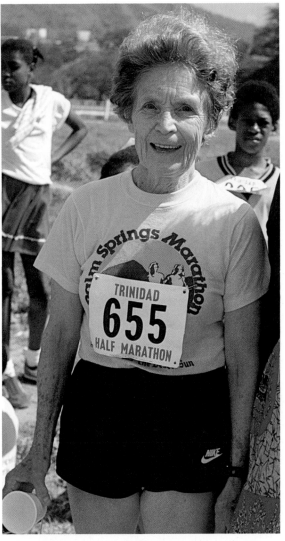

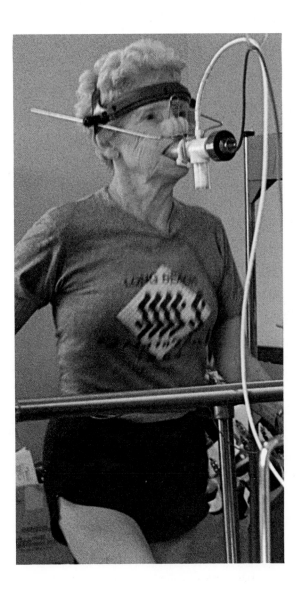

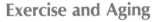
Mavis Lindgren, at age 81, has the heart and lungs of a woman 58 years younger.

Exercise and Aging

Exercise is one of the health habits receiving renewed attention today for its effects upon the aging process.

Aging is complex. It is a continuum that begins at birth and is both a psychological and physical condition, influenced by life-style, environment, and heredity.

There is an amazing similarity between the changes that occur with aging and the changes that accompany inactivity and weightlessness. The ability of the heart and lungs to transport oxygen to the muscles is decreased, body fat increases while muscle tissue decreases, bones lose their minerals, bowel function is decreased, and immune-system function

decreases. Can a regular program of exercise lessen the biological functional changes that normally occur as a person ages? Does the similarity of physiological changes that occur with inactivity and aging mean that exercise can forestall the aging process?

Most researchers who have tried to answer this question have focused on work capacity, or $VO_{2 max}$ (46,47). $VO_{2 max}$, the ability of the body to take in oxygen from the environment, transport it, and use it for muscle movement, is seen by many as the single best variable to define the changes that occur with aging.

$VO_{2 max}$ normally declines eight to ten percent per decade in persons age 30 and over. Researchers are now showing that this "normal" decrease can be lessened through regular cardiovascular exercise such as brisk walking, jogging, swimming, or bicycling (47). Healthy people in their 50s who exercise regularly have VO_2 max values 20–30 percent higher than those of young sedentary men. Middle-aged and old-master athletes who train for competition have VO_2 max values 50 percent above those of ex-athletes of the same age who have stopped training (46).

In general, aerobic capacity, or VO_2 max values, can be improved at all ages. As Mavis Lindgren and others have shown, inactive elderly persons who start regular exercise programs can recapture more than 40 years' worth of their VO_2 max capacity. No medicine currently exists that comes close to this proven power of exercise, and probably never will.

In other words, it appears that much of the human deterioration that we attribute to aging is simply a manifestation of deconditioning caused by inactivity. Physical activity can help counteract the decrease in function that occurs with increase of age and help with the troublesome symptoms accompanying the aging process.

It is well established that in contrast to machines, which wear out more rapidly the more they are used, the tissues and organs of humans grow stronger and more durable in response to increased use. Exercise training can help slow the deterioration in structure and function of the cardiovascular system, skeletal muscles, bones, tendons, and ligaments, while protecting against cardiovascular disease, diabetes, obesity, and osteoporosis. There is even preliminary evidence that physically trained elderly persons do not experience the usual decline in reaction time performance to various mental tasks.

As Albert Schweitzer once wrote, "The tragedy of life is what dies inside a man while he lives." A life lived actively gives the brightest promise for us to enjoy the "later best years for which the first were made."

HEALTH-PROMOTION INSIGHT
Nutrition and the Immune System

The Immune System

The body has an amazing array of internal bodyguards, called the **immune system,** to counter the vast army of invisible enemies that continually beseige the system. (See figure 15.11). These specialized **white blood cells** cleanse the lungs of foreign particles, rid the bloodstream of infectious bacteria and viruses, and destroy cancer cells (48).

The body has about one trillion white blood cells, originating in the bone marrow. Cells leave the bone marrow and are further developed in the thymus, spleen, tonsils, and lymphatic system. These cells include the phagocytes that consume bacteria and viruses, and lymphocytes, called T cells and B cells. Together these white blood cells identify and destroy all substances that are not part of the normal human body.

Aging and the Immune System

Differences in the immune systems of young and elderly subjects are striking (49). The **thymus,** an important organ that helps T cells mature, is much smaller in the elderly than in young adults. The number of T cells also declines with age. The B cells are not able to multiply as readily or produce as many antibodies.

This decline in immune-system function is thought to be related to many of the diseases from which the elderly suffer. Infections are common among the very old, striking the lungs, urinary tract, abdominal area, and other sites. Cancer is more prevalent among the elderly and may be related to the decline in ability of the immune system to identify and destroy cancer cells. Rheumatic diseases, ulcers, liver disease, infections of the tissues around the teeth, allergies, and kidney infections are other diseases found among the elderly that are associated with failing immune systems.

Nutrition and the Immune System

Can an optimal diet help to preserve the functioning of the immune system in the elderly? Can the elderly prevent their immune systems from failing by eating properly? On the other hand, does malnutrition or an improper diet hasten the decline of the immune system? Many people—lay public and health professional alike—believe that diet plays an important role in immune-system function and resistance to infection.

It is clear from various studies that malnutrition or inadequate intake of calories and nutrients can lead to an impaired immune system, with an increase in infectious disease (50). Researchers have shown

FIGURE 15.11

About one trillion strong, our white blood cells constitute a highly specialized army of defenders, the most important of which are depicted here in a typical battle against a formidable enemy.

Virus

Needing help to spring to life, a virus is little more than a package of genetic information that must commandeer the machinery of a host cell to permit its own replication.

Macrophage

Housekeeper and frontline defender, this cell engulfs and digests debris that washes into the bloodstream. Encountering a foreign organism, it summons helper T cells to the scene.

Helper T Cell

As a commander in chief of the immune system, it identifies the enemy and rushes to the spleen and lymph nodes, where it stimulates the production of other cells to fight the infection.

Killer T cell

Recruited and activated by helper T cells, it specializes in killing cells of the body that have been invaded by foreign organisms, as well as cells that have turned cancerous.

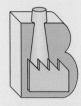

B cell

Biologic arms factory, it resides in the spleen or the lymph nodes, where it is induced to replicate by helper T cells and then to produce potent chemical weapons called antibodies.

Antibody

Engineered to target a specific invader, this Y-shaped protein molecule is rushed to the infection site, where it either neutralizes the enemy or tags it for attack by other cells or chemicals.

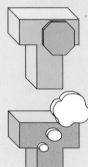

Suppressor T cell

A third type of T cell, it is able to slow down or stop the activities of B cells and other T cells, playing a vital role in calling off the attack after an infection has been conquered.

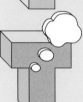

Memory cell

Generated during an initial infection, this defense cell may circulate in the blood or lymph for years, enabling the body to respond more quickly to subsequent infections.

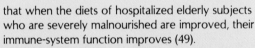

that when the diets of hospitalized elderly subjects who are severely malnourished are improved, their immune-system function improves (49).

Results from animal studies have suggested that high-fat diets accelerate the decline of the immune system as well as shorten the life span (49). In addition, when rats are fed a diet restricted in Calories, immune function and longevity are improved. However, these studies have not yet been duplicated in humans, and it must not be assumed that these results would be the same for humans.

The use of single nutrients such as vitamin C and zinc to stimulate immune function has received much attention (51,52,53). Many studies have shown that vitamin C is important for many aspects of immune function. However, most of these studies have been done in the laboratory with animals, and further research is needed with humans. There is no evidence to suggest that supplementation with large doses of vitamin C will prevent colds and flus.

There is clear indication that zinc deficiency markedly impairs the immune response in humans. In one study, low dietary zinc intake was associated with depression of the immune system (51). A large number of elderly people consume inadequate amounts of zinc. As described in chapter 11, foods high in zinc include wheat germ, seeds, whole-grain cereals, nuts, legumes, low-fat cheeses, and low-fat meats, especially turkey. Eating more of these foods may help increase the amount of zinc in the body of the elderly person, helping to improve immune function.

Overnutrition appears to be harmful to the immune system (54). For example, obesity and excessive intake of polyunsaturated fatty acids, iron, zinc, and vitamin E suppress the immune system. Also, deficiencies of most vitamins and minerals are associated with reduced immune-system function.

The topic of nutrition and immunology is an exciting one, and much more will be learned in the future. For now, a balanced, moderate diet appears to be the best guide and practice to ensure that the immune system is nourished properly.

SUMMARY

1. Statistics indicate that the elderly (those 65 years and older), are the fastest growing minority in the U.S. today. By the year 2030, 21 percent of the total U.S. population will be elderly.

2. Unfortunately, most studies reveal that despite improved life expectancy, the number of years elderly individuals live with disease and disability is increasing. However, there appears to be a large variation between elderly individuals, with some having optimal life-styles, living actively and independently into their ninth and tenth decades.

3. As a person ages, many changes take place in the body that are important from a nutritional point of view. This includes decrease in lean body weight, loss of taste and smell, periodontal bone loss, decrease in gastrointestinal function, loss in visual and auditory function, loss of bone mineral mass, mental impairment, decrease in heart and lung fitness, decreased ability to metabolize drugs, increased chronic disease, neuromuscular changes, urinary incontinence, and decrease in liver and kidney function.

4. In addition to limitations imposed by normal physiological decline and chronic disease conditions, many psychological, social, and economic factors influence the nutritional status in the elderly.

5. Community feeding programs can greatly assist in providing the elderly with an adequate diet.

6. Several national surveys of the dietary habits of the elderly show that in general, the intake of most vitamins and minerals decreases with age in this country.

7. Little is known regarding optimal nutritional requirements for the elderly and how they differ from those for younger adults. Information from research on the special needs of the elderly for energy, fats, carbohydrates, protein, minerals, and vitamins was reviewed.

8. If we keep winning the fight against heart disease and other chronic diseases, the possibility exists that a high percentage of people will live into old age, reaching the theoretical limits of biological longevity.

9. Osteoporosis is an age-related disorder characterized by decreased bone mass and increases susceptibility to fractures. The mainstays of prevention and treatment of osteoporosis are estrogen replacement, adequate calcium intake, and appropriate exercise.

10. The elderly are prescribed more drugs than any other segment of the U.S. population. These drugs can affect nutrient absorption and utilization by the body.

11. There is an amazing similarity between the changes that occur with aging and the changes that accompany inactivity. Elderly individuals who exercise regularly can possess the heart and lung fitness of people much younger than themselves.

12. As a person ages, immune-system function decreases. Malnutrition or inadequate intake of nutrients can hasten the decline of the immune system.

REFERENCES

1. Brody, J. A., D. B. Brock, and T. F. Williams. 1987. Trends in the Health of the Elderly Population. *Annual Review of Public Health* 8:211–34.

2. U.S. Bureau of the Census. 1983. Current Population Reports, Series P-23, No. 128, America in Transition: An Aging Society. Washington, D.C.: U.S. Government Printing Office.

3. National Center for Health Statistics: Health, United States, 1986. DHHS Pub. No. (PHS) 87–1232. Public Health Service. Washington, D.C.: U.S. Government Printing Office.

4. Riggs, B. L., and L. J. Melton. 1986. Involutional Osteoporosis. *New England Journal of Medicine* 314:1676–1684.

5. Ray, W. A., et al. 1987. Impact of Growing Numbers of the Very Old on Medicaid Expenditures for Nursing Homes: A Multi-State, Population-Based Analysis. *American Journal of Public Health* 77:699–703.

6. Board of Trustees Report. 1986. A Proposal for Financing Health Care of the Elderly. *Journal of the American Medical Association* 256:3379–3382.

7. American Dietetic Association Reports. 1987. Nutrition, Aging, and the Continuum of Health Care: Technical Support Paper. *Journal of the American Dietetic Association* 87:345–47.

8. Taubman, L. B. 1986. Theories of Aging. *Resident & Staff Physician* (April):31–37.

9. Rowe, J. W. 1985. Health Care of the Elderly. *New England Journal of Medicine* 312:827–35.

10. Shephard, R. J. 1986. Nutrition and the Physiology of Aging. In *Nutrition, Aging, and Health*, E. A. Young, ed. New York: Alan R. Liss, Inc.

11. Institute of Food Technologists' Expert Panel on Food Safety & Nutrition. 1986. *Food Technology* (September):81–88.

12. Crapo, P. A. 1982. Nutrition in the Aged. In *Clinical Internal Medicine in the Aged*, R. W. Schrier, ed. Philadelphia: W. B. Saunders Co.

13. Geissler, C. A., and J. F. Bates. 1984. The Nutritional Effects of Tooth Loss. *American Journal of Clinical Nutrition* 39:478–89.

14. Lowenstein, F. W. 1986. Nutritional Requirements of the Elderly. In *Nutrition, Aging, and Health*, E. A. Young, ed. New York: Alan R. Liss, Inc.

15. Morrow, F. D. 1986. Assessment of Nutritional Status in the Elderly: Application and Interpretation of Nutritional Biochemistries. *Clinical Nutrition* 5(3):112-20.

16. Eckstein, D., and T. Hesla. 1983. Nutritional Care of the Elderly. *Clinical Nutrition* 2(6):19-23.

17. American Dietetic Association Reports. 1984. ADA Takes Proactive Stance, Testifies on Older Americans Act Reauthorization. *Journal of the American Dietetic Association* 84:822-35.

18. Pao, E. M., S. J. Mickle, and M. C. Burk. 1985. One-day and 3-day Nutrient Intakes by Individuals — Nationwide Food Consumption Survey Findings, Spring 1977. *Journal of the American Dietetic Association* 85:313-24.

19. Pennington, J. A. T., et al. 1986. Mineral Content of Foods and Total Diets: The Selected Minerals in Foods Survey, 1982 to 1984. *Journal of the American Dietetic Association* 86:876-91.

20. Bowman, B. B., and I. H. Rosenberg. 1982. Assessment of the Nutritional Status of the Elderly. *American Journal of Clinical Nutrition* 35:1142-1151.

21. Kergoat, M. I., et al. 1987. Discriminant Biochemical Markers for Evaluating and Nutritional Status of Elderly Patients in Long-Term Care. *American Journal of Clinical Nutrition* 46:849-61.

22. Hartz, S. C., and T. Blumberg. 1986. Use of Vitamin and Mineral Supplements by the Elderly. *Clinical Nutrition* 5(3):130-36.

23. Fanelli, M. T., and K. J. Stevenhagen. 1985. Characterizing Consumption Patterns by Food Frequency Methods: Core Foods and Variety of Foods in Diets of Older Americans. *Journal of the American Dietetic Association* 85:1570-1576.

24. Lee, S. L. 1984. Nutrition Services for Adults and the Elderly. *Clinical Nutrition* 3(3):109-120.

25. Russell, R. M. 1983. Evaluating the Nutritional Status of the Elderly. *Clinical Nutrition* 2(6):4-8.

26. Suter, P. M., and R. M. Russell. 1987. Vitamin Requirements of the Elderly. *American Journal of Clinical Nutrition* 45:501-12.

27. Schneider, E. L., et al. 1986. Recommended Dietary Allowances and the Health of the Elderly. *New England Journal of Medicine* 314:157-60.

28. Bidlack, W. R., A. Kirsch, and M. S. Meskin. 1986. Nutrition Requirements of the Elderly. *Food Technology* (February): 61-70.

29. Holic, M. F. 1986. Vitamin D Requirements for the Elderly. *Clinical Nutrition* 5:121-29.

30. Munro, H. N., et al. 1987. Protein Nutriture of a Group of Free-Living Elderly. *American Journal of Clinical Nutrition* 46:586-92.

31. Schneider, E. L., and T. D. Reed. 1985. Life Extension. *New England Journal of Medicine* 312:1159-1168.

32. Freis, J. 1980. Aging, Natural Death, and the Compression of Morbidity. *New England Journal of Medicine* 33:130-35.

33. Kaplan, G. A., et al. 1987. Mortality among the Elderly in the Alameda County Study: Behavioral and Demographic Risk Factors. *Journal of Public Health* 77:307-12.

34. Snowdon, D. A. 1983. Epidemiology of Aging: Seventh-day Adventists — A Bellwether for Future Progress. In *Intervention in the Aging Process, Part A: Quantification, Epidemiology, and Clinical Research.* Alan R. Liss Publishers.

35. Masoro, E. J. 1984. Food Restriction and the Aging Process. *Journal of the American Geriatrics Society* 32(4):296-300.

36. National Institutes of Health. 1984. Consensus Conference: Osteoporosis. *Journal of the American Medical Association* 252:799-802.

37. Kiel, D. P., et al. 1987. Hip Fracture and the Use of Estrogens in Postmenopausal Women: The Framingham Study. *New England Journal of Medicine* 317:1169-1174.

38. Riis, B., K. Thomsen, and C. Christiansen. 1987. Does Calcium Supplementation Prevent Postmenopausal Bone Loss? *New England Journal of Medicine* 316:173-77.

39. Dawson-Hughes, B., P. Jacques, and C. Shipp. 1987. Dietary Calcium Intake and Bone Loss from the Spine in Health Postmenopausal Women. *American Journal of Clinical Nutrition* 46:685-87.

40. Nordin, B. E. C., et al. 1985. A Prospective Trial of the Effect of Vitamin D Supplementation on Metacarpal Bone Loss in Elderly Women. *American Journal of Clinical Nutrition* 42:470-74.

41. Smith, E. L., and C. Gilligan. 1987. Effects of Inactivity and Exercise on Bone. *Physician and Sports Medicine* 15(11):91-104.

42. Pirnay, F., et al. 1987. Bone Mineral Content and Physical Activity. *International Journal of Sports Medicine* 8:331-35.

43. Drinkwater, B. L., et al. 1984. Bone Mineral Content of Amenorrheic and Eumenorrheic Athletes. *New England Journal of Medicine* 311:277-81.

44. Gryfe, C. I., and B. M. Gryfe. 1984. Drug Therapy of the Aged: The Problem of Compliance and the Roles of Physicians and Pharmacists. *Journal of the American Geriatrics Society* 32(4):301-306.

45. Lamy, P. P. 1983. Nutrition, Drugs, and the Elderly. *Clinical Nutrition* 2(6):9-14.

46. Pollock, M. L., et al. 1987. Effect of Age and Training on Aerobic Capacity and Body Consumption of Master Athletes. *Journal of Applied Physiology* 62:725-31.

47. Larson, E. B., and R. A. Bruce. 1987. Health Benefits of Exercise in an Aging Society. *Archives of International Medicine* 147:353-56.

48. Jaret, P. 1986. Our Immune System: The Wars Within. *National Geographic* (June):702-34.

49. Lipschitz, D. A. 1986. The Role of Nutrition in Age-Related Changes in Hematopoiesis and Immunocompetence. In *Nutrition, Aging, and Health,* E. A. Young, ed. New York: Alan R. Liss, Inc.

50. Keusch, G. T., and M. J. G. Farthing. 1986. Nutrition and Infection. *Annual Review of Nutrition* 6:131-54.

51. Bogden, J. D., et al. 1987. Zinc and Immunocompetence in the Elderly: Baseline Data on Zinc Nutriture and Immunity in Unsupplemented Subjects. *American Journal of Clinical Nutrition* 46:101-109.

52. Bendich, A. 1987. Vitamin C and Immune Responses. *Food Technology* (November):112-14.

53. Koller, L. D., et al. 1987. Immune Dysfunction in Rats Fed a Diet Deficient in Copper. *American Journal of Clinical Nutrition* 45:997-1006.

54. Chandra, R. 1988. *Nutrition and Immunology, Contemporary Issues in Clinical Nutrition 11.* New York: Alan R. Liss.

HEALTH-PROMOTION ACTIVITY 15.1
Living to Your Biological Life Span

Some researchers claim that humans are genetically programmed to live up to 110 years if all obstacles, primarily infectious and chronic diseases, are removed. This nutrition textbook has outlined many principles to guide you in decreasing your risk of heart disease, cancer, diabetes, high blood pressure, osteoporosis, and infectious diseases. Accidents also are a concern, especially for college-age people. Review these principles, and summarize below *ten major guidelines to help you live out your maximum life span.* In other words, what are ten guidelines to help you avoid the various diseases that might prevent you from living to 110 years of age?

1.
2.
3.
4.
5.
6.
7.
8.
9.
10.
Comments

HEALTH-PROMOTION ACTIVITY 15.3
Choosing Attractive Recipes for the Elderly

In table 15.2, many practical suggestions for improving the nutrient intake of the elderly were listed. Locate a recipe book, and find a recipe that you feel would be desirable to a very old person who has diminished taste and smell senses. Write the recipe below, and describe why you feel this recipe would be attractive and readily eaten by a very old person.

Recipe:

Why this recipe will be attractive to a very old person:

HEALTH-PROMOTION ACTIVITY 15.2
Improving Mineral Intake of the Elderly

In table 15.3, the average intake of various minerals and vitamins by the elderly in this country are compared with the RDA. Average intake of several of the minerals is low. Choose two of these minerals and, referring to chapter 11, find five foods for each mineral that would help the elderly person to improve intake. Try to find foods that are not only high in the mineral, but also attractive and desirable for use by the elderly.

Mineral #1 _____

Food #1 _____

Food #2 _____

Food #3 _____

Food #4 _____

Food #5 _____

Mineral #2 _____

Food #1 _____

Food #2 _____

Food #3 _____

Food #4 _____

Food #5 _____

A P P E N D I X

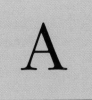

List of Selected Nutrient Tables and Figures

B

Food Composition Tables

This comprehensive food composition table was prepared with the Food Processor II nutrition system software program (ESHA Research, P.O. Box 13028, Salem, Oregon, 97309). This professional-level nutrition system is based on the latest United States Department of Agriculture data, more than 350 additional sources of information, and more than three years of research. With the kind permission of ESHA Research, 30 nutrients for more than 1,350 items are outlined in this appendix.

Common abbreviations used within the food composition table are outlined below. Blanks in the tables represent no available data or lack of reliable data. Zeros mean that the food has been analyzed, and there is no nutrient content.

Many factors influence the levels of nutrients in foods. These include the method of processing; length and method of storage; food-preparation techniques; the season of the year; exposure to heat, air, and/or light; and many other factors (see chapter 9). Therefore, all nutrient data in the following table should be regarded as an approximation of the actual nutrient content of the food.

The food composition table contains the following sections, with foods listed within each in alphabetical order.

Abbreviations

A-Car	Vitamin A — carotene (from plant sources)
A-Pre	Vitamin A — preformed (from animal sources)
A-Tot	Vitamin A — total
avg	average
BV/bkd val	baked value
bkd	baked
bev	beverage
bld	boiled
bttld	bottled
brd/brdd	breaded
braisd	braised
brld	broiled
btr/buttr	butter
btr/batr	batter
btr frd	batter fried
buttr	butter
cal	kcalories
calc	calcium
carb	carbohydrate
cbs	cubes
cd	curd
chick	chicken
choc	chocolate
chol	cholesterol
chnk	chunky
chp/chpd	chopped
chz	cheese
cinn	cinnamon

ckd	cooked	hm rec	home recipe
cnd	canned	home rec	home recipe
comm	commercial	icng	icing
crm	cream	in	inch
crmchz	cream cheese	inst	instant
conc	concentrate	lsl	Island (dressing)
cond	condensed	jc/jce	juice
Cu	copper	jr	junior
dm/diam	diameter	KFC	Kentucky Fried Chicken
diet	diet pack	2L	two layer
(low sodium for canned goods; low calorie for other)		LL	Loma Linda (veg foods)
		lem	lemon
drnk/drk	drink	lg/lrg	large
dnk	drink	liq	liquid
drnd	drained	lt/lite	light
drssng	dressing	ln	lean
drum	drumstick	ln&ft	lean and fat
ea	each	L&F	lean and fat
enr	enriched	lo-cal	low calorie
env/envl	envelope	lowMst	low moisture
fill	filling	lo-mst	low moisture
flr frd	flour fried	loMoist	low moisture
flvr/flvrd	flavor(ed)	marg	margarine
fort	fortified	msh/mshd	mashed
f/ fr/	from	mayo	mayonnaise
fol	folacin, folic acid	McD	McDonald's
frd	fried	meas	measure
fz/fzn/frzn	frozen	med	medium
frsh	fresh	MF	Morningstar Farms brand
frst/fstg	frosting	Mg	magnesium
F-sat	saturated fats	mlk	milk
F-tot	total fat	mono	monounsaturated fats
halvs	halves	mt	meat
hvy	heavy	mx	mix
		mxd	mixed

BEVERAGES

Qty	Name	Wgt G	Wtr G	Cal	Prot G	Carb G	Fiber G	F-Tot G	F-Sat G	Mono G	Poly G	Chol Mg	A-Car RE	A-Pre RE	A-Tot RE
1 cup	Carob flavor mix-prep/mlk	256	215	195	8.20	22.6	0.200	8.20	5.08	2.36	0.310	33.0	—	—	76.0
1 cup	Hot cocoa-with whole milk	250	204	218	9.10	25.8	0.200	9.05	5.61	2.65	0.330	33.0	5.00	80.0	85.0
1 cup	Coffee-brewed	240	238	2.00	0.135	1.08	0.020	0.011	0.005	0	0.005	0	0	0	0
1 cup	Coffee-instant-prepared	240	238	2.00	0.271	0.949	0	0.011	0.005	0	0.005	0	0	0	0
1 cup	Cappuchino coffee fr/mix	256	237	82.7	0.533	14.3	—	2.80	2.44	0.164	0.051	—	0	0	0
1 cup	Swiss mocha coffee-fr/mix	251	236	68.0	0.667	11.2	0.251	2.53	2.15	0.145	0.045	0	0	0	0
1 oz.	Coffee substitute-dry-prp	28.3	28.0	1.42	0.016	0.299	—	0.016	0.002	0.001	0.006	0	0	0	0
1 cup	Cola beverage-regular	247	221	101	0	25.7	0	0	0	0	0	0	0	0	0
1 cup	Diet cola-w/aspartame	237	236	1.33	0	0.200	0	0	0	0	0	0	0	0	0
1 cup	Club soda	237	237	0	0	0	0	0	0	0	0	0	0	0	0
1 cup	Cream soda	247	214	127	0	32.9	0	0	0	0	0	0	0	0	0
1 cup	Sego-liquid diet drink	256	125	180	8.80	27.2	0	4.0	0	0.060	1.72	1.50	0	300	300
1 cup	Sego-Lite-liq.diet drink	256	125	120	8.80	16.0	0	2.40	0.358	0.389	0.904	—	0	300	300
1 cup	Nutrament liquid diet	256	125	240	10.7	34.7	0	6.67	0.993	1.08	2.51	—	0	353	353
1 cup	Diet soda-avg assorted	237	236	1.33	0	0.200	0	0	0	0	0	0	0	0	0
1 cup	Egg nog-commercial	254	189	342	9.68	34.4	0	19.0	11.3	5.67	0.860	149	33.0	170	203

Note: Mcg = μg

Na	sodium	shrd	shredded
natrl	natural	skm	skim
ovn	oven	slc/sl	slice
ovn rst	oven roasted	slt/sltd	salted
ovn rstd	oven roasted	sml/sm	small
oz	ounce	sol	solids
panto	pantothenic acid	sprd	spread
p/pr	proof	sprs	spears
pce	piece	stm	steamed
phos	phosphorus	str/strn	strained
pkg	package	stwd/stewd	stewed
pkt	packet	swt/swtn	sweetened
poly	polyunsaturated fats	swtnd	sweetened
potas	potassium	syrp	syrup
prep/prp	prepared	2L	two layer
preprd	prepared	thd/thwd	thawed
pressur	pressurized	tom	tomato
pressrzd	pressurized	tst/tstd	toasted
prot	protein	unckd	uncooked
prt	part	unenr	unenriched
prtwhlwt	part whole wheat	unprep	unprepared
pwdr/pwder	powder	unswt	unsweetened
rais	raisins	unswtnd	unsweetened
RDA	Recommended Dietary Allowance	vacpac	vacuum pack
		W	Worthington (veg. foods)
rec	recipe	W	white (bread,corn,etc.)
reg	regular	wgt	weight
RNI	Recommended Nutrient Intake	wht/wte	white
		whl	whole
rst/rstd	roasted	WW/whl wt	whole wheat
RTS	ready-to-serve	w/	with
san/sand	sandwich	wo/	without
sce	sauce	/	or, per, divided by
sds	seeds	wtr	water
sel	selenium		
sft	soft		

B1 Mg	B2 Mg	B3 Mg	B6 Mg	B12 Mcg	Fol. Mcg	Panto Mg	Vit-C Mg	Vit-E Mg	Calc Mg	Cu Mg	Iron Mg	Mg Mg	Phos Mg	Potas Mg	Sel Mcg	Na Mg	Zinc Mg
0.095	0.394	0.297	0.118	0.870	12.2	0.765	2.30	—	291	0.023	0.670	33.0	228	370	—	132	0.930
0.102	0.435	0.365	0.107	0.870	12.0	0.808	2.40	0.222	298	0.085	0.780	56.0	270	480	3.05	123	1.22
0	0.020	0.533	0	0	0.270	0.002	0	0	4.07	0.016	0.976	13.5	2.71	130	0.108	5.42	0.040
0	0.003	0.687	0	0	0	0.003	0	0	8.14	0.010	0.122	9.00	8.14	86.8	0	8.14	0.068
0.020	0.008	0.429	0	0	0	0.013	0	—	9.33	0.036	0.200	12.0	34.7	159	—	139	0.107
0.005	0.005	0.345	0	0	0	0.008	0	9.33	0.080	0.320	12.0	38.7	159	—	—	48.0	0.200
	0.000	0.061	—	0	—	—	—	—	0.787	0.003	0.019	1.10	2.05	6.77	—	1.10	0.009
0	0	0	0	0	0	0	0	0	6.00	0.027	0.080	2.00	30.7	2.67	0	10.00	0.033
0.012	0.055	0	0	0	0	0	0	0	8.00	0.038	0.073	2.67	20.0	0	0	14.0	0.187
0	0	0	0	0	0	0	0	0	11.3	0.100	0.099	2.67	0	4.00	0	50.0	0.240
0	0	0	0	0	0	0	0	12.7	0.020	0.127	2.00	0	2.67	—	—	28.7	0.160
0.300	0.340	4.00	0.400	1.20	80.0	2.00	12.0	6.00	200	0.400	3.60	80.0	200	480	—	288	3.00
0.300	0.340	4.00	0.400	1.20	80.0	2.00	12.0	6.00	200	0.400	3.60	80.0	200	480	—	288	3.00
0.350	0.397	4.67	0.467	1.40	93.3	2.33	14.0	7.00	233	0.467	4.20	93.3	233	333	—	167	3.50
0	0	0	0	0	0	0	0	0	9.33	0.059	0.095	1.67	25.3	4.67	0	21.3	0.067
0.086	0.483	0.267	0.127	1.14	2.00	1.06	3.81	0.200	330	0.079	0.510	47.0	278	420	5.00	138	1.17

Qty	Name	Wgt G	Wtr G	Cal	Prot G	Carb G	Fiber G	F-Tot G	F-Sat G	Mono G	Poly G	Chol Mg	A-Car RE	A-Pre RE	A-Tot RE
1 cup	Fruit flavored soda pop	248	221	113	0	28.0	0	0	0	0	0	0	0	0	0
1 cup	Fruit punch drink fr/fzn	247	218	113	0.100	29.0	—	0	0.002	0.002	0.005	0	2.70	0	2.70
1 cup	Gatorade	230	228	39.0	0	10.5	0	0	0	0	0	0	0	0	0
1 cup	Ginger ale	244	223	82.7	0.067	21.3	0	0	0	0	0	0	0	0	0
1 cup	Grape soda-carbonated	248	220	107	0	27.8	0	0	0	0	0	0	0	0	0
1 cup	Grape drink-non carbonate	250	221	112	0	34.7	0.253	0.040	0.008	0.002	0.005	0	0.270	0	0.270
1 cup	Kefir	233	191	160	9.30	8.80	0	4.50	2.91	1.23	0.125	10.0	20.0	135	155
1 cup	Koolade w/nutrasweet	240	239	4.00	0	0	0	0	0	0	0	0	0	0	0
1 cup	Koolade w/sugar added	240	239	100	0	25.0	0	0	0	0	0	0	0	0	0
1 cup	Lemon-lime soda	245	220	99.3	0	25.6	0	0	0	0	0	0	0	0	0
1 cup	Lemonade flvr drk fr/dry	266	237	113	0	28.8	0	0.100	0.045	0.005	0.011	0	0	0	0
1 cup	Lemonade drink from dry	264	237	102	0	26.9	0	0.003	0	0	0.003	0	0	0	0
1 cup	Lemonade-prep from frozen	248	221	100	0.150	26.0	0.292	0.100	0.015	0.005	0.032	0	5.30	0	5.30
1 cup	Limeade-prep/from frozen	247	220	102	0.100	27.1	0.292	0.054	0.005	0.005	0.015	0	0.100	0	0.100
1 cup	Vanilla milkshake	226	169	251	7.84	40.6	0.152	6.72	4.21	1.95	0.251	25.6	8.00	64.0	72.0
1 cup	Orange drink/carbonated	248	217	118	0	30.5	0	0	0	0	0	0	0	0	0
1 cup	Root beer	247	220	101	0.067	26.1	0	0	0	0	0	0	0	0	0
1 cup	Pineapple grapefruit drnk	250	220	117	0.600	29.0	0	0.200	0.015	0.025	0.070	0	8.80	0	8.80
1 cup	Pineapple orange drink	250	217	125	3.10	29.4	0	0.240	0.027	0.042	0.047	0	133	0	133
1 cup	Tonic water/Quinine water	244	222	83.3	0	21.5	0	0	0	0	0	0	0	0	0
1 cup	Tea-brewed	240	239	2.00	0.010	0.539	0	0.017	0.005	0.003	0.009	0	0	0	0
1 cup	Tea from instant-unswtnd	237	236	2.00	0	0.400	0	0.015	0.004	0.003	0.008	0	0	0	—
1 cup	Tea from instant-sweetnd	262	238	86.0	0	22.1	0	0.015	0.004	0.003	0.008	0	0	0	0
1 cup	Tea & lemon-diet-prep/dry	238	236	5.00	0.100	1.30	0	0	0	0	0.002	0	0	0	0
1 cup	Tea & lemon inst-prepared	238	237	4.00	0.100	1.10	0	0	0	0	0.002	0	0	0	0
1 cup	Water	237	237	0	0	0	0	0	0	0	0	0	0	0	0
8 oz.	Water-bottled-Perrier	227	227	0	0	0	0	0	0	0	0	0	0	0	0
1 cup	Gin, rum, vodka, whiskey 80p	224	143	508	0	0.240	0	0	0	0	0	0	0	0	0
1 cup	Gin, rum, vodka, whiskey 86p	224	143	560	0	0.244	0	0	0	0	0	0	0	0	0
1 cup	Gin, rum, vodka, whiskey 90p	224	139	588	0	0.052	0	0	0	0	0	0	0	0	0
1 cup	Beer	237	219	97.3	0.600	8.80	0.475	0	0	0	0	0	0	0	0
1 cup	Light beer	236	225	66.7	0.472	3.07	0.167	0	0	0	0	0	0	0	0
1 cup	Brandy	224	172	548	0	84.0	0	0	0	0	0	0	0	0	0
1 cup	Champagne	238	205	182	0.360	5.00	0	0	0	0	0	0	0	0	0
1 oz.	Liqueur-coffee-53 proof	28.3	8.79	94.9	0	13.3	0	0.055	0.030	0.006	0.030	0	0	0	0
1 oz.	Liqueur-coffee+cream-34pr	28.3	13.2	92.9	0.784	5.91	0	4.46	2.74	1.27	0.189	—	—	—	—
1 oz.	Liqueur-de menthe-72proof	28.3	8.02	105	0	11.8	0	0.057	0.004	0.005	0.048	0	0	0	0
1 ea.	Bloody mary-5 fl oz drink	148	127	116	0.800	4.80	0.850	0.100	0.015	0.019	0.038	0	51.0	0	51.0
1 cup	Bourbon and soda	232	202	210	0	0	0	0	0	0	0	0	0	0	0
1 ea.	Daiquiri-2 fl oz drink	60.0	41.9	111	0	4.10	0.020	0.030	0.004	0.004	0.010	0	0	0	0
1 ea.	Manhattan-2 fl oz drink	57.0	37.7	128	0	1.80	0	0	0	0	0	0	0	0	0
1 ea.	Martini-2.5 fl oz drink	70.0	47.3	156	0	0.200	0	0	0	0	0	0	0	0	0
1 ea.	Pina colada-4.5 fl oz drk	141	91.8	262	0.600	39.9	0	2.60	1.23	0.228	0.491	0	0.300	0	0.300
1 ea.	Screwdriver-7 fl oz drink	213	178	174	1.20	18.4	0.100	0.100	0.013	0.017	0.021	0	13.3	0	13.3
1 ea.	Tequila sunrise-5.5 oz dnk	172	137	189	0.600	14.7	0.100	0.200	0.021	0.029	0.040	0	16.6	0	16.6
1 ea.	Tom collins-7.5 fl oz dnk	222	203	121	0.100	3.00	0	0.030	0.007	0.002	0.013	0	0	0	0
1 ea.	Whiskey sour-3 fl oz dnk	90.0	69.4	123	0.200	5.00	0	0.100	0.017	0.005	0.040	0	0.700	0	0.700
1 ea.	Whiskey sour/liq mx-3.5 oz	106	77.0	158	0	13.8	0	0.019	0.005	0.001	0.013	0	1.40	0	1.40
1 ea.	Whiskey sour from dry mix	103	71.2	169	0.100	16.4	0	0.010	0.003	0.001	0.006	0	0.500	0	0.500
1 ea.	Pina colada-cnd-6.8 oz	222	122	525	1.30	61.3	0.090	16.9	14.6	0.981	0.304	0	0.900	0	0.900
1 cup	Dessert wine-dry	236	171	298	0.472	9.68	0	0	0	0	0	0	0	0	0
1 cup	Dessert wine-sweet	236	171	362	0.472	27.8	0	0	0	0	0	0	0	0	0
1 cup	Wine red	236	209	170	0.458	4.12	0	0	0	0	0	0	0	0	0
1 cup	Wine rosé	236	210	168	0.458	3.44	0	0	0	0	0	0	0	0	0
1 cup	Wine-dry white	238	213	158	0.240	1.44	0	0	0	0	0	0	0	0	0
1 cup	Wine-medium white	236	211	160	0.236	1.83	0	0	0	0	0	0	0	0	0
1 cup	Vermouth-dry	240	185	288	0.240	13.2	0	0	0	0	0	0	0	0	0
1 cup	Vermouth-sweet	240	185	372	0.120	38.2	0	0	0	0	0	0	0	0	0

B1 Mg	B2 Mg	B3 Mg	B6 Mg	B12 Mcg	Fol. Mcg	Panto Mg	Vit-C Mg	Vit-E Mg	Calc Mg	Cu Mg	Iron Mg	Mg Mg	Phos Mg	Potas Mg	Sel Mcg	Na Mg	Zinc Mg
0	0	0.013	0	0	0	0	0	0	10.00	0.041	0.174	2.67	1.33	13.3	0	32.0	0.181
0.025	0.032	0.052	0.015	0	2.30	0.020	108	—	9.00	0.074	0.220	6.00	2.00	31.0	—	11.0	0.090
—	—	—	—	0	—	—	—	0	23.0	—	—	—	0	23.0	—	123	—
0	0	0	0	0	0	0	0	0	8.00	0.044	0.440	2.00	0.667	3.33	—	16.7	0.122
0	0	0	0	0	0	0	0	0	8.00	0.055	0.207	2.67	0	2.00	—	38.0	0.173
0.079	0.010	0.065	0.015	0	0.664	0.010	85.4	—	2.70	0.030	0.412	5.00	3.00	13.3	2.00	16.0	0.279
0.450	0.440	0.300	0.087	0.900	20.0	—	6.00	—	350	0.140	0.500	28.0	319	205	4.00	50.0	0.900
0	0	0	0	0	0	0	6.00	0	0	0.004	0	0.240	0	0	0	0	0
0	0	0	0	0	0	0	6.00	0	0	0	0	0	0	0	0	0	0
0	0	0.037	0	0	0	0	0	0	6.00	0.029	0.167	1.33	0.667	2.67	0	27.3	0.120
0	0.003	0	0	0	0	0	34.0	—	29.0	0.027	0.040	3.00	3.00	1.00	—	19.0	0.070
0.005	—	0.034	0.008	0	3.50	0.016	8.50	—	71.0	—	0.150	3.00	34.0	33.0	—	13.0	0.100
0.015	0.052	0.040	0.015	0	5.50	0.032	9.80	—	4.00	0.005	0.410	2.50	5.00	38.0	0.075	2.00	0.050
0.005	0.005	0.054	0.027	0	6.00	0.061	6.60	—	3.00	0.028	0.060	15.0	3.00	32.0	0.075	0.010	0.027
0.102	0.412	0.419	0.118	0.808	7.36	0.944	1.76	0.560	275	0.115	0.208	28.0	231	394	—	186	0.808
0	0	0	0	0	0	0	0	0	12.7	0.037	0.153	2.67	2.67	6.00	—	30.7	0.253
0	0	0	0	0	0	0	0	0	12.7	0.017	0.123	2.67	1.33	2.00	—	32.7	0.173
0.075	0.040	0.668	0.105	0	26.2	0.133	115	0.041	18.0	0.113	0.770	15.0	14.0	154	—	34.0	0.150
0.075	0.048	0.518	0.118	0	27.2	0.143	56.2	0.040	13.0	0.103	0.670	14.0	10.0	116	—	9.00	0.140
0	0	0	0	0	0	0	0	0	3.33	—	0.165	0.667	0	0.667	—	10.00	—
0	0.034	0.100	0	0	12.4	0.001	0	0	0	0.024	0.054	6.74	1.35	89.0	0.150	6.74	0.054
0	0.005	0.008	0.088	0	0.700	0.026	0	0	5.00	0.019	0.047	5.00	3.00	47.0	0.250	8.00	0.071
0	0.040	0.090	0	0	5.00	0.023	0	0	1.00	0.006	0.040	3.00	3.00	49.0	0.250	1.00	0.020
0	0.012	0.062	—	0	4.60	—	0	—	5.00	0.017	0.150	4.00	2.00	41.0	—	24.0	0.070
0	0.019	0.090	—	0	—	—	0	0	5.00	0.019	0.020	4.00	2.00	49.0	—	14.0	0.080
0	0	0	0	0	0	0	0	0	5.00	0.014	0.010	2.00	0	1.00	0	7.00	0.060
0	0	0	0	0	0	0	0	0	307	0	0	1.18	0	0	3.54	0	—
0	0	0	0	0	0	0	0	0	0	0.132	0.080	0	0	8.00	0	0	0
0.016	0.012	0.028	0	0	0	0	0	0	0	0.048	0.092	0	9.20	4.40	—	2.40	0.092
0	0	0	0	0	0	0	0	0	0	0.124	0.076	0	0	6.80	—	0	0
0.014	0.062	1.07	0.119	0.040	14.3	0.137	0	0	12.0	0.021	0.071	13.3	29.3	59.3	2.37	12.7	0.047
0.021	0.071	0.927	0.080	0.013	9.80	0.085	0	0	12.0	0.057	0.095	11.8	28.7	42.7	2.37	6.67	0.071
0.016	0.016	0.028	—	0	0	—	0	0	20.0	0.068	0.092	—	8.00	8.00	—	8.00	0.156
0	0.024	0.160	0.048	0	0.360	0.072	0	0	13.0	0.016	0.778	20.2	16.0	190	—	14.6	0.224
0.001	0.003	0.041	—	—	0	0	0	—	0.545	0.011	0.016	0.545	1.64	8.18	—	2.18	0.005
0	0.016	0.022	—	—	0	0.025	0	—	4.22	0.011	0.036	0.603	13.9	9.05	—	25.9	0.048
0	0	0.001	0	0	0	0	0	—	0	0.023	0.023	0	0	0	—	1.70	—
0.050	0.033	0.642	0.107	0	19.6	0.241	20.4	—	10.0	0.102	0.550	11.0	21.0	216	—	332	0.140
0.006	0	0.042	0	0	0	0	0	0	8.00	—	—	2.00	4.00	4.00	—	32.0	0.180
0.008	0.001	0.025	0.004	0	1.20	0.010	1.00	—	2.00	0.026	0.090	1.00	4.00	13.0	—	3.00	0.040
0.006	0.003	0.053	0	0	0.100	0.005	0	0	1.00	0.016	0.050	0.024	4.00	15.0	—	2.00	0.030
0.001	0.002	0.011	0.004	0	0.200	0.004	0	0	1.00	0.004	0.060	1.00	2.00	13.0	—	2.00	0.010
0.039	0.020	0.166	—	0	14.4	—	6.70	—	11.0	0.116	0.310	—	10.0	100	—	9.00	0.190
0.136	0.032	0.345	0.075	0	74.8	0.271	66.5	—	16.0	0.079	0.170	17.0	29.0	325	—	2.00	0.090
0.065	0.028	0.327	0.086	0	58.0	0.210	33.2	—	10.0	0.072	0.470	12.0	17.0	178	—	7.00	0.110
0.007	0.002	0.031	0.007	0	1.50	0.013	3.80	—	10.0	—	—	3.00	1.00	18.0	—	39.0	0.170
0.192	0.005	0.111	0.020	0	4.60	0.041	11.4	—	5.00	0.027	0.070	4.00	6.00	48.0	—	10.0	0.050
0.012	0.006	0.021	0	0	0	0.008	1.70	—	1.00	0.010	0.080	1.00	6.00	19.0	—	66.0	0.060
0.004	0	0.021	0	0	0	0.010	0.500	—	47.0	0.034	0.080	4.00	5.00	4.00	—	48.0	0.050
—	—	—	—	—	—	—	—	—	1.00	—	0.070	—	—	184	—	158	—
0.042	0.042	0.502	0	0	0.940	0.076	0	0	18.8	0.106	0.566	21.2	21.2	218	—	21.2	0.166
0.042	0.042	0.502	0	0	0.940	0.076	0	0	18.8	0.106	0.476	21.2	22.0	218	—	21.2	0.166
0.012	0.066	0.190	0.080	0.032	4.80	0.082	0	0	18.4	0.048	1.02	30.0	32.0	262	—	12.6	0.220
0.010	0.036	0.174	0.058	0.020	2.52	0.066	0	0	20.0	0.038	0.896	22.8	34.0	234	—	10.6	0.146
0.004	0.012	0.160	0.048	0	0.460	0.058	0	0	22.0	0.024	0.780	14.0	14.0	146	—	10.0	0.160
0.010	0.012	0.158	0.032	0	0.460	0.050	0	0	20.8	0.030	0.708	25.2	32.0	188	—	12.0	0.156
—	—	0.096	0.020	0	—	—	0	0	16.8	0.144	0.816	12.0	16.0	96.0	—	40.0	0.084
—	—	0.096	0.010	0	—	—	0	0	14.4	0.096	0.840	9.60	14.0	72.0	—	68.0	0.072

DAIRY PRODUCTS AND EGGS

Qty	Name	Wgt G	Wtr G	Cal	Prot G	Carb G	Fiber G	F-Tot G	F-Sat G	Mono G	Poly G	Chol Mg	A-Car RE	A-Pre RE	A-Tot RE
1 oz.	American cheese-processed	28.3	11.1	107	6.37	0.456	0	8.97	5.65	2.57	0.283	27.3	10.1	72.9	83.0
1 oz.	American cheese spread	28.3	13.5	83.0	5.23	2.51	0	6.10	3.83	1.78	0.182	16.2	6.07	48.6	54.7
1 oz.	Blue cheese	28.3	12.0	101	6.18	0.668	0	8.25	5.37	2.24	0.233	21.3	0	65.8	65.8
1 oz.	Brick cheese	28.3	11.7	106	6.50	0.800	0	8.52	5.39	2.47	0.223	27.3	5.77	81.3	87.1
1 oz.	Brie cheese	28.3	13.7	96.2	5.95	0.132	0	7.95	5.01	2.32	0.253	28.3	0	57.7	57.7
1 oz.	Camembert cheese	28.3	14.7	86.1	5.68	0.132	0	6.96	4.38	2.02	0.207	20.2	4.05	67.8	71.9
1 oz.	Caraway cheese	28.3	11.1	108	7.23	0.881	0	8.38	5.50	2.38	0.243	25.3	3.95	79.1	83.0
1 oz.	Cheddar cheese	28.3	10.4	115	7.15	0.364	0	9.52	6.05	2.69	0.273	30.4	5.77	81.3	87.1
1 oz.	Cheshire cheese	28.3	10.7	111	6.70	1.38	0	8.79	5.76	2.48	0.253	29.4	7.09	62.8	69.9
1 oz.	Colby cheese	28.3	10.8	113	6.82	0.739	0	9.21	5.80	2.66	0.273	27.3	5.06	73.9	79.0
1 cup	Cottage cheese-crmd-sm cd	210	166	215	26.2	5.63	0	8.93	5.99	2.70	0.290	31.0	0.600	100	101
1 cup	Cottage cheese-crmd-lg cd	225	178	235	28.0	6.00	0	9.60	6.42	2.90	0.310	34.0	2.00	106	108
1 cup	Cottage cheese w/fruit	226	163	279	22.4	30.1	0	7.68	4.86	2.19	0.240	25.0	1.00	80.0	81.0
1 cup	Cottage cheese-dry curd	145	116	123	25.0	2.68	0	0.610	0.396	0.160	0.022	10.0	0.600	11.4	12.0
1 cup	Cottage cheese-lowfat 2%	226	179	205	31.1	8.20	0	4.36	2.76	1.24	0.130	19.0	1.20	43.8	45.0
1 cup	Cottage cheese-lowfat 1%	226	186	164	28.0	6.15	0	2.30	1.46	0.660	0.070	10.0	0.100	24.9	25.0
1 oz.	Cream cheese	28.3	15.3	100	2.13	0.759	0	10.0	6.31	2.82	0.364	31.4	0	126	126
1 oz.	Edam cheese	28.3	11.8	102	7.17	0.410	0	7.90	5.04	2.33	0.192	25.3	4.56	68.3	72.9
1 oz.	Feta cheese	28.3	15.6	75.9	4.56	1.17	0	6.28	4.29	1.33	0.172	25.3	1.52	34.9	36.4
1 oz.	Fontina cheese	28.3	10.7	111	7.35	0.445	0	8.75	5.51	2.49	0.476	33.4	0	101	101
1 oz.	Gjetost cheese	28.3	3.80	134	2.77	12.3	0	8.43	5.50	2.26	0.273	25.3	0	75.9	75.9
1 oz.	Gorgonzola cheese	28.3	11.1	112	7.09	0	0	9.11	5.57	2.43	0.506	25.3	0	104	104
1 oz.	Gouda cheese	28.3	11.8	102	7.16	0.638	0	7.83	5.05	2.23	0.192	32.4	3.04	46.6	49.6
1 oz.	Gruyere cheese	28.3	9.41	118	8.56	0.101	0	9.18	5.43	2.89	0.496	31.4	3.04	96.2	99.2
1 oz.	Liederkranz cheese	28.3	15.0	88.1	5.06	0	0	8.10	5.37	2.23	0.233	21.3	0	92.1	92.1
1 oz.	Limburger cheese	28.3	13.7	94.2	5.75	0.142	0	7.69	4.81	2.47	0.142	26.3	0	116	116
1 oz.	Monterey jack cheese	28.3	11.6	107	7.03	0.192	0	8.69	5.50	2.38	0.243	26.3	0	82.0	82.0
1 oz.	Mozzarella-part skim-reg	28.3	15.3	72.9	7.09	0.790	0	4.66	2.91	1.30	0.132	16.2	0	50.6	50.6
1 oz.	Mozzarella-whl milk-reg	28.3	15.3	81.0	5.58	0.638	0	5.83	3.78	1.88	0.223	22.3	0	68.8	68.8
1 oz.	Muenster cheese	28.3	11.9	105	6.50	0.324	0	8.54	5.49	2.50	0.192	27.3	2.73	88.4	91.1
1 oz.	Neufchatel cheese	28.3	17.6	74.9	2.86	0.840	0	6.79	4.25	1.94	0.182	22.3	10.1	65.8	75.9
1 oz.	Parmesan cheese-grated	28.3	5.02	131	11.9	1.07	0	8.62	5.48	2.53	0.202	22.3	5.47	44.1	49.6
1 oz.	Pimento processed cheese	28.3	11.1	107	6.35	0.496	0	8.95	5.64	2.56	0.283	27.3	5.06	82.0	87.1
1 oz.	Ricotta cheese-part skim	28.3	21.1	39.2	3.23	1.45	0	2.25	1.39	0.656	0.074	8.76	2.30	29.7	32.0
1 oz.	Ricotta cheese-whole milk	28.3	20.3	49.3	3.19	0.862	0	3.68	2.35	1.03	0.109	14.3	1.84	36.2	38.0
1 oz.	Romano cheese	28.3	8.76	111	9.13	1.04	0	7.74	4.91	2.25	0.169	29.4	4.35	36.1	40.5
1 oz.	Roquefort cheese	28.3	11.2	106	6.19	0.577	0	9.06	5.53	2.43	0.516	26.3	0	96.2	96.2
1 oz.	Swiss cheese	28.3	10.5	108	8.14	0.972	0	7.90	5.10	2.09	0.283	26.3	0	72.9	72.9
1 oz.	Swiss processed cheese	28.3	12.0	96.2	7.10	0.607	0	7.07	4.61	2.02	0.182	24.3	2.02	63.8	65.8
1 cup	Chocolate milk-whole	250	206	210	7.92	25.9	0.150	8.48	5.26	2.48	0.310	31.0	8.80	64.2	73.0
1 cup	Chocolate milk 1%	250	211	160	8.10	26.1	0.150	2.50	1.54	0.750	0.090	7.00	1.00	147	148
1 Tbs	Frzn/liq coffee whitener	15.0	11.6	20.4	0.150	1.71	0	1.50	1.40	0.016	0.000	0	1.38	0	1.38
1 Tbs	Cream-half & half	15.1	12.2	19.7	0.447	0.650	0	1.74	1.08	0.502	0.064	5.56	1.75	14.4	16.2
1 Tbs	Cream-coffee/table	15.0	11.1	29.3	0.405	0.549	0	2.89	1.81	0.837	0.107	9.94	2.56	24.7	27.3
1 Tbs	Sour cream-cultured	14.4	10.2	30.8	0.454	0.614	0	3.01	1.88	0.869	0.112	6.38	3.06	24.9	28.0
1 Tbs	Sour cream-imitation	14.4	10.2	29.9	0.345	0.956	0	2.81	2.56	0.084	0.008	0	0	0	0
1 Tbs	Light whipping cream-liq.	14.9	9.49	43.7	0.324	0.442	0	4.62	2.89	1.36	0.132	16.6	3.19	40.9	44.1
1 Tbs	Heavy whipping cream-liq.	14.9	8.58	51.3	0.305	0.415	0	5.50	3.42	1.59	0.204	20.4	1.50	61.1	62.6
1 Tbs	Whipped cream	7.44	4.29	25.7	0.152	0.207	0	2.75	1.71	0.794	0.102	10.2	0.750	30.6	31.3
1 ea.	Egg white-cooked	33.0	26.1	16.0	3.35	0.410	0	0	0	0	0	0	0	0	0
1 ea.	Egg yolk-cooked	17.0	7.82	63.0	2.79	0.040	0	5.60	1.72	2.92	0.063	262	0	95.0	95.0
1 ea.	Fried egg (in butter)	46.0	33.1	95.0	5.37	0.530	0	6.41	2.41	2.40	0.700	278	0	94.0	94.0
1 ea.	Hard cooked egg	50.0	37.3	79.0	6.07	0.600	0	5.58	1.67	2.23	0.720	274	0	78.0	78.0
1 tsp	Hard-cooked egg-chopped	2.83	2.11	4.48	0.344	0.034	0	0.317	0.095	0.126	0.041	15.5	0	4.42	4.42
1 ea.	Poached egg	50.0	37.1	79.0	6.04	0.600	0	5.55	1.67	2.22	0.720	273	0	78.0	78.0
1 ea.	Hard cooked egg	50.0	37.3	79.0	6.07	0.600	0	5.58	1.67	2.23	0.720	274	0	78.0	78.0
1 ea.	Scrambled egg-milk-butter	64.0	46.7	95.0	6.00	1.37	0	7.08	3.01	2.75	0.760	282	0	102	102
1 Tbs	Dried egg white-powder	6.69	0.571	25.1	5.51	0.299	0	0.002	0	0	0	0	0	0	0
1 Tbs	Egg substitute-frozen	15.0	11.0	24.0	1.69	0.480	0	1.67	0.290	0.365	0.935	0.250	20.2	0	20.2

B1 Mg	B2 Mg	B3 Mg	B6 Mg	B12 Mcg	Fol. Mcg	Panto Mg	Vit-C Mg	Vit-E Mg	Calc Mg	Cu Mg	Iron Mg	Mg Mg	Phos Mg	Potas Mg	Sel Mcg	Na Mg	Zinc Mg
0.008	0.101	0.020	0.020	0.199	2.43	0.139	0	0.181	176	0.008	0.111	6.58	214	46.6	3.69	411	0.945
0.014	0.124	0.037	0.033	0.114	2.02	0.196	0	0.181	161	0.009	0.092	8.10	204	69.9	3.04	386	0.790
0.008	0.109	0.292	0.048	0.349	10.1	0.496	0	0.181	152	0.011	0.091	6.83	111	73.9	1.01	401	0.759
0.004	0.101	0.033	0.018	0.360	6.07	0.083	0	0.181	193	0.007	0.132	7.19	130	38.5	3.12	161	0.743
0.020	0.149	0.109	0.068	0.474	18.2	0.198	0	0.181	52.6	0.060	0.142	6.07	53.7	43.5	1.01	180	0.709
0.008	0.140	0.181	0.065	0.372	17.8	0.392	0	0.181	111	0.006	0.095	6.07	99.2	53.7	1.70	239	0.683
0.009	0.130	0.052	0.021	0.078	2.02	0.055	0	0.181	193	0.049	0.101	6.07	141	28.3	1.01	198	0.893
0.008	0.107	0.023	0.021	0.237	5.06	0.118	0	0.181	207	0.009	0.199	7.80	148	28.3	4.08	178	0.936
0.013	0.084	0.023	0.021	0.304	4.05	0.081	0	0.181	184	0.060	0.061	6.07	133	27.3	1.01	200	0.810
0.004	0.107	0.026	0.022	0.237	5.06	0.061	0	0.181	196	0.012	0.219	7.09	131	36.4	2.02	173	0.881
0.044	0.342	0.265	0.141	1.31	26.0	0.447	0.001	1.34	126	0.059	0.295	11.0	277	177	12.6	850	0.802
0.050	0.370	0.300	0.140	1.31	27.0	0.447	0.001	1.35	135	0.059	0.255	11.0	297	190	13.5	911	0.800
0.038	0.292	0.226	0.120	1.12	22.0	0.380	0.001	1.45	108	0.045	0.250	9.00	236	151	13.5	915	0.660
0.036	0.206	0.225	0.119	1.20	21.0	0.236	0	0.928	46.0	0.029	0.330	6.00	151	47.0	12.1	19.0	0.680
0.054	0.418	0.325	0.172	1.61	30.0	0.547	0	1.45	155	0.063	0.360	14.0	340	217	13.6	918	0.950
0.047	0.373	0.289	0.154	1.43	28.0	0.486	0	1.45	138	0.045	0.320	12.0	302	193	13.6	918	0.860
0.005	0.057	0.029	0.013	0.121	3.75	0.078	0	0.181	23.3	0.004	0.342	2.02	30.4	34.4	1.01	85.0	0.329
0.010	0.111	0.023	0.022	0.440	5.06	0.081	0	0.181	210	0.010	0.127	8.49	154	53.7	1.01	277	1.07
0.040	0.233	0.294	0.016	0.304	3.04	0.081	0	0.010	142	0.009	0.183	5.47	97.2	18.2	1.01	320	0.823
0.006	0.059	0.044	0.024	0.304	3.04	0.081	0	0.181	158	0.060	0.061	4.05	172	25.3	1.01	—	1.00
0.009	0.101	0.233	0.078	0.304	1.01	0.081	0	0.181	114	0.111	0.132	8.10	128	40.5	1.01	172	0.958
0.010	0.091	0.202	0.040	0.263	9.11	0.496	0	0.181	151	0.010	0.121	8.10	123	26.3	1.01	519	0.577
0.009	0.096	0.018	0.023	0.440	6.07	0.097	0	0.181	200	0.060	0.071	8.10	157	34.4	1.01	235	1.11
0.017	0.080	0.030	0.023	0.460	3.04	0.161	0	0.181	291	0.060	0.061	4.05	174	23.3	1.01	96.2	1.01
0.010	0.182	0.101	0.044	0.263	34.4	0.496	0	0.181	111	0.009	0.121	6.88	101	68.8	1.01	395	0.709
0.023	0.145	0.046	0.024	0.299	16.2	0.338	0	0.181	143	0.060	0.040	6.07	112	36.4	1.01	230	0.607
0.004	0.112	0.023	0.016	0.304	3.04	0.081	0	0.181	215	0.009	0.204	8.10	128	23.3	8.16	154	0.857
0.005	0.087	0.030	0.020	0.235	2.63	0.022	0	0.181	185	0.007	0.061	7.09	133	24.3	1.01	134	0.838
0.004	0.070	0.024	0.016	0.187	2.02	0.018	0	0.181	149	0.008	0.051	5.06	106	19.2	8.10	107	0.709
0.004	0.092	0.029	0.016	0.423	3.44	0.055	0	0.181	206	0.009	0.127	8.10	135	38.5	8.10	180	0.854
0.004	0.056	0.036	0.012	0.076	3.04	0.162	0	0.181	21.3	0.043	0.081	2.02	39.5	33.4	1.01	114	0.152
0.013	0.110	0.090	0.030	0.425	2.02	0.151	0	0.181	395	0.011	0.273	14.3	232	30.4	1.01	535	1.01
0.008	0.101	0.022	0.020	0.199	2.02	0.139	0.010	0.181	176	0.008	0.121	6.07	214	46.6	3.75	410	0.850
0.006	0.052	0.022	0.006	0.083	1.61	0.046	0	0.181	77.1	0.010	0.126	0.496	51.7	35.4	0.576	35.4	0.379
0.004	0.055	0.030	0.012	0.096	1.61	0.046	0	0.183	58.7	0.010	0.108	3.23	44.8	29.6	0.519	23.9	0.328
0.011	0.106	0.022	0.026	0.425	2.02	0.127	0	0.181	306	0.060	0.233	12.1	218	26.3	2.83	344	1.01
0.011	0.168	0.211	0.035	0.184	14.2	0.497	0	0.181	190	0.010	0.174	8.25	123	26.3	1.01	519	0.577
0.006	0.104	0.026	0.024	0.481	1.82	0.124	0	0.181	275	0.009	0.051	10.1	173	31.4	4.93	74.9	1.11
0.004	0.079	0.011	0.010	0.352	2.02	0.075	0	0.181	222	0.008	0.172	8.10	219	61.8	3.75	393	1.03
0.092	0.405	0.313	0.100	0.835	12.0	0.738	2.28	0.222	280	0.085	0.600	33.0	251	417	3.05	149	1.02
0.095	0.415	0.317	0.102	0.855	12.0	0.755	2.32	0.073	287	0.073	0.600	33.0	256	425	8.37	152	1.02
0	0	0	0	0	0	0	0	—	1.38	—	0.005	0.032	9.62	28.6	0.421	11.9	0.002
0.005	0.023	0.012	0.006	0.050	0.344	0.044	0.130	0.017	15.9	0.011	0.011	1.56	14.4	19.6	0.117	6.13	0.077
0.005	0.022	0.009	0.005	0.033	0.344	0.041	0.114	0.023	14.4	0.016	0.006	1.31	12.0	18.2	0.082	5.94	0.041
0.005	0.021	0.010	0.002	0.043	1.56	0.052	0.124	0.094	16.7	0.016	0.009	1.63	12.2	20.7	0.081	7.69	0.043
0	0	0	0	0	0	0	0	0	0.375	0.007	0.001	—	6.38	23.1	—	14.7	0
0.004	0.019	0.006	0.004	0.029	0.563	0.039	0.091	0.094	10.4	0.016	0.004	1.06	9.12	14.4	0.087	5.13	0.037
0.003	0.016	0.006	0.004	0.027	0.625	0.038	0.086	0.094	9.62	0.016	0.004	1.06	9.31	11.2	0.087	5.56	0.034
0.002	0.008	0.003	0.002	0.013	0.313	0.019	0.043	0.047	4.81	0.008	0.002	0.531	4.66	5.59	0.044	2.78	0.017
0.002	0.090	0.128	0.001	0.018	4.00	0.080	0	0	4.00	0.013	0.010	3.00	4.00	45.0	4.44	50.0	0.060
0.036	0.071	0.012	0.050	0.550	19.4	0.753	0	0.415	26.0	0.035	0.950	3.00	86.0	15.0	7.96	9.00	0.550
0.040	0.130	0.026	0.050	0.581	22.5	0.763	0	0.390	28.0	0.033	0.930	6.20	90.0	62.0	12.0	113	0.760
0.037	0.143	0.030	0.057	0.657	24.5	0.864	0	0.530	28.0	0.033	1.04	6.10	90.0	65.0	12.0	65.0	0.720
0.002	0.008	0.002	0.003	0.037	1.40	0.049	0	0.030	1.58	0.002	0.059	0.354	5.10	3.69	0.679	3.69	0.041
0.035	0.127	0.026	0.051	0.616	24.0	0.860	0	0.385	28.0	0.015	1.04	6.00	90.0	65.0	12.1	146	0.720
0.037	0.143	0.030	0.057	0.657	24.5	0.864	0	0.530	28.0	0.033	1.04	6.10	90.0	65.0	12.0	65.0	0.720
0.039	0.180	0.042	0.058	0.638	22.0	0.819	0.130	0.550	54.0	0.033	0.930	7.40	109	90.0	12.0	112	0.780
0.002	0.155	0.048	0.002	0.035	6.38	0.131	0	—	6.00	—	0.016	4.81	6.00	74.6	—	82.8	0.011
0.018	0.058	0.025	0.020	0.112	4.00	0.249	0	0.050	11.0	—	0.297	—	10.7	32.0	—	30.0	0.147

DAIRY PRODUCTS AND EGGS (continued)

Qty	Name	Wgt G	Wtr G	Cal	Prot G	Carb G	Fiber G	F-Tot G	F-Sat G	Mono G	Poly G	Chol Mg	A-Car RE	A-Pre RE	A-Tot RE
1 Tbs	Egg substitute-liquid	15.7	13.0	13.2	1.88	0.101	0	0.519	0.104	0.141	0.251	0.188	33.9	0	33.9
1 oz.	Egg substitute-powder	28.3	1.09	125	15.6	6.12	0	3.66	1.05	1.50	0.482	162	34.6	0	34.6
1 cup	Evaporated milk-skim-cnd	255	201	200	19.0	29.0	0	0.520	0.310	0.158	0.016	10.0	0	300	300
1 cup	Evaporated milk-whole-cnd	252	186	340	17.0	25.0	0	19.6	11.6	5.88	0.620	74.0	15.0	121	136
1 cup	Ice cream-regular-vanilla	133	80.9	269	4.80	31.7	0	14.3	8.29	4.14	0.530	59.0	15.0	118	133
1 cup	Ice cream-rich-vanilla	148	87.2	349	4.13	32.0	0	23.7	14.7	6.84	0.880	88.0	25.0	194	219
1 cup	Ice cream-soft serve	173	103	377	7.04	38.3	0	22.5	13.5	6.68	0.980	153	20.0	179	199
1 cup	Inst breakfast w/whl milk	281	244	280	15.0	34.4	0	8.15	5.07	2.35	0.300	33.0	183	68.0	251
1 Tbs	Instant nonfat dry milk	4.25	0.168	15.2	1.49	2.22	0	0.032	0.020	0.008	0.001	0.750	0	30.2	30.2
1 cup	1% lowfat milk	244	220	102	8.03	11.7	0	2.54	1.61	0.750	0.100	10.0	2.50	142	145
1 cup	2% lowfat milk	244	218	121	8.12	11.7	0	4.78	2.92	1.35	0.170	22.0	5.00	135	140
1 cup	Skim milk	245	222	86.0	8.35	11.9	0	0.440	0.287	0.116	0.016	4.00	0	149	149
1 cup	Whole milk	244	215	150	8.03	11.4	0	8.15	5.07	2.35	0.300	33.0	8.10	67.9	76.0
1 cup	Buttermilk	245	221	99.0	8.11	11.7	0	2.16	1.34	0.620	0.080	9.00	2.00	18.0	20.0
1 cup	Swtned condensed milk-cnd	306	83.2	982	24.2	166	0	26.6	16.8	7.43	1.03	104	27.0	221	248
1 cup	Carob flavor mix-powder	64.0	1.86	240	1.07	59.7	1.07	0.107	0.021	0.037	0.043	0	—	—	—
1 cup	Chocolate milk-whole	250	206	210	7.92	25.9	0.150	8.48	5.26	2.48	0.310	31.0	8.80	64.2	73.0
1 cup	Hot cocoa-with whole milk	250	204	218	9.10	25.8	0.200	9.05	5.61	2.65	0.330	33.0	5.00	80.0	85.0
1 cup	Egg nog-commercial	254	189	342	9.68	34.4	0	19.0	11.3	5.67	0.860	149	33.0	170	203
1 cup	Kefir	233	191	160	9.30	8.80	0	4.50	2.91	1.23	0.125	10.0	20.0	135	155
1 cup	Malted milk powder/natrl	336	6.72	1392	37.0	254	4.80	27.2	14.1	6.86	4.05	64.0	0	304	304
1 cup	Malted milk drink-natural	265	215	237	10.4	27.3	0.300	9.80	5.96	2.78	0.557	37.0	8.50	85.5	94.0
1 cup	Vanilla milkshake	226	169	251	7.84	40.6	0.152	6.72	4.21	1.95	0.251	25.6	8.00	64.0	72.0
1 cup	Ovaltine drink-malt flvr	265	228	228	9.93	29.0	0.030	8.33	5.19	2.45	0.330	33.0	234	67.0	301
1 cup	Goat milk	244	212	168	8.68	10.9	0	10.1	6.51	2.71	0.360	28.0	0	137	137
1 cup	Human milk	246	215	171	2.53	17.0	0	10.8	4.94	4.08	1.22	34.0	10.0	147	157
1 cup	Soybean milk	263	242	87.0	7.90	5.80	0	4.00	0.509	0.745	2.08	0	10.5	0	10.5
1 cup	Yogurt-coffee/vanilla	227	202	193	11.2	31.3	0	2.83	1.84	0.772	0.091	11.4	4.00	26.0	30.0
1 cup	Yogurt-lowfat with fruit	227	169	231	9.92	43.0	0.270	2.45	1.58	0.670	0.070	10.0	3.10	21.9	25.0
1 cup	Yogurt-lowfat-plain	227	193	144	11.9	16.0	0	3.46	2.27	0.970	0.100	14.0	4.50	31.5	36.0
1 cup	Yogurt-nonfat milk	227	193	127	13.0	17.4	0	0.408	0.263	0.112	0.012	4.00	0.500	4.50	5.00

FAST FOODS, SANDWICHES

Qty		Wgt G	Wtr G	Cal	Prot G	Carb G	Fiber G	F-Tot G	F-Sat G	Mono G	Poly G	Chol Mg	A-Car RE	A-Pre RE	A-Tot RE
1 ea.	KFC-chicken breast/orig	95.0	49.0	236	23.9	7.40	0.100	12.3	3.40	5.20	12.3	86.7	0	5.70	5.70
1 ea.	KFC-chick side-brst/orig	69.0	26.8	199	16.2	7.10	0.100	11.7	3.18	4.84	2.74	69.8	0	4.20	4.20
1 ea.	KFC-chicken drum/original	47.0	25.0	117	12.1	2.60	0.100	6.50	1.68	2.65	1.56	63.0	0	2.70	2.70
1 ea.	KFC-chicken thigh/originl	88.0	43.5	257	18.4	6.50	0.100	17.5	4.36	7.12	4.14	109	0	5.40	5.40
1 ea.	KFC-chicken wing/original	42.0	18.3	136	9.60	4.20	0.200	9.10	2.31	3.90	2.20	54.6	0	2.70	2.70
1 ea.	KFC-2-pce dinner/combo	341	216	661	32.6	47.8	1.00	37.8	8.44	14.0	11.2	172	0	76.5	76.5
1 ea.	KFC-2-pce dinner/dark	346	223	643	35.1	46.2	0.800	35.2	7.81	12.8	10.6	180	0	76.5	76.5
1 ea.	KFC-2-pce dinner/white	322	205	604	30.4	48.3	1.00	32.1	7.26	11.7	9.82	133	0	76.5	76.5
1 ea.	KFC-chicken breast/crispy	104	40.5	297	23.6	13.6	0.100	16.4	4.32	6.93	3.91	78.8	0	6.30	6.30
1 ea.	KFC-chicken side-breast/C	84.0	32.7	286	17.2	14.1	0.200	17.8	4.85	7.36	4.18	65.1	0	5.10	5.10
1 ea.	KFC-chicken drum/crispy	58.0	29.5	155	13.3	5.10	0.100	9.00	2.30	3.67	2.16	65.5	0	3.60	3.60
1 ea.	KFC-chicken thigh/crispy	107	48.1	343	20.4	12.6	0.200	23.4	6.37	9.52	5.54	109	0	6.60	6.60
1 ea.	KFC-chicken wing/crispy	53.0	18.8	201	11.2	8.70	0.100	13.5	3.70	5.80	3.30	58.7	0	3.30	3.30
1 ea.	KFC-2-pce combo dinner	371	222	902	36.2	58.4	1.00	48.2	11.9	18.3	13.7	176	0	76.5	76.5
1 ea.	KFC-2-pce dinner/dark	375	233	765	38.3	54.7	1.00	53.7	10.5	16.2	12.6	183	0	76.5	76.5
1 ea.	KFC-2-pce dinner/white	348	207	755	33.0	59.9	1.00	42.6	10.3	16.2	12.4	132	0	76.5	76.5
1 ea.	KFC-serving of coleslaw	91.0	68.9	121	0.900	12.7	0.500	7.50	1.11	2.00	3.90	7.18	22.0	11.0	33.0
1 ea.	KFC-svg mashed potatoes	85.0	68.9	64.0	1.50	12.2	0.340	0.900	0.240	0.200	0.440	0.200	0	5.40	5.40
1 ea.	Biscuit-bacon+egg+cheese	145	59.7	483	16.5	33.2	0.200	31.6	9.26	12.6	2.96	263	0	196	196
1 ea.	Biscuit with sausage-McD	121	39.1	467	12.1	35.3	0.400	30.9	11.7	13.9	3.73	48.0	0	18.0	18.0
1 ea.	Biscuit & sausage&egg-McD	175	75.1	585	19.8	36.4	0.100	39.9	14.5	16.6	4.57	285	0	126	126

B1 Mg	B2 Mg	B3 Mg	B6 Mg	B12 Mcg	Fol. Mcg	Panto Mg	Vit-C Mg	Vit-E Mg	Calc Mg	Cu Mg	Iron Mg	Mg Mg	Phos Mg	Potas Mg	Sel Mcg	Na Mg	Zinc Mg
0.017	0.047	0.017	0.000	0.047	—	0.424	0	—	8.31	—	0.329	—	19.0	51.7	—	27.7	0.204
0.062	0.493	0.162	0.040	—	—	—	0.198	—	90.7	—	0.879	—	133	210	—	224	—
0.114	0.796	0.400	0.140	0.610	22.0	1.88	3.00	0.226	738	0.188	0.700	68.0	497	845	3.20	293	2.18
0.120	0.800	0.488	0.126	0.410	18.0	1.61	4.74	0.454	657	0.328	0.480	60.0	510	764	3.16	267	1.94
0.052	0.329	0.134	0.061	0.625	3.00	0.654	0.700	0.492	176	0.027	0.120	18.0	134	257	9.31	116	1.41
0.044	0.283	0.115	0.053	0.537	2.00	0.562	0.610	0.518	151	0.030	0.100	16.0	115	221	8.01	108	1.21
0.080	0.448	0.178	0.095	0.996	9.00	1.07	0.920	0.605	236	0.035	0.430	25.0	199	338	12.6	153	1.99
0.393	0.463	5.20	0.502	1.97	112	2.77	29.3	7.72	301	0.585	8.00	113	243	370	3.05	286	3.95
0.018	0.074	0.038	0.015	0.170	2.13	0.137	0.237	—	52.3	0.020	0.013	5.00	41.9	72.5	0.725	23.3	0.191
0.095	0.407	0.212	0.105	0.898	12.0	0.788	2.37	0.073	300	0.061	0.120	34.0	235	381	8.37	123	0.963
0.095	0.403	0.210	0.105	0.888	12.0	0.781	2.32	0.080	297	0.073	0.120	33.0	232	377	5.66	122	0.963
0.088	0.343	0.216	0.098	0.926	14.0	0.806	2.40	0.001	302	0.049	0.100	28.0	247	406	11.6	126	0.915
0.093	0.395	0.205	0.102	0.871	12.0	0.766	2.29	0.100	291	0.085	0.120	33.0	228	370	3.05	120	0.940
0.083	0.377	0.142	0.083	0.537	12.2	0.674	2.40	0.172	285	0.024	0.120	25.8	219	371	2.52	257	1.03
0.275	1.27	0.640	0.156	1.36	34.0	2.30	7.96	0.650	868	0.673	0.580	78.0	775	1136	3.16	389	2.88
0.005	—	0.485	0.080	—	—	—	—	—	—	—	2.93	—	—	—	—	64.0	—
0.092	0.405	0.313	0.100	0.835	12.0	0.738	2.28	0.222	280	0.085	0.600	33.0	251	417	3.05	149	1.02
0.102	0.435	0.365	0.107	0.870	12.0	0.808	2.40	0.222	298	0.085	0.780	56.0	270	480	3.05	123	1.22
0.086	0.483	0.267	0.127	1.14	2.00	1.06	3.81	0.200	330	0.079	0.510	47.0	278	420	5.00	138	1.17
0.450	0.440	0.300	0.087	0.900	20.0	—	6.00	—	350	0.140	0.500	28.0	319	205	4.00	50.0	0.900
1.70	3.09	17.6	1.38	2.56	155	—	9.60	—	1008	0.672	2.48	320	1200	2544	—	1648	3.36
0.199	0.588	1.31	0.188	1.03	21.9	0.766	2.90	0.222	354	0.066	0.270	52.0	303	529	3.05	223	—
0.102	0.412	0.419	0.118	0.808	7.36	0.944	1.76	0.560	275	0.115	0.208	28.0	231	394	—	186	0.808
0.670	1.16	11.9	0.748	0.871	29.0	0.766	30.0	0.222	371	0.084	4.49	47.0	308	576	3.05	201	1.08
0.117	0.337	0.676	0.112	0.159	2.00	0.756	3.15	—	326	0.081	0.120	34.0	270	499	—	122	0.730
0.034	0.089	0.435	0.027	0.111	13.0	0.549	12.3	2.44	79.0	—	0.070	8.00	34.0	126	—	42.0	0.420
0.020	0.080	0.500	0.280	0	28.0	0.280	0	—	55.0	—	0.800	57.0	126	340	—	55.0	0.400
0.095	0.456	0.243	0.102	1.20	23.0	1.25	1.70	—	388	0.090	0.159	36.0	306	497	5.00	150	1.88
0.084	0.404	0.216	0.091	1.06	21.0	1.11	1.50	—	345	0.090	0.160	31.0	325	442	3.00	125	1.68
0.100	0.486	0.259	0.111	1.28	25.0	1.34	1.82	—	415	0.090	0.180	40.0	326	531	5.45	159	2.02
0.109	0.531	0.281	0.120	1.40	28.0	1.46	2.00	—	452	0.066	0.204	43.0	354	579	8.00	173	2.20

B1 Mg	B2 Mg	B3 Mg	B6 Mg	B12 Mcg	Fol. Mcg	Panto Mg	Vit-C Mg	Vit-E Mg	Calc Mg	Cu Mg	Iron Mg	Mg Mg	Phos Mg	Potas Mg	Sel Mcg	Na Mg	Zinc Mg
0.080	0.110	7.57	0.313	0.398	7.80	0.540	1.90	0.960	29.8	0.047	1.17	27.7	205	267	11.3	631	0.720
0.060	0.080	5.66	0.200	0.455	6.40	0.387	1.40	0.950	50.1	0.042	0.980	19.1	151	176	8.20	558	0.774
0.040	0.090	2.38	0.085	0.405	4.20	0.221	1.00	0.700	12.1	0.038	0.800	12.6	95.0	122	6.40	207	1.29
0.080	0.160	4.03	0.167	0.968	8.60	0.563	1.80	0.700	34.2	0.070	1.45	21.6	169	217	12.0	566	1.65
0.030	0.040	2.28	0.097	0.316	3.80	0.199	0.850	0.550	21.6	0.038	0.680	9.77	76.0	86.0	4.90	302	0.580
0.240	0.270	8.36	0.471	1.44	41.3	1.06	36.6	3.51	126	0.199	3.78	63.6	344	684	25.5	1536	—
0.250	0.320	8.46	0.459	1.53	41.7	1.08	36.6	3.66	116	0.199	3.90	66.4	363	720	27.0	1441	3.47
0.220	0.190	10.0	0.504	0.925	39.1	0.885	36.6	3.76	142	0.171	3.31	61.1	326	643	21.7	1528	—
0.110	0.110	7.89	0.302	0.478	10.8	0.281	2.10	1.38	62.2	0.062	1.29	29.3	218	244	11.3	584	—
0.120	0.130	5.37	0.237	0.541	8.50	0.304	1.70	1.13	56.8	0.059	1.12	21.2	157	188	8.20	564	—
0.070	0.110	3.07	0.157	0.434	5.90	0.174	1.20	0.700	11.0	0.041	0.950	14.0	100	147	6.40	263	1.32
0.120	0.190	5.35	0.171	0.973	11.0	0.567	2.20	1.04	49.0	0.086	1.49	24.1	185	228	12.0	549	1.73
0.060	0.090	2.94	0.112	0.336	5.30	0.278	1.10	0.850	15.5	0.021	0.650	11.6	77.0	100	4.90	312	0.673
0.310	0.350	10.3	0.490	1.46	45.2	1.14	36.6	4.15	135	1.63	6.40	67.9	361	729	25.5	1529	—
0.320	0.380	10.4	0.535	1.56	45.8	1.04	36.6	4.00	130	0.391	4.09	70.3	383	776	27.0	1480	3.58
0.310	0.290	10.4	0.556	1.03	42.7	0.881	36.6	4.24	143	1.60	6.03	65.0	333	689	21.7	1544	2.08
0.030	0.020	0.190	0.081	0.046	10.9	0.100	31.7	1.53	31.8	0.018	0.530	10.6	23.0	132	2.02	225	0.146
0.010	0.020	0.760	0.110	0.063	10.8	0.212	4.90	0.440	15.6	0.043	0.460	14.9	44.0	232	0.760	268	0.170
0.300	0.430	2.32	0.102	1.06	43.5	1.19	1.60	0.840	2.00	0.073	2.57	19.9	461	232	—	1269	1.55
0.560	0.220	3.39	0.121	0.520	12.1	0.460	1.00	0.627	82.0	0.073	2.05	17.2	353	231	—	1147	1.31
0.530	0.490	3.85	0.193	1.33	35.0	1.50	1.45	0.887	119	0.105	3.43	23.9	476	312	—	1301	2.10

Qty	Name	Wgt G	Wtr G	Cal	Prot G	Carb G	Fiber G	F-Tot G	F-Sat G	Mono G	Poly G	Chol Mg	A-Car RE	A-Pre RE	A-Tot RE
1 ea.	'Egg McMuffin'- McD	138	70.7	340	18.5	31.0	0.138	15.8	5.87	4.99	1.52	259	16.0	129	145
1 ea.	Sausage McMuffin-McD	115	43.4	427	17.6	30.0	0.400	26.3	10.1	11.0	2.97	59.0	0	114	114
1 ea.	Sausage McMuffin+egg-McD	165	78.2	517	22.9	32.2	0.300	32.9	12.7	13.8	3.65	287	0	198	198
1 ea.	'Big Mac'- McDonalds	200	96.4	570	24.6	39.2	0.612	35.0	11.5	12.7	7.60	83.0	38.0	0	38.0
1 ea.	Cheeseburger-McD	114	51.5	318	15.1	28.5	0.230	16.0	6.66	6.12	1.09	40.0	19.0	48.0	67.0
1 ea.	Chicken McNuggets-McD	18.2	8.83	53.8	3.18	2.45	0.037	3.37	0.850	1.80	0.332	10.4	0	4.50	4.50
1 ea.	'Filet of Fish' sandwich	143	63.3	435	14.7	35.9	0.139	25.7	5.56	8.64	9.45	46.6	13.0	15.0	28.0
1 ea.	Hamburger-McD	100	45.6	263	12.4	28.3	0.306	11.3	4.43	5.07	0.980	29.1	5.00	9.00	14.0
1 ea.	Quarter-Pounder/McDonalds	160	79.0	427	24.6	29.3	0.664	23.5	9.11	10.7	1.72	80.0	8.00	15.0	23.0
1 ea.	Quarter-Pounder w/cheese	186	89.5	525	29.6	30.5	0.664	31.6	12.8	12.4	1.86	107	35.0	93.0	128
1 cup	Macaroni & cheese-recipe	200	116	430	17.0	40.0	1.20	22.0	9.80	7.40	3.60	44.0	13.0	219	232
1 pce	Meat loaf-beef & 1/3pork	87.0	51.3	212	14.9	4.56	0.043	14.7	5.49	6.30	1.18	96.8	8.40	17.2	25.6
1 ea.	Burrito-bean	174	95.7	322	13.1	47.1	8.22	9.92	3.76	3.35	2.20	15.0	17.6	40.1	57.7
1 ea.	Burrito-beef & bean	175	955	390	21.0	40.0	5.00	17.5	6.80	6.72	2.29	52.0	17.6	40.1	57.7
1 ea.	Burrito-beef	177	86.7	463	28.9	32.4	1.58	25.4	9.89	10.3	2.42	89.0	13.9	41.0	54.9
1 ea.	Burrito-deluxe combinatn	198	110	424	21.6	41.0	4.93	20.8	8.70	7.83	2.44	58.2	16.9	65.1	82.0
1 ea.	Beef Enchilada	120	78.5	292	13.1	15.6	1.97	13.8	5.27	5.13	2.24	37.8	41.1	41.3	82.4
1 ea.	Cheese enchilada	120	73.2	330	13.2	16.0	1.97	17.8	9.17	5.49	2.31	43.0	46.9	121	168
1 ea.	Chicken enchilada	120	80.4	269	14.3	15.6	1.97	10.5	3.78	3.59	2.52	38.5	41.1	45.5	86.5
1 ea.	Enchirito	207	135	441	23.0	24.2	5.46	22.4	9.64	8.14	2.74	67.0	60.0	80.5	141
1 ea.	Chicken taco	78.0	43.7	172	15.4	10.1	1.12	8.34	2.62	2.56	2.33	45.4	6.80	26.7	33.5
1 ea.	Beef taco	78.0	40.6	207	13.6	10.1	1.12	13.2	4.85	4.88	1.91	44.5	6.76	20.5	27.3
1 ea.	Tostada w/refried beans	157	108	212	9.77	26.2	6.93	8.69	3.56	2.50	2.34	15.1	33.8	40.0	73.8
1 ea.	Beef & bean tostada-fancy	192	129	332	18.4	20.2	3.95	20.7	9.38	7.15	2.61	61.6	54.4	77.4	132
1 ea.	Tostada w/beans/chicken	157	105	249	19.4	18.7	3.70	11.4	4.37	3.54	2.85	53.1	33.8	46.7	80.5
5 ea.	Onion rings-frozen-heated	50.0	14.2	202	2.67	19.1	0.425	13.3	4.30	5.42	2.55	0	11.3	0	11.3
1 pce	Pizza-cheese-15inch-1/8th	120	55.2	290	15.0	39.0	2.16	9.00	4.10	2.60	1.30	56.0	60.0	46.0	106
1 pce	Thick crst pizza-1/2 10in	210	92.4	519	24.4	75.6	4.19	14.1	6.19	4.22	2.20	77.0	—	—	—
1 cup	Chicken salad w/celery	156	81.9	532	21.0	2.58	0.600	49.0	8.12	14.4	24.0	95.0	3.80	57.6	61.2
1 cup	Egg salad	183	120	438	18.8	2.88	0.021	38.8	8.35	13.2	13.5	838	0	257	257
1 cup	Ham salad spread	240	150	518	20.8	25.5	0.300	37.2	12.1	17.3	6.47	88.0	6.00	36.0	42.0
1 cup	Macaroni salad-no cheese	141	86.3	371	2.68	17.5	1.33	33.1	5.06	9.47	17.2	24.4	4.82	34.9	39.7
1 cup	Potato salad w/mayo+eggs	250	190	358	6.70	27.9	3.70	20.5	3.60	6.20	9.34	170	37.0	46.0	83.0
1 cup	Tuna salad	205	129	375	33.0	19.0	2.46	19.0	3.30	4.90	9.20	80.0	8.00	45.0	53.0
1 cup	Waldorf salad	142	82.6	424	3.62	13.1	3.62	41.7	5.61	11.2	23.1	21.7	10.0	31.0	41.0
1 ea.	Avocado cheese san/WhlWt	209	122	459	15.8	38.6	10.6	29.3	9.14	11.9	6.20	31.7	70.0	90.4	160
1 ea.	Avocado cheese san/partWW	195	116	432	14.4	33.0	5.81	28.6	8.72	11.8	5.96	31.7	70.0	90.4	160
1 ea.	Bacon L&T sand/whole wht	149	78.7	355	13.1	33.9	8.73	19.8	5.35	7.65	5.74	21.4	41.3	8.35	49.7
1 ea.	Grilled cheese san/WhlWt	131	49.8	420	19.5	32.8	7.92	24.8	12.9	7.88	2.57	54.7	20.2	193	214
1 ea.	Grilled cheese san/firm-w	127	47.4	425	18.2	33.2	1.79	24.3	12.9	7.78	2.38	54.7	20.2	193	214
1 ea.	Cheeseburger	112	51.5	300	15.0	28.0	1.40	15.0	7.30	5.60	1.00	44.0	18.5	46.5	65.0
1 ea.	Chicken patty sandwich	157	81.6	436	24.8	33.8	1.35	22.5	6.13	9.50	5.40	68.0	0	16.0	16.0
1 ea.	Chicken salad san/WholeWt	114	49.8	321	12.1	32.7	8.11	17.1	3.20	5.18	7.75	25.1	0.950	16.9	17.8
1 ea.	Chicken salad san/firm-W	110	47.4	326	10.8	33.1	1.98	16.6	3.12	5.08	7.56	25.1	0.900	16.9	17.8
1 ea.	Corn dog	111	49.9	330	10.0	27.3	0.100	20.0	8.40	10.0	1.40	37.0	0	0.300	0.300
1 ea.	Corned beef&swiss on rye	147	66.0	429	27.3	25.4	3.31	23.8	9.42	8.15	4.99	85.1	0	84.7	84.7
1 ea.	Engl mfn (egg/chees/bacon)	138	67.6	360	18.0	31.0	1.54	18.0	8.00	8.00	0.700	213	18.0	142	160
1 ea.	Egg salad san/firm WhlWht	125	58.2	346	11.5	32.8	7.93	20.1	4.09	6.44	7.97	215	0	72.6	72.6
1 ea.	Egg salad san/firm white	121	54.1	351	10.3	33.2	1.79	19.6	4.01	6.34	7.78	215	0	72.6	72.6
1 ea.	Fish sandwich-reg w/chees	140	60.2	420	16.2	38.5	1.30	22.6	6.30	6.90	7.70	56.0	12.0	13.0	25.0
1 ea.	Ham sandwich-whole wheat	136	71.5	283	18.2	32.8	7.94	9.79	2.38	3.66	2.98	29.0	0	4.47	4.47
1 ea.	Ham sandwich-firm white	132	69.2	288	16.9	33.2	1.81	9.31	2.30	3.56	2.79	29.0	0	4.47	4.47
1 ea.	Ham & swiss san/on rye	145	73.9	350	23.8	26.0	3.32	16.5	6.99	5.30	3.11	55.4	0	76.8	76.8
1 ea.	Ham & cheese san/firm wht	161	80.3	395	23.2	33.7	1.81	18.3	7.95	6.13	3.08	56.4	10.1	77.4	87.5
1 ea.	Ham salad san/firm white	135	63.4	371	10.8	38.8	1.86	19.2	4.95	7.36	6.02	27.4	1.50	17.3	18.8
1 ea.	Hamburger with bun	98.0	45.1	245	12.0	0	1.30	11.0	4.40	5.30	0.500	32.0	5.00	9.00	14.0
1 ea.	Hotdog/frankfurter & bun	85.0	45.3	260	8.40	21.1	1.20	15.3	5.30	7.00	1.80	22.9	0	0.300	0.300
1 ea.	Patty melt-GroundBeef/rye	177	79.5	567	31.8	24.7	3.30	37.9	14.1	13.9	6.52	107	10.1	129	139
1 ea.	Peanut btrjam-WholeWheat	114	33.1	368	13.7	49.6	9.86	15.5	2.96	7.05	4.56	0	0.200	0.600	0.800

B1 Mg	B2 Mg	B3 Mg	B6 Mg	B12 Mcg	Fol. Mcg	Panto Mg	Vit-C Mg	Vit-E Mg	Calc Mg	Cu Mg	Iron Mg	Mg Mg	Phos Mg	Potas Mg	Sel Mcg	Na Mg	Zinc Mg
0.470	0.442	3.77	0.211	0.750	30.0	0.773	1.38	0.423	226	0.120	2.93	25.8	322	168	12.0	885	1.92
0.700	0.250	4.14	0.150	0.679	23.0	0.529	1.27	0.383	168	0.069	2.25	23.8	186	215	—	942	1.68
0.840	0.500	4.46	0.198	1.37	33.0	1.40	0.160	0.550	196	0.116	3.47	29.9	288	294	—	1044	2.36
0.480	0.380	7.20	0.265	1.80	21.0	0.286	3.00	0.827	203	0.182	4.90	38.4	314	249	40.0	979	4.69
0.300	0.240	4.33	0.115	0.908	21.0	0.333	2.05	0.280	169	0.108	2.84	22.9	205	157	29.0	730	2.60
0.027	0.023	1.25	0.063	0.060	1.83	0.155	0.350	0.029	1.88	0.008	0.208	4.38	47.2	50.3	1.26	85.3	0.148
0.360	0.230	3.00	0.095	0.820	20.0	0.222	2.15	0.930	133	0.097	2.47	26.8	229	150	35.0	800	0.890
0.310	0.220	4.08	0.122	0.806	17.0	0.296	1.80	0.200	84.0	0.099	2.85	19.4	126	142	26.0	506	2.09
0.350	0.320	7.20	0.266	1.88	23.0	0.531	2.56	0.267	98.0	0.169	4.30	37.0	249	322	31.0	718	5.11
0.370	0.410	7.07	0.233	2.15	23.0	0.601	2.79	0.373	255	0.175	4.84	40.7	382	341	34.6	1195	—
0.200	0.400	1.80	0.050	0.298	10.3	0.392	1.00	3.52	362	0.094	1.80	36.8	322	240	28.0	1086	1.20
0.189	0.190	3.07	0.192	1.64	8.31	0.491	1.33	0.347	33.0	0.113	1.39	17.8	128	238	14.2	—	—
0.257	0.226	2.40	1.01	0.160	55.0	0.313	5.00	1.62	181	0.315	2.53	75.8	243	427	22.3	1030	2.37
0.257	0.293	4.36	0.727	1.59	47.6	0.627	5.00	1.67	165	0.255	2.70	61.0	274	388	23.0	516	3.30
0.260	0.364	6.42	0.295	2.72	34.5	0.590	3.39	1.84	148	0.198	2.87	47.2	306	363	28.5	382	5.80
0.270	0.320	4.44	0.666	1.48	51.3	0.569	6.60	1.90	183	0.279	2.75	64.0	289	433	23.1	537	—
0.070	0.163	2.09	0.152	1.02	11.1	0.304	8.98	2.19	255	0.085	1.77	36.0	159	193	12.0	157	2.25
0.065	0.210	0.646	0.094	0.386	15.2	0.308	8.00	2.19	457	0.059	1.37	36.7	260	135	11.1	311	1.50
0.076	0.154	3.22	0.205	0.245	11.6	0.505	8.98	2.16	256	0.069	1.52	36.0	170	176	10.7	160	—
0.111	0.273	3.12	0.696	1.56	33.4	0.569	14.8	2.73	376	0.235	2.99	70.0	303	449	16.7	463	4.04
0.039	0.119	4.17	0.236	0.198	14.0	0.532	0.552	0.590	86.9	0.037	0.899	22.8	156	158	7.87	145	1.34
0.030	0.134	2.49	0.158	1.36	13.3	0.231	0.552	0.624	85.0	0.062	1.29	22.7	141	183	9.94	141	2.89
0.063	0.138	0.845	1.01	0.317	47.1	0.413	5.92	1.49	177	0.273	1.93	62.4	195	422	63.5	—	—
0.078	0.243	2.94	0.668	1.66	36.8	0.606	6.10	1.79	186	0.244	2.16	51.9	247	442	69.3	—	—
0.072	0.190	4.53	0.732	0.436	33.9	0.795	3.43	1.51	162	0.186	1.69	48.0	242	358	67.1	—	—
0.140	0.070	1.80	0.037	0	6.50	0.115	0.700	0.345	15.5	0.040	0.850	9.50	40.0	65.0	0.425	188	0.210
0.340	0.290	4.20	0.041	0.480	39.6	0.158	2.00	0.360	220	0.243	1.60	36.0	216	230	18.0	699	1.81
0.678	0.589	—	—	—	—	—	—	—	290	0.350	1.30	53.0	318	368	—	1132	2.60
0.068	0.156	6.50	0.348	0.230	8.14	0.970	1.90	22.0	32.6	0.208	1.31	22.2	160	274	13.1	—	—
0.120	0.451	0.157	0.182	1.97	74.2	2.66	0	12.1	93.9	0.240	3.39	21.4	282	211	40.1	428	2.24
1.04	0.288	5.02	0.359	1.83	2.50	0.745	14.0	11.3	19.0	0.174	1.42	23.3	286	359	30.0	2187	2.64
0.098	0.068	0.669	0.069	0	7.30	0.216	3.24	16.3	27.4	0.208	1.14	11.5	50.1	162	6.87	—	—
0.193	0.150	2.23	0.353	0.385	16.8	1.34	24.9	27.3	48.0	0.295	1.63	39.0	130	635	13.0	1323	0.780
0.060	0.140	13.3	0.487	3.59	41.0	0.642	6.00	22.4	31.0	0.326	2.50	42.5	281	531	112	877	1.16
0.103	0.063	0.367	0.156	0	19.0	0.317	5.76	15.5	44.2	0.409	0.982	41.3	87.7	279	4.77	246	0.690
0.346	0.369	4.18	0.357	0.304	90.6	1.39	10.5	2.99	279	0.483	3.52	105	353	608	55.0	660	—
0.358	0.401	4.02	0.289	0.304	75.8	1.11	10.5	2.46	299	0.379	3.09	65.8	274	562	30.6	—	—
0.406	0.225	4.29	0.214	0.330	55.3	0.825	12.6	2.14	59.9	0.325	3.00	75.5	260	315	50.7	—	—
0.263	0.350	2.72	0.171	0.403	44.9	0.797	0.010	1.97	404	0.262	2.61	78.3	610	219	53.6	—	—
0.327	0.408	2.52	0.063	0.403	28.1	0.565	0.010	1.36	437	0.116	2.10	27.0	500	169	28.2	—	—
0.260	0.240	3.70	0.112	0.884	20.4	0.324	1.00	0.783	135	0.105	2.30	22.3	174	219	28.2	672	2.53
0.289	0.258	9.21	0.368	0.198	17.9	0.783	3.61	0.540	44.0	0.101	1.87	29.8	173	194	19.4	2732	1.00
0.265	0.186	4.31	0.222	0.057	42.6	0.768	0.687	7.49	59.2	0.297	2.73	70.8	223	197	49.6	—	—
0.329	0.244	4.11	0.114	0.057	25.8	0.536	0.687	6.88	92.4	0.151	2.23	19.7	113	147	24.2	—	—
0.280	0.170	3.27	0.110	0.580	2.00	0.195	3.00	1.24	34.0	0.090	1.94	22.0	303	164	3.50	1252	1.44
0.227	0.407	3.65	0.136	1.57	25.2	0.596	0	3.42	331	0.241	3.98	32.0	310	174	25.7	1045	—
0.460	0.500	3.71	0.152	0.828	35.0	0.730	1.00	1.27	197	0.121	3.10	27.6	290	201	12.0	832	1.86
0.278	0.262	2.72	0.178	0.492	58.8	1.20	0.002	4.84	75.3	0.323	3.28	70.5	255	180	56.8	—	—
0.342	0.320	2.52	0.070	0.492	42.0	0.973	0.002	4.23	109	0.177	2.78	19.4	144	130	31.4	—	—
0.322	0.266	3.30	0.098	0.840	23.8	0.476	2.80	2.22	132	0.098	1.85	29.4	223	274	35.0	667	0.952
0.786	0.286	5.52	0.398	0.425	43.8	0.791	14.2	1.90	59.3	0.312	2.96	77.7	313	333	57.8	—	—
0.850	0.344	5.32	0.290	0.425	27.0	0.559	14.2	1.29	92.5	0.166	2.45	26.6	202	283	32.4	—	—
0.750	0.404	4.52	0.341	0.906	25.2	0.621	14.2	1.57	325	0.143	1.99	34.8	376	342	33.0	1336	—
0.858	0.445	5.34	0.310	0.622	29.4	0.698	14.2	1.47	269	0.174	2.56	33.2	416	329	36.1	—	—
0.572	0.280	3.74	0.114	0.457	24.1	0.494	3.50	3.96	89.8	0.161	2.29	19.9	145	167	28.8	—	—
0.230	0.240	3.80	0.117	0.774	16.3	0.284	1.00	0.588	56.0	0.095	2.20	18.6	107	202	24.9	463	2.00
0.286	0.186	2.48	0.074	0.580	16.8	0.372	11.7	0.352	58.7	0.106	1.71	12.6	82.7	113	13.9	745	1.19
0.254	0.447	6.08	0.309	2.81	25.7	0.729	0.008	2.50	228	0.207	3.33	40.1	423	410	36.0	—	—
0.284	0.181	5.97	0.229	0	61.9	0.738	0.402	2.65	62.0	0.442	3.02	108	274	308	48.7	559	1.89

FAST FOODS, SANDWICHES (continued)

Qty	Name	Wgt G	Wtr G	Cal	Prot G	Carb G	Fiber G	F-Tot G	F-Sat G	Mono G	Poly G	Chol Mg	A-Car RE	A-Pre RE	A-Tot RE
1 ea.	Peanut btr&jam-firm white	110	30.7	373	12.5	50.0	3.73	15.0	2.88	6.95	4.37	0	0.200	0.600	0.800
1 ea.	Reuben sandwich-grilled	233	141	480	28.2	29.0	4.79	27.8	10.2	9.96	6.24	85.1	1.40	132	133
1 ea.	Roast beef san/firm white	132	65.5	312	18.0	32.6	1.79	11.7	2.66	3.82	4.49	29.7	0	8.40	8.40
1 ea.	Tuna salad san/firm white	126	58.1	335	13.8	37.2	2.40	14.6	2.75	4.26	6.71	25.4	2.00	19.6	21.6
1 ea.	Turkey san/firm white	132	66.7	303	18.3	32.4	1.79	10.8	2.21	3.29	4.57	28.6	0	8.35	8.35
1 ea.	Turkey ham san-firm white	132	70.1	285	16.5	33.5	1.81	9.44	2.32	2.95	3.26	34.5	0	4.50	4.50
1 ea.	TurkeyHam & cheese on rye	145	75.4	347	21.6	25.8	3.32	17.7	7.55	5.17	3.57	61.9	10.1	76.8	86.9
1 ea.	Turkey Ham&cheese-part WW	151	77.5	361	22.7	28.0	3.14	18.1	7.63	5.47	3.48	61.9	10.1	77.4	87.5

FATS AND OILS

Qty	Name	Wgt G	Wtr G	Cal	Prot G	Carb G	Fiber G	F-Tot G	F-Sat G	Mono G	Poly G	Chol Mg	A-Car RE	A-Pre RE	A-Tot RE
1 Tbs	Butter	14.2	2.26	102	0.121	0.009	0	11.5	7.19	3.32	0.425	31.1	11.6	95.2	107
1 Tbs	Butter-unsalted	14.2	2.26	102	0.121	0.009	0	11.5	7.19	3.32	0.425	31.1	11.6	95.2	107
1 Tbs	Bacon fat	14.0	0.028	126	0	0	0	14.0	4.95	6.73	1.65	84.0	0	0.300	0.300
1 Tbs	Beef fat/tallow-drippings	12.8	0.026	115	0	0	0	12.8	6.38	5.35	0.512	13.9	0	0.031	0.031
1 Tbs	Chicken fat	12.8	0.026	115	0	0	0	12.8	3.82	5.75	2.69	10.9	0	21.9	21.9
1 Tbs	Duck Fat	12.8	0.026	115	0	0	0	12.8	4.26	6.31	1.66	12.8	0	—	—
1 Tbs	Lard	12.8	0	116	0	0	0	12.8	5.02	5.78	1.44	12.2	0	0	0
1 Tbs	Mutton tallow	12.8	0.026	115	0	0	0	12.8	6.06	5.20	1.00	13.1	0	—	—
1 Tbs	Turkey fat	12.8	0.026	115	0	0	0	12.8	3.77	5.49	2.96	13.1	0	—	—
1 Tbs	Vegetable shortening	12.8	0	113	0	0	0	12.8	3.21	5.71	3.36	0	0	0	0
1 Tbs	Margarine-imit-soft/40%ft	14.2	8.26	49.1	0.0711	0.055	0	5.50	1.09	2.22	1.96	0	0	141	141
1 Tbs	Margarine-reg-hard-80%fat	14.2	2.23	102	0.127	0.127	0	11.4	2.24	5.07	3.60	0	0	141	141
1 Tbs	Margarine sprd-hard-60%ft	14.1	5.23	76.2	0.085	0	0	8.59	1.99	3.66	2.55	0	0	140	140
1 Tbs	Coconut oil	13.6	0	120	0	0	0	13.6	11.8	0.794	0.244	0	0	0	0
1 Tbs	Corn oil	13.6	0	120	0	0	0	13.6	1.73	3.29	8.00	0	0	0	0
1 Tbs	Cottonseed oil	13.6	0	120	0	0	0	13.6	3.52	2.43	7.06	0	0	0	0
1 Tbs	Olive oil	13.5	0	119	0	0	0	13.5	1.82	9.94	1.13	0	0	0	0
1 Tbs	Palm oil	13.6	0	120	0	0	0	13.6	6.69	5.04	1.27	0	0	0	0
1 Tbs	Palm kernal oil	13.6	0	120	0	0	0	13.6	11.1	1.55	0.212	0	0	0	0
1 Tbs	Peanut oil	13.5	0	119	0	0	0	13.5	2.27	6.24	4.32	0	0.006	0	0.006
1 Tbs	Rapeseed oil-30% erucic	13.6	0	120	0	0	0	13.6	0.756	8.50	3.77	0	0	0	0
1 Tbs	Safflower oil	13.6	0	120	0	0	0	13.6	1.24	1.65	10.1	0	0	0	0
1 Tbs	Sesame oil	13.6	0	120	0	0	0	13.6	1.93	5.41	5.69	0	0.006	0	0.006
1 Tbs	Soybean oil	13.6	0	120	0	0	0	13.6	2.03	5.86	5.13	0	0	0	0
1 Tbs	Soybean/cottonseed oil	13.6	0	120	0	0	0	13.6	2.45	4.02	6.56	0	0	0	0
1 Tbs	Sunflower oil	13.6	0	120	0	0	0	13.6	1.41	2.66	8.94	0	0	0	0
1 Tbs	Blue cheese salad dressng	15.3	4.95	77.2	0.737	1.13	0.012	8.00	1.51	1.89	4.26	4.13	0	10.0	10.0
1 Tbs	Ceasar's salad dressing	11.5	4.32	51.0	1.08	0.272	0.018	5.15	0.885	3.52	0.470	13.8	0.200	4.55	4.75
1 Tbs	French dressing	15.6	5.47	82.6	0.087	1.00	0.119	8.81	1.36	3.91	3.42	0	0.006	0	0.006
1 Tbs	French dressing-lo cal	16.3	12.2	24.1	0.037	1.94	0.044	1.56	0.196	0.293	0.975	0	0.006	0	0.006
1 Tbs	Italian dressing	14.7	4.99	68.6	0.094	1.50	0.031	8.81	1.27	3.63	3.13	0	2.94	0	2.94
1 Tbs	Italian dressing-lo cal	15.0	12.9	15.8	0.012	0.725	0.044	0.625	0.091	0.257	0.222	0.875	0.006	0	0.006
1 Tbs	Mayonnaise (soybean)	13.8	2.06	98.6	0.150	0.375	0	10.9	1.67	3.14	5.69	8.13	0	11.6	11.6
1 Tbs	Imitation mayonnaise	15.0	9.45	35.0	0	2.00	0	3.00	0.500	0.700	1.60	4.00	0	0	0
1 Tbs	Salad dressing/mayo-type	14.7	5.88	57.2	0.131	3.51	0	4.90	0.725	1.31	2.64	3.75	0	9.69	9.69
1 Tbs	Mayo type dressing-lo cal	15.0	9.45	34.7	0.037	2.40	0	2.88	0.518	0.837	1.39	3.63	0	10.3	10.3
1 Tbs	Ranch style salad drssng	14.9	5.21	54.4	0.449	0.688	0	5.64	0.840	2.42	2.13	5.82	0	10.7	10.7
1 Tbs	Russian salad dressing	15.3	5.28	75.6	0.244	1.63	0.044	7.81	1.12	1.81	4.50	9.94	10.6	0	10.6
1 Tbs	1000 island dressing	15.6	7.19	58.9	0.144	2.38	0.031	5.58	0.944	1.29	3.09	4.00	0.438	13.4	13.9
1 Tbs	1000 isl. dressing-lo cal	15.3	10.6	24.3	0.119	2.47	0.181	1.63	0.206	0.408	0.919	1.81	0.438	13.6	14.0
1 Tbs	Vinegar & oil dressing	16.0	7.52	70.0	0	0	0	8.00	1.50	2.40	3.90	0	0	0	0

B1 Mg	B2 Mg	B3 Mg	B6 Mg	B12 Mcg	Fol. Mcg	Panto Mg	Vit-C Mg	Vit-E Mg	Calc Mg	Cu Mg	Iron Mg	Mg Mg	Phos Mg	Potas Mg	Sel Mcg	Na Mg	Zinc Mg
0.348	0.239	5.77	0.121	0	45.1	0.506	0.402	2.04	95.2	0.296	2.51	57.2	164	257	23.3	455	—
0.247	0.431	3.80	0.241	1.57	26.6	0.673	11.6	3.51	358	0.335	5.20	43.7	328	313	26.4	—	—
0.358	0.316	5.48	0.213	1.46	26.7	0.632	0.002	1.19	92.3	0.171	3.15	24.8	168	309	26.7	—	—
0.327	0.243	5.81	0.146	0.897	33.7	0.468	1.50	9.06	92.8	0.199	2.56	24.7	144	210	—	—	—
0.334	0.268	7.20	0.229	1.15	26.4	0.643	0.002	3.66	89.0	0.148	2.16	25.4	203	234	26.0	—	—
0.355	0.366	5.28	0.185	1.28	27.3	0.943	0.002	2.84	93.5	0.193	3.56	28.4	214	244	26.8	—	—
0.257	0.423	4.48	0.231	1.48	26.1	1.02	0	3.23	226	0.169	3.15	33.1	428	319	26.1	—	—
0.311	0.441	5.34	0.245	1.48	31.7	1.04	0.002	3.22	256	0.243	3.74	46.9	459	296	—	—	—

B1 Mg	B2 Mg	B3 Mg	B6 Mg	B12 Mcg	Fol. Mcg	Panto Mg	Vit-C Mg	Vit-E Mg	Calc Mg	Cu Mg	Iron Mg	Mg Mg	Phos Mg	Potas Mg	Sel Mcg	Na Mg	Zinc Mg
0.001	0.005	0.006	0.000	0.000	0.425	0	0.228	3.38	0.004	0.023	0.281	3.25	3.69	0.094	96.7	0.007	—
0.001	0.005	0.006	0.000	0.000	0.425	0	0.228	3.38	0.004	0.023	0.281	3.25	3.69	0.094	96.7	0.007	—
—	—	—	0	—	—	—	1.00	—	—	—	—	—	—	—	140	—	—
0.000	0.000	0.000	0.000	0.000	0.000	—	0	0.375	0.125	—	0.026	—	1.69	0.063	—	0.063	—
—	—	—	0	—	0	—	0	0.350	—	—	—	—	—	—	—	—	—
—	—	—	0	—	0	—	0	—	—	—	—	—	—	—	—	—	—
0	0	0	0	0	0	—	0	0.167	0.008	0.004	0	0.002	0.375	0.002	0	0.002	0.014
—	—	—	0	—	0	—	0	—	—	—	—	—	—	—	—	—	—
—	—	—	0	—	0	—	0	—	—	—	—	—	—	—	—	—	—
0	0	0	0	0	0	—	0	—	—	0	—	0	0	0	0	0	0.006
0.001	0.003	0.002	0.001	0.008	0.101	0.007	0.014	0.750	2.50	0.006	0	0.156	1.94	3.56	0.035	136	0.014
0.001	0.005	0.003	0.001	0.013	0.169	0.012	0.023	1.56	4.25	0.024	0.008	0.369	3.25	6.00	0.142	134	0.028
0.001	0.004	0.002	0.001	0.009	0.117	0.008	0.016	1.16	2.95	0.018	0	0.257	2.27	4.21	0.106	140	0.021
—	—	—	0	0	—	—	0	0.225	0.005	—	—	—	0.012	—	—	—	—
0	0	0	0	0	0.000	—	0	11.3	0	0.001	0.001	0	0.125	0.250	0	0	0.001
—	—	—	0	0	0	—	—	4.81	—	—	—	—	—	—	—	—	—
0	0	0	0	0	0.000	—	0	1.81	0.024	0.009	0.052	0.001	0.188	0	—	0	0.008
—	—	—	0	—	0	—	0	2.61	—	—	0.001	—	0.021	—	—	—	—
—	—	—	—	—	—	—	0	—	—	—	—	—	—	—	—	—	—
0	0	0	0	0	0.000	—	0	3.38	0.012	0.001	0.004	0.005	0	0	—	0	0.001
—	—	—	—	—	—	—	0	—	—	—	—	—	—	—	—	—	—
0	0	0	0	0	0	—	0	7.19	0	0.018	0	—	0	0	—	—	0.026
0	0	0	0	0	0	—	0	3.94	0	0.018	0	—	—	—	—	—	0.026
0	0	0	0	0	0.000	—	0	8.81	0.006	0.054	0.003	0.003	0.063	0	0	—	0.025
0	0	0	0	0	0.000	—	0	7.81	0	—	0	—	0	0	—	0	0.025
0	0	0	0	0	0	—	0	8.81	0	0	0	0	0	0	2.50	0	—
0.002	0.015	0.015	0.006	0	4.38	0.056	0.306	1.13	12.4	0.001	0.031	11.3	11.0	6.00	0.112	8.31	0.038
0.003	0.010	0.081	0.008	0.560	2.10	0.042	0.622	0.822	18.0	0.007	0.097	1.03	16.1	6.81	0.585	—	—
0.000	0.000	0.000	0.002	0	0	—	—	4.38	1.96	—	0.063	1.60	1.00	1.94	—	184	0.012
0.000	0.000	0.000	0	0	0.000	—	—	0.813	5.63	—	0.063	—	4.88	2.94	—	299	0.029
0.000	0.000	0.000	0.002	0	0	—	—	4.38	1.44	0.001	0.031	0.029	0.750	2.19	0	71.9	0.001
0.000	0.000	0.000	0	0	0.000	—	—	0.306	0.313	—	0.031	—	0.750	2.25	—	118	0
0.002	0.006	0.001	0.004	—	0.375	0.036	0	1.02	2.75	0.020	0.081	0.178	3.88	4.88	0.475	78.1	0.165
0	0	0	0	—	0.010	—	0	—	0	—	0	—	0	2.00	—	75.0	—
0.001	0.004	0.000	0.002	0	0.000	—	—	1.00	2.06	—	0.031	0.294	3.81	1.31	—	104	0
0.002	0.005	0.000	—	0	0.000	—	—	0.600	2.81	—	0.031	—	4.38	1.44	—	74.6	0.016
0.005	0.021	0.010	0.007	0.041	0.791	0.053	0.092	2.50	14.9	0.021	0.039	1.55	12.5	19.7	0.589	65.2	0.054
0.007	0.007	0.094	0.005	0	0.000	—	0.938	3.81	2.94	—	0.094	—	5.69	24.1	—	133	0.066
0.003	0.005	0.031	0.003	0	0.600	0.034	0.500	2.75	1.94	0.042	0.094	0.875	2.63	17.6	—	109	0.025
0.003	0.004	0.031	0.002	0	0.000	—	0.438	0.800	1.69	0.016	0.094	0.875	2.63	17.3	—	153	0
0	0	0	0	0	—	—	0	—	0	—	0	—	0	1.00	—	0	—

FRUIT

Qty	Name	Wgt G	Wtr G	Cal	Prot G	Carb G	Fiber G	F-Tot G	F-Sat G	Mono G	Poly G	Chol Mg	A-Car RE	A-Pre RE	A-Tot RE
1 ea.	Apple w/peel 2.75in diam	138	116	80.0	0.270	21.0	3.87	0.490	0.100	0.021	0.145	0	7.40	0	7.40
1 cup	Apple juice-canned/bottld	248	218	116	0.150	29.0	0.744	0.280	0.047	0.012	0.082	0	0.200	0	0.200
1 cup	Applesauce-unsweetened	244	216	106	0.400	27.5	4.40	0.120	0.020	0.005	0.034	0	7.00	0	7.00
1 cup	Applesauce-sweetened	255	203	195	0.470	51.0	4.20	0.470	0.077	0.018	0.138	0	2.80	0	2.80
3 ea.	Apricots-fresh-pitted-ea	106	91.6	51.0	1.48	11.8	2.02	0.410	0.029	0.180	0.082	0	277	0	277
1 cup	Apricots-cnd-jce pack-cup	248	215	119	1.56	30.6	3.95	0.090	0.007	0.042	0.017	0	419	0	419
1 cup	Apricots-cnd-lt syrup-cup	253	209	160	1.35	41.7	2.85	0.120	0.008	0.053	0.025	0	334	0	334
1 cup	Apricot halves-dried-cup	130	40.4	310	4.75	80.0	11.8	0.594	0.041	0.260	0.119	0	941	0	941
1 cup	Apricot nectar-canned	251	213	141	0.920	36.1	1.26	0.220	0.015	0.095	0.043	0	330	0	330
1 ea.	Avocado-average	201	149	324	3.99	14.9	5.63	30.8	4.90	19.3	3.93	0	123	0	123
1 ea.	Banana (peeled weight)	114	84.7	105	1.18	26.7	2.83	0.547	0.211	0.047	0.101	0	9.20	0	9.20
1 cup	Blackberries-fresh	144	123	74.0	1.04	18.4	9.72	0.560	0.250	0.120	0.140	0	23.7	0	23.7
1 cup	Blueberries-fresh	145	123	82.0	0.970	20.5	4.42	0.550	0.040	0.170	0.340	0	14.5	0	14.5
1 cup	Boysenberries-frozen	132	113	66.0	1.46	16.1	5.15	0.350	0.161	0.077	0.090	0	8.90	0	8.90
1 ea.	Cantaloupe melon-each	534	480	188	4.70	44.6	5.34	1.50	0.240	0.280	0.480	0	1722	0	1722
1 cup	Sour cherries-frozen	155	135	72.0	1.42	17.1	2.10	0.680	0.135	0.186	0.285	0	135	0	135
1 cup	Sweet cherries-fresh-cup	145	117	104	1.74	24.0	2.20	1.39	0.313	0.380	0.419	0	31.0	0	31.0
1 cup	Cranberries-whole-raw	95.0	82.2	46.0	0.370	12.0	4.00	0.190	0.023	0.051	0.109	0	4.40	0	4.40
1 cup	Cranberry juice cocktail	253	215	145	0.080	36.0	0.759	0.130	0.015	0.034	0.074	0	1.00	0	1.00
1 cup	Cranberry-apple juice	253	218	169	0.138	43.0	0.630	1.33	0.230	0.061	0.399	0	0.200	0	0.200
1 cup	Cranberry sauce-cnd/strnd	277	168	419	0.550	108	5.90	0.420	0.050	0.112	0.240	0	5.50	0	5.50
1 cup	Currants black fresh	112	91.8	71.0	1.57	17.2	9.74	0.450	0.038	0.065	0.200	0	26.0	0	26.0
1 cup	Dates-chopped-cup	178	40.0	489	3.50	131	14.5	0.800	0.348	0.239	0.048	0	8.90	0	8.90
10 ea.	Dates-whole-each	83.0	18.7	228	1.63	61.0	6.76	0.373	0.162	0.111	0.022	0	4.00	0	4.00
3 ea.	Figs-medium-fresh-each	150	119	111	1.14	28.8	5.58	0.450	0.090	0.099	0.216	0	21.3	0	21.3
1 cup	Fruit cocktail-juice pack	248	217	115	1.13	29.4	2.58	0.030	0.005	0.007	0.015	0	76.0	0	76.0
1 cup	Fruit cocktail-lite syrup	252	213	145	1.01	37.6	2.52	0.180	0.025	0.035	0.078	0	52.4	0	52.4
1 cup	Fruit punch drink-cnd	253	223	118	0.136	30.1	0	0.056	0.005	0.005	0.008	0	3.60	0	3.60
1 cup	Fruit salad-cnd juice pck	248	214	124	1.28	32.4	4.16	0.060	0.010	0.012	0.028	0	149	0	149
1 cup	Grape drink-non carbonate	250	221	112	0	34.7	0.253	0.040	0.008	0.002	0.005	0	0.270	0	0.270
1 ea.	Grapefruit half-pink/red	123	112	37.0	0.680	9.45	1.60	0.120	0.017	0.016	0.030	0	31.8	0	31.8
1 cup	Grapefruit juice-unsw-cnd	247	223	93.0	1.29	22.1	0.668	0.240	0.032	0.032	0.057	0	2.00	0	2.00
1 cup	Grapefruit juice-fresh	247	223	96.0	1.24	22.7	0.988	0.250	0.035	0.032	0.059	0	2.40	0	2.40
1 cup	Grape juice-bottled/cnd	253	213	155	1.41	37.9	1.26	0.190	0.063	0.008	0.056	0	2.00	0	2.00
1 cup	Grapefruit juice-unsw-cnd	247	223	93.0	1.29	22.1	0.668	0.240	0.032	0.032	0.057	0	2.00	0	2.00
1 cup	Grapefruit jce-swtnd/cnd	250	218	115	1.45	27.8	0.668	0.230	0.030	0.030	0.053	0	2.00	0	2.00
1 cup	Grapes-Thompson-sdls-cup	160	129	114	1.06	28.4	2.64	0.920	0.302	0.031	0.270	0	11.7	0	11.7
10 ea.	Grapes-Tokay/Empr-each	57.0	45.9	40.0	0.378	10.1	0.940	0.328	0.107	0.013	0.096	0	4.00	0	4.00
1 cup	Honeydew melon-cubes	170	152	60.0	0.770	15.6	1.84	0.170	0.028	0.032	0.050	0	6.80	0	6.80
1 pce	Honeydew melon (1/10th)	129	116	45.0	0.590	11.8	1.40	0.130	0.021	0.024	0.038	0	5.00	0	5.00
1 ea.	Lemon-fresh fruit wo/peel	58.0	51.6	17.0	0.640	5.41	1.19	0.170	0.023	0.006	0.052	0	2.00	0	2.00
1 cup	Lemon peel	96.0	78.3	48.0	1.44	15.4	4.80	0.320	0.032	0.016	0.080	0	4.80	0	4.80
1 cup	Lemon juice-bottled	244	226	52.0	0.980	15.8	0.732	0.700	0.093	0.027	0.207	0	4.00	0	4.00
1 cup	Lemon juice-fresh	244	221	60.0	0.920	21.1	0.854	0.700	0.093	0.027	0.207	0	5.00	0	5.00
1 cup	Lemonade-prep from frozen	248	221	100	0.150	26.0	0.292	0.100	0.015	0.005	0.032	0	5.30	0	5.30
1 cup	Lemonade drink from dry	264	237	102	0	26.9	0	0.003	0	0	0.003	0	0	0	0
1 cup	Lemonade-lo cal-from dry	238	236	5.00	0.050	1.25	0	0	0	0	0	0	0	0	0
1 ea.	Lime-fresh fruit wo/peel	67.0	59.2	20.0	0.470	7.06	0.540	0.130	0.015	0.013	0.037	0	0.700	0	0.700
1 cup	Lime juice-bottled	246	228	50.0	1.00	16.0	0.861	1.00	0.064	0.054	0.157	0	4.00	0	4.00
1 cup	Limeade-prep/from frozen	247	220	102	0.100	27.1	0.292	0.054	0.005	0.005	0.015	0	0.100	0	0.100
1 cup	Loganberries-fresh	149	126	104	2.27	19.4	9.25	0.463	0.213	0.101	0.119	0	11.9	0	11.9
1 ea.	Loquats-raw	9.90	8.58	5.00	0.040	1.20	—	0.020	0.004	0.001	0.009	0	15.1	0	15.1
1 cup	Mandarin oranges-canned	252	209	155	1.00	41.0	4.25	0.100	0.011	0.018	0.019	0	212	0	212
1 cup	Mango-fresh-slices	165	135	108	0.850	28.1	2.48	0.450	0.109	0.167	0.084	0	642	0	642
1 cup	Orange juice-fresh	248	219	111	1.74	25.8	0.992	0.500	0.060	0.089	0.099	0	50.0	0	50.0
1 cup	Orange juice frozen conc.	284	164	452	6.80	108	3.99	0.587	0.068	0.108	0.116	0	78.7	0	78.7
1 cup	Orange peel-grated	96.0	69.6	80.0	1.44	24.0	4.80	0.160	0.016	0.032	0.032	0	40.0	0	40.0
1 ea.	Orange-california navel	140	122	65.0	1.44	16.3	3.00	0.130	0.015	0.024	0.025	0	25.6	0	25.6
1 ea.	Orange-florida	151	132	69.0	1.06	17.4	3.23	0.320	0.038	0.059	0.063	0	30.2	0	30.2

B1 Mg	B2 Mg	B3 Mg	B6 Mg	B12 Mcg	Fol. Mcg	Panto Mg	Vit-C Mg	Vit-E Mg	Calc Mg	Cu Mg	Iron Mg	Mg Mg	Phos Mg	Potas Mg	Sel Mcg	Na Mg	Zinc Mg
0.023	0.019	0.106	0.066	0	3.90	0.084	7.80	0.655	10.0	0.057	0.250	6.00	10.0	159	0.500	1.00	0.050
0.052	0.042	0.248	0.074	0	0.590	0.001	2.30	0.010	17.0	0.055	0.920	8.00	17.0	295	0.400	7.00	0.070
0.032	0.061	0.459	0.063	0	2.44	0.232	2.90	0.472	7.00	0.063	0.290	7.00	18.0	183	0.400	5.00	0.060
0.030	0.070	0.500	0.066	0	1.50	0.133	4.00	0.472	10.0	0.110	1.00	7.00	18.0	156	0.400	8.00	0.100
0.032	0.042	0.636	0.057	0	9.10	0.254	10.6	0.944	15.0	0.094	0.580	8.00	21.0	313	—	1.00	0.280
0.045	0.047	0.853	0.180	0	5.00	0.226	12.2	2.21	30.0	0.134	0.744	24.0	50.0	409	—	9.00	0.270
0.040	0.051	0.769	0.137	0	4.30	0.233	6.90	2.21	28.0	0.200	0.990	21.0	34.0	349	—	10.0	0.270
0.011	0.197	3.90	0.204	0	13.4	0.981	3.10	8.11	59.4	0.557	6.13	59.4	152	1790	—	11.0	0.966
0.023	0.035	0.653	0.160	0	3.30	0.070	2.00	0.700	18.0	0.183	0.960	13.0	23.0	286	—	8.00	0.230
0.217	0.245	3.86	0.563	0	124	1.95	15.9	2.69	21.8	0.527	2.01	78.6	83.0	1204	0	21.0	0.860
0.051	0.114	0.616	0.659	0	24.0	0.296	10.3	0.274	7.00	0.119	0.353	32.4	22.0	451	1.14	1.00	0.190
0.043	0.058	0.576	0.084	0	48.9	0.346	30.2	0.864	46.0	0.202	0.800	29.0	30.0	282	—	0	0.390
0.070	0.073	0.700	0.052	0	9.30	0.135	20.0	2.72	9.00	0.088	0.240	7.00	15.0	129	0	9.00	0.160
0.070	0.049	1.01	0.074	0	83.6	0.330	4.10	0.340	36.0	0.106	1.12	21.0	36.0	183	—	2.00	0.290
0.192	0.112	3.06	0.614	0	160	0.684	226	0.748	58.0	0.224	1.12	38.0	90.0	1650	0	48.0	0.854
0.068	0.053	0.212	0.104	0	7.00	0.276	2.60	—	20.0	0.140	0.820	13.0	25.0	192	—	1.00	0.160
0.073	0.087	0.580	0.052	0	8.39	0.184	10.2	1.30	21.0	0.138	0.565	16.0	28.0	325	0	1.00	0.090
0.029	0.019	0.095	0.062	0	2.00	0.208	12.8	0.950	7.00	0.055	0.190	5.00	8.00	67.0	—	1.00	0.120
0.020	0.020	0.090	0.050	0	0.500	0.170	90.0	0.300	8.00	0.033	0.380	5.00	5.00	45.0	—	5.00	0.177
0.012	0.051	0.151	0.060	0	0.380	0.123	81.3	0.015	18.0	0.020	0.152	5.00	7.00	68.0	0.400	5.00	0.100
0.042	0.058	0.277	0.050	0	2.50	0.247	5.50	0.450	11.0	0.055	0.610	8.00	17.0	72.0	—	80.0	0.085
0.056	0.056	0.336	0.074	0	3.90	0.446	203	1.12	61.0	0.096	1.53	27.0	66.0	361	—	2.00	0.300
0.160	0.178	3.92	0.342	0	29.0	1.39	0	—	58.0	0.513	2.14	63.0	70.0	1161	3.38	5.00	0.520
0.075	0.083	1.83	0.159	0	13.5	0.648	0	—	27.0	0.239	1.00	29.4	33.0	541	1.58	2.33	0.242
0.090	0.075	0.600	0.171	0	4.50	0.450	3.00	—	54.0	0.105	0.540	24.0	21.0	348	3.39	3.00	0.210
0.030	0.040	0.999	0.128	0	1.50	0.153	6.80	2.17	20.0	0.154	0.530	17.0	34.0	235	0	10.0	0.210
0.045	0.048	0.958	0.106	0	1.20	0.154	4.90	2.17	16.0	0.176	0.730	14.0	28.0	225	0	15.0	0.210
0.056	0.058	0.053	0	0	3.13	0.035	74.9	—	19.0	0.129	0.517	5.44	2.72	63.9	—	55.8	0.313
0.028	0.034	0.882	—	0	—	—	8.20	1.86	28.0	0.124	0.620	20.0	36.0	288	—	14.0	0.360
0.079	0.010	0.065	0.015	0	0.664	0.010	85.4	—	2.70	0.030	0.412	5.00	3.00	13.3	2.00	16.0	0.279
0.042	0.025	0.235	0.052	0	15.0	0.348	46.8	0.307	13.0	0.054	0.148	10.0	11.0	158	1.06	0	0.090
0.104	0.049	0.571	0.049	0	25.6	0.321	72.0	0.320	17.0	0.094	0.494	24.0	27.0	378	0.500	2.00	0.220
0.099	0.049	0.494	0.109	0	52.0	0.467	93.9	0.450	22.0	0.082	0.490	30.0	37.0	400	0.500	2.00	0.130
0.066	0.094	0.663	0.164	0	6.50	0.104	0.200	0.071	22.0	0.071	0.607	24.0	27.0	334	2.50	8.00	0.130
0.104	0.049	0.571	0.049	0	25.6	0.321	72.0	0.320	17.0	0.094	0.494	24.0	27.0	378	0.500	2.00	0.220
0.100	0.060	0.800	0.050	0	25.9	0.325	67.0	0.320	20.0	0.120	0.900	24.0	28.0	405	0.500	5.00	0.150
0.147	0.091	0.480	0.176	0	11.2	0.038	17.3	1.04	17.0	0.272	0.410	10.0	21.0	296	15.4	3.00	0.090
0.052	0.032	0.171	0.063	0	3.99	0.014	6.20	0.371	6.10	0.096	0.146	3.50	7.50	105	5.49	1.07	0.032
0.131	0.031	1.02	0.100	0	51.0	0.352	42.1	0.170	10.0	0.070	0.120	12.0	17.0	461	—	17.0	0.147
0.099	0.023	0.774	0.076	0	38.7	0.267	32.0	0.129	8.00	0.053	0.090	9.00	13.0	350	—	13.0	0.110
0.023	0.012	0.058	0.046	0	7.00	0.110	30.7	0.540	15.0	0.021	0.350	1.60	9.00	80.0	6.97	1.00	0.064
0.064	0.080	0.384	0.160	0	—	0.304	123	—	128	—	0.800	16.0	16.0	160	6.72	0	—
0.100	0.022	0.481	0.105	0	24.6	0.222	61.0	0.536	26.0	0.090	0.310	22.0	21.0	248	0.490	50.0	0.150
0.073	0.024	0.244	0.124	0	31.5	0.251	112	0.536	18.0	0.071	0.080	16.0	14.0	303	0.490	2.00	0.120
0.015	0.052	0.040	0.015	0	5.50	0.032	9.80	—	4.00	0.005	0.410	2.50	5.00	38.0	0.075	2.00	0.050
0.005	—	0.034	0.008	0	3.50	0.016	8.50	—	71.0	—	0.150	3.00	34.0	33.0	—	13.0	0.100
0	0	0	0	0	0	0	5.86	—	51.0	0.017	0.097	2.50	23.2	0.750	—	7.25	0.063
0.020	0.013	0.134	0.029	0	5.50	0.145	19.5	—	22.0	0.044	0.400	3.70	12.0	68.0	0.134	1.00	0.070
0.080	0.010	0.400	0.066	0	19.5	0.162	16.0	—	30.0	0.074	0.600	16.0	25.0	185	0.490	39.0	0.150
0.005	0.005	0.054	0.027	0	6.00	0.061	6.60	—	3.00	0.028	0.060	15.0	3.00	32.0	0.075	0.010	0.027
0.075	0.051	1.25	0.097	0	38.8	0.364	52.2	0.448	44.8	0.209	0.955	32.8	38.8	216	—	1.49	0.507
0.002	0.002	0.018	—	0	0.100	—	2.00	0.004	0.030	1.00	3.00	26.0	—	0	0	—	—
0.130	0.110	1.10	0.172	0	20.0	0.375	50.0	1.26	18.0	0.125	0.900	22.0	25.0	197	2.00	15.0	0.075
0.096	0.094	0.964	0.221	0	31.0	0.264	45.7	1.85	17.0	0.182	0.210	15.0	18.0	257	—	3.00	0.260
0.223	0.074	0.992	0.099	0	109	0.476	124	0.790	27.0	0.109	0.500	27.0	42.0	496	0.490	2.00	0.124
0.795	0.181	2.04	0.443	0	441	1.59	392	1.91	90.7	0.440	0.995	97.3	161	1915	1.99	8.00	0.511
0.112	0.080	0.864	0.176	0	—	0.464	131	—	160	—	0.800	16.0	16.0	208	—	0	—
0.122	0.056	0.406	0.097	0	47.2	0.350	80.3	0.336	56.0	0.078	0.168	15.0	27.0	250	0.200	1.00	0.084
0.151	0.060	0.604	0.077	0	26.1	0.378	68.0	0.363	65.0	0.059	0.130	15.0	18.0	254	0.302	1.00	0.120

FRUIT (continued)

Qty	Name	Wgt G	Wtr G	Cal	Prot G	Carb G	Fiber G	F-Tot G	F-Sat G	Mono G	Poly G	Chol Mg	A-Car RE	A-Pre RE	A-Tot RE
1 ea.	Orange-valencia	121	104	59.0	1.26	14.4	2.60	0.360	0.042	0.067	0.073	0	27.8	0	27.8
1 cup	Orange sections-fresh	180	156	85.0	1.69	21.2	3.85	0.220	0.027	0.041	0.045	0	37.0	0	37.0
1 cup	Orange grapefruit jce-cnd	247	219	105	1.48	25.4	0.494	0.240	0.027	0.042	0.047	0	29.3	0	29.3
1 ea.	Papaya-whole-fresh	304	270	117	1.86	29.8	5.17	0.430	0.131	0.116	0.094	0	612	0	612
1 cup	Papaya-slices-fresh	140	124	60.0	0.860	13.7	2.38	0.200	0.060	0.053	0.043	0	282	0	282
1 cup	Papaya nectar-canned	250	213	142	0.430	36.3	1.50	0.380	0.118	0.103	0.088	0	27.7	0	27.7
1 cup	Passion fruit jce-purple	247	211	126	0.960	33.6	0.800	0.120	—	—	—	0	177	0	177
1 ea.	Peaches-fresh-2.5in diam	87.0	76.3	37.0	0.610	9.64	1.60	0.080	0.009	0.030	0.039	0	47.0	0	47.0
1 cup	Peach slices-fresh	170	149	73.0	1.19	18.9	3.13	0.160	0.017	0.058	0.077	0	91.0	0	91.0
1 cup	Peaches-cnd-juice pk-cup	248	217	109	1.57	28.7	3.28	0.080	0.010	0.030	0.040	0	94.0	0	94.0
1 cup	Peaches-cnd-lt syrup-cup	251	213	136	1.13	36.5	4.70	0.080	0.008	0.030	0.038	0	88.8	0	88.8
1 cup	Peach halves-ckd from dry	258	201	200	3.00	50.8	3.70	0.630	0.067	0.230	0.304	0	50.8	0	50.8
1 cup	Peach nectar-canned	249	213	134	0.670	34.7	1.49	0.050	0.005	0.020	0.027	0	64.3	0	64.3
1 ea.	Pears-Bartlett-166g each	166	139	98.0	0.650	25.1	4.80	0.660	0.037	0.139	0.156	0	3.30	0	3.30
1 ea.	Pears-Bosc-141g each	141	118	85.0	0.550	21.0	4.00	0.520	0.050	0.100	0.100	0	3.00	0	3.00
1 ea.	Pears-D'Anjou-200g each	200	168	120	0.780	30.0	5.80	0.660	0.050	0.200	0.200	0	4.00	0	4.00
1 cup	Pear slices-fresh	165	138	97.0	0.650	24.9	4.80	0.660	0.036	0.139	0.155	0	3.30	0	3.30
1 cup	Pears-cnd-juice pack-cup	248	215	123	0.850	32.1	5.00	0.160	0.010	0.035	0.037	0	1.40	0	1.40
1 cup	Pears-cnd-lite syrup-cup	251	212	144	0.480	38.1	5.25	0.080	0.005	0.015	0.018	0	0	0	0
3 ea.	Pear halves-dried	52.5	14.0	138	0.984	36.6	5.73	0.330	0.018	0.069	0.078	0	0.180	0	0.180
1 cup	Pear nectar-canned	250	210	149	0.270	39.4	1.80	0.030	0.003	0.008	0.008	0	0.100	0	0.100
1 ea.	Persimmon-native-sml-raw	25.0	16.1	33.0	0.200	8.38	0.380	0.100	—	—	—	0	—	—	—
1 cup	Pineapple chunks-fresh	155	134	76.0	0.600	19.2	2.70	0.660	0.050	0.074	0.226	0	4.00	0	4.00
1 cup	Pineapple-canned-jce pack	250	209	150	1.04	39.2	2.48	0.210	0.015	0.025	0.073	0	9.50	0	9.50
1 cup	Pineapple-cnd-light syrup	252	216	131	0.900	33.9	2.38	0.290	0.023	0.033	0.101	0	3.70	0	3.70
1 cup	Pineapple juice-fr/frozen	250	216	129	1.00	31.9	0.750	0.080	0.005	0.008	0.025	0	2.50	0	2.50
1 cup	Pineapple juice-cnd-unsw	250	214	140	0.800	34.4	0.750	0.200	0.013	0.023	0.070	0	1.20	0	1.20
1 cup	Pineapple grapefruit drnk	250	220	117	0.600	29.0	0	0.200	0.015	0.025	0.070	0	8.80	0	8.80
1 cup	Pineapple orange drink	250	217	125	3.10	29.4	0	0.240	0.027	0.042	0.047	0	133	0	133
1 ea.	Plum-medium 2-1/8in diam	66.0	56.2	36.0	0.520	8.59	1.28	0.410	0.032	0.268	0.088	0	21.3	0	21.3
1 cup	Plum slices-fresh	165	141	91.0	1.30	21.5	3.20	1.02	0.081	0.067	0.221	0	53.3	0	53.3
1 cup	Plums-cnd-jce pack-cup	252	212	146	1.30	38.2	4.00	0.060	0.005	0.035	0.013	0	254	0	254
1 cup	Plums-cnd-lite syrup-cup	252	209	158	0.930	41.0	3.95	0.260	0.020	0.174	0.058	0	66.6	0	66.6
5 ea.	Prunes-dried	42.0	13.6	100	1.09	26.3	5.90	0.215	0.017	0.143	0.047	0	83.5	0	83.5
1 cup	Prunes-cooked from dry	212	148	227	2.48	59.5	15.0	0.488	0.040	0.322	0.106	0	64.9	0	64.9
1 cup	Prune juice-bottled	256	208	181	1.55	44.7	3.00	0.080	0.008	0.054	0.018	0	0.900	0	0.900
1 cup	Pummelo-raw sections	190	169	71.0	1.44	18.3	0.912	0.080	—	—	—	0	0	0	0
1 ea.	Quince-raw	92.0	77.2	53.0	0.370	14.1	1.56	0.090	0.009	0.033	0.046	0	3.70	0	3.70
1 cup	Raisins-seedless-pkd meas	165	25.4	494	5.32	131	14.4	0.760	0.248	0.030	0.223	0	1.30	0	1.30
1 cup	Golden sdls raisins-pkd	165	24.7	498	5.60	131	14.4	0.760	0.249	0.031	0.223	0	7.30	0	7.30
1 cup	Raspberries-fresh	123	107	60.0	1.11	14.2	7.68	0.680	0.023	0.065	0.385	0	16.0	0	16.0
1 cup	Raspberries-frozen-thawed	250	182	255	1.74	65.4	11.5	0.390	0.013	0.038	0.223	0	15.0	0	15.0
1 cup	Raspberry juice-fresh	240	—	98.0	0.400	25.6	—	0	0	0	0	0	24.0	0	24.0
1 cup	Rhubarb-raw-diced	122	114	26.0	1.09	5.53	3.17	0.240	0.008	0.009	0.218	0	12.2	0	12.2
1 cup	Strawberries-fresh	149	136	45.0	0.910	10.5	3.28	0.550	0.030	0.077	0.277	0	4.00	0	4.00
1 cup	Strawberries-frozen	149	134	52.0	0.630	13.6	3.23	0.160	0.009	0.022	0.080	0	6.60	0	6.60
1 cup	Strawberries-fzn/thwd/swt	255	187	245	1.36	66.1	5.53	0.330	0.018	0.046	0.163	0	6.10	0	6.10
1 ea.	Tangerine-fresh	84.0	73.6	37.0	0.530	9.39	1.70	0.160	0.018	0.029	0.031	0	77.3	0	77.3
1 cup	Tangerine sections-fresh	195	171	86.0	1.23	21.8	3.90	0.360	0.043	0.066	0.072	0	179	0	179
1 cup	Tangerines-cnd-lite syrup	252	209	154	1.13	41.0	4.03	0.250	0.030	0.045	0.100	0	212	0	212
1 cup	Tangerine juice-cnd/swtnd	249	217	125	1.25	29.9	0.750	0.500	0.032	0.043	0.062	0	105	0	105
1 cup	Watermelon-diced/pieces	160	146	50.0	0.990	11.5	0.640	0.680	0.100	0.125	0.351	0	58.5	0	58.5
1 pce	Watermelon-1x10in diam	482	441	152	2.97	34.6	1.93	2.06	0.300	0.200	1.00	0	176	0	176

B1 Mg	B2 Mg	B3 Mg	B6 Mg	B12 Mcg	Fol. Mcg	Panto Mg	Vit-C Mg	Vit-E Mg	Calc Mg	Cu Mg	Iron Mg	Mg Mg	Phos Mg	Potas Mg	Sel Mcg	Na Mg	Zinc Mg
0.105	0.048	0.332	0.076	0	46.7	0.303	58.7	0.291	48.0	0.045	0.110	12.0	21.0	217	0.242	0	0.070
0.157	0.072	0.508	0.108	0	82.8	0.450	95.8	0.396	72.0	0.081	0.187	18.0	25.0	326	0.200	0.001	0.398
0.138	0.074	0.830	0.057	0	20.0	0.346	71.9	0.220	20.0	0.188	1.10	24.0	35.0	390	2.20	7.00	0.180
0.082	0.097	1.03	0.058	0	48.0	0.663	188	—	72.0	0.049	0.300	31.0	16.0	780	—	8.00	0.220
0.038	0.045	0.473	0.027	0	26.0	0.305	92.0	—	33.0	0.022	0.300	14.0	12.0	247	—	9.00	0.100
0.015	0.010	0.375	0.023	0	5.20	0.135	7.50	—	24.0	0.033	0.860	8.00	1.00	78.0	—	14.0	0.380
—	0.324	3.61	—	0	—	—	73.6	—	9.00	—	0.590	35.0	31.0	343	—	7.00	—
0.015	0.036	0.861	0.016	0	3.00	0.148	5.70	0.870	4.00	0.059	0.096	6.00	10.0	171	0.348	0	0.120
0.029	0.070	1.68	0.031	0	5.80	0.289	11.2	1.64	9.00	0.116	0.187	11.0	20.0	335	0.680	1.00	0.183
0.020	0.042	1.44	0.047	0	8.20	1.25	8.80	4.32	15.0	0.124	0.720	18.0	43.0	317	0.750	11.0	0.260
0.023	0.063	1.49	0.048	0	8.20	0.126	5.90	4.32	9.00	0.131	0.900	12.0	27.0	244	0.750	13.0	0.226
0.013	0.054	3.92	0.098	0	0.200	0.467	9.50	2.50	23.0	0.302	3.37	35.0	99.0	825	1.37	6.00	0.464
0.007	0.035	0.717	0.026	0	2.30	0.063	13.1	0.251	13.0	0.172	0.473	11.0	16.0	101	0	10.0	0.200
0.033	0.066	0.166	0.030	0	12.1	0.116	6.60	0.825	19.0	0.188	0.415	9.00	18.0	208	0.990	1.00	0.200
0.030	0.060	0.100	0.025	0	10.0	0.099	6.00	0.701	16.0	0.160	0.400	7.60	16.0	176	0.840	0.010	0.170
0.040	0.080	0.200	0.036	0	14.0	0.140	8.00	0.994	22.0	226	0.500	10.8	22.0	250	1.20	0.010	0.241
0.033	0.066	0.165	0.030	0	18.0	0.116	6.60	0.825	19.0	0.186	0.412	9.00	18.0	207	0.990	10.0	0.220
0.027	0.027	0.496	0.035	0	5.00	0.136	4.00	1.00	22.0	0.131	0.710	17.0	29.0	238	0.502	10.0	0.220
0.025	0.040	0.387	0.035	0	3.00	0.055	1.90	1.00	13.0	0.123	0.703	11.0	17.0	165	0.502	13.0	0.210
0.004	0.076	0.720	0.003	0	6.30	0.108	3.69	0.810	17.7	0.195	1.10	17.4	30.9	280	0.900	3.00	0.204
0.005	0.033	0.320	0.030	0	2.00	0.045	2.70	0.091	11.0	0.168	0.647	6.00	7.00	33.0	—	8.00	0.160
—	—	—	—	0	2.00	—	16.5	—	7.00	—	0.630	—	7.00	78.0	—	0	—
0.143	0.056	0.651	0.135	0	16.4	0.248	23.9	0.163	11.0	0.171	0.574	21.0	11.0	175	0.852	2.00	0.120
0.238	0.048	0.710	0.189	0	12.0	0.734	23.8	0.125	35.0	0.215	0.700	35.0	15.0	305	1.60	3.00	0.250
0.229	0.063	0.736	0.186	0	11.9	0.252	19.0	0.125	36.0	0.260	0.980	40.0	17.0	266	1.51	3.00	0.290
0.175	0.050	0.500	0.185	0	64.0	0.313	30.0	0.050	28.0	0.225	0.750	23.0	20.0	340	—	3.00	0.290
0.138	0.055	0.643	0.240	0	57.7	0.250	26.7	0.050	43.0	0.225	0.650	34.0	20.0	335	0.900	3.00	0.275
0.075	0.040	0.668	0.105	0	26.2	0.133	115	0.041	18.0	0.113	0.770	15.0	14.0	154	—	34.0	0.150
0.075	0.048	0.518	0.118	0	27.2	0.143	56.2	0.040	13.0	0.103	0.670	14.0	10.0	116	—	9.00	0.140
0.028	0.063	0.330	0.053	0	3.20	0.120	6.30	0.566	3.00	0.028	0.070	4.00	7.00	114	0	0.400	0.066
0.071	0.158	0.825	0.134	0	9.50	0.300	15.8	1.42	6.00	0.071	0.170	11.0	17.0	284	0	1.00	0.160
0.058	0.149	1.19	0.097	0	7.50	0.234	7.00	0.520	25.0	0.136	0.856	20.0	38.0	388	0	3.00	0.277
0.040	0.098	0.748	0.068	0	6.40	0.181	1.10	1.52	24.0	0.096	2.16	13.0	33.0	233	0	50.0	0.190
0.034	0.068	0.825	0.111	0	1.70	0.193	1.40	1.05	21.5	0.180	1.04	19.0	33.0	313	0	1.50	0.222
0.051	0.212	1.53	0.462	0	0.100	0.227	6.20	2.33	49.0	0.409	2.35	43.0	74.0	708	0	4.00	0.509
0.041	0.179	2.01	0.558	0	1.00	0.240	10.6	0.520	31.0	0.174	3.02	36.0	64.0	707	0	10.0	0.538
0.065	0.051	0.418	0.068	0	—	—	116	—	7.00	0.091	0.220	12.0	32.0	411	—	2.00	0.150
0.018	0.028	0.184	0.037	0	—	0.075	13.8	—	10.0	0.120	0.640	7.00	16.0	181	—	4.00	—
0.257	0.145	1.35	0.411	0	6.60	0.074	5.50	0.483	81.0	0.510	3.46	54.0	159	1239	9.00	19.0	0.528
0.013	0.315	1.88	0.533	0	5.50	0.231	5.20	0.200	87.0	0.599	2.95	57.0	190	1231	17.3	20.0	0.528
0.037	0.111	1.11	0.070	0	32.5	0.295	30.8	0.369	27.0	0.091	0.701	22.0	15.0	187	—	0	0.566
0.048	0.113	1.50	0.085	0	65.0	0.375	41.3	0.185	38.0	0.263	1.62	32.0	43.0	285	—	3.00	0.450
—	0.400	—	—	0	—	—	36.0	—	58.0	—	20.0	—	28.0	—	—	—	—
0.024	0.037	0.366	0.029	0	8.70	0.104	9.80	0.244	105	0.026	0.268	14.0	17.0	351	—	5.00	0.122
0.030	0.098	0.343	0.088	0	28.0	0.507	84.5	0.300	21.0	0.073	0.566	16.0	28.0	247	0	2.00	0.194
0.033	0.055	0.688	0.042	0	28.0	0.161	61.4	0.317	23.0	0.073	1.12	16.0	20.0	220	0	3.00	0.190
0.041	0.130	1.02	0.077	0	42.0	0.275	106	0.540	28.0	0.051	1.50	18.0	33.0	250	0	8.00	0.153
0.088	0.018	0.134	0.056	0	17.1	0.168	25.9	0.269	12.0	0.024	0.084	10.0	8.00	132	0.570	1.00	0.380
0.205	0.043	0.312	0.131	0	40.0	0.390	60.1	0.624	27.0	0.055	0.200	24.0	20.0	305	1.32	3.00	0.882
0.130	0.110	1.10	0.112	0	34.0	0.320	50.0	0.870	18.0	0.111	0.930	19.0	25.0	197	0.500	15.0	0.604
0.149	0.050	0.249	0.080	0	7.86	0.924	54.8	0.867	45.0	0.062	0.500	20.0	35.0	443	0.500	2.00	0.075
0.128	0.032	0.320	0.230	0	3.40	0.339	15.4	0.160	13.0	0.051	0.272	17.0	14.0	186	0	3.00	0.112
0.386	0.096	0.964	0.694	0	10.4	1.02	46.5	0.482	38.0	0.154	0.822	52.0	41.0	560	0	10.0	0.340

GRAIN, BREADS, CEREALS

Qty	Name	Wgt G	Wtr G	Cal	Prot G	Carb G	Fiber G	F-Tot G	F-Sat G	Mono G	Poly G	Chol Mg	A-Car RE	A-Pre RE	A-Tot RE
1 ea.	Bagel-plain 3.5 inch diam	68.0	21.8	180	7.00	34.7	0.748	1.00	0.171	0.286	0.400	0	0	0	0
1 ea.	Egg bagel-3.5 inch diam.	68.0	21.8	180	7.45	34.7	0.748	1.00	0.171	0.286	0.400	44.0	0	7.00	7.00
1 pce	Banana nut bread-1/2in sl	50.0	22.5	161	2.74	22.4	1.17	7.06	1.45	2.57	2.59	32.2	1.80	9.20	10.9
1 cup	Barley-whole-cooked	200	22.0	200	5.50	44.0	4.60	1.60	0.300	0.200	0.900	0	0	0	0
1 cup	Barley-pearled-cooked	200	144	196	4.60	44.0	4.40	0.560	0.084	0.056	0.252	0	0	0	0
1 ea.	Biscuit-homemade	28.0	7.73	100	2.00	12.8	0.410	4.85	1.20	2.00	1.30	0.100	0	3.00	3.00
1 ea.	Biscuit-from mix	28.0	8.01	94.4	2.10	13.7	0.400	3.10	0.800	1.40	0.900	0.100	1.00	3.00	4.00
1 Tbs	Wheat bran	2.25	0.259	4.75	0.360	1.39	0.959	0.103	0.014	0.012	0.049	0	0	0	0
1 oz.	Rice bran	28.3	2.75	78.2	3.77	14.4	3.26	5.44	1.47	1.96	1.90	0	0	0	0
1 cup	Bran Buds cereal	84.0	2.35	217	11.7	63.9	23.3	2.00	0.356	0.348	1.14	0	0	1112	1112
1 cup	Bran Chex cereal	49.0	1.13	156	5.10	39.0	9.00	1.40	0.249	0.244	0.795	0	10.7	0	10.7
1 cup	40% Bran flakes-Kelloggs	39.0	1.25	125	4.90	30.5	5.40	0.741	0.139	0.139	0.418	0	0	522	522
1 cup	40% Bran flakes Post	47.0	1.41	152	5.30	37.0	6.40	0.752	0.168	0.168	0.336	0	0	629	629
1 ea.	Bran muffin-recipe	45.0	15.7	125	3.00	19.0	2.83	6.00	1.40	1.60	2.30	24.0	19.5	10.5	30.0
1 ea.	Cornmeal muffin-fr/mix	45.0	13.5	145	3.00	22.0	1.60	6.00	1.70	2.30	1.40	42.0	5.50	10.5	16.0
1 pce	Cracked wheat bread-slice	25.0	8.80	65.0	2.32	12.5	1.14	0.870	0.170	0.237	0.314	0	0	0	0
1 pce	French bread 5x2.5 in.pce	35.0	11.9	100	3.30	17.7	0.620	1.36	0.293	0.440	0.455	0	0	0	0
1 pce	Italian bread slice	30.0	9.54	83.0	2.70	16.9	0.330	0.264	0.040	0.020	0.106	0	0	0	0
1 pce	Mixed grain bread-slice	25.0	9.35	65.0	2.00	12.0	0.963	0.930	0.176	0.226	0.360	0	0	0.100	0.100
1 pce	Oatmeal bread (slice)	25.0	9.25	65.0	2.09	12.0	0.675	1.10	0.204	0.391	0.452	0	0	0	0
1 ea.	Pita pocket bread	60.0	18.7	165	6.23	33.0	0.613	0.880	0.100	0.100	0.400	0	0	0	0
1 pce	Raisin bread-25grm slice	25.0	8.25	68.0	1.90	13.2	0.600	0.990	0.226	0.358	0.370	0	0.050	0.020	0.070
1 pce	Rye bread-light-piece	25.0	9.25	65.0	2.12	12.0	0.800	0.913	0.200	0.300	0.320	0	0	0	0
1 pce	Pumpernickel bread-slice	32.0	11.8	80.0	2.93	15.4	1.26	1.10	0.200	0.300	0.500	0	0	0	0
1 pce	Bread-partWhlWt-28grm pce	28.0	10.4	72.0	2.65	13.1	1.30	1.15	0.241	0.450	0.278	0	0	0.100	0.100
1 pce	White bread-firm-33g slce	33.0	12.2	88.0	2.73	16.1	0.600	1.29	0.407	0.472	0.305	0	0	0.100	0.100
1 pce	White bread-28grm slice	28.0	10.4	75.0	2.32	13.7	0.500	1.10	0.345	0.401	0.259	0	0	0.100	0.100
1 pce	White bread-28grms-tstd	24.0	6.72	78.0	2.34	14.1	0.500	1.10	0.349	0.403	0.261	0	0	0.100	0.100
1 pce	White bread-25grm slice	25.0	9.25	65.0	2.07	12.2	0.450	0.980	0.308	0.358	0.231	0	0	0.100	0.100
1 pce	White bread-20grm slice	20.0	7.40	55.0	1.66	10.0	0.353	0.784	0.247	0.286	0.185	0	0	0.100	0.100
1 pce	Whole wheat bread-35g pce	35.0	13.4	85.6	3.37	15.9	2.98	1.53	0.447	0.524	0.401	0	0	0.100	0.100
1 pce	Whole wheat bread-35g-tst	29.0	8.41	81.0	3.50	14.7	2.98	1.41	0.420	0.493	0.377	0	0	0.100	0.100
1 pce	Whole wheat bread-28g pce	28.0	10.7	70.0	3.00	12.7	2.38	1.22	0.363	0.425	0.325	0	0	0.100	0.100
1 cup	Croutons/dry bread cubes	30.0	2.10	111	3.90	21.7	0.090	1.10	0.410	0.400	0.260	0	0	0.100	0.100
1 cup	Bread crumbs-dry grated	100	7.00	390	13.0	73.0	4.04	5.00	1.50	1.60	1.00	5.00	0	0	0
1 cup	Bread crumbs soft	45.0	16.6	120	3.73	22.0	1.22	1.76	0.600	0.600	0.400	0	0	0.100	0.100
1 cup	Bread stuffing prep f/dry	140	46.2	500	9.10	49.8	1.30	30.5	6.10	13.3	9.60	0	0	273	273
1 cup	Bread stuffng w/egg-moist	203	124	420	8.80	40.0	1.30	25.6	5.30	11.3	8.00	67.0	0	256	256
1 ea.	Bread sticks wo/salt coat	10.00	0.500	38.4	1.20	7.53	0.150	0.290	0.091	0.105	0.068	0	0	0	0
1 ea.	Bread sticks w/salt coat	35.0	1.75	106	3.30	20.3	0.500	1.10	0.345	0.400	0.260	0	0	0	0
1 cup	Brown rice-cooked	195	137	232	4.88	49.7	2.80	1.17	0.312	0.390	0.409	0	0	0	0
1 cup	Buckwheat flour-dark	98.0	11.8	338	11.5	70.6	8.00	2.50	0.482	0.833	0.900	0	0	0	0
1 ea.	Buckwheat pancakes fr/mix	27.0	15.7	55.0	2.00	6.00	1.30	2.00	0.900	0.900	0.500	20.0	0	17.0	17.0
1 cup	Bulgar wheat-cooked	135	75.6	246	9.50	44.3	7.07	0.950	0.432	0.108	0.432	0	0	0	0
1 ea.	Cinnamon bun small	50.0	13.5	158	3.00	26.0	1.57	5.00	1.54	2.01	1.10	0	0	189	189
1 ea.	Hamburger bun	45.0	15.3	129	3.71	22.5	1.21	2.36	0.563	0.900	0.675	0	0	0.300	0.300
1 ea.	Hotdog bun	40.0	13.6	115	3.30	20.0	1.08	2.10	0.500	0.800	0.600	0	0	0.300	0.300
1 cup	Alpha Bits cereal	28.0	0.364	111	2.20	24.6	0.300	0.600	0.100	0.192	0.295	0	0	375	375
1 cup	Apple Jacks cereal	28.0	0.644	110	1.50	25.7	0.200	0.100	0.035	0.025	0.035	0	0	375	375
1 cup	Buc Wheats cereal	37.3	—	147	2.67	32.0	2.67	1.33	0.187	0.153	0.627	0	0	909	909
1 cup	C.W. Post cereal-plain	97.0	2.23	432	8.70	69.4	2.20	15.2	11.3	1.72	1.42	0	0	1284	1284
1 cup	C.W. Post cereal w/raisns	103	4.02	446	8.89	73.9	2.40	14.7	11.0	1.67	1.38	0	0	1364	1364
1 cup	Cap'n Crunch cereal	37.0	0.925	156	1.90	29.9	0.925	3.40	2.23	0.440	0.540	0	5.30	0	5.30
1 cup	Cap'n Crunch-pnut butter	35.0	0.630	154	2.50	26.5	0.400	4.50	1.90	1.37	1.01	0	0	0	0
1 cup	Cap'n Crunchberries	35.0	0.910	146	1.80	28.5	0.400	2.90	1.93	0.380	0.470	0	0	0	0
1 cup	Cheerios cereal	23.0	1.15	89.0	3.44	15.7	0.897	1.44	0.246	0.492	0.575	0	0	304	304
1 cup	Cocoa Krispies cereal	36.0	0.900	139	1.90	32.0	0.200	0.500	0.150	0.150	0.200	0	0	477	477
1 cup	Cocoa Pebbles cereal	31.3	0.658	130	1.49	27.3	0	1.64	0.060	0.045	0.060	0	0	421	421
1 cup	Corn Bran cereal	36.0	0.900	124	2.50	30.4	6.84	1.30	0.163	0.325	0.731	0	—	—	—

B1 Mg	B2 Mg	B3 Mg	B6 Mg	B12 Mcg	Fol. Mcg	Panto Mg	Vit-C Mg	Vit-E Mg	Calc Mg	Cu Mg	Iron Mg	Mg Mg	Phos Mg	Potas Mg	Sel Mcg	Na Mg	Zinc Mg
0.258	0.197	2.40	0.030	0	16.3	0.267	0	1.80	20.0	0.115	2.10	15.0	61.0	65.0	21.0	300	0.612
2.58	0.197	2.40	0.030	0.065	16.3	0.267	0	1.80	20.0	0.115	2.10	18.0	61.0	65.0	5.00	300	0.612
0.095	0.082	0.776	0.126	0.077	10.5	0.209	1.30	0.392	17.8	0.089	0.830	14.2	47.8	104	5.82	—	—
0.120	0.040	2.10	0.139	0	12.0	0.373	0	1.70	19.0	0.470	1.55	33.0	170	170	27.0	1.00	1.16
0.049	0.022	1.70	0.087	0	10.0	0.250	0	0.425	6.00	0.130	1.17	12.4	112	72.0	22.0	2.00	1.15
0.080	0.080	0.800	0.013	—	2.00	0.107	0.001	1.30	48.0	0.020	0.700	6.00	36.0	32.0	0.400	195	0.153
0.122	0.108	0.851	0.013	0.045	1.70	0.090	0.001	0.780	59.0	0.031	0.581	6.80	129	57.0	0.400	265	0.179
0.018	0.008	0.607	0.031	0	5.80	0.054	0	0.121	2.59	0.031	0.244	11.4	27.9	25.6	2.25	0.375	0.292
0.641	0.071	8.45	0.936	0	11.1	0.825	0	4.22	21.5	0.075	5.50	23.4	393	424	9.07	0	0.138
1.10	1.30	14.8	1.50	0	297	1.63	45.0	3.00	56.0	0.890	13.4	267	729	1404	5.68	516	11.1
0.600	0.260	8.60	0.900	2.60	173	0.501	26.0	1.67	29.0	0.387	7.80	126	327	394	5.40	455	2.14
0.507	0.591	6.86	0.702	2.07	138	0.098	0	1.42	19.0	0.289	11.2	71.0	192	248	8.00	363	5.15
0.620	0.721	8.30	0.846	2.50	166	0.098	0	1.40	21.0	0.321	7.47	102	296	251	10.4	431	2.50
0.110	0.130	1.30	0.010	0.130	9.00	0.210	3.00	1.90	60.0	0.047	1.40	34.0	125	99.0	8.60	189	0.370
0.090	0.090	0.800	0.040	0.130	5.00	0.374	0.001	2.00	30.0	0.022	1.30	11.0	128	31.0	4.83	291	0.340
0.095	0.095	0.843	0.023	0	12.0	0.151	0.001	0.225	16.0	0.067	0.666	12.0	32.0	34.0	14.1	106	0.350
0.160	0.120	1.40	0.019	0	13.0	0.126	0.001	0.100	39.0	0.051	1.08	7.30	30.0	32.0	8.30	203	0.221
0.123	0.070	1.00	0.016	0	11.0	0.114	0	0.080	5.00	0.060	0.800	7.00	23.0	22.0	7.11	176	0.205
0.100	0.100	1.10	0.026	0	16.3	0.158	0.001	0.312	27.0	0.071	0.800	12.3	55.0	56.0	11.0	106	0.300
0.115	0.066	0.850	0.004	0	0.800	0.039	0	0.055	15.0	0.055	0.700	8.50	31.0	39.0	8.00	124	0.245
0.274	0.130	2.32	0.014	0	12.0	0.256	0	0.428	49.0	0.108	1.45	15.6	60.0	71.0	18.0	339	0.501
0.082	0.155	1.02	0.008	0	9.00	0.108	0.001	0.200	25.0	0.043	0.775	6.25	22.0	59.0	7.50	92.0	0.155
0.102	0.080	0.828	0.024	0	9.80	0.111	0	0.050	20.0	0.048	0.680	8.00	36.0	51.0	8.50	175	0.380
0.109	0.166	1.06	0.051	0	15.6	0.153	0	0.365	23.0	0.087	0.877	22.0	71.0	141	11.2	277	0.400
0.129	0.089	1.26	0.031	0	12.6	0.119	0.001	0.080	35.0	0.067	0.974	12.9	51.5	39.3	10.9	151	0.294
0.155	0.102	1.24	0.011	0	11.6	0.142	0.001	0.018	41.6	0.046	0.938	6.93	35.6	36.9	10.4	170	0.205
0.131	0.087	1.05	0.009	0	9.80	0.122	0.001	0.016	35.3	0.039	0.796	5.88	30.2	31.3	8.90	144	0.173
0.100	0.088	1.06	0.008	0	9.70	0.121	0.001	0.016	35.3	0.040	0.850	5.90	30.0	31.0	8.47	142	0.175
0.118	0.078	0.938	0.009	0	8.90	0.108	0.001	0.014	31.5	0.035	0.710	5.30	27.0	28.0	7.50	129	0.155
0.094	0.062	0.750	0.007	0	7.00	0.086	0.001	0.011	25.0	0.028	0.568	4.20	21.6	22.4	6.00	103	0.124
0.123	0.073	1.34	0.065	0	20.0	0.258	0.001	0.327	25.0	0.119	1.19	32.5	91.0	62.0	23.1	222	0.588
0.093	0.068	1.26	0.058	0	14.0	0.239	0.001	0.310	23.0	0.111	1.11	30.0	86.0	58.0	21.5	209	0.580
0.100	0.059	1.09	0.052	0	15.6	0.206	0.001	0.265	20.0	0.096	0.970	26.0	74.0	50.0	18.5	180	0.500
0.105	0.105	1.44	0.007	0	3.48	0.093	0.001	0.156	37.0	0.060	1.08	9.30	57.0	52.0	4.00	399	0.180
0.350	0.350	4.80	0.023	0	28.0	0.310	0	0.520	122	0.200	4.10	31.0	141	152	12.0	736	0.500
0.212	0.140	1.69	0.015	0	15.8	0.194	0.001	0.322	57.0	0.063	1.28	9.45	48.6	50.0	13.5	231	0.279
0.170	0.200	2.50	0.017	0	14.0	0.241	0	1.00	92.0	0.300	2.20	30.0	136	126	9.00	1254	0.546
0.100	0.183	1.62	0.036	18.0	20.0	0.245	0.010	2.00	81.0	0.304	2.03	44.6	134	118	15.0	1023	0.780
0.006	0.007	0.100	0.002	0	1.10	0.014	0.000	0.027	2.80	0.011	0.090	2.00	9.90	9.20	2.50	70.0	0.057
0.020	0.030	0.300	0.007	0	4.00	0.050	0.001	0.090	16.0	0.040	0.300	7.00	31.0	33.0	9.00	548	0.200
0.176	0.039	2.73	0.294	0	10.0	0.684	0	1.40	23.4	0.197	1.17	72.2	142	137	26.0	0	1.05
0.578	0.155	2.75	0.405	0	125	1.42	0	7.75	32.0	0.686	2.50	135	298	490	9.00	1.00	2.65
0.040	0.050	0.200	0.060	0.054	5.50	0.084	0.001	1.22	59.0	0.092	0.400	18.0	91.0	66.0	2.40	125	0.500
0.080	0.050	4.10	0.070	0	18.0	0.224	0	0.476	27.0	0.600	2.87	57.0	263	151	14.7	3.00	2.81
0.080	0.090	1.20	0.017	0	18.0	0.235	0	0.210	27.0	0.080	0.900	14.0	51.0	62.0	13.0	195	0.452
0.220	0.148	1.78	0.016	0	16.6	0.238	0.001	0.190	61.0	0.074	1.34	8.55	49.5	63.0	12.5	271	0.408
0.196	0.132	1.58	0.014	0	14.8	0.212	0.001	0.185	54.0	0.066	1.19	7.60	44.0	56.0	11.1	241	0.363
0.400	0.400	5.00	0.500	1.50	100	0.146	—	—	8.00	0.070	1.80	17.0	51.0	110	10.1	219	1.50
0.400	0.400	5.00	0.500	0	100	0.100	15.0	—	3.00	0.099	4.50	6.00	30.0	23.0	9.56	125	3.70
0.900	1.02	12.0	1.20	3.60	—	—	36.0	—	80.0	0.107	10.8	32.0	80.0	—	3.17	313	0.400
1.30	1.50	17.1	1.70	5.10	342	—	—	—	47.0	0.376	15.4	67.0	224	198	11.0	167	1.64
1.30	1.50	18.1	1.90	5.50	364	—	—	—	51.0	0.398	16.4	74.0	232	260	11.6	160	1.64
0.660	0.710	8.64	1.00	2.30	238	5.04	0	—	6.00	0.044	9.83	15.0	47.0	48.0	2.96	278	4.01
0.600	0.700	8.97	1.04	2.30	244	4.77	—	—	7.00	0.042	9.10	19.0	49.0	57.0	2.96	268	3.79
0.590	0.670	8.14	0.927	2.50	128	2.99	—	—	11.0	0.042	9.04	14.0	47.0	49.0	2.21	243	3.56
0.320	0.320	4.00	0.400	1.20	4.80	0.268	12.0	—	38.4	0.114	3.60	31.2	109	82.0	9.00	246	0.632
0.500	0.500	6.30	0.600	0	127	0.098	19.0	—	6.00	0.034	2.30	12.0	47.0	53.0	7.68	275	1.90
0.448	0.448	5.52	0.597	1.64	112	—	—	—	5.97	0.070	1.94	13.4	23.9	52.2	—	152	1.64
0.380	0.700	10.9	0.858	1.39	232	4.31	—	—	41.0	—	12.2	18.0	52.0	70.0	1.36	310	4.00

Qty	Name	Wgt G	Wtr G	Cal	Prot G	Carb G	Fiber G	F-Tot G	F-Sat G	Mono G	Poly G	Chol Mg	A-Car RE	A-Pre RE	A-Tot RE
1 cup	Corn Chex cereal	28.0	0.532	111	2.00	24.9	0.500	0.100	0.125	0.250	0.562	0	14.3	0	14.3
1 cup	Corn flakes Kellogg's	22.4	0.672	88.0	1.84	19.5	0.321	0.068	0.008	0.016	0.040	0	0	300	300
1 cup	Corn Flakes-Post Toasties	22.4	0.672	88.0	1.84	19.5	0.321	0.068	0.008	0.016	0.084	0	0	300	300
1 cup	Corn grits-enr-yellow-dry	156	15.6	579	13.7	124	3.00	1.80	0.217	0.434	0.976	0	68.6	0	68.6
1 cup	Corn grits-enr-yellow-ckd	242	206	146	3.50	31.4	0.750	0.500	0.003	0.121	0.294	0	14.5	0	14.5
1 cup	Corn grits-enr-white-ckd	242	206	146	3.50	31.4	0.750	0.500	0.003	0.121	0.294	0	0	0	0
1 cup	Cracklin'Oat Bran cereal	60.0	2.22	229	5.50	41.1	9.06	8.80	2.10	2.30	3.50	0	0	794	794
1 cup	Cream of rice cereal-ckd	244	213	126	2.10	28.1	1.40	0.100	0.030	0.030	0.040	0	0	0	0
1 cup	Cream of Wheat cereal-ckd	244	210	140	3.60	29.0	0.640	0.600	0.100	0.100	0.200	0	0	0	0
1 cup	Crispy Wheat 'N Raisins	43.0	3.05	150	3.00	35.1	2.00	0.700	0.126	0.095	0.398	0	0	569	569
1 cup	Farina-enriched-cooked	233	205	116	3.40	24.6	0.622	0.200	0.030	0.023	0.100	0	0	0	0
1 cup	Fortified Oat flakes	48.0	1.49	177	9.00	34.7	1.20	0.700	0.133	0.252	0.287	0	0	636	636
1 cup	Froot Loops cereal	28.0	0.700	111	1.70	25.0	0.300	1.00	0.200	0.100	0.100	0	0	375	375
1 cup	Frosted Rice Krispies	28.0	0.728	109	1.30	25.7	1.00	0.100	0.030	0.030	0.040	0	0	375	375
1 cup	Fruity Pebbles cereal	32.0	0.928	131	1.26	27.9	0	1.71	0.583	0.480	0.651	0	0	429	429
1 cup	Fruit & Fiber w/apples	56.0	—	180	6.00	44.0	8.00	2.00	0.300	0.300	1.10	0	0	750	750
1 cup	Fruit & Fiber w/dates	56.0	—	180	6.00	42.0	8.00	2.00	0.300	0.300	1.10	0	0	756	756
1 cup	Fruitful Bran cereal	45.3	—	147	4.00	36.0	5.33	0	0	0	0	0	0	504	504
1 cup	Golden Grahams cereal	39.0	0.780	150	2.20	33.2	2.30	1.50	1.03	0.130	0.210	0	0	516	516
1 cup	Granola-Nature Valley	113	4.52	503	11.5	75.5	7.46	19.6	13.3	2.82	2.82	0	8.10	0	8.10
1 cup	Granola cereal-homemade	122	4.03	595	15.0	67.3	8.05	33.1	5.84	9.37	17.2	0	4.30	0	4.30
1 cup	Grape Nuts cereal	114	3.65	404	13.2	93.4	6.04	0.440	0.020	0.020	0.400	0	0	1526	1526
1 cup	Grape Nuts flakes cereal	32.0	1.09	117	3.43	26.5	1.83	0.343	0.057	0.039	0.106	0	0	429	429
1 cup	Honey & Nut Corn flakes	37.3	1.49	151	2.40	31.1	0.400	2.00	0.260	0.667	0.961	0	0	500	500
1 cup	Honey Nut Cheerios cereal	33.0	1.06	125	3.60	26.5	0.920	0.800	0.130	0.310	0.300	0	0	437	437
1 cup	Honey Bran cereal	35.0	0.875	119	3.10	28.6	3.90	0.700	0.125	0.122	0.398	0	0	463	463
1 cup	Honey Comb cereal	22.0	0.308	86.0	1.30	19.6	0.300	0.400	0.059	0.115	0.205	0	0	291	291
1 cup	King Vitamin cereal	21.0	0.378	85.0	1.10	17.8	0.100	1.20	0.740	0.160	0.200	0	0	717	717
1 cup	Kix cereal	19.0	0.608	73.0	1.67	15.6	0.267	0.467	0.120	0.110	0.167	0	0	250	250
1 cup	Life cereal	44.0	1.98	162	8.10	31.5	1.40	0.800	0.110	0.228	0.380	0	0	0	0
1 cup	Lucky Charms cereal	32.0	0.896	125	2.90	26.1	0.704	1.20	0.220	0.430	0.490	0	0	424	424
1 cup	Malt-O-Meal cereal-ckd	240	211	122	3.60	25.9	0.640	0.240	0.038	0.032	0.120	0	0	0	0
1 cup	Maypo cereal-cooked	240	198	171	5.87	31.9	0.933	2.40	—	—	—	0	0	703	703
1 cup	Most cereal	52.0	2.39	175	7.40	39.6	6.45	0.600	0.082	0.171	0.285	0	0	2754	2754
1 cup	Nutri-Grain Barley	41.0	1.19	153	4.50	33.9	2.40	0.300	0.045	0.030	0.135	0	0	540	540
1 cup	Nutri-Grain Corn	42.0	1.22	160	3.40	35.5	2.60	1.00	0.125	0.250	0.562	0	0	556	556
1 cup	Nutri-Grain Rye	40.0	1.32	144	3.50	33.9	3.05	0.300	0.052	0.082	0.136	0	0	530	530
1 cup	Nutri-Grain Wheat	44.0	1.32	158	3.80	37.2	2.80	0.500	0.100	0.080	0.320	0	0	583	583
1 cup	Oatmeal cereal-prepared	234	199	145	6.00	25.2	2.10	2.40	0.440	0.840	1.00	0	3.80	0	3.80
1 cup	Inst Oatmeal-plain-f/pkt	236	202	139	5.87	24.1	2.13	2.27	0.400	0.800	0.933	0	0	604	604
1 cup	Instant Oatmeal w/apples	170	132	154	4.46	30.1	1.60	1.83	0.343	0.686	0.800	0	0	497	497
1 cup	Inst Oatmeal w/bran/raisn	223	178	181	5.60	34.7	3.66	2.17	0.343	0.800	0.914	0	0	547	547
1 cup	Inst Oatmeal w/maple	177	132	186	5.26	36.5	1.60	2.17	0.343	0.800	0.914	0	0	515	515
1 cup	Inst Oatmeal w/cinn/spice	184	135	202	5.49	40.1	1.60	2.17	0.343	0.800	0.914	0	0	543	543
1 cup	Inst Oatmeal w/rais/spice	181	135	184	4.91	36.3	1.71	2.06	0.343	0.686	0.800	0	0	503	503
1 cup	100% Bran cereal	66.0	1.98	178	8.30	48.1	19.5	3.30	0.590	0.574	1.87	0	0	0	0
1 cup	100% Natural cereal	112	2.46	540	12.1	72.0	5.60	24.1	16.2	4.60	2.16	0	8.00	0	8.00
1 cup	100% Natural-w/apples	104	1.98	478	10.7	69.8	4.80	19.5	15.5	1.83	1.34	0	8.00	0	8.00
1 cup	100% Natural w/rais/dates	110	3.85	496	11.2	72.4	4.20	20.3	13.7	3.72	1.71	0	8.00	0	8.00
1 cup	Product 19 cereal	33.0	0.990	126	3.20	27.4	0.430	0.200	0.010	0.010	0.117	0	0	1769	1769
1 cup	Puffed rice cereal	14.0	0.420	55.0	0.882	12.6	0.112	0.100	0.030	0.030	0.040	0	0	0	0
1 cup	Puffed Wheat cereal	12.0	0.360	44.0	1.80	9.50	2.30	0.100	0.019	0.016	0.065	0	0	0	0
1 cup	Quisp cereal	30.0	0.600	124	1.50	25.0	0.400	2.20	1.48	0.260	0.310	0	—	—	—
1 cup	Raisin Bran-Kellogg's	49.0	4.07	160	4.00	40.0	5.90	0.800	0.155	0.135	0.417	0	0	500	500
1 cup	Raisin Bran Post	56.0	5.15	174	5.30	42.9	6.30	1.08	0.200	0.200	0.400	0	0	750	750
1 cup	Raisins-Rice & Rye cereal	46.0	3.91	155	2.60	39.3	0.500	0.100	0.030	0.025	0.040	0	0	467	467
1 cup	Ralston cereal-cooked	253	218	134	5.50	28.2	3.30	0.800	0.131	0.131	0.400	0	0	0	0
1 cup	Rice Chex cereal	25.3	0.659	100.0	1.33	22.5	1.64	0.892	0.267	0.267	0.357	0	1.47	0	1.47
1 cup	Rice Krispies-Kelloggs	29.0	0.580	112	1.90	24.8	0.090	0.200	0.015	0.015	0.080	0	0	388	388

B1 Mg	B2 Mg	B3 Mg	B6 Mg	B12 Mcg	Fol. Mcg	Panto Mg	Vit-C Mg	Vit-E Mg	Calc Mg	Cu Mg	Iron Mg	Mg Mg	Phos Mg	Potas Mg	Sel Mcg	Na Mg	Zinc Mg
0.400	0.070	5.00	0.500	1.50	100	0.046	15.0	—	3.00	0.024	1.80	4.00	11.0	23.0	1.00	271	0.100
0.294	0.340	4.00	0.408	0	80.0	0.040	12.0	0.094	0.800	0.015	1.44	2.40	14.4	20.8	0.800	281	0.048
0.294	0.340	4.00	0.408	0	80.0	0.040	0	0.094	0.800	0.015	0.560	2.40	9.60	26.4	0.800	238	0.048
1.00	0.590	7.73	0.229	0	7.00	0.544	0	1.28	3.00	0.178	6.10	42.0	114	213	11.8	1.00	0.640
0.240	0.150	1.96	0.058	0	2.00	0.082	0	0.368	1.00	0.029	1.55	11.0	29.0	54.0	4.60	0	0.175
0.240	0.150	1.96	0.058	0	2.00	0.082	0	0.368	1.00	0.029	1.55	11.0	29.0	54.0	4.60	0	0.175
0.800	0.900	10.6	1.10	0	212	0.666	32.0	—	40.0	0.336	3.80	116	241	355	5.10	402	3.20
0.100	0	1.00	0.066	0	8.00	0.162	0	—	8.00	0.083	0.400	8.00	42.0	49.0	8.64	2.00	0.390
0.240	0.070	1.50	0.024	0	9.20	0.174	0	0.312	54.0	0.068	10.9	12.0	43.0	46.0	26.8	5.00	0.347
0.600	0.600	7.60	0.800	2.30	40.0	0.205	—	—	71.0	0.129	6.80	35.0	117	174	3.30	204	0.510
0.190	0.120	1.28	0.023	0	6.00	0.130	0	0.298	4.00	0.026	1.17	4.00	28.0	30.0	25.6	1.00	0.160
0.600	0.700	0.390	0.900	2.50	169	0.201	—	—	68.0	0.255	13.7	58.0	176	343	6.80	429	1.50
0.400	0.400	5.00	0.500	0	100	0.103	15.0	—	3.00	0.060	4.50	7.00	24.0	26.0	7.29	145	3.70
0.400	0.400	5.00	0.500	0	100	0.128	15.0	0.052	1.00	0.071	1.80	5.00	27.0	21.0	6.53	240	0.310
0.457	0.457	5.71	0.571	1.71	114	—	—	—	3.43	0.041	2.06	9.14	19.4	24.0	—	179	1.71
0.750	0.850	10.0	1.00	3.00	200	—	—	—	20.0	0.320	9.00	120	300	—	—	390	3.00
0.750	0.850	10.0	1.00	3.00	200	—	—	—	20.0	0.400	9.00	120	200	—	—	340	3.00
0.500	0.567	6.67	0.667	2.00	133	—	—	—	13.3	0.267	10.8	80.0	200	200	—	320	5.00
0.500	0.600	6.90	0.700	2.10	—	0.169	21.0	—	24.0	0.311	6.20	16.0	56.0	86.0	—	476	0.340
0.390	0.190	0.830	0.317	0	85.0	0.931	0	1.00	71.0	0.367	3.78	116	354	389	10.0	232	2.19
0.730	0.310	2.14	0.428	0	99.0	0.736	1.00	1.00	76.0	0.699	4.84	141	494	612	10.0	12.0	4.47
1.60	1.60	20.0	2.00	6.00	400	0.850	0	—	44.0	0.376	4.92	76.0	284	380	10.1	788	2.48
0.457	0.457	5.71	0.571	1.71	114	0.334	—	—	12.6	0.131	5.14	35.4	96.0	113	20.3	249	0.651
0.533	0.533	6.67	0.667	0	133	0.107	20.0	—	4.00	—	2.40	8.00	17.3	48.0	2.77	300	0.147
0.400	0.500	5.80	0.600	1.70	3.60	0.222	17.0	—	23.0	0.231	5.20	39.0	122	115	14.9	299	0.870
0.500	0.500	6.20	0.600	1.90	23.0	0.197	19.0	—	16.0	0.167	5.60	46.0	132	151	—	202	0.900
0.300	0.300	3.90	0.400	1.20	78.0	0.086	—	—	4.00	0.038	1.40	8.00	22.0	70.0	2.57	166	1.20
0.092	1.06	12.9	1.18	4.12	286	0.042	33.0	9.00	—	0.028	12.7	7.00	—	26.0	—	161	0.160
0.267	0.267	3.33	0.333	1.00	1.75	—	10.0	—	23.3	0.031	5.40	8.00	26.0	29.0	—	226	0.167
0.950	1.00	11.6	0.046	0	37.0	0.488	—	0.159	154	0.236	11.6	55.0	238	197	—	229	1.55
0.400	0.500	5.60	0.600	1.70	—	0.203	17.0	—	36.0	0.110	5.10	27.0	88.0	66.0	7.57	227	0.560
0.480	0.240	5.80	0.019	0	4.80	0.139	0	—	5.00	0.026	9.60	14.0	24.0	31.0	8.00	2.00	0.168
0.667	0.800	9.33	0.867	2.80	9.33	0.339	28.0	—	125	0.159	8.40	50.7	248	211	12.0	8.00	1.49
2.80	3.10	36.7	3.70	11.0	734	—	110	—	79.0	0.291	33.0	103	361	340	—	276	2.80
0.500	0.600	7.20	0.700	2.20	145	—	22.0	—	11.0	0.246	1.45	32.0	126	108	6.23	277	5.40
0.500	0.600	7.40	0.750	2.20	148	—	22.0	0	1.00	0.122	0.890	27.0	120	98.0	12.0	276	5.50
0.500	0.600	7.00	0.700	2.10	141	—	21.0	—	8.00	0.137	1.13	31.0	104	72.0	1.08	272	5.30
0.600	0.700	7.70	0.800	2.30	155	—	23.0	11.6	12.0	0.238	1.24	34.0	164	120	13.6	299	5.80
0.260	0.050	0.300	0.047	0	9.50	0.468	0	0.400	20.0	0.129	1.59	56.0	178	132	20.2	1.00	1.15
0.707	0.387	7.32	0.989	0	200	0.472	0	0.893	217	0.159	8.43	68.0	177	132	17.3	380	1.33
0.549	0.320	5.86	0.797	0	157	0.403	0	1.14	181	0.137	6.94	58.3	134	122	13.1	254	1.11
0.640	0.720	9.28	0.870	0	177	0.519	0.011	1.14	198	0.325	8.70	65.1	235	270	15.3	282	1.54
0.606	0.366	6.11	0.842	0	166	0.361	0.011	1.14	185	0.136	7.26	58.3	163	117	15.0	320	1.14
0.640	0.389	6.47	0.878	0	175	0.438	0.011	1.14	197	0.136	7.60	58.3	167	119	15.1	320	1.11
0.583	0.411	6.25	0.851	0	171	0.427	0.011	1.14	189	0.160	7.52	58.3	152	171	14.7	257	1.26
1.60	1.80	20.9	2.10	6.30	200	1.27	63.0	2.66	46.0	1.04	8.12	312	801	824	6.16	457	5.74
0.340	0.604	2.40	2.55	0	33.2	0.896	0	1.08	196	0.496	3.30	135	416	552	12.9	48.0	2.53
0.330	0.580	1.88	0.107	0	17.0	1.09	—	1.00	157	0.423	2.89	71.0	350	513	10.5	52.0	2.00
0.300	0.640	2.08	0.165	0	45.0	0.939	—	1.00	160	0.484	3.12	124	347	538	9.00	47.0	2.11
1.70	2.00	23.3	2.30	7.00	466	0.177	70.0	—	4.00	0.092	21.0	12.0	47.0	51.0	—	378	0.500
0.015	0.014	0.420	0.011	0	2.66	0.045	—	0.012	1.00	0.024	0.150	3.50	14.0	16.0	0.480	0.420	0.144
0.020	0.030	1.30	0.020	0	4.00	0.062	0	0.140	3.00	0.049	0.570	17.0	43.0	42.0	1.00	0	0.296
0.540	0.760	5.80	0.909	2.58	8.00	0.038	—	—	9.00	0.010	6.31	12.0	25.0	45.0	—	241	0.180
0.507	0.573	6.67	0.667	2.00	133	0.130	0	1.41	25.0	0.280	24.0	73.0	200	307	3.96	293	5.00
0.737	0.851	10.0	1.02	3.00	200	0.140	0	1.40	27.0	0.310	9.01	96.0	237	349	4.00	370	3.01
0.500	0.600	6.30	0.600	1.90	125	—	0	—	10.0	—	5.60	20.0	50.0	144	4.60	350	4.70
0.200	0.180	2.05	0.114	0.109	18.0	0.329	0	1.40	14.0	0.200	1.64	59.0	148	153	20.0	4.00	1.42
0.357	0.267	4.45	0.445	1.33	89.3	0.089	13.3	0.003	3.47	0.067	1.60	6.24	25.3	29.3	2.69	211	0.347
0.400	0.400	5.00	0.500	0	100	0.198	15.0	0.081	4.00	0.071	1.80	10.0	34.0	30.0	5.00	340	0.480

Qty	Name	Wgt G	Wtr G	Cal	Prot G	Carb G	Fiber G	F-Tot G	F-Sat G	Mono G	Poly G	Chol Mg	A-Car RE	A-Pre RE	A-Tot RE
1 cup	Roman Meal cereal-cooked	241	200	148	6.53	33.1	7.47	0.933	0.131	0.108	0.440	0	0	0	0
1 cup	Shredded Wheat cereal	42.7	2.13	153	4.65	33.9	4.67	1.07	0.152	0.152	0.457	0	0	0	0
1 ea.	Shredded wheat-lg biscuit	19.0	1.22	65.0	2.05	11.0	1.95	0.300	0.050	0.050	0.150	0	0	0	0
1 cup	Special K cereal	21.3	0.427	83.3	4.20	16.0	0.200	0.075	0.023	0.023	0.029	0	0	286	286
1 cup	Sugar Corn Pops cereal	28.0	0.952	108	1.40	25.6	0.100	0.100	0.012	0.025	0.056	0	0	375	375
1 cup	Sugar Frosted flakes	35.0	1.05	133	1.80	31.7	0.460	0.100	0.125	0.250	0.563	0	0	463	463
1 cup	Sugar Smacks cereal	37.3	1.12	141	2.67	32.9	0.427	0.667	0.133	0.133	0.267	0	0	500	500
1 cup	Super Golden Crisp cereal	33.0	0.495	123	2.10	29.8	0.620	0.300	0	0	0.118	0	0	437	437
1 cup	Tasteeos cereal	24.0	0.504	94.0	3.10	19.0	0.840	0.700	0.162	0.242	0.285	0	0	318	318
1 cup	Team cereal	42.0	1.60	164	2.70	36.0	0.400	0.700	0.151	0.181	0.309	0	0	556	556
1 cup	Total cereal	33.0	1.32	116	3.30	26.0	2.40	0.700	0.118	0.118	0.354	0	0	1769	1769
1 cup	Trix cereal	28.0	0.700	108	1.50	24.9	0.184	0.400	0.200	0.100	0.100	0	0	375	375
1 cup	Waffelos cereal	30.0	0.750	121	1.70	25.9	0.400	1.30	—	—	—	0	0	397	397
1 cup	Wheat & Raisin Chex	54.0	3.78	185	5.10	43.0	3.60	0.400	0.120	0.100	0.160	0	0.030	0	0.030
1 cup	Wheat Chex cereal	46.0	1.15	169	4.50	37.8	3.40	1.10	0.180	0.180	0.550	0	0	0	0
1 Tbs	Wheat germ toasted	7.06	0.297	26.9	2.06	3.51	0.189	0.769	0.131	0.109	0.458	0	0	0	0
1 cup	Wheatena cereal-ckd	243	208	135	5.00	28.7	3.30	1.10	0.180	0.180	0.550	0	0	0	0
1 cup	Wheaties cereal	29.0	1.45	101	2.80	23.1	2.50	0.520	0.070	0.050	0.240	0	0	388	388
1 cup	Whole grain wheat-ckd	150	129	84.1	2.85	17.1	3.60	6.01	1.20	0.901	3.60	0	0	0	0
1 cup	Whole wheat cereal-cooked	242	203	151	4.90	23.0	3.90	0.700	0.098	0.081	0.330	0	0	0	0
1 oz.	Corn chips	28.3	0.283	157	2.02	16.2	0.304	9.11	1.82	3.44	3.75	0	11.1	0	11.1
1 cup	Corn flour	117	14.0	431	9.10	89.9	1.60	3.04	0.380	0.760	1.71	0	40.0	0	40.0
1 ea.	Corn fritter-recipe	45.0	21.6	116	2.71	13.0	1.83	6.25	1.04	2.59	2.22	34.2	8.00	9.80	—
1 ea.	Corn tortilla-enr-reg-6in	30.0	13.5	65.0	2.00	13.0	1.23	1.02	0.101	0.305	0.612	0	8.00	0	8.00
1 cup	Cornmeal-degermed-enr/dry	138	16.6	502	10.9	108	4.00	1.66	0.200	0.400	0.900	0	61.0	0	61.0
1 ea.	Cornmeal muffin-recipe	45.0	14.8	145	3.00	21.0	1.60	5.00	1.50	2.20	1.40	23.0	4.50	10.5	15.0
1 Tbs	Cornstarch	8.00	0.960	29.0	0.025	7.00	0.100	0.048	0.005	0.010	0.022	0	0	0	0
1 oz.	Cottonseed flour-lowfat	28.3	1.96	93.8	14.2	10.3	0.689	0.399	0.088	0.063	0.164	0	12.3	0	12.3
1 pce	Armenian cracker bread	7.00	0.280	29.2	1.16	4.72	0.915	0.582	0.104	0.170	0.280	0	0.350	0	0.350
5 ea.	Cheese crackers	5.00	0.190	25.0	0.480	2.70	0.011	1.51	0.450	0.600	0.150	3.00	0.250	2.25	2.50
2 ea.	Graham crackers	14.0	0.630	60.0	1.04	10.8	1.40	1.46	0.400	0.600	0.400	0	0	0	0
3 ea.	Round crackers-like Ritz	9.00	0.297	45.0	0.620	6.40	0.240	2.90	0.600	1.20	0.300	0	0	0	0
3 ea.	Rye wafers-whole grain	21.0	1.05	82.5	1.50	15.0	3.13	1.50	0.450	0.600	0.450	0	0	0	0
3 ea.	Saltine crackers	9.00	0.387	37.5	0.825	6.60	0.043	0.825	0.375	0.300	0.150	3.00	0	0	0
3 ea.	Sesame crackers	9.00	0.360	45.0	0.900	5.47	0.210	2.17	0.330	0.900	0.825	0	0.300	0	0.300
1 oz.	Oyster crackers-33 per oz	28.3	1.22	120	2.70	20.0	0.170	3.31	1.50	1.20	0.601	0	0	0	0
3 ea.	Triscuit crackers	13.5	0.540	63.0	1.20	9.30	0.615	2.25	0.750	0.900	0.600	0	0	0	0
5 ea.	Wheat cracker thin	10.0	0.300	43.8	1.12	6.25	0.750	1.75	0.625	0.625	0.500	0	0	0	0
3 ea.	Whole wheat crackers	12.0	0.480	52.5	1.35	7.50	0.900	2.25	0.750	0.900	0.600	0	0	0	0
1 oz.	Doritos-nacho flavor	28.3	0.283	141	2.23	18.3	0.405	6.88	1.42	2.57	2.81	0	12.9	0	12.9
1 cup	Egg noodles-cooked	160	112	200	6.60	37.3	1.50	2.00	0.500	0.600	0.600	50.0	0	34.0	34.0
1 ea.	English muffin-enr/plain	57.0	23.9	140	4.51	26.2	1.54	1.10	0.300	0.200	0.300	0	0	0	0
1 ea.	English muffin-sourdough	56.0	24.1	129	4.50	25.2	1.54	1.10	0.300	0.200	0.300	0	0	0	0
1 cup	Rye flour-dark	128	408	17.4	89.6	15.4	2.30	0.418	0.627	1.05	0	0	0	0	—
1 cup	White flour-enr-unsifted	125	15.0	455	13.1	95.1	3.50	1.25	0.200	0.100	0.550	0	0	0	0
1 cup	White flour-enr-sifted	115	13.8	419	12.1	87.5	3.22	1.15	0.184	0.092	0.506	0	0	0	0
1 cup	Gluten flour	140	11.9	529	58.0	66.1	0.600	2.70	—	—	—	0	0	0	0
1 cup	Self-rising flour-enr.	125	14.4	440	12.0	93.0	3.50	1.25	0.200	0.100	0.550	0	0	0	0
1 cup	Whole wheat flour	120	14.4	400	16.0	85.2	12.5	2.40	0.336	0.276	1.13	0	0	0	0
1 ea.	Flour tortilla 8 in diam	35.4	9.52	105	2.58	19.3	0.955	2.69	0.404	1.15	1.02	0	0	0	0
1 pce	French toast-recipe	65.0	34.4	123	4.88	15.4	0.768	4.47	1.07	1.40	1.10	73.0	2.00	55.0	57.0
1 ea.	Granola bar	28.0	0.980	127	2.92	18.3	—	5.50	—	—	—	—	1.00	0	1.00
1 cup	Macaroni-ckd firm-hot	130	82.7	190	6.50	39.1	1.04	0.650	0.091	0.078	0.273	0	0	0	0
1 cup	Macaroni-ckd tender-hot	140	101	155	5.00	32.0	1.12	0.650	0.077	0.070	0.240	0	0	0	0
1 cup	Macaroni-ckd tender-cold	105	75.6	115	3.75	24.0	0.840	0.413	0.058	0.053	0.180	0	0	0	0
1 cup	Chow mein noodles-dry	45.0	4.95	220	5.90	26.1	0.050	11.0	2.10	7.30	0.400	5.00	0	0	0
1 cup	Egg noodles-cooked	160	112	200	6.60	37.3	1.50	2.00	0.500	0.600	0.600	50.0	0	34.0	34.0
1 pce	Oatmeal bread (slice)	25.0	9.25	65.0	2.09	12.0	0.675	1.10	0.204	0.391	0.452	0	0	0	0
1 ea.	Pancakes-plain-homeRecipe	27.0	13.5	60.0	2.00	9.00	0.720	2.00	0.500	0.800	0.500	16.0	0	10.0	10.0

B1 Mg	B2 Mg	B3 Mg	B6 Mg	B12 Mcg	Fol. Mcg	Panto Mg	Vit-C Mg	Vit-E Mg	Calc Mg	Cu Mg	Iron Mg	Mg Mg	Phos Mg	Potas Mg	Sel Mcg	Na Mg	Zinc Mg
0.240	0.120	3.09	0.113	0	24.0	0.372	—	0.960	29.3	0.321	2.12	109	216	303	9.33	2.67	1.79
0.105	0.120	2.23	0.108	0	21.1	0.352	0	0.607	16.5	0.281	1.80	55.5	149	153	2.00	4.00	1.40
0.055	0.050	0.865	0.048	0	9.50	0.154	—	0.180	7.50	0.095	0.595	32.0	68.5	62.0	1.00	0.500	0.475
0.300	0.300	3.75	0.375	0	74.7	0.112	11.3	—	6.00	0.096	3.37	12.0	41.3	36.7	17.0	199	2.77
0.400	0.400	5.00	0.500	0	100	0.062	15.0	—	1.00	0.060	1.80	2.00	28.0	17.0	1.70	103	1.50
0.500	0.500	6.20	0.600	0	124	0.062	19.0	—	1.00	0.074	2.20	3.00	26.0	22.0	2.45	284	0.050
0.493	0.573	6.67	0.667	0	133	0.167	20.0	—	4.00	0.105	2.40	17.3	41.3	56.0	—	100.0	0.373
0.400	0.500	5.80	0.600	1.70	116	0.121	0	—	7.00	0.090	2.10	20.0	60.0	123	34.3	29.0	1.70
0.300	0.400	4.20	0.400	1.30	9.00	0.118	13.0	—	11.0	0.141	3.80	26.0	96.0	71.0	—	183	0.690
0.550	0.630	7.40	0.800	2.20	—	0.309	22.0	—	6.00	0.216	2.57	19.0	65.0	71.0	6.02	259	0.580
1.70	2.00	23.3	2.30	7.00	466	0.208	70.0	—	56.0	0.142	21.0	37.0	137	123	3.85	409	0.780
0.400	0.400	4.90	0.500	1.50	—	0.082	15.0	—	6.00	0.044	4.50	6.00	19.0	26.0	2.05	179	0.130
0.400	0.500	5.30	0.500	1.60	3.00	0.053	—	16.0	8.00	0.034	4.80	6.00	244	26.0	—	125	0.240
0.500	0.600	7.10	0.700	2.20	143	0.157	2.00	0.097	—	0.283	7.70	53.0	163	174	4.10	306	1.19
0.600	0.170	8.10	0.800	2.40	162	0.223	24.0	0.097	18.0	0.269	7.30	58.0	182	174	4.14	308	1.23
0.118	0.058	0.395	0.071	0	29.6	0.103	0	1.94	3.13	0.106	0.544	22.6	80.9	66.9	7.13	0.250	1.18
0.020	0.050	1.34	0.046	0	17.0	0.191	0	1.43	11.0	0.126	1.36	49.0	146	187	27.0	5.00	1.68
0.400	0.400	5.10	0.500	1.50	9.00	0.205	15.0	0.612	44.0	0.134	4.60	32.0	100	108	2.50	363	0.650
0.120	0.030	1.20	0.093	0	18.0	0.300	0	1.06	9.01	0.150	0.901	35.1	90.1	87.1	18.3	3.00	1.32
0.170	0.120	2.15	0.135	0	26.0	0.404	0	0.677	17.0	0.201	1.50	54.0	167	171	19.0	1.00	1.16
0.040	0.051	0.405	0.040	0	3.04	—	1.01	1.82	35.4	0.076	0.506	21.3	52.6	52.6	2.58	236	0.445
0.234	0.070	1.64	0.070	0	19.9	0.643	0	1.23	7.00	0.234	2.10	124	142	140	3.80	1.00	2.92
0.115	0.068	0.986	0.026	0.082	17.0	0.359	1.80	3.67	10.0	0.055	0.711	13.6	51.3	95.8	4.63	167	0.295
0.050	0.030	0.400	0.090	0	5.70	0.047	0	0.361	42.0	0.005	0.600	19.0	55.0	43.0	2.70	1.00	0.357
0.610	0.360	4.80	0.345	0	29.0	0.800	0	2.94	8.00	0.100	5.93	64.9	137	166	9.45	1.00	1.15
0.110	0.110	0.900	0.041	0.130	5.00	0.374	0.001	2.00	66.0	0.025	0.900	11.0	59.0	57.0	4.86	169	0.310
0	0.006	0	—	0	—	—	0	—	—	0.004	0.040	0.160	2.00	0	0.250	0	0.002
0.592	0.112	1.15	0.217	0	—	0.126	0.699	—	135	0.332	3.56	203	450	499	—	9.98	3.29
0.015	0.010	0.262	0.006	0	3.00	0.045	0.400	0.082	5.32	0.020	0.112	10.2	0.250	—	0.425	—	0.225
0.025	0.020	0.200	0.005	0	—	—	0	—	5.50	0.015	0.175	1.30	8.50	8.50	0.450	56.0	0.036
0.020	0.030	0.600	0.011	0	1.80	0.072	0	—	6.00	0.030	0.367	6.00	20.0	36.0	1.54	86.0	0.113
0.030	0.030	0.300	0.002	0	1.00	—	0	—	9.00	0.020	0.300	2.00	18.0	12.0	0.765	90.0	0.051
0.090	0.045	0.750	0.040	0	15.0	—	0	—	10.5	0.060	0.750	24.0	66.0	97.5	7.32	172	2.40
0.045	0.037	0.450	0.005	0	1.50	0.024	0	—	2.25	0.015	0.375	2.32	9.00	12.7	0.600	116	0.068
0.045	0.030	0.225	—	0	3.75	0.056	0	0.106	15.0	0.022	0.300	12.7	10.5	—	—	81.0	0.094
0.100	0.140	1.50	0.010	0.010	8.01	0.060	0	—	4.01	0.045	1.20	5.01	25.0	34.1	1.90	357	0.200
—	—	—	—	0	—	—	0	—	—	—	—	—	—	—	0.378	—	—
0.050	0.037	0.500	0.012	0	3.75	—	0	—	3.75	—	0.375	8.75	18.8	21.3	0.600	86.2	0.300
0.030	0.045	0.600	0.015	0	4.50	0.043	0	0.034	4.50	0.099	0.360	12.0	33.0	46.5	0.636	88.5	0.349
0.040	0.030	0.405	0.105	0	—	—	0	1.06	17.2	0.081	0.405	13.2	99.2	110	2.58	108	0.425
0.220	0.130	1.90	0.011	0.435	6.60	0.250	0	0.110	16.0	0.132	2.60	28.0	94.0	70.0	30.4	3.00	1.08
0.262	0.182	2.14	0.023	0	18.2	0.250	0	0.800	96.0	0.176	1.70	10.8	67.0	331	11.5	378	0.410
0.220	0.140	2.20	0.023	0	15.0	0.250	0	0.800	112	0.176	1.40	10.8	67.0	331	11.5	254	0.410
0.559	0.250	3.51	0.416	0	100	1.40	0	3.53	46.0	0.538	4.21	107	573	543	45.0	2.00	2.81
0.799	0.496	6.61	0.050	0	20.0	0.544	0	1.67	20.0	0.159	5.50	26.3	109	119	38.0	2.50	0.825
0.735	0.457	6.08	0.046	0	18.4	0.501	0	1.54	18.4	0.146	5.06	24.2	100	109	35.0	2.30	0.759
—	—	—	—	—	—	—	0	—	56.0	—	—	—	196	84.0	—	3.00	—
0.799	0.496	6.61	0.050	0	20.0	0.544	0	1.67	331	0.159	5.50	26.3	583	113	38.0	1349	0.825
0.660	0.144	5.16	0.384	0	58.0	1.30	0	3.11	49.0	0.466	5.16	168	446	444	96.0	3.60	2.96
0.127	0.078	1.20	0.014	0	15.6	0.091	0	0.661	21.2	0.046	0.549	11.5	58.8	35.0	8.00	134	0.269
0.153	0.173	1.09	0.036	0.274	18.0	0.434	0.280	0.457	79.0	0.063	1.08	12.0	82.0	96.0	10.0	189	0.474
0.080	0.030	0.200	—	—	23.0	—	0	—	17.5	—	0.907	—	79.0	99.0	—	85.0	1.00
0.234	0.130	1.82	0.104	0	4.00	0.139	0	0.020	14.0	0.130	2.10	18.0	85.0	103	15.0	1.30	0.610
0.200	0.110	1.50	0.088	0	4.00	0.118	0	0.020	11.0	0.125	1.74	18.0	70.0	85.0	15.0	1.00	0.588
0.150	0.083	1.13	0.066	0	3.00	0.089	0	0.015	8.30	0.105	1.31	11.6	53.0	64.0	7.00	0.750	0.390
0.050	0.030	0.600	0.031	0	10.0	—	0	—	14.0	—	0.400	—	41.0	33.0	19.0	450	0.100
0.220	0.130	1.90	0.011	0.435	6.60	0.250	0	0.110	16.0	0.132	2.60	28.0	94.0	70.0	30.4	3.00	1.08
0.115	0.066	0.850	0.004	0	0.800	0.039	0	0.055	15.0	0.055	0.700	8.50	31.0	39.0	8.00	124	0.245
0.060	0.070	0.500	0.023	0.054	3.70	0.110	0.001	1.32	27.0	0.016	0.500	6.90	38.0	33.0	2.43	115	0.226

GRAIN, BREADS, CEREALS (continued)

Qty	Name	Wgt G	Wtr G	Cal	Prot G	Carb G	Fiber G	F-Tot G	F-Sat G	Mono G	Poly G	Chol Mg	A-Car RE	A-Pre RE	A-Tot RE
1 ea.	Pancakes-plain-from/mix	27.0	14.6	60.0	2.00	8.00	0.720	2.00	0.500	0.900	0.500	16.0	1.00	6.00	7.00
1 ea.	Whole wheat pancakes-5 in	52.0	29.6	94.0	3.65	14.1	1.80	2.79	0.775	1.01	0.737	30.1	0.600	24.7	25.3
1 cup	Popcorn-plain-air popped	8.00	0.320	30.0	1.00	6.00	1.45	0.400	0.064	0.180	0.155	0	1.00	0	1.00
1 cup	Popcorn-ckd in oil/salted	11.0	0.330	55.0	0.900	6.00	1.45	3.10	0.500	1.40	1.20	0	2.00	0	2.00
10 ea.	Pretzel-dutch twist	160	4.00	650	15.1	128	3.60	5.71	1.14	2.28	1.71	0	0	0	0
10 ea.	Pretzels-thin twists	60.0	1.80	240	6.00	48.0	1.34	2.00	0.400	0.800	0.600	0	0	0	0
10 ea.	Pretzels-thin sticks	3.00	0.075	10.0	0.283	2.40	0.067	0.107	0.019	0.038	0.038	0	0	0	0
1 pce	Raisin bread-25grm slice	25.0	8.25	68.0	1.90	13.2	0.600	0.990	0.226	0.358	0.370	0	0.050	0.020	0.070
1 pce	Raisin Bread toasted	21.0	5.04	68.0	1.90	13.0	0.600	0.990	0.226	0.358	0.370	0	0.050	0.020	0.070
1 cup	Brown rice-cooked	195	137	232	4.88	49.7	2.80	1.17	0.312	0.390	0.409	0	0	0	0
1 cup	White rice-converted-ckd	175	128	186	3.70	40.8	0.650	0.100	0.020	0.020	0.040	0	0	0	0
1 cup	White rice-regular-cooked	205	149	223	4.10	49.6	0.650	0.205	0.062	0.062	0.082	0	0	0	0
1 cup	White rice-instant-prepd	165	120	180	3.63	39.9	0.330	0.190	0.057	0.057	0.076	0	0	0	0
1 cup	Wild rice-cooked	200	152	184	7.20	38.0	5.12	0.400	0.106	0.094	0.140	0	0	0	0
1 ea.	Dinner rolls-commercial	28.0	9.04	85.0	2.00	14.0	0.760	2.00	0.500	0.800	0.600	0.001	0	0.300	0.300
1 ea.	Dinner roll-homemade	35.0	9.10	120	3.00	20.0	0.945	3.00	0.800	—	—	—	—	—	—
1 ea.	Hard roll white	50.0	12.5	155	5.00	30.0	0.830	2.00	0.400	0.500	0.600	0	0	0	0
1 ea.	Rye roll dark	28.4	10.5	79.0	2.53	14.1	1.00	1.47	0.366	0.519	0.469	0	0	0	0
1 ea.	Submarine roll/hoagie	135	41.8	400	11.0	72.0	2.24	8.00	1.80	3.00	2.20	0	0	0	0
1 ea.	Whole wheat roll	35.0	13.3	88.0	3.34	15.5	3.86	1.95	0.552	0.711	0.503	2.74	0	1.00	1.00
1 ea.	Rye roll dark	28.4	10.5	79.0	2.53	14.1	1.00	1.47	0.366	0.519	0.469	0	0	0	0
1 cup	Spaghetti-ckd firm-hot	130	82.7	190	6.50	39.1	1.04	0.650	0.091	0.078	0.273	0	0	0	0
1 cup	Spaghetti-ckd tender-hot	140	101	155	5.00	32.0	1.12	0.550	0.077	0.070	0.240	0	0	0	0
1 cup	Whole wheat spaghetti-ckd	123	82.9	151	6.64	32.5	3.75	0.492	0.069	0.057	0.232	0	0	0	0
1 cup	Stove Top stuffing-prep	216	144	352	—	41.4	—	17.8	10.0	—	1.40	42.0	0	214	214
1 ea.	Taco shell-13.6 gram size	13.6	0.544	59.0	1.11	9.40	0.880	2.72	0.247	0.742	1.48	0	0.600	0	0.600
1 oz.	Tortilla chips	28.3	1.13	141	2.23	17.0	0.405	7.59	1.08	3.12	3.09	0	0.709	0	0.709
1 ea.	Waffles homemade	75.0	27.6	245	6.90	25.7	1.60	12.6	4.00	4.90	2.60	102	1.50	37.5	39.0
1 ea.	Waffles-prepared from mix	75.0	31.5	205	6.90	27.0	1.60	8.00	2.70	2.90	1.50	59.0	1.00	48.0	49.0
1 ea.	Frozen waffle	35.0	14.0	98.0	2.03	14.6	0.103	3.30	1.11	1.20	0.619	20.0	0	131	131
1 cup	Rolled wheat-cooked	240	192	142	4.20	32.1	4.19	0.700	0.098	0.081	0.330	0	0	0	0
1 cup	Whole grain wheat-ckd	150	129	84.1	2.85	17.1	3.60	6.01	1.20	0.901	3.60	0	0	0	0
1 cup	Wheat-sprouted	106	47.1	236	7.97	48.4	6.07	1.42	0.200	0.164	0.672	0	6.40	0	6.40
5 ea.	Wheat cracker thin	10.0	0.300	43.8	1.12	6.25	0.750	1.75	0.625	0.625	0.500	0	0	0	0
1 grm	Whole grain wheat	1.000	0.100	3.30	0.131	0.704	0.100	0.026	0.004	0.003	0.012	0	0	0	0
1 cup	Whole grain wheat-ckd	150	129	84.1	2.85	17.1	3.60	6.01	1.20	0.901	3.60	0	0	0	0

HERBS AND SPICES

Qty	Name	Wgt G	Wtr G	Cal	Prot G	Carb G	Fiber G	F-Tot G	F-Sat G	Mono G	Poly G	Chol Mg	A-Car RE	A-Pre RE	A-Tot RE
1 tsp	Allspice	2.00	0.170	5.33	0.123	1.44	0.433	0.173	0.050	0.013	0.047	0	1.07	—	—
1 tsp	Basil - dried	1.50	0.096	3.67	0.217	0.913	0.267	0.060	—	—	—	0	14.1	0	14.1
1 tsp	Black pepper	2.13	0.224	5.43	0.234	1.38	0.280	0.070	0.028	0.029	0.033	0	0.400	0	0.400
1 tsp	Caraway seed	2.23	0.190	7.33	0.440	1.11	0.450	0.327	0.013	0.160	0.073	0	0.800	0	0.800
1 tsp	Cayenne/red pepper	1.77	0.143	5.67	0.213	1.000	0.800	0.307	0.057	0.050	0.147	0	73.7	0	73.7
1 tsp	Chili powder	2.50	0.195	8.00	0.307	1.37	0.557	0.420	0.100	0.100	0.200	0	87.3	0	87.3
1 tsp	Chives-fresh	1.000	0.920	0.333	0.013	0.043	0.007	0.003	0.001	0.001	0.002	0	4.67	0	4.67
1 tsp	Cinnamon	2.27	0.215	5.90	0.088	1.81	0.553	0.072	0.015	0.011	0.012	0	0.600	0	0.600
1 tsp	Cloves-ground	2.20	0.152	7.00	0.130	1.35	0.210	0.440	0.097	0.167	0.133	0	1.17	0	1.17
1 tsp	Cumin seed	2.00	0.162	7.33	0.357	0.883	0.210	0.447	—	—	—	0	2.53	0	2.53
1 tsp	Curry powder	2.10	0.199	6.00	0.267	1.22	0.343	0.290	0.017	0.227	0.030	0	2.07	0	2.07
1 tsp	Dill weed dried	1.03	0.075	2.67	0.207	0.577	0.123	0.047	—	—	—	0	—	—	—
1 ea.	Garlic cloves	3.00	1.76	4.47	0.191	0.992	0.050	0.015	0.003	0.000	0.007	0	0	0	0
1 tsp	Garlic powder	2.80	0.182	9.33	0.470	2.04	0.053	0.020	0.007	0.001	0.010	0	0	0	0
1 tsp	Ginger-ground	1.80	0.169	6.33	0.150	1.27	0.107	0.107	0.033	0.017	0.023	0	0.267	0	0.267
1 tsp	Marjoram-dried	0.567	0.043	1.67	0.070	0.343	0.103	0.040	—	—	—	0	4.57	0	4.57

B1 Mg	B2 Mg	B3 Mg	B6 Mg	B12 Mcg	Fol. Mcg	Panto Mg	Vit-C Mg	Vit-E Mg	Calc Mg	Cu Mg	Iron Mg	Mg Mg	Phos Mg	Potas Mg	Sel Mcg	Na Mg	Zinc Mg
0.090	0.120	0.800	0.010	0.054	3.00	0.084	0.001	0.300	36.0	0.016	0.700	6.90	71.0	43.0	2.43	160	0.226
0.093	0.088	0.726	0.307	0.174	9.02	0.295	0.232	1.30	51.6	0.071	0.817	22.4	95.0	102	12.8	150	0.519
0.030	0.010	0.200	0.016	0	3.00	—	0	—	1.00	0.022	0.200	23.0	22.0	20.0	1.04	0.500	0.223
0.010	0.020	0.100	0.016	0	3.00	—	0	—	3.00	0.033	0.270	25.0	31.0	19.0	1.04	86.0	0.285
0.500	0.400	7.01	0.030	0	26.0	0.480	0	1.23	41.6	0.230	3.15	38.4	150	160	53.0	2580	1.73
0.190	0.150	2.60	0.011	0	10.0	0.040	0	0.462	16.0	0.088	1.20	14.6	55.0	61.0	20.0	966	0.419
0.009	0.008	0.131	0.001	0	0.488	0.009	0	0.023	0.780	0.004	0.059	0.720	2.73	3.00	1.01	48.0	0.032
0.082	0.155	1.02	0.008	0	9.00	0.108	0.001	0.200	25.0	0.043	0.775	6.25	22.0	59.0	7.50	92.0	0.155
0.060	0.155	1.02	0.007	0	8.00	0.108	0.001	0.200	25.0	0.043	0.800	6.25	22.0	59.0	7.50	92.0	0.155
0.176	0.039	2.73	0.294	0	10.0	0.684	0	1.40	23.4	0.197	1.17	72.2	142	137	26.0	0	1.05
0.190	0.020	2.10	0.175	0	6.70	0.457	0	0.472	33.0	0.250	1.40	11.1	100	75.0	16.6	9.00	0.562
0.223	0.021	2.05	0.103	0	4.10	0.472	0	0.462	20.5	0.166	2.87	22.6	57.4	57.4	19.5	0	0.841
0.215	0.016	1.65	0.016	0	7.00	0.070	0	0.215	4.95	0.129	1.32	16.5	31.0	0	11.6	0	0.643
0.220	0.320	3.20	2.62	0	70.0	7.72	0	4.00	10.0	0.076	2.20	65.6	170	110	5.60	4.00	2.34
0.142	0.091	1.10	0.012	0	10.8	0.154	0.001	0.150	33.0	0.023	0.810	6.00	44.0	36.0	7.40	155	0.223
0.120	0.120	1.20	0.012	0	12.0	0.165	0	0.160	16.0	0.056	1.10	9.80	36.0	41.0	9.70	98.0	0.317
0.200	0.120	1.70	0.017	0	17.0	0.155	0	0.080	24.0	0.080	1.40	14.0	46.0	49.0	13.8	313	0.438
0.117	0.121	1.02	0.028	0	12.2	0.133	0	0.273	28.4	0.060	0.809	13.3	48.4	81.7	9.70	254	0.274
0.540	0.330	4.50	0.086	0	48.6	0.667	0	0.220	100	0.135	3.80	31.0	115	128	32.0	683	1.17
0.120	0.073	1.31	0.064	0.007	19.7	0.260	0.001	0.533	24.6	0.116	1.17	31.7	89.6	61.1	22.6	217	0.580
0.117	0.121	1.02	0.028	0	12.2	0.133	0	0.273	28.4	0.060	0.809	13.3	48.4	81.7	9.70	254	0.274
0.234	0.130	1.82	0.104	0	9.10	0.139	0	0.039	14.3	0.130	2.08	18.0	84.5	103	15.0	1.30	0.611
0.200	0.110	1.50	0.088	0	8.00	0.118	0	0.020	11.0	0.125	1.74	18.0	70.0	85.0	15.0	1.00	0.588
0.210	0.086	1.54	0.868	0	25.0	0.590	0	1.16	18.5	0.185	1.06	43.0	106	200	27.7	16.0	0.910
0.300	0.260	3.00	0.120	0.040	44.0	0.680	2.00	—	82.0	0.166	2.34	26.0	124	206	—	1264	0.544
0.001	0.012	0.247	0.027	0	2.20	0.025	0	0.247	26.0	0.002	0.258	8.60	33.0	25.0	1.20	62.0	0.216
0.010	0.020	0.202	0.081	0	0.515	0.015	0.001	1.06	83.0	0.111	1.01	22.3	74.9	30.4	2.58	142	0.425
0.180	0.240	1.50	0.031	0.100	13.0	0.242	0.001	2.20	154	0.053	1.50	16.5	135	129	13.5	445	0.652
0.140	0.230	0.900	0.029	0.100	4.00	0.242	0.001	2.20	179	0.062	1.20	14.0	257	146	13.7	515	0.515
0.154	0.185	1.85	0.093	0.050	1.00	0.124	0.001	1.00	29.0	0.021	1.70	7.30	134	73.0	3.06	242	0.288
0.170	0.070	2.20	0.078	0	27.0	0.365	0	1.24	19.0	0.500	1.70	58.0	182	202	20.0	2.00	1.96
0.120	0.030	1.20	0.093	0	18.0	0.300	0	1.06	9.01	0.150	0.901	35.1	90.1	87.1	18.3	3.00	1.32
0.246	0.177	3.35	0.289	0	44.0	1.13	3.00	2.50	31.0	0.286	2.37	90.0	222	188	34.4	18.0	1.83
0.050	0.037	0.500	0.012	0	3.75	—	0	—	3.75	—	0.375	8.75	18.8	21.3	0.600	86.2	0.300
0.005	0.001	0.043	0.005	0	0.730	0.014	0	0.046	0.410	0.007	0.032	1.60	3.68	3.70	0.565	0.030	0.061
0.120	0.030	1.20	0.093	0	18.0	0.300	0	1.06	9.01	0.150	0.901	35.1	90.1	87.1	18.3	3.00	1.32

B1 Mg	B2 Mg	B3 Mg	B6 Mg	B12 Mcg	Fol. Mcg	Panto Mg	Vit-C Mg	Vit-E Mg	Calc Mg	Cu Mg	Iron Mg	Mg Mg	Phos Mg	Potas Mg	Sel Mcg	Na Mg	Zinc Mg
0.002	0.001	0.057	—	0	—	—	0.783	—	13.3	—	0.141	2.67	2.33	21.0	0.060	1.67	0.020
0.002	0.005	0.104	—	0	—	—	0.920	—	31.7	0.020	0.630	6.13	7.33	51.3	—	0.667	0.087
0.002	0.005	0.024	0	0	—	—	0	—	9.33	0.024	0.617	4.00	3.67	27.0	0.107	1.000	0.030
0.009	0.008	0.081	—	0	—	—	—	—	15.3	0.028	0.363	5.67	12.7	30.3	0.201	0.333	0.124
0.006	0.016	0.154	—	0	—	—	1.35	—	2.67	—	0.138	2.67	5.33	35.7	—	0.667	0.044
0.009	0.020	0.197	—	0	1.25	—	1.60	—	7.00	—	0.357	4.50	7.67	48.0	0.747	25.3	0.068
0.001	0.001	0.004	0.002	0	—	—	0.433	—	0.667	—	0.013	—	0.333	2.00	—	—	—
0.002	0.003	0.029	0.020	0	—	—	0.647	—	28.0	0.005	0.867	1.27	1.37	11.3	0.340	0.600	0.045
0.003	0.006	0.032	—	0	—	1.78	—	14.3	0.001	0.227	5.93	2.33	24.3	—	—	5.33	0.093
0.013	0.007	0.092	—	0	—	—	0.153	—	18.7	—	1.33	7.33	10.00	35.7	—	3.33	0.096
0.005	0.006	0.073	—	0	—	0	0.240	—	10.00	0.022	0.620	5.33	7.33	32.3	—	1.000	0.087
0.004	0.003	0.029	0.015	0	—	—	—	0.017	16.7	0.005	0.500	4.33	5.33	36.7	—	2.00	0.033
0.006	0.003	0.021	0.100	0	0.092	—	0.935	0.000	5.42	0.008	0.051	0.750	4.60	12.0	0.747	0.510	0.265
0.013	0.004	0.019	0.567	0	1.67	—	0.003	0.001	2.33	0.021	0.077	1.67	11.7	31.0	1.77	0.667	0.074
0.001	0.003	0.093	—	0	0.333	—	0	—	2.00	0.009	0.207	3.33	2.67	22.7	—	0.667	0.083
0.002	0.002	0.023	—	0	—	—	0.290	—	12.0	0.006	0.470	2.00	1.67	8.67	—	0.333	0.020

HERBS AND SPICES (continued)

Qty	Name	Wgt G	Wtr G	Cal	Prot G	Carb G	Fiber G	F-Tot G	F-Sat G	Mono G	Poly G	Chol Mg	A-Car RE	A-Pre RE	A-Tot RE
1 tsp	Nutmeg-ground	2.33	0.145	12.3	0.137	1.15	0.093	0.847	0.607	0.077	0.007	0	0.233	0	0.233
1 tsp	Onion powder	2.17	0.108	5.00	0.220	1.75	0.123	0.023	0.005	0.004	0.010	0	0	0	0
1 tsp	Oregano-ground	1.50	0.105	4.67	0.167	0.967	0.223	0.153	0.040	0.010	0.080	0	10.4	0	10.4
1 tsp	Paprika	2.30	0.218	6.67	0.340	1.28	0.480	0.297	0.017	0.017	0.200	0	139	0	139
1 tsp	Parsley-freeze dried	0.117	0.002	0.333	0.037	0.049	0.047	0.006	0.001	0.000	0.003	0	7.42	0	7.42
1 tsp	Parsley-fresh-chopped	1.25	1.10	0.417	0.027	0.086	0.081	0.004	0.000	0.000	0.002	0	6.50	0	6.50
1 tsp	Poppyseed	2.93	0.199	15.7	0.530	0.697	0.183	1.31	0.143	0.187	0.903	0	0	0	0
1 tsp	Pumpkin pie spice	1.87	0.159	6.33	0.107	1.29	0.277	0.237	—	—	—	0	0.500	0	0.500
1 tsp	Rosemary-dried	1.10	0.102	3.67	0.053	0.703	0.193	0.167	—	—	—	0	3.43	0	3.43
1 tsp	Sage-ground	0.667	0.053	2.00	0.070	0.407	0.120	0.083	0.047	0.013	0.013	0	3.93	0	3.93
1 tsp	Salt	5.50	0	0	0	0	0	0	0	0	0	0	0	0	0
1 tsp	Salt substitute-Morton	2.00	0	0	0	0.033	0	0	0	0	0	0	0	0	0
1 tsp	Light salt-Morton	6.00	0	0	0	0	0	0	0	0	0	0	0	0	0
1 ea.	No-salt pkt-Norclf Thayer	0.750	0	0	0	0	0	0	0	0	0	0	0	0	0
1 tsp	Tarragon-ground	1.60	0.123	4.67	0.363	0.803	0.120	0.117	—	—	—	0	6.73	0	6.73
1 tsp	Thyme-ground	1.43	0.112	4.00	0.130	0.917	0.267	0.107	0.040	0.007	0.017	0	5.43	0	5.43
1 tsp	Turmeric-ground	2.27	0.258	8.00	0.177	1.47	0.153	0.223	—	—	—	0	0.033	0	0.033
1 tsp	White pepper	2.37	0.270	7.00	0.247	1.62	0.103	0.050	0.021	0.021	0.024	0	0.000	0	0.000

LEGUMES, NUTS, SEEDS

Qty	Name	Wgt G	Wtr G	Cal	Prot G	Carb G	Fiber G	F-Tot G	F-Sat G	Mono G	Poly G	Chol Mg	A-Car RE	A-Pre RE	A-Tot RE
1 cup	Almonds-dried-chopped	130	5.75	766	25.9	26.5	9.60	67.9	6.43	44.1	14.2	0	0	0	0
1 cup	Almonds-dried-sliced	94.0	4.15	554	18.8	19.2	7.03	49.1	4.65	31.9	10.3	0	0	0	0
1 cup	Almonds-dried-whole	142	6.28	837	28.3	29.0	10.8	74.1	7.03	48.2	15.6	0	0	0	0
1 cup	Almonds-dry rstd-salted	138	4.14	810	22.5	33.4	11.3	71.2	6.75	46.2	15.0	0	0	0	0
1 cup	Almonds-oil rstd-salted	157	4.71	970	32.0	24.9	11.2	90.5	8.58	58.8	19.0	0	0	0	0
1 Tbs	Almond butter-plain	15.6	0.156	98.9	2.36	3.31	0.762	9.25	0.875	6.00	1.94	0	0	0	0
1 cup	Black beans-cooked	171	113	225	15.0	41.0	15.4	0.800	0.100	0.100	0.500	0	1.00	0	1.00
1 cup	Red kidney beans-dry-ckd	185	126	226	15.1	41.1	15.0	0.930	0.107	0.107	0.640	0	1.00	0	1.00
1 cup	Lima beans-dry-cooked	190	122	260	16.1	49.0	10.3	0.944	0.202	0.070	0.472	0	0	0	0
1 cup	Navy beans-dry-cooked	190	131	225	15.0	40.0	13.0	1.12	0.100	0.100	0.700	0	0	0	0
1 cup	Pinto beans-dry-cooked	180	119	265	15.0	49.0	19.5	0.800	0.100	0.100	0.500	0	1.00	0	1.00
1 cup	Refried beans-canned	290	209	295	18.0	51.0	22.0	3.00	0.400	0.600	1.40	0	0	0	0
1 cup	Soybeans-dry-cooked	180	128	235	19.8	19.5	2.90	10.2	1.30	1.90	5.30	0	5.00	0	5.00
1 cup	White beans-dry-cooked	185	128	218	14.5	39.0	14.1	1.12	0.136	0.083	0.650	0	0	0	0
1 cup	Black-eyed peas-ckd f/dry	250	200	190	12.8	34.5	10.8	0.800	0.314	0.052	0.410	0	3.00	0	3.00
1 cup	Black walnuts-chopped	125	5.45	759	30.4	15.1	10.6	70.7	4.54	15.9	46.9	0	37.0	0	37.0
1 cup	Brazil nuts-dry-unsalted	140	4.68	919	20.1	17.9	12.5	92.7	22.6	32.2	33.8	0	0.100	0	0.100
1 cup	Filberts/hazelnuts-whole	135	7.32	853	17.6	20.7	9.20	84.5	6.20	66.3	8.10	0	9.00	0	9.00
1 Tbs	Caraway seed	6.70	0.569	22.0	1.32	3.34	1.35	0.980	0.040	0.480	0.220	0	2.40	0	2.40
1 cup	Cashews-dry rstd-salted	137	2.33	787	21.0	44.8	8.10	63.5	12.6	37.4	10.7	0	0	0	0
1 cup	Cashews-dry rstd-unsalted	137	2.33	787	21.0	44.8	8.10	63.5	12.6	37.4	10.7	0	0	0	0
1 cup	Cashews-oil rstd-salted	130	5.07	748	21.0	37.1	8.00	62.7	12.4	36.9	10.6	0	0	0	0
1 Tbs	Cashew butter	16.0	0.480	94.0	2.81	4.41	0.850	7.91	1.56	4.66	1.34	0	0	0	0
1 Tbs	Celery seed	6.00	0.362	25.5	1.17	2.69	0.780	1.64	0.141	1.03	0.243	0	0.300	0	0.300
1 cup	Chestnuts-roasted	143	57.9	350	4.53	75.7	18.5	3.15	0.592	1.09	1.24	0	3.50	0	3.50
1 pce	Coconut-raw piece-2.5x2in	45.0	21.1	159	1.50	6.85	6.12	15.1	13.4	0.641	0.165	0	0	0	0
1 cup	Coconut-grated-fresh	80.0	37.6	283	2.66	12.2	11.2	26.8	23.8	1.14	0.293	0	0	0	0
1 cup	Coconut shredded/swtd pkg	93.0	11.7	466	2.68	44.3	14.5	33.0	29.3	1.41	0.361	0	0	0	0
1 Tbs	Coriander seed	5.00	0.445	15.0	0.620	2.75	1.46	0.890	0.050	0.680	0.090	0	0	0	0
1 Tbs	Cumin seed	6.00	0.486	22.0	1.07	2.65	0.630	1.34	—	—	—	0	7.60	0	7.60
1 cup	Filberts/hazelnuts-chpd	115	6.23	727	15.0	17.6	7.40	72.0	5.30	56.5	6.90	0	7.70	0	7.70
1 cup	Garbanzo/chickpeas cooked	163	97.8	270	15.0	45.0	8.63	3.75	0.400	0.900	1.90	0	4.10	0	4.10
1 cup	Great northern beans-ckd	180	124	210	14.0	38.2	11.9	1.10	0.140	0.140	0.640	0	0	0	0
1 oz.	Hickory nuts	28.3	0.751	187	3.60	5.17	0.918	18.3	2.00	9.60	6.22	0	—	—	—

B1 Mg	B2 Mg	B3 Mg	B6 Mg	B12 Mcg	Fol. Mcg	Panto Mg	Vit-C Mg	Vit-E Mg	Calc Mg	Cu Mg	Iron Mg	Mg Mg	Phos Mg	Potas Mg	Sel Mcg	Na Mg	Zinc Mg
0.008	0.001	0.030	—	0	—	—	—	—	4.33	0.023	0.070	4.33	5.00	8.00	0.267	0.333	0.050
0.009	0.001	0.014	0.033	0	3.00	0.032	0.317	—	8.00	0.067	0.057	2.67	7.00	20.0	—	1.000	0.050
0.005	—	0.093	—	0	—	—	1.000	—	23.7	—	0.660	4.00	3.00	25.0	—	0.333	0.067
0.015	0.040	0.353	—	0	—	—	1.63	0.188	4.07	0.014	0.543	4.27	8.00	54.0	0.253	0.767	0.093
0.001	0.003	0.012	0.002	0	1.79	0.003	0.175	0.017	0.167	0.000	0.062	0.417	0.667	7.33	0.007	0.417	0.007
0.001	0.001	0.009	0.002	0	2.29	0.004	1.12	0.021	1.62	0.001	0.077	0.542	0.500	6.71	0.006	0.500	0.009
0.025	0.005	0.029	0.013	0	—	—	0	0.323	42.3	0.063	0.276	9.67	25.0	20.7	—	0.667	0.300
0.002	0.003	0.102	—	0	—	—	0.437	—	12.7	—	0.367	2.53	2.33	12.3	—	1.000	0.044
0.006	—	0.011	—	0	—	—	0.673	—	14.0	0.001	0.322	2.43	0.667	11.0	—	0.667	0.036
0.005	0.002	0.038	—	0	—	—	0.217	—	11.0	0.005	0.187	3.00	0.667	7.00	—	0	0.031
0	0	0	0	0	0	0	0	0	14.0	0.001	0.006	1.80	3.00	0.333	—	2132	0.021
0	0	0	0	0	0	0	0	0	10.00	0	0	0	9.33	933	—	0	0
0	0	0	0	0	0	0	0	0	3.00	0	0	4.00	0	1500	—	1100	0
0	0	0	0	0	0	0	0	0	—	—	—	—	—	385	—	0	—
0.004	0.021	0.143	—	0	—	—	—	—	18.3	0.014	0.517	5.67	5.00	48.3	0.033	1.000	0.062
0.007	0.006	0.071	—	0	—	—	—	—	27.0	0.013	1.77	3.00	3.00	11.7	0.100	0.667	0.089
0.003	0.005	0.117	—	0	0.407	—	0.587	—	4.00	—	0.940	4.33	6.00	57.3	—	1.000	0.100
0.001	0.003	0.005	—	0	—	—	—	—	6.33	—	0.340	2.00	4.00	1.67	—	0.003	0.027

B1 Mg	B2 Mg	B3 Mg	B6 Mg	B12 Mcg	Fol. Mcg	Panto Mg	Vit-C Mg	Vit-E Mg	Calc Mg	Cu Mg	Iron Mg	Mg Mg	Phos Mg	Potas Mg	Sel Mcg	Na Mg	Zinc Mg
0.274	1.01	4.37	0.147	0	76.3	0.612	0.780	27.6	346	1.23	4.76	384	676	952	5.20	14.3	3.80
0.198	0.732	0.316	0.106	0	55.2	0.443	0.564	20.0	250	0.886	3.44	278	489	688	3.76	10.0	2.75
0.300	1.11	4.77	0.160	0	83.3	0.669	0.850	30.2	378	1.34	5.20	420	738	1034	6.67	15.0	4.15
0.179	0.827	3.89	0.102	0	88.1	0.351	1.00	29.0	389	1.69	5.25	419	756	1063	5.52	1076	6.76
0.204	1.55	5.50	0.132	0	100	0.399	1.10	32.0	367	1.92	6.02	477	859	1073	6.28	1223	7.69
0.021	0.096	0.449	0.012	10.2	0	0.040	0.112	3.13	42.1	0.141	0.578	47.4	81.7	118	0.625	1.75	0.477
0.430	0.050	0.900	0.190	0	84.0	0.216	0	1.03	47.0	0.992	2.90	136	239	608	13.7	1.00	1.30
0.203	0.106	1.36	0.119	0	115	0.410	0.010	1.15	53.0	0.546	6.66	82.0	236	710	0.350	4.00	2.03
0.250	0.114	1.34	0.293	0	170	0.660	0	6.20	55.0	0.426	5.90	78.8	293	1163	4.60	4.01	2.08
0.268	0.130	1.27	0.724	0	108	0.842	0	2.05	95.0	0.627	5.10	89.1	281	790	6.50	13.0	2.01
0.330	0.160	0.700	0.330	0	137	0.407	0	0.900	86.0	0.474	5.40	93.0	296	882	10.8	3.00	2.20
0.140	0.160	1.40	3.25	0.141	106	0.606	17.0	1.45	141	0.789	5.10	171	245	1141	13.6	1228	3.43
0.385	0.155	1.15	0.500	0	76.0	0.491	0	11.8	132	1.21	4.90	1.40	321	972	4.70	4.00	2.11
0.263	0.130	1.27	0.705	0	105	0.502	0	2.00	93.0	0.576	5.00	81.0	273	770	3.12	13.0	1.90
0.400	0.100	1.00	0.140	0	142	0.415	0	—	43.0	0.800	3.30	117	238	573	47.0	20.0	3.22
0.271	0.136	0.863	0.698	0	82.5	0.789	1.00	3.15	72.5	1.28	3.84	253	580	655	22.0	1.30	4.28
1.40	0.171	2.27	0.351	0	5.60	0.330	1.00	10.7	246	2.48	4.76	315	840	840	1518	2.00	6.42
0.675	0.149	1.54	0.826	0	97.0	1.55	1.40	32.3	253	2.04	4.41	385	421	601	4.32	3.50	3.24
0.026	0.025	0.242	—	0	—	—	—	—	46.0	0.085	1.09	17.0	38.0	91.0	0.603	1.00	0.372
0.274	0.274	1.92	0.351	0	95.0	1.67	0	10.2	62.0	3.04	8.22	356	671	774	28.0	877	7.67
0.274	0.274	1.92	0.351	0	95.0	1.67	0	10.2	62.0	3.04	8.22	356	671	774	28.0	21.0	7.67
0.551	0.228	2.34	0.325	0	88.0	1.55	0	10.4	53.0	2.82	5.33	332	554	689	3.51	814	6.18
0.050	0.030	0.256	0.040	0	10.9	0.192	0	0.093	7.00	0.350	0.085	41.0	73.0	87.0	0.452	2.00	0.830
0.030	0.030	0.300	—	0	—	—	1.03	—	114	—	2.70	28.6	33.0	90.0	—	10.5	0.417
0.347	0.250	1.92	0.711	0	100	0.792	37.2	—	42.0	0.725	1.30	47.0	153	846	—	3.00	0.815
0.030	0.009	0.243	0.024	0	11.9	0.135	1.50	0.329	6.30	0.196	1.09	14.0	51.0	160	6.30	9.00	0.495
0.053	0.016	0.432	0.043	0	21.1	0.240	2.60	0.560	12.0	0.348	1.94	26.0	90.0	285	11.2	16.0	0.880
0.029	0.019	0.441	0.289	0	8.90	0.754	0.600	0	14.0	0.291	1.79	47.0	100	313	12.0	244	1.69
0.012	0.014	0.106	—	0	—	—	—	—	35.0	—	0.816	17.0	20.0	63.0	—	2.00	0.235
0.038	0.020	0.275	—	0	—	—	0.460	—	56.0	—	3.98	22.0	30.0	107	—	10.0	0.288
0.575	0.127	1.31	0.704	0	82.6	1.32	1.20	27.5	216	1.74	3.76	328	359	512	3.68	3.00	2.76
0.180	0.095	0.900	0.386	0	108	0.748	0	1.92	85.0	0.766	5.30	77.0	291	503	—	11.0	2.84
0.250	0.130	1.30	0.398	0	74.0	0.555	0	1.95	90.0	0.558	4.90	76.0	266	749	3.76	13.0	1.72
—	—	—	0		—	—	—	—	17.0	0.210	0.599	48.9	94.8	124		0	1.22

LEGUMES, NUTS, SEEDS (continued)

Qty	Name	Wgt G	Wtr G	Cal	Prot G	Carb G	Fiber G	F-Tot G	F-Sat G	Mono G	Poly G	Chol Mg	A-Car RE	A-Pre RE	A-Tot RE
1 cup	Lentils-dry-cooked	200	144	215	16.0	38.0	8.70	0.800	0.100	0.200	0.500	0	4.00	0	4.00
1 cup	Macadamias-dried	134	3.86	940	11.1	18.4	7.00	98.8	14.8	78.0	1.70	0	1.20	0	1.20
1 cup	Macadamias-oilrstd-salted	134	2.24	962	9.73	17.3	7.00	103	15.4	80.9	1.77	0	1.20	0	1.20
1 cup	Mxd nuts rstd-salted	137	2.40	814	23.7	34.7	11.0	70.5	9.45	43.0	14.8	0	2.10	0	2.10
1 cup	Mxd nuts-oil rstd-salted	142	2.88	876	23.8	30.4	11.4	80.0	12.4	45.0	18.9	0	2.80	0	2.80
1 cup	Mxd nuts-oil rstd-unsaltd	142	2.88	876	23.8	30.4	11.4	80.0	12.4	45.0	18.9	0	2.80	0	2.80
1 Tbs	Peanut butter-unsalted	16.1	0.322	95.3	4.59	2.56	1.15	8.25	1.38	4.00	2.50	0	0	0	0
1 Tbs	Peanut butter-regular	16.1	0.322	95.3	4.59	2.56	1.15	8.25	1.38	4.00	2.50	0	0	0	0
1 cup	Peanuts-raw with skins	149	8.36	842	37.6	26.9	12.1	70.9	10.3	36.7	23.4	0	2.39	0	2.39
1 cup	Peanuts-dried-unsalted	146	9.71	827	37.5	23.6	12.7	71.8	9.96	35.6	22.7	0	0	0	0
1 cup	Peanuts-oil rstd-salted	145	2.90	841	38.8	26.8	12.7	71.3	9.93	35.5	22.6	0	0	0	0
1 cup	Peanuts-oil rstd-unsalted	145	2.90	841	38.8	26.8	12.7	71.3	9.93	35.5	22.6	0	0	0	0
1 cup	Black-eyed peas-ckd f/dry	250	200	190	12.8	34.5	10.8	0.800	0.314	0.052	0.410	0	3.00	0	3.00
1 cup	Peas-split-dry-cooked	200	141	230	16.0	42.0	9.80	0.600	0.250	0.100	0.300	0	8.00	0	8.00
1 cup	Pecans-dried-chopped	119	5.71	794	9.22	21.7	7.20	80.5	6.45	50.2	20.0	0	15.2	0	15.2
1 cup	Pecans-dried-halves	108	5.18	720	8.37	19.7	6.54	73.1	5.85	45.6	18.1	0	13.8	0	13.8
1 cup	Pecans dry rstd-salted	118	1.30	779	9.42	26.4	7.17	76.7	6.12	47.9	19.0	0	14.6	0	14.6
1 cup	Pecans oil rstd-salted	110	4.62	754	7.65	17.7	6.66	78.3	6.28	48.8	19.4	0	3.50	0	3.50
1 oz.	Pine nuts-pignola-dried	28.3	1.90	146	6.81	4.03	0.499	14.4	2.21	5.41	6.05	0	0	0	0
1 oz.	Pine nuts-pinyon-dried	28.3	1.67	161	3.28	5.47	2.07	17.3	2.64	6.51	7.29	0	0.799	0	0.799
1 cup	Pistachios-dried-noshells	128	4.95	739	26.3	31.8	6.38	61.9	7.85	41.9	9.37	0	30.0	0	30.0
1 cup	Pistachios-dry rst-salted	128	2.69	776	19.1	35.2	7.06	67.6	8.56	45.7	10.3	0	29.7	0	29.7
1 Tbs	Poppyseed	8.80	0.598	47.0	1.59	2.09	0.550	3.93	0.430	0.560	2.71	0	0	0	0
1 Tbs	Pumpkin kernls-dry-unsltd	8.62	0.597	46.7	2.12	1.54	0.469	3.96	0.750	1.23	1.81	0	3.28	0	3.28
1 Tbs	Pumpkin kernls-rst-sltd	14.2	1.01	74.1	4.68	1.91	0.563	5.98	1.13	1.86	2.72	0	5.51	0	5.51
1 Tbs	Sesame seed kernals-dried	9.38	0.451	55.1	2.47	0.881	0.644	5.14	0.719	1.94	2.25	0	0.063	0	0.063
1 cup	Soybeans-dry-cooked	180	128	235	19.8	19.5	2.90	10.2	1.30	1.90	5.30	0	5.00	0	5.00
1 Tbs	Sunflower seed butter	16.0	0.197	92.7	3.15	4.39	1.10	7.64	0.800	1.46	5.04	0	0.800	0	0.800
1 Tbs	Sunflower seeds-dry	9.00	0.482	51.3	2.05	1.69	0.756	4.46	0.467	0.850	2.95	0	0.450	0	0.450
1 Tbs	Sunflower seeds-dry rst	8.00	0.096	46.6	1.55	1.92	0.675	3.98	0.417	0.762	2.63	0	0.394	0	0.394
1 Tbs	Sunflower seeds-oil rst	8.44	0.219	51.9	1.80	1.24	0.625	4.85	0.508	0.925	3.20	0	0.394	0	0.394
1 cup	Black walnuts-chopped	125	5.45	759	30.4	15.1	10.6	70.7	4.54	15.9	46.9	0	37.0	0	37.0
1 cup	English walnuts-chopped	120	4.38	770	17.2	22.0	8.40	74.2	6.70	17.0	47.0	0	14.8	0	14.8

MEAT AND RELATED PRODUCTS—BEEF

Qty	Name	Wgt G	Wtr G	Cal	Prot G	Carb G	Fiber G	F-Tot G	F-Sat G	Mono G	Poly G	Chol Mg	A-Car RE	A-Pre RE	A-Tot RE
3 oz.	Beef chuck-pot rstd ln&ft	85.0	36.6	325	22.0	0	0	26.0	10.8	11.7	0.901	87.1	0	3.00	3.00
3 oz.	Beef chuck-pot rstd lean	85.0	45.1	233	25.9	0	0	12.3	5.35	5.76	0.411	90.6	0	2.00	2.00
3 oz.	Beef round-pot rstd ln&ft	85.0	45.9	220	25.0	0	0	13.0	4.80	5.70	0.500	81.0	0	2.40	2.40
3 oz.	Beef round-pot rstd lean	85.0	48.5	191	27.3	0	0	8.72	2.94	3.71	0.327	81.8	0	1.09	1.09
3 oz.	Ground beef (10% fat)	85.0	47.6	230	21.0	0	0	16.0	6.20	6.90	0.600	74.0	0	1.00	1.00
3 oz.	Ground beef (21% fat)	85.0	45.9	245	20.0	0	0	17.8	6.90	7.70	0.700	76.0	0	1.00	1.00
1 oz.	Beef-thin sliced lunchmt	28.3	19.8	35.1	6.20	0.081	0	0.891	0.364	0.391	0.040	12.1	0	0	0
3 oz.	Beef rib-oven rst-ln&fat	85.0	39.1	315	19.0	0	0	26.0	10.8	11.4	0.901	72.0	0	3.00	3.00
3 oz.	Beef rib-oven rst-ln only	85.0	48.5	209	24.0	0	0	12.5	5.02	5.16	0.418	68.0	0	2.00	2.00
3 oz.	Beef round-oven rst-ln&ft	85.0	48.5	205	23.0	0	0	12.0	4.90	5.40	0.500	62.0	0	2.40	2.40
3 oz.	Beef rump roast-lean&fat	85.0	48.5	205	23.0	0	0	12.0	4.90	5.40	0.500	62.0	0	4.00	4.00
3 oz.	Beef rump roast-lean only	85.0	53.6	153	25.2	0	0	5.67	2.15	2.38	0.227	58.9	0	2.00	2.00
3 oz.	Sirloin steak-lean & fat	85.0	45.1	240	23.0	0	0	15.0	6.40	6.90	0.600	77.0	0	5.00	5.00
3 oz.	Sirloin steak-lean part	85.0	50.2	177	26.0	0	0	7.09	3.07	3.31	0.354	75.6	0	4.72	4.72
3 oz.	T-bone steak-lean & fat	85.0	45.1	401	16.7	0	0	36.6	15.6	16.8	1.47	65.5	0	6.90	6.90
3 oz.	T-bone steak-lean part	85.0	50.2	189	25.7	0	0	18.4	7.99	8.61	0.922	83.0	0	3.07	3.07
3 oz.	Beef liver fried	85.0	47.6	185	23.0	7.00	0	7.00	2.50	3.60	1.30	410	0	9125	9125
3 oz.	Corned beef-canned	85.0	50.2	185	22.0	0	0	10.0	4.20	4.90	0.400	80.0	0	6.00	6.00
.5 cup	Corned beef hash-canned	110	74.1	101	9.10	10.9	0.595	5.00	2.12	2.45	0.229	66.0	0	0	0

0.140	0.120	1.12	0.220	0	64.0	0.620	0	1.16	50.0	0.500	4.20	60.0	238	498	6.63	26.0	2.30
0.469	0.147	2.87	0.381	0	91.0	1.23	0	22.0	94.0	0.397	3.23	155	182	493	—	7.00	2.29
0.285	0.146	2.71	0.333	0	79.0	1.08	0	19.0	60.0	0.402	2.41	157	268	441	—	348	1.47
0.274	0.274	6.44	0.406	0	69.0	1.65	0.600	11.0	96.0	1.75	5.07	308	596	817	31.5	917	5.21
0.707	0.315	7.19	0.341	0	118	1.77	0.700	11.0	153	2.36	4.56	334	659	825	11.5	926	7.22
0.707	0.315	7.19	0.341	0	118	1.77	0.700	11.0	153	2.36	4.56	334	659	825	11.5	16.0	7.22
0.024	0.017	2.17	0.063	0	13.2	0.148	0	1.03	5.31	0.094	0.292	28.2	60.3	110	1.37	2.75	0.471
0.024	0.017	2.17	0.063	0	13.2	0.148	0	1.16	5.31	0.094	0.292	28.2	60.3	110	1.38	65.0	0.471
1.70	0.194	25.7	0.597	0	161	3.13	0	24.5	94.0	1.06	3.13	270	493	1037	10.4	11.9	4.63
0.969	0.191	20.7	0.432	0	153	4.04	0	14.6	85.0	1.46	4.72	263	559	1047	10.8	23.0	4.78
0.425	0.146	21.5	0.577	0	153	3.03	0	14.5	125	1.85	2.78	273	734	1020	10.7	626	9.60
0.425	1.46	21.5	0.577	0	153	3.03	0	14.5	125	1.85	2.78	273	734	1020	10.8	22.0	9.60
0.400	0.100	1.00	0.140	0	142	0.415	0	—	43.0	0.800	3.30	117	238	573	47.0	20.0	3.22
0.280	0.180	1.80	0.133	0	16.0	0.770	0	1.55	23.0	0.440	3.40	70.0	178	592	19.0	26.0	1.91
1.01	0.152	1.06	0.224	0	46.6	2.03	2.31	3.70	43.0	1.41	2.53	152	346	466	6.06	1.10	6.51
0.916	0.138	0.958	0.203	0	42.3	1.84	2.16	3.40	39.0	1.28	2.30	138	314	423	5.50	1.00	5.91
0.375	0.146	1.07	0.208	0	48.3	2.07	2.43	3.68	41.7	1.46	2.58	158	358	437	13.8	921	6.71
0.335	0.123	0.875	0.180	0	38.0	0.454	0.532	3.42	37.0	1.32	2.32	156	323	395	110	832	6.05
0.230	0.054	1.01	0.080	0	19.2	0.256	0.599	1.70	7.39	0.290	2.61	66.9	144	170	—	0.998	1.21
0.352	0.063	1.24	0.080	0	19.2	0.256	0.599	1.70	2.30	0.293	0.868	66.9	9.98	178	—	20.0	1.22
1.05	0.223	1.38	0.270	0	74.2	0.900	0	6.67	173	1.52	8.68	2.20	644	1399	12.6	7.70	1.72
0.541	0.315	1.80	0.270	0	74.0	0.900	0	6.35	90.0	1.55	4.06	166	609	1242	12.6	998	1.74
0.075	0.015	0.086	0.040	0	—	—	0	0.968	127	0.189	0.827	29.0	75.0	62.0	—	2.00	0.900
0.018	0.028	0.151	0.008	0	4.94	0.007	0.000	0.938	3.69	0.120	1.29	46.1	101	69.6	—	1.56	0.644
0.016	0.041	0.225	0.013	0	7.19	0.012	0	1.00	6.10	0.196	2.12	75.7	163	114	—	81.6	1.06
0.067	0.008	0.439	0.074	0	9.38	0.064	0	0.216	12.3	—	0.731	32.6	72.7	38.2	—	3.69	0.962
0.385	0.155	1.15	0.500	0	76.0	0.491	0	11.8	132	1.21	4.90	1.40	321	972	4.70	4.00	2.11
0.047	0.041	0.851	0.176	0	34.0	0.190	0.430	4.72	19.5	0.293	0.760	59.0	118	12.0	9.77	0.480	0.847
0.206	0.022	0.405	0.114	0	21.2	0.126	0.001	1.82	10.4	0.157	0.609	31.9	63.4	62.0	0.250	0.250	0.456
0.008	0.020	0.564	0.087	0	17.0	0.095	0.100	2.32	5.63	0.146	0.304	10.3	92.4	68.0	5.84	0.237	0.423
0.027	0.024	0.349	0.101	0	19.7	0.111	0.119	2.69	4.75	0.152	0.566	10.7	96.1	40.7	6.13	0.250	0.440
0.271	0.136	0.863	0.698	0	82.5	0.789	1.00	3.15	72.5	1.28	3.84	253	580	655	22.0	1.30	4.28
0.458	0.178	1.25	0.670	0	79.2	0.757	3.84	4.00	113	1.65	2.93	203	380	602	8.88	12.0	3.28

0.060	0.190	2.00	0.255	2.61	4.00	0.609	0	0.108	11.0	0.212	2.50	12.8	163	163	23.6	53.0	5.09
0.068	0.961	2.33	0.255	2.87	4.00	0.719	0	0.123	11.0	0.212	3.15	15.3	200	223	27.5	60.0	5.11
0.060	0.210	3.30	0.340	2.80	4.00	0.730	0	0.367	5.00	0.139	2.80	22.0	217	248	23.0	43.0	5.12
0.065	0.218	3.27	0.349	2.85	4.00	0.720	0	0.246	4.36	0.142	2.94	22.9	231	262	25.1	43.6	5.45
0.040	0.180	4.40	0.238	2.60	3.40	0.340	0	0.535	9.01	0.106	1.80	21.2	134	256	14.4	65.0	4.90
0.030	0.160	4.90	0.238	2.60	3.42	0.340	0	0.536	9.01	0.090	2.10	20.4	144	248	14.3	70.0	5.10
0.023	0.054	1.50	0.094	0.729	1.62	0.162	0	0.027	3.64	0.027	0.607	5.40	47.2	116	2.70	470	1.13
0.060	0.160	3.10	0.204	1.72	4.00	0.482	0	0.204	8.00	0.136	2.00	17.0	145	246	20.1	54.0	4.93
0.070	0.181	3.76	0.280	1.69	4.00	0.520	0	0.161	7.00	0.144	2.40	23.8	177	375	21.7	63.0	5.13
0.070	0.140	3.00	0.258	2.62	3.70	0.663	0	0.324	5.00	0.110	1.60	21.0	177	308	20.0	50.0	5.60
0.070	0.140	3.00	0.204	2.16	4.00	0.431	0	0.187	5.00	0.110	1.60	23.8	177	308	23.6	50.0	4.93
0.079	0.147	3.17	0.280	2.84	4.00	0.719	0	0.153	3.40	0.119	1.70	24.7	193	337	27.5	52.0	5.04
0.100	0.230	3.30	0.294	2.77	3.00	0.474	0	0.590	9.01	0.153	2.60	21.0	186	306	18.0	53.0	4.93
0.106	0.260	3.66	0.280	2.35	7.09	0.719	0	0.390	9.45	0.161	2.83	23.6	208	343	20.1	56.7	5.60
0.067	0.137	3.48	0.228	1.13	1.43	0.301	0	0.695	6.90	0.006	2.21	17.8	141	185	16.7	40.2	2.99
0.079	0.195	4.97	0.319	1.53	2.54	0.513	0	0.465	10.2	0.101	2.66	24.6	205	288	16.9	63.5	5.32
0.180	3.52	12.3	0.312	87.1	150	4.85	23.0	1.38	9.01	2.19	5.30	21.6	392	309	40.8	90.1	5.19
0.020	0.200	2.90	0.089	1.63	5.30	0.340	0	0.663	17.0	0.204	3.70	12.7	90.1	51.0	4.67	802	3.70
0.061	0.201	2.30	0.205	0.770	7.35	0.320	4.00	0.044	14.5	0.158	2.20	1.50	73.5	220	2.10	677	2.19

MEAT AND RELATED PRODUCTS—BEEF (continued)

Qty	Name	Wgt G	Wtr G	Cal	Prot G	Carb G	Fiber G	F-Tot G	F-Sat G	Mono G	Poly G	Chol Mg	A-Car RE	A-Pre RE	A-Tot RE
1 oz.	Beef-dried-chipped	28.3	13.6	57.1	9.45	0	0	1.57	0.709	0.787	0.079	18.1	0	0.118	0.118
1 cup	Beef & veg stew-recipe	245	201	220	16.0	15.0	3.40	11.0	4.40	4.50	0.500	71.0	569	0	569
1 cup	Beef stew canned	245	202	194	14.2	17.8	1.30	7.60	3.10	3.11	0.350	15.0	262	0	262
1 ea.	Burrito-beef & bean	175	955	390	21.0	40.0	5.00	17.5	6.80	6.72	2.29	52.0	17.6	40.1	57.7
1 ea.	Beef & bean tostada-fancy	192	129	332	18.4	20.2	3.95	20.7	9.38	7.15	2.61	61.6	54.4	77.4	132
1 cup	Beef+macaroni+tom sce-rec	226	181	189	10.0	25.2	2.32	5.78	2.10	2.33	0.413	22.4	111	0	111
2 oz.	Sandwich spread-pork&beef	56.7	34.2	132	4.35	6.77	0	9.83	3.40	4.31	1.44	22.7	0	3.78	3.78
1 ea.	Beef Enchilada	120	78.5	292	13.1	15.6	1.97	13.8	5.27	5.13	2.24	37.8	41.1	41.3	82.4
1 ea.	Frankfurter-beef-2oz each	57.0	30.8	184	6.43	1.36	0	16.8	6.82	8.18	0.660	27.0	0	0	0
1 ea.	Frankfurter-bf&prk-2oz ea	57.0	30.7	183	6.43	1.46	0	16.6	6.13	7.79	1.56	29.0	0	0	0
1 Tbs	Beef gravy-homemade	16.9	14.5	18.9	0.272	0.749	0.029	1.60	0.790	0.577	0.068	1.08	0	0	0
1 ea.	Beef pot pie fr/frozen	234	129	426	16.4	39.4	0.900	22.5	5.93	9.70	5.60	41.0	136	51.0	187
1 ea.	Beef taco	78.0	40.6	207	13.6	10.1	1.12	13.2	4.85	4.88	1.91	44.5	6.76	20.5	27.3

MEAT AND RELATED PRODUCTS—CHICKEN

Qty	Name	Wgt G	Wtr G	Cal	Prot G	Carb G	Fiber G	F-Tot G	F-Sat G	Mono G	Poly G	Chol Mg	A-Car RE	A-Pre RE	A-Tot RE
3 oz.	Chicken meat-all-fried	85.0	48.9	187	26.0	1.44	0.006	7.78	2.09	2.85	1.82	79.6	0	15.2	15.2
3 oz.	Chicken meat-all-roasted	85.0	54.3	162	24.6	0	0	6.32	1.74	2.26	1.44	75.9	0	13.4	13.4
3 oz.	Chicken meat-all-stewed	85.0	56.8	151	23.2	0	0	5.70	1.57	2.03	1.31	70.5	0	12.8	12.8
3 oz.	Boned chicken w/broth-cnd	85.0	58.4	141	18.5	0	0	6.77	1.87	2.68	1.49	52.7	0	28.7	28.7
3 oz.	Chicken-dark meat-roasted	85.0	53.7	174	23.3	0	0	8.26	2.26	3.03	1.93	79.0	0	18.2	18.2
3 oz.	Chicken-light meat-roastd	85.0	55.1	147	26.3	0	0	3.83	1.08	1.31	0.832	71.7	0	7.29	7.29
1 ea.	Chick breast+skin-batr fr	140	72.2	364	34.8	12.6	0.050	18.5	4.93	7.64	4.31	119	0	28.0	28.0
1 ea.	Chick breast+skin-roastd	98.0	61.2	193	29.2	0	0	7.63	2.15	2.97	1.63	83.0	0	26.0	26.0
1 ea.	Chick breast w/skin-stewd	220	146	404	60.2	0	0	16.3	4.58	6.38	3.48	166	0	52.0	52.0
1 ea.	Chick breast-noskin-fried	86.0	51.8	161	28.8	0.440	0	4.05	1.11	1.48	0.920	78.0	0	6.00	6.00
1 ea.	Chick breast-no skin-rstd	86.0	56.2	142	26.7	0	0	3.00	0.870	1.07	0.660	73.0	0	5.00	5.00
1 ea.	Chick breast meat-stewed	190	130	288	55.0	0	0	5.76	1.62	1.96	1.26	146	0	12.0	12.0
1 ea.	Chick drumstick-battr frd	72.0	38.0	193	15.8	6.00	0.020	11.3	2.98	4.63	2.73	62.0	0	19.0	19.0
1 ea.	Chick drumstick-roasted	52.0	32.6	112	14.1	0	0	5.80	1.58	2.21	1.30	48.0	0	15.0	15.0
1 ea.	Chick drum-meatonly-fried	42.0	26.1	82.0	12.0	0	0	3.39	0.890	1.24	0.830	40.0	0	8.00	8.00
1 ea.	Chick drum-no skin-rstd	44.0	29.3	76.0	12.5	0	0	2.49	0.650	0.820	0.600	41.0	0	8.00	8.00
1 ea.	Chick thigh+skin-battrfrd	86.0	44.3	238	18.6	7.80	0.030	14.2	3.79	5.77	3.36	80.0	0	25.0	25.0
1 ea.	Chick thigh+skin-roasted	62.0	36.8	153	15.5	0	0	9.60	2.86	3.81	2.12	58.0	0	30.0	30.0
1 ea.	Chick thigh-noskin-fried	52.0	30.8	113	14.6	0.610	0.010	5.36	1.45	1.99	1.26	53.0	0	11.0	11.0
1 ea.	Chick thigh-noskin-roastd	52.0	32.7	109	13.5	0	0	5.66	1.57	2.16	1.29	49.0	0	10.4	10.4
1 ea.	Chick wing-flour fried	32.0	15.6	103	8.36	0.760	0.010	7.09	1.94	2.84	1.58	26.0	0	12.0	12.0
1 ea.	Chick wing-roasted	34.0	18.7	99.0	9.13	0	0	6.63	1.85	2.60	1.41	29.0	0	16.0	16.0
1 ea.	Chick wing-noskin-fried	20.0	12.0	42.0	6.03	0	0.010	1.83	0.500	0.620	0.410	17.0	0	4.00	4.00
1 ea.	Chick wing-meat only-rstd	21.0	13.2	43.0	6.40	0	0	1.71	0.470	0.550	0.370	18.0	0	4.00	4.00
1 ea.	Chicken gizzards-simmered	22.0	14.8	34.0	6.00	0.250	0	0.806	0.229	0.204	0.234	42.6	0	12.0	12.0
1 ea.	Chicken hearts-simmered	3.30	2.14	6.00	0.872	0.003	0	0.260	0.074	0.066	0.076	8.00	0	0.270	0.270
1 ea.	Chicken livers-simmered	20.0	13.7	31.3	4.87	0.176	0	1.09	0.369	0.269	0.179	126	0	983	983
1 pce	Chicken roll light meat	28.5	19.6	45.0	5.55	0.695	0	2.09	0.575	0.840	0.455	14.0	0	7.00	7.00
1 ea.	Chicken frankfurter-45g	45.0	25.9	115	5.82	3.06	0	8.76	2.49	3.81	1.82	45.0	0	17.0	17.0
1 cup	Chicken a la king-frozen	224	152	255	25.0	8.00	1.33	14.0	5.30	5.50	2.60	50.0	20.0	144	164
1 cup	Chicken & noodles-frozen	260	185	289	19.9	22.8	0.200	12.0	3.40	4.73	2.60	73.3	0	135	135
1 cup	Chicken chow mein-canned	250	222	95.0	7.00	18.0	5.00	1.00	0.100	0.100	0.800	8.00	8.50	19.5	28.0
1 cup	Chicken curry-recipe	225	186	203	17.5	5.07	0.261	12.1	2.73	5.12	3.41	42.3	0.667	101	102
1 ea.	Chicken pot pie fr/frozen	230	131	430	14.9	41.2	1.70	23.0	7.60	11.5	4.90	40.0	113	3.00	116
0.5 cup	Chicken salad w/celery	78.0	40.9	266	10.5	1.29	0.300	24.5	4.06	7.22	12.0	47.5	1.90	28.8	30.6
1 ea.	Chicken patty sandwich	157	81.6	436	24.8	33.8	1.35	22.5	6.13	9.50	5.40	68.0	0	16.0	16.0
1 ea.	Tostada w/beans/chicken	157	105	249	19.4	18.7	3.70	11.4	4.37	3.54	2.85	53.1	33.8	46.7	80.5
1 ea.	Chicken taco	78.0	43.7	172	15.4	10.1	1.12	8.34	2.62	2.56	2.33	45.4	6.80	26.7	33.5
1 ea.	Chicken enchilada	120	80.4	269	14.3	15.6	1.97	10.5	3.78	3.59	2.52	38.5	41.1	45.5	86.5

B1 Mg	B2 Mg	B3 Mg	B6 Mg	B12 Mcg	Fol. Mcg	Panto Mg	Vit-C Mg	Vit-E Mg	Calc Mg	Cu Mg	Iron Mg	Mg Mg	Phos Mg	Potas Mg	Sel Mcg	Na Mg	Zinc Mg
0.020	0.091	1.06	0.057	0.520	1.54	0.119	0	0.117	5.51	0.091	0.906	10.6	113	55.9	2.02	1202	1.62
0.150	0.170	4.70	0.276	1.60	37.0	0.298	17.0	2.15	29.0	0.186	2.90	40.0	184	613	15.0	292	5.29
0.067	0.123	2.43	0.202	1.59	31.0	0.288	7.00	0.931	23.0	0.149	3.18	39.0	56.0	417	13.3	992	4.23
0.257	0.293	4.36	0.727	1.59	47.6	0.627	5.00	1.67	165	0.255	2.70	61.0	274	388	23.0	516	3.30
0.078	0.243	2.94	0.668	1.66	36.8	0.606	6.10	1.79	186	0.244	2.16	51.9	247	442	69.3	—	—
0.191	0.169	3.51	0.299	0.765	23.2	0.531	15.8	0.774	30.4	0.330	2.39	37.0	118	562	10.0	974	—
0.098	0.076	0.983	0.068	0.643	1.51	0.227	0	—	7.56	0.076	0.454	3.78	34.0	60.5	—	575	0.567
0.070	0.163	2.09	0.152	1.02	11.1	0.304	8.98	2.19	255	0.085	1.77	36.0	159	193	12.0	157	2.25
0.029	0.058	1.44	0.060	0.940	2.00	0.195	14.0	0.240	7.00	0.030	0.760	7.00	47.0	90.0	5.00	584	1.21
0.113	0.068	1.50	0.080	0.740	2.00	0.195	15.0	0.240	6.00	0.050	0.660	7.00	49.0	95.0	5.00	639	1.05
0.006	0.007	0.167	0.002	0.037	0.902	0.004	0	0.046	1.11	0.013	0.057	0.241	3.00	9.12	0.230	49.0	0.012
0.180	0.150	3.05	0.267	1.30	17.0	0.285	2.00	0.054	20.0	0.106	3.60	6.40	121	14.0	11.6	1093	2.64
0.030	0.134	2.49	0.158	1.36	13.3	0.231	0.552	0.624	85.0	0.062	1.29	22.7	141	183	9.94	141	2.89

B1 Mg	B2 Mg	B3 Mg	B6 Mg	B12 Mcg	Fol. Mcg	Panto Mg	Vit-C Mg	Vit-E Mg	Calc Mg	Cu Mg	Iron Mg	Mg Mg	Phos Mg	Potas Mg	Sel Mcg	Na Mg	Zinc Mg
0.072	0.168	8.20	0.407	0.292	6.07	0.990	0	0.486	14.6	0.064	1.15	23.1	174	219	11.1	77.2	1.90
0.059	0.151	7.78	0.395	0.279	4.86	0.942	0	0.468	12.8	0.057	1.03	21.3	166	207	11.1	72.9	1.79
0.042	0.139	5.20	0.225	0.188	4.86	0.632	0	0.425	12.1	0.052	0.990	17.6	128	153	10.4	59.5	1.69
0.013	0.110	5.38	0.299	0.252	2.22	0.725	1.80	0.341	12.0	0.035	1.32	10.2	94.6	117	6.59	428	1.28
0.062	0.193	5.57	0.304	0.267	6.68	1.03	0	0.468	12.8	0.068	1.13	20.0	152	204	11.1	79.0	2.38
0.055	0.098	10.6	0.510	0.292	3.04	0.826	0	0.468	12.8	0.043	0.905	23.1	183	210	9.84	65.6	1.05
0.161	0.204	14.7	0.600	0.410	8.00	1.15	0	1.10	28.0	0.084	1.75	34.0	258	282	11.7	385	1.33
0.065	0.117	12.5	0.540	0.320	3.00	0.917	0	0.624	14.0	0.049	1.04	27.0	210	240	11.7	69.0	1.00
0.090	0.254	17.2	0.640	0.460	6.00	1.20	0	1.00	28.0	0.096	2.02	48.0	344	390	17.0	136	2.12
0.068	0.108	12.7	0.550	0.310	4.00	0.894	0	0.330	14.0	0.046	0.980	27.0	212	237	10.5	68.0	0.930
0.060	0.098	11.8	0.516	0.292	3.44	0.830	0	0.312	0	0.042	0.894	24.9	196	220	9.97	64.0	0.860
0.080	0.226	17.0	0.640	0.440	6.00	1.09	0	0.500	24.0	0.082	1.68	44.0	314	356	16.8	118	1.84
0.081	0.155	3.67	0.200	0.200	6.00	0.725	0	0.340	12.0	0.055	0.970	14.0	106	134	6.90	194	1.67
0.036	0.112	3.12	0.180	0.170	4.00	0.630	0	0.286	6.00	0.040	0.690	12.0	91.0	119	7.10	47.0	1.49
0.032	0.099	2.58	0.170	0.140	4.00	0.554	0	0.250	5.00	0.034	0.550	10.0	78.0	105	5.70	40.0	1.35
0.033	0.103	2.67	0.170	0.150	4.00	0.574	0	0.242	5.00	0.035	0.570	11.0	81.0	108	5.70	42.0	1.40
0.102	0.195	4.92	0.230	0.240	8.00	0.845	0	0.474	16.0	0.071	1.24	18.0	134	165	8.50	248	1.75
0.042	0.131	3.95	0.190	0.180	4.00	0.687	0	0.341	8.00	0.048	0.830	14.0	108	137	8.50	52.0	1.46
0.046	0.133	3.70	0.200	0.170	4.00	0.668	0	0.286	7.00	0.047	0.760	14.0	103	134	7.12	49.0	1.45
0.038	0.120	3.39	0.180	0.160	4.00	0.616	0	0.286	6.00	0.042	0.680	12.0	95.0	124	7.12	46.0	1.34
0.019	0.044	2.14	0.130	0.090	1.00	0.280	0	0.176	5.00	0.020	0.400	6.00	48.0	57.0	3.70	25.0	0.560
0.014	0.044	2.26	0.140	0.100	1.000	0.305	0	0.055	5.00	0.019	0.430	7.00	51.0	62.0	1.33	28.0	0.620
0.009	0.026	1.45	0.120	0.070	1.00	0.198	0	0.024	3.00	0.011	0.230	4.00	33.0	42.0	3.75	18.0	0.420
0.010	0.027	1.54	0.120	0.070	1.00	0.210	0	0.138	3.00	0.011	0.240	4.00	35.0	44.0	3.90	19.0	0.450
0.006	0.054	0.874	0.026	0.043	11.7	0.158	0.364	—	2.00	0.024	0.913	4.40	34.0	39.0	2.58	15.0	0.963
0.002	0.024	0.092	0.011	0.240	2.64	0.087	0.059	0.010	0.614	0.016	0.298	0.660	7.00	4.00	—	2.00	0.240
0.031	0.350	0.890	0.117	3.87	154	1.08	3.17	0.289	2.86	0.074	1.70	4.14	62.4	28.0	6.14	10.1	0.867
0.018	0.037	1.50	0.154	0.097	0.900	0.275	0	0.157	12.0	0.010	0.275	5.00	44.5	64.5	2.97	165	0.205
0.030	0.052	1.39	0.090	0.580	2.30	0.154	0	0.175	43.0	0.020	0.900	8.00	48.0	38.0	4.30	616	1.00
0.160	0.160	5.50	0.163	0.020	6.60	0.440	0	0.500	46.0	0.200	1.20	18.0	182	307	7.00	895	0.920
0.087	0.167	4.27	0.136	0.547	8.13	0.509	1.33	0.133	144	0.209	3.60	34.3	164	196	29.3	971	2.47
0.050	0.100	1.00	0.093	0.051	12.0	0.156	13.0	0.900	45.0	0.200	1.30	14.0	85.0	418	1.32	725	1.30
0.070	0.153	6.80	0.235	0.322	3.53	0.541	0.095	1.37	20.0	0.144	1.35	16.1	149	273	7.73	647	—
0.167	0.167	3.93	0.460	0.230	29.0	1.10	1.00	4.00	30.0	0.130	3.10	30.1	177	16.0	11.5	907	1.22
0.034	0.078	3.25	0.174	0.115	4.07	0.485	0.950	11.0	16.3	0.104	0.657	11.1	80.0	137	6.53	—	—
0.289	0.258	9.21	0.368	0.198	17.9	0.783	3.61	0.540	44.0	0.101	1.87	29.8	173	194	19.4	2732	1.00
0.072	0.190	4.53	0.732	0.436	33.9	0.795	3.43	1.51	162	0.186	1.69	48.0	242	358	67.1	—	—
0.039	0.119	4.17	0.236	0.198	14.0	0.532	0.552	0.590	86.9	0.037	0.899	22.8	156	158	7.87	145	1.34
0.076	0.154	3.22	0.205	0.245	11.6	0.505	8.98	2.16	256	0.069	1.52	36.0	170	176	10.7	160	—

MEAT AND RELATED PRODUCTS—LAMB

Qty	Name	Wgt G	Wtr G	Cal	Prot G	Carb G	Fiber G	F-Tot G	F-Sat G	Mono G	Poly G	Chol Mg	A-Car RE	A-Pre RE	A-Tot RE
3 oz.	Lamb arm chop-brsd-ln+fat	85.0	37.4	297	27.0	0	0	20.2	9.31	8.10	1.21	104	0	2.70	2.70
3 oz.	Lamb loin chop-brld L+F	85.0	45.9	250	23.4	0	0	17.0	7.76	6.80	1.06	82.9	0	2.13	2.13
3 oz.	Lamb loin chop brld/lean	85.0	51.9	186	25.2	0	0	7.97	3.46	3.19	0.532	79.7	0	1.33	1.33
3 oz.	Lamb cutlet-grilled	85.0	54.4	189	23.6	0	0	9.01	5.13	4.60	0.708	89.1	0	0.300	0.300
3 oz.	Leg of lamb-lean w/fat	85.0	50.2	205	22.0	0	0	13.0	5.60	4.90	0.800	78.0	0	2.00	2.00
3 oz.	Leg of lamb-lean only	85.0	54.4	163	23.3	0	0	7.00	2.80	2.56	0.466	76.0	0	1.00	1.00
3 oz.	Lamb rib roast-lean & fat	85.0	40.0	315	18.0	0	0	26.0	12.1	10.6	1.50	77.0	0	2.00	2.00
3 oz.	Lamb shoulder roast-w/fat	85.0	41.7	297	27.0	0	0	20.2	9.32	8.10	1.21	104	0	0.300	0.300
3 oz.	Lamb shoulder roast-lean	85.0	41.7	239	30.1	0	0	12.4	5.13	4.60	0.708	104	0	0.300	0.300

MEAT AND RELATED PRODUCTS—PORK

Qty	Name	Wgt G	Wtr G	Cal	Prot G	Carb G	Fiber G	F-Tot G	F-Sat G	Mono G	Poly G	Chol Mg	A-Car RE	A-Pre RE	A-Tot RE
1 pce	Bacon-regular-cooked	6.33	0.817	36.3	1.93	0.037	0	3.12	1.11	1.50	0.367	5.33	0	0	0
1 ea.	Bacon L&T sand/soft white	135	72.6	333	11.0	29.5	2.33	18.9	5.15	7.41	5.46	21.4	41.3	8.35	49.7
1 pce	Beerwurst/beer salami-prk	23.0	14.1	55.0	3.27	0.470	0	4.32	1.44	2.06	0.540	13.0	0	0	0
1 pce	Bologna-beef & pork	28.4	15.4	89.0	3.31	0.790	0	8.01	3.03	3.80	0.680	15.6	0	0	0
1 pce	Bologna-cured pork	23.0	13.9	57.0	3.52	0.170	0	4.57	1.58	2.25	0.490	14.0	0	0	0
1 pce	Canadian bacon-cooked	23.5	14.6	43.0	5.65	0.315	0	1.96	0.660	0.940	0.185	13.5	0	0	0
1 ea.	Frankfurter-bf&prk-2oz ea	57.0	30.7	183	6.43	1.46	0	16.6	6.13	7.79	1.56	29.0	0	0	0
1 ea.	Frankfurter-bf&pork-reg	45.0	24.3	145	5.08	1.15	0	13.1	4.84	6.15	1.23	22.9	0	0	0
3 oz.	Ham-canned-heated	85.0	56.6	142	17.8	0.413	0	7.17	2.39	3.46	0.765	34.6	0	0	0
3 oz.	Ham-canned-unheated	85.0	60.5	123	15.3	0	0	6.32	2.08	3.04	0.644	32.2	0	0	0
1 pce	Ham-chopped-canned	21.0	12.8	50.0	3.37	0.060	0	3.95	1.32	1.93	0.430	10.0	0	0	0
1 pce	Ham-chopped-packaged	21.0	12.8	49.0	3.37	0.059	0	3.95	1.32	1.92	0.430	10.5	0	0	0
1 pce	Ham & cheese roll/loaf	28.5	16.5	73.5	4.71	0.405	0	5.75	2.13	2.63	0.620	16.5	2.50	18.0	20.5
1 pce	Ham-lunchmeat-extra lean	28.3	20.0	37.5	5.50	0.275	0	1.40	0.460	0.665	0.136	13.3	0	0	0
1 pce	Ham-lunchmeat-regular	28.3	18.3	51.5	5.00	0.880	0	3.00	0.960	1.40	0.343	16.0	0	0	0
3 oz.	Ham roasted-lean w/fat	85.0	49.7	207	18.3	0	0	14.3	5.08	6.68	1.54	52.2	0	0	0
3 oz.	Ham roasted-lean only	85.0	56.0	133	21.3	0	0	4.68	1.57	2.15	0.536	46.8	0	0	0
0.5 cup	Ham salad spread	120	75.1	259	10.4	12.7	0.150	18.6	6.05	8.65	3.23	44.0	3.00	18.0	21.0
1 ea.	Ham salad san/part WhlWht	125	59.7	339	10.6	32.8	3.19	18.9	4.62	7.32	5.97	27.4	1.50	17.3	18.8
1 ea.	Ham sandwich on rye bread	116	63.3	242	15.7	25.0	3.32	8.56	1.89	3.21	2.82	29.0	0	3.87	3.87
1 ea.	Ham sandwich-part WhlWt	122	65.5	256	16.7	27.2	3.14	9.03	1.97	3.51	2.74	29.0	0	4.47	4.47
1 ea.	Ham & cheese san/part WW	151	76.7	363	23.1	27.7	3.14	18.0	7.62	6.08	3.02	56.4	10.1	77.4	87.5
1 ea.	Ham & swiss san/on rye	145	73.9	350	23.8	26.0	3.32	16.5	6.99	5.30	3.11	55.4	0	76.8	76.8
1 pce	Keilbasa sausage	26.0	14.0	81.0	3.45	0.560	0	7.06	2.58	3.36	0.800	17.0	0	0	0
1 ea.	Knockwurst sausage-link	68.0	37.7	209	8.08	1.20	0	18.9	6.94	8.71	1.98	39.0	0	0	0
1 pce	Pepperoni sausage-SmSlice	5.50	1.49	27.2	1.15	0.156	0	2.42	0.887	1.16	0.240	1.90	0	0	0
1 pce	Pork breakfast strips-ckd	11.3	3.05	52.0	3.28	0.120	0	4.17	1.45	1.86	0.640	12.0	0	0	0
0.5 cup	Pork & beans-tom sce-cnd	127	90.5	155	7.80	24.0	8.50	3.30	1.20	1.35	0.350	5.00	16.5	0	16.5
3 oz.	Pork liver-braised	85.0	54.7	141	22.1	3.20	0	3.74	1.20	0.530	0.901	302	0	4592	4592
3 oz.	Pork loin chop-brsd-ln&ft	85.0	37.3	313	23.1	0	0	23.7	8.58	10.9	2.67	87.4	0	2.52	2.52

B1 Mg	B2 Mg	B3 Mg	B6 Mg	B12 Mcg	Fol. Mcg	Panto Mg	Vit-C Mg	Vit-E Mg	Calc Mg	Cu Mg	Iron Mg	Mg Mg	Phos Mg	Potas Mg	Sel Mcg	Na Mg	Zinc Mg
0.054	0.216	5.94	0.144	1.57	2.75	0.450	0	0.188	21.6	0.108	2.02	15.4	178	263	14.4	62.1	3.91
0.096	0.223	5.85	0.123	1.97	19.0	0.520	0	0.131	17.0	0.115	1.49	22.3	172	289	12.5	65.9	3.31
0.106	0.239	5.85	0.133	2.13	20.6	0.561	0	0.141	15.9	0.124	1.73	24.2	193	320	13.6	71.8	3.57
0.128	0.255	5.07	0.187	1.70	3.00	0.595	0	0.136	8.00	0.162	1.87	23.8	204	323	14.7	64.0	3.57
0.090	0.247	5.50	0.170	1.52	2.80	0.510	0	0.068	8.00	0.139	1.73	19.5	162	273	14.5	57.0	3.79
0.093	0.233	5.36	0.187	1.62	3.00	0.595	0	0.061	7.00	0.155	1.75	19.6	175	288	14.7	58.0	3.89
0.080	0.180	5.50	0.128	1.70	2.60	0.425	0	0.102	19.0	0.127	1.40	17.2	139	224	9.66	60.0	2.90
0.054	0.216	5.94	0.136	1.48	2.60	0.425	0	0.187	21.0	0.108	2.02	15.4	178	263	14.5	62.0	3.91
0.053	0.230	5.31	0.187	1.48	2.66	0.595	0	0.085	21.0	0.127	2.30	19.2	197	287	14.7	64.0	4.20

B1 Mg	B2 Mg	B3 Mg	B6 Mg	B12 Mcg	Fol. Mcg	Panto Mg	Vit-C Mg	Vit-E Mg	Calc Mg	Cu Mg	Iron Mg	Mg Mg	Phos Mg	Potas Mg	Sel Mcg	Na Mg	Zinc Mg
0.044	0.018	0.463	0.017	0.110	0.333	0.067	2.13	0.032	0.667	0.011	0.108	1.67	21.3	30.7	1.01	101	0.207
0.422	0.253	3.71	0.102	0.330	34.9	0.553	12.6	1.46	80.5	0.165	2.22	22.2	138	253	—	—	—
0.127	0.044	0.748	0.080	0.200	1.00	0.113	6.70	0.156	—	0.012	0.170	3.00	24.0	58.0	1.00	285	0.400
0.049	0.039	0.731	0.050	0.380	1.00	0.080	6.00	0.139	3.00	0.020	0.430	3.00	26.0	51.0	3.00	289	0.550
0.120	0.036	0.897	0.060	0.210	1.10	0.166	8.10	0.113	3.00	0.017	0.180	3.00	33.0	65.0	2.90	272	0.470
0.191	0.046	1.61	0.105	0.180	1.00	0.121	5.00	0.120	2.50	0.012	0.190	5.00	69.0	90.5	5.55	359	0.395
0.113	0.068	1.50	0.080	0.740	2.00	0.195	15.0	0.240	6.00	0.050	0.660	7.00	49.0	95.0	5.00	639	1.05
0.090	0.054	1.18	0.060	0.580	1.58	0.154	11.8	0.190	4.74	0.039	0.520	6.00	38.7	75.0	4.00	504	0.830
0.814	0.213	4.28	0.340	0.705	4.25	0.532	19.4	0.400	6.07	0.066	0.911	16.4	188	298	21.2	908	1.97
0.747	0.196	3.90	0.391	0.680	5.10	0.389	21.4	0.400	4.86	0.066	0.765	13.4	176	284	21.2	1086	1.57
0.112	0.035	0.672	0.070	0.150	1.20	0.030	8.00	0.085	1.00	0.010	0.200	3.00	29.0	60.0	3.50	287	0.380
0.112	0.035	0.700	0.067	0.147	1.00	0.095	0.378	0.105	1.50	0.010	0.199	2.73	29.0	59.5	3.00	286	0.384
0.170	0.053	0.980	0.075	0.230	1.47	0.148	7.10	0.054	16.5	0.021	0.260	4.50	71.5	83.0	1.75	381	0.565
0.264	0.063	1.37	0.130	0.212	1.15	0.132	7.45	0.067	2.00	0.021	0.215	4.82	62.0	99.0	3.00	405	0.545
0.244	0.071	1.49	0.096	0.235	0.850	0.126	7.85	0.142	2.00	0.028	0.280	5.40	70.0	94.0	3.00	373	0.605
0.551	0.188	3.79	0.323	0.547	2.55	0.389	0	0.442	6.07	0.070	0.741	16.4	182	243	21.2	1009	1.97
0.578	0.216	4.27	0.400	0.595	3.40	0.423	0	0.400	6.07	0.074	0.802	18.8	193	269	22.8	1129	2.19
0.520	0.144	2.51	0.179	0.915	1.25	0.372	7.00	5.65	9.50	0.087	0.710	11.6	143	179	15.0	1093	1.32
0.520	0.254	3.78	0.154	0.457	26.1	0.448	3.50	4.04	76.6	0.203	2.36	31.8	177	172	29.8	—	—
0.744	0.300	4.50	0.316	0.425	23.4	0.497	14.2	1.38	49.3	0.134	1.94	24.7	203	311	28.1	—	—
0.798	0.318	5.36	0.330	0.425	29.0	0.513	14.2	1.37	79.3	0.208	2.52	38.5	234	287	33.4	—	—
0.806	0.419	5.38	0.350	0.625	31.4	0.652	14.2	1.55	256	0.216	2.64	45.1	447	334	37.1	—	—
0.750	0.404	4.52	0.341	0.906	25.2	0.621	14.2	1.57	325	0.143	1.99	34.8	376	342	33.0	1336	—
0.059	0.056	0.749	0.050	0.420	1.00	0.210	6.00	0.148	11.0	0.030	0.380	4.00	38.0	70.0	1.50	280	0.520
0.233	0.095	1.86	0.110	0.800	2.00	0.220	18.0	0.388	7.00	0.040	0.620	8.00	67.0	136	3.00	687	1.13
0.017	0.014	0.272	0.014	0.138	—	0.103	0.000	0.020	0.550	0.004	0.077	0.880	6.55	19.1	0.080	112	0.137
0.084	0.042	0.860	0.040	0.200	0.333	0.104	4.93	0.057	1.67	0.017	0.223	3.00	30.0	52.7	1.37	238	0.417
0.100	0.040	0.750	0.100	0	30.5	0.117	2.50	0.765	69.0	0.280	2.30	45.0	117	268	7.50	590	1.30
0.219	1.87	7.17	0.485	15.9	139	4.06	20.0	3.58	8.50	0.539	15.2	11.9	205	128	24.0	42.0	5.71
0.517	0.256	5.08	0.311	0.671	3.59	0.489	0.240	0.587	7.19	0.092	0.982	16.8	169	293	15.7	55.1	2.58

MEATS AND RELATED PRODUCTS—PORK (continued)

Qty	Name	Wgt G	Wtr G	Cal	Prot G	Carb G	Fiber G	F-Tot G	F-Sat G	Mono G	Poly G	Chol Mg	A-Car RE	A-Pre RE	A-Tot RE
3 oz.	Pork loin chop-brsd-Lean	85.0	43.4	232	28.0	0	0	12.4	4.28	5.58	1.52	89.7	0	2.32	2.32
3 oz.	Pork loin chop-brld-ln&ft	85.0	42.4	269	23.4	0	0	18.8	6.84	8.63	2.15	82.1	0	2.54	2.54
3 oz.	Pork loin chop-brld-lean	85.0	48.5	196	27.2	0	0	8.91	3.07	4.02	1.07	83.9	0	2.36	2.36
3 oz.	Pork loin chop-fried-L&F	85.0	38.6	319	19.8	0	0	26.0	9.37	11.9	2.96	87.9	0	2.58	2.58
3 oz.	Pork loin chop-fried-lean	85.0	45.9	226	24.5	0	0	13.6	4.65	6.09	1.69	90.1	0	2.03	2.03
3 oz.	Pork leg-roasted-lean&fat	85.0	45.4	250	21.0	0	0	18.0	6.40	8.10	2.00	79.0	0	2.00	2.00
3 oz.	Pork rib roast-lean & fat	85.0	43.4	270	21.0	0	0	20.0	7.25	9.21	2.30	69.0	0	2.60	2.60
1 ea.	Pork sausage link-ckd	13.0	5.80	48.0	2.55	0.130	0	4.05	1.40	1.81	0.500	11.0	0	0	0
1 pce	Pork sausage patty-ckd	27.0	12.0	100	5.31	0.280	0	8.41	2.92	3.75	1.03	22.0	0	0	0
3 oz.	Pork shlder-brsd-lean&fat	85.0	39.6	293	22.8	0	0	21.7	7.90	10.0	2.43	93.1	0	2.60	2.60
3 oz.	Pork spareribs-cooked	85.0	34.4	338	24.7	0	0	25.8	9.99	12.1	2.98	103	0	2.55	2.55
1 pce	Salami-pork & beef	28.3	17.0	71.5	3.94	0.640	0	5.70	2.29	2.60	0.570	18.4	0	0	0
0.5 cup	Sandwich spread-pork&beef	120	72.4	280	9.20	14.3	0	20.8	7.20	9.12	3.04	48.0	0	8.00	8.00
1 ea.	Smoked link sausage-pork	68.0	26.7	265	15.1	1.43	0	21.6	7.70	9.95	2.55	46.0	0	0	0
1 pce	Turkey ham	28.5	20.5	36.5	5.40	0.425	0	1.50	0.475	0.375	0.375	16.0	0	0	0

MEAT AND RELATED PRODUCTS—TURKEY

Qty	Name	Wgt G	Wtr G	Cal	Prot G	Carb G	Fiber G	F-Tot G	F-Sat G	Mono G	Poly G	Chol Mg	A-Car RE	A-Pre RE	A-Tot RE
3 oz.	Turkey meat rstd-all type	85.0	55.3	145	24.9	0	0	4.22	1.39	0.881	1.21	65.0	0	0	0
3 oz.	Turkey dark meat-roasted	85.0	53.7	159	24.3	0	0	6.14	2.06	1.39	1.84	72.3	0	0	0
3 oz.	Turkey white meat-roasted	85.0	56.4	133	25.5	0	0	2.73	0.875	0.480	0.729	58.9	0	0	0
3 oz.	Ground turkey-cooked	85.0	51.0	191	22.1	0	0	11.1	3.83	4.59	2.72	71.4	0	0	0
3 oz.	Turkey breast-barbecued	85.0	59.5	121	19.4	0	0	4.25	1.29	1.46	0.850	48.6	0	0	0
3 oz.	Turkey breast-hickory smk	85.0	59.5	106	17.9	1.82	0	3.34	0.860	1.03	0.860	39.5	0	0	0
1 ea.	Turkey gizzards-cooked	67.0	43.8	109	19.7	0.397	0	2.60	0.744	0.504	0.749	155	0	37.0	37.0
1 ea.	Turkey hearts-cooked	16.0	10.3	28.0	4.28	0.329	0	0.975	0.280	0.190	0.282	36.1	0	1.30	1.30
1 ea.	Turkey livers-cooked	75.0	49.2	127	18.0	2.57	0	4.46	1.41	1.12	1.06	469	0	2806	2806
3 oz.	Turkey & gravy fr/frozen	85.0	72.3	56.9	5.00	3.92	0.258	2.23	0.725	0.839	0.419	15.6	0	10.8	10.8
3 oz.	Turkey frzn/roastd-seasnd	85.0	57.8	130	18.0	3.00	0	5.00	1.60	1.00	1.40	45.0	0	0	0
1 ea.	Turkey patty-breaded/frd	64.0	32.0	181	9.00	10.0	0.030	11.5	3.00	4.80	3.00	40.0	0	7.00	7.00
3 oz.	Turkey loaf-breast meat	85.0	61.2	92.1	19.1	0	0	1.34	0.420	0.382	0.240	34.8	0	0	0
3 oz.	Turkey roll-light meat	85.0	60.0	124	15.8	0.448	0	6.10	1.70	2.12	1.48	35.8	0	0	0
3 oz.	Turkey roll-light & dark	85.0	59.7	125	15.4	1.79	0	5.91	1.72	1.95	1.51	46.3	0	0	0
1 pce	Bologna-turkey	28.5	18.8	56.5	3.89	0.275	0	4.30	1.48	1.85	1.22	28.0	0	0	0
1 pce	Turkey breakfast sausage	28.0	16.8	65.0	6.20	0	0	4.25	1.59	1.84	1.22	23.0	0	0	0
1 ea.	Turkey frankfurter-45g ea	45.0	28.3	102	6.43	0.670	0	8.28	2.70	3.30	2.12	39.0	0	17.0	17.0
1 pce	Turkey ham	28.5	20.5	36.5	5.40	0.425	0	1.50	0.475	0.375	0.375	16.0	0	0	0
1 pce	Turkey pastrami	28.5	20.5	37.0	5.25	0.435	0	1.76	0.515	0.580	0.450	15.0	0	0	0
1 pce	Salami-turkey	28.5	18.8	55.5	4.64	0.155	0	3.91	1.13	1.29	1.00	23.0	0	0	0
1 oz.	Smoked turkey sausage	28.3	18.7	55.7	4.56	0.304	0	4.02	1.32	1.61	1.06	19.2	0	0	0
1 oz.	Turkey summer sausage	28.3	18.7	50.6	4.86	0.304	0	3.44	1.17	1.41	0.918	22.3	0	0	0
1 Tbs	Turkey gravy-canned	14.9	13.2	7.63	0.387	0.762	0.015	0.313	0.092	0.134	0.073	0.313	0	0	0
1 ea.	Turkey pot pie frozen	233	133	416	14.8	38.2	0.900	22.6	7.50	6.00	6.90	20.0	141	4.00	145
1 ea.	Turkey san/part Whl Wheat	122	63.0	271	18.2	26.4	3.12	10.5	1.87	3.25	4.51	28.6	0	8.35	8.35
1 ea.	Turkey san/soft white	122	63.0	277	17.5	27.6	1.52	10.4	2.08	3.15	4.47	28.6	0	8.35	8.35
1 ea.	Turkey ham sandwich-rye	116	64.1	239	15.3	25.3	3.32	8.69	1.90	2.60	3.29	34.5	0	3.90	3.90
1 ea.	Turkey ham san-part WhlWt	122	66.4	253	16.3	27.5	3.14	9.16	1.98	2.90	3.20	34.5	0	4.50	4.50
1 ea.	Turkey ham san-soft white	122	66.5	259	15.7	28.7	1.54	9.06	2.19	2.80	3.16	34.5	0	4.50	4.50
1 ea.	Turkey Ham & cheese on rye	145	75.4	347	21.6	25.8	3.32	17.7	7.55	5.17	3.57	61.9	10.1	76.8	86.9
1 ea.	Turkey Ham&cheese-part WW	151	77.5	361	22.7	28.0	3.14	18.1	7.63	5.47	3.48	61.9	10.1	77.4	87.5
1 ea.	Turkey ham & chz/sft whte	151	77.5	367	22.0	29.2	1.54	18.0	7.84	5.38	3.45	61.9	10.1	77.4	87.5

B1 Mg	B2 Mg	B3 Mg	B6 Mg	B12 Mcg	Fol. Mcg	Panto Mg	Vit-C Mg	Vit-E Mg	Calc Mg	Cu Mg	Iron Mg	Mg Mg	Phos Mg	Potas Mg	Sel Mcg	Na Mg	Zinc Mg
0.585	0.303	5.91	0.387	0.711	4.64	0.597	0.309	0.424	7.73	0.107	1.19	20.1	203	356	18.9	63.4	3.17
0.850	0.232	4.25	0.340	0.604	4.30	0.501	0.254	0.464	3.91	0.065	0.689	21.5	180	305	14.8	59.6	1.64
0.977	0.262	4.71	0.402	0.630	5.08	0.588	0.340	0.304	4.25	0.070	0.782	25.5	208	357	15.5	66.1	1.90
0.869	0.234	4.38	0.332	0.655	4.25	0.859	0.258	0.644	4.25	0.068	0.715	22.0	182	309	12.5	61.2	1.66
1.06	0.281	5.12	0.425	0.621	5.10	0.674	0.340	0.463	4.32	0.076	0.850	27.2	226	387	15.5	72.4	2.04
0.539	0.265	3.89	0.331	0.595	8.50	0.500	0.300	0.446	5.00	0.085	0.850	18.0	210	280	13.3	50.0	2.43
0.500	0.237	4.17	0.300	0.476	6.80	0.577	0.260	0.496	8.50	0.063	0.757	16.0	190	313	13.3	37.0	1.67
0.096	0.033	0.587	0.040	0.220	0.870	0.094	0.200	0.041	4.00	0.018	0.160	2.00	24.0	47.0	3.79	168	0.330
0.200	0.069	1.22	0.090	0.470	1.80	0.195	0.500	0.086	9.00	0.038	0.340	5.00	50.0	97.0	7.88	349	0.680
0.460	0.261	4.43	0.230	0.587	3.40	0.472	0.300	0.360	6.00	0.117	1.40	16.0	162	286	15.7	74.0	3.43
0.347	0.325	4.66	0.298	0.918	3.41	0.639	0	0.281	39.9	0.121	1.57	20.4	222	272	13.4	79.3	3.91
0.068	0.106	1.00	0.059	1.03	0.565	0.240	3.40	0.193	3.68	0.065	0.755	4.25	32.6	56.0	3.50	302	0.605
0.208	0.160	2.08	0.144	1.36	3.20	0.480	0	—	16.0	0.160	0.960	8.00	72.0	128	—	1216	1.20
0.476	0.175	3.08	0.240	1.11	2.00	0.530	1.00	0.218	20.0	0.050	0.790	13.0	110	228	9.00	1020	1.92
0.020	0.075	1.38	0.079	0.645	2.00	0.325	0	0.182	2.50	0.034	0.780	6.00	69.0	81.5	2.25	274	0.790

B1 Mg	B2 Mg	B3 Mg	B6 Mg	B12 Mcg	Fol. Mcg	Panto Mg	Vit-C Mg	Vit-E Mg	Calc Mg	Cu Mg	Iron Mg	Mg Mg	Phos Mg	Potas Mg	Sel Mcg	Na Mg	Zinc Mg
0.053	0.155	4.63	0.389	0.316	6.07	0.802	0	0.375	21.3	0.080	1.51	22.5	181	254	21.9	60.1	2.64
0.053	0.211	3.10	0.304	0.316	7.90	1.09	0	0.544	27.3	0.136	1.99	20.7	174	247	22.5	66.8	3.80
0.052	0.110	5.81	0.456	0.316	4.86	0.576	0	0.055	16.4	0.036	1.14	23.7	187	259	21.9	54.1	1.73
0.068	0.230	5.11	0.221	1.91	2.38	0.262	0.009	0.298	24.7	0.060	1.41	17.0	164	201	25.5	97.8	2.93
0.030	0.091	8.29	0.334	0.486	3.04	0.298	0.003	0.273	6.07	0.027	0.364	21.3	225	173	21.3	474	1.06
0.030	0.091	8.35	0.334	0.577	3.04	0.298	0.003	0.273	3.04	0.182	0.607	21.3	240	179	21.3	632	0.911
0.022	0.219	2.06	0.079	1.28	36.0	0.568	1.06	—	10.2	0.116	3.64	12.5	86.0	141	7.80	37.0	2.79
0.011	0.141	0.520	0.051	1.14	12.6	0.436	0.276	—	2.10	0.100	1.10	3.53	33.0	29.0	—	9.00	0.843
0.039	1.07	4.46	0.391	35.6	499	4.47	1.39	—	8.00	0.420	5.85	11.3	204	146	20.0	48.0	2.32
0.020	0.108	1.53	0.085	0.069	1.32	0.168	0	0.198	12.0	0.017	0.791	6.83	68.9	52.1	1.75	471	0.595
0.040	0.140	5.30	0.238	0.280	5.44	0.500	0	0.320	4.00	0.070	1.40	20.0	207	253	7.10	578	2.37
0.064	0.122	1.47	0.128	0.140	2.50	0.260	0	0.640	9.00	0.035	1.41	12.0	173	176	3.50	512	1.50
0.034	0.090	7.08	0.306	1.72	4.40	0.502	0	0.100	6.00	0.046	0.340	17.0	194	236	7.00	1217	0.961
0.075	0.191	5.92	0.336	0.269	2.98	0.433	0	0.045	34.3	0.030	1.07	13.4	155	212	7.16	413	1.31
0.078	0.240	4.06	0.336	0.269	2.98	0.433	0	0.045	26.9	0.060	1.13	14.9	142	228	8.36	495	1.69
0.015	0.047	1.05	0.050	0.420	1.40	0.097	0.000	0.139	23.5	0.008	0.435	4.00	37.0	56.5	2.50	249	0.495
0.030	0.080	1.42	0.080	0.500	1.00	0.096	—	0.150	5.00	0.030	0.520	6.00	52.0	76.0	2.60	191	0.970
0.037	0.080	1.70	0.095	0.585	2.30	0.154	0.010	0.175	58.0	0.022	0.770	7.70	83.0	88.0	4.30	454	1.00
0.020	0.075	1.38	0.079	0.645	2.00	0.325	0	0.182	2.50	0.034	0.780	6.00	69.0	81.5	2.25	274	0.790
0.022	0.075	1.24	0.082	0.575	2.00	0.097	0.000	0.190	2.50	0.022	0.405	5.00	71.0	77.5	2.50	284	0.730
0.029	0.075	1.11	0.070	0.990	2.63	0.097	0.000	0.190	5.50	0.027	0.465	4.50	36.5	62.5	2.50	267	0.625
0.020	0.061	1.17	0.061	0.567	1.01	0.097	—	0.152	5.06	0.030	0.415	5.06	37.5	59.7	2.63	222	0.719
0.030	0.121	1.42	0.081	1.16	1.01	0.097	—	0.152	4.05	0.040	0.537	6.07	68.8	65.8	2.63	308	0.729
0.003	0.012	0.194	—	—	—	—	0	—	0.625	—	0.104	—	—	—	—	—	—
0.170	0.170	3.80	0.460	0.200	24.0	1.10	3.50	3.00	64.0	0.289	2.10	25.0	137	138	28.4	1000	1.50
0.282	0.242	7.24	0.269	1.15	28.4	0.597	0.002	2.75	75.8	0.190	2.23	37.3	235	239	27.0	—	—
0.286	0.238	6.82	0.225	1.15	22.8	0.603	0.002	1.40	76.4	0.134	1.87	23.3	192	223	23.0	—	—
0.249	0.322	4.46	0.211	1.28	23.7	0.881	0	2.94	50.3	0.161	3.04	26.5	214	273	22.5	986	—
0.303	0.340	5.32	0.225	1.28	29.3	0.897	0.002	2.93	80.3	0.235	3.63	40.3	245	249	27.8	—	—
0.307	0.336	4.90	0.181	1.28	23.7	0.903	0.002	2.78	80.9	0.179	3.28	26.3	203	233	23.8	—	—
0.257	0.423	4.48	0.231	1.48	26.1	1.02	0	3.23	226	0.169	3.15	33.1	428	319	26.1	—	—
0.311	0.441	5.34	0.245	1.48	31.7	1.04	0.002	3.22	256	0.243	3.74	46.9	459	296	—	—	—
0.315	0.437	4.92	0.201	1.48	26.1	1.04	0.002	3.07	257	0.187	3.39	32.9	416	280	—	—	—

Qty	Name	Wgt	Wtr G	Cal	Prot G	Carb G	Fiber G	F-Tot G	F-Sat G	Mono G	Poly G	Chol Mg	A-Car RE	A-Pre RE	A-Tot RE
3 oz.	Bass-baked/broiled	85.0	57.8	167	18.3	5.70	0	3.40	0.729	1.04	1.05	62.1	0	32.8	32.8
3 oz.	Bluefish-baked/broiled	85.0	57.8	135	22.3	0	0	6.97	1.50	3.10	1.72	53.6	0	12.8	12.8
3 oz.	Bluefish-fried	85.0	51.7	174	19.3	4.00	0	8.33	1.82	3.69	2.09	51.0	0	12.8	12.8
3 oz.	Cod-baked w/butter	85.0	62.9	112	19.6	0	0	2.81	0.330	0.220	0.441	51.0	0	25.5	25.5
3 oz.	Cod-batter fried	85.0	51.9	169	16.7	6.38	0	8.76	3.29	4.68	0.724	46.8	0	0.255	0.255
3 oz.	Cod broiled	85.0	54.9	97.0	21.0	0	0	0.936	0.842	0.561	1.12	51.0	0	51.0	51.0
3 oz.	Cod-steamed	85.0	67.4	70.6	15.8	0	0	0.765	0.200	0.122	0.435	51.0	0	0.255	0.255
3 oz.	Fried fish cakes fr/frzn	85.0	45.0	181	7.77	13.8	1.19	10.5	2.55	4.17	3.57	76.5	0	16.6	16.6
1 ea.	Fish sandwich-reg w/chees	140	60.2	420	16.2	38.5	1.30	22.6	6.30	6.90	7.70	56.0	12.0	13.0	25.0
1 ea.	Fish sticks	28.0	14.6	70.0	6.00	4.00	0.010	3.00	0.800	1.40	0.800	26.0	0	5.00	5.00
3 oz.	Sole/Flounder-bkd w/marg.	85.0	62.1	120	16.0	0	0	6.00	1.20	2.30	1.90	55.0	0	69.0	69.0
3 oz.	Sole/Flounder-fried	85.0	51.0	189	14.9	7.61	0	7.65	2.04	3.57	2.04	45.1	0	10.2	10.2
3 oz.	Sole/Flounder-steamed	85.0	66.3	78.2	17.0	0	0	0.995	0.332	0.221	0.442	44.2	0	8.50	8.50
3 oz.	Haddock-breaded/fried	85.0	51.9	175	17.0	7.00	0.030	9.01	2.40	3.90	2.40	75.0	0	23.0	23.0
3 oz.	Haddock-smoked/steamed	85.0	60.9	85.9	19.8	0	0	0.765	0.168	0.168	0.335	74.0	0	5.10	5.10
3 oz.	Halibut-brld-buttr+lemJce	85.0	57.0	140	20.0	0	0	6.00	3.30	1.60	0.700	62.0	4.60	169	174
3 oz.	Halibut-steamed-pacific	85.0	66.4	111	20.2	0	0	3.23	0.425	1.13	0.995	62.1	0	22.7	22.7
3 oz.	Herring-pickled	85.0	50.5	190	17.3	0	0	12.8	4.30	4.60	3.10	85.0	0	33.0	33.0
3 oz.	Herring-smoked/kippered	85.0	51.9	179	18.9	0	0	11.0	2.45	6.12	2.15	68.0	0	9.36	9.36
3 oz.	Herring-canned w/liquid	85.0	53.6	177	16.9	0	0	11.6	2.58	6.46	2.27	82.5	0	33.2	33.2
3 oz.	Mackerel-fried	85.0	42.5	117	13.4	0	0	9.61	2.90	2.69	3.73	76.5	0	10.2	10.2
3 oz.	Mackerel-Atlantic-cooked	85.0	52.4	201	18.5	0	0	11.0	3.88	3.25	3.31	80.8	0	137	137
3 oz.	Mackerel-canned	85.0	56.1	155	17.2	0	0	10.7	3.78	3.17	3.23	79.9	0	59.5	59.5
3 oz.	Ocean perch-breaded/fried	85.0	50.2	185	16.0	7.00	0	11.0	2.60	4.60	2.80	66.0	0	23.0	23.0
3 oz.	Pollock steamed	85.0	65.5	84.2	19.8	0	0	0.765	0.085	0.085	0.425	63.8	0	0.255	0.255
3 oz.	Salmon-broiled or baked	85.0	57.0	140	21.0	0	0	5.00	1.20	2.40	1.40	60.0	0	87.1	87.1
3 oz.	Salmon-smoked	85.0	50.2	150	18.0	0	0	8.00	2.60	3.90	0.700	51.0	0	77.0	77.0
3 oz.	Salmon-Atlantic-canned	85.0	54.1	173	18.5	0	0	6.51	2.03	3.00	0.572	51.0	0	15.3	15.3
3 oz.	Salmon-canned pink w/liq	85.0	60.4	120	17.0	0	0	5.00	0.901	1.50	2.10	34.0	0	18.0	18.0
3 oz.	Salmon-Sockeye-canned	85.0	57.2	128	19.1	0	0	5.70	0.638	0.919	2.93	42.5	0	59.5	59.5
1 oz.	Sardines-Atlantic-cnd/drn	28.3	17.6	58.4	6.67	0	0	3.14	0.700	1.23	0.967	28.3	0	18.7	18.7
1 oz.	Sardines-Atlantic-cnd+liq	28.3	14.5	88.2	5.84	0	0	6.92	1.59	2.83	2.21	34.0	0	15.6	15.6
1 oz.	Sardines-Pacific-canned	28.3	17.6	56.7	6.52	0	0	3.12	0.697	1.23	0.961	34.0	0	5.10	5.10
1 oz.	Sardines-cnd/tomato Sauce	28.3	18.2	55.8	5.30	0.482	0	3.46	0.771	1.36	1.07	28.3	0	5.67	5.67
1 oz.	Sardines cnd in mustard	28.3	18.2	55.6	5.33	0.482	0	3.40	1.07	1.05	1.15	28.3	0	2.55	2.55
3 oz.	Snapper-baked	85.0	59.5	91.9	20.4	0	0	1.30	0.413	0.264	0.582	51.0	0	10.2	10.2
3 oz.	Lemon sole-steamed	85.0	65.7	77.4	17.5	0	0	0.765	0.230	0.153	0.306	51.0	0	10.2	10.2
3 oz.	Swordfish broiled w/buttr	85.0	54.9	148	23.8	0	0	5.10	2.10	1.58	0.310	51.0	0	528	528
3 oz.	Trout-brld w/buttr+lemJce	85.0	53.6	175	21.0	0.010	0	9.01	4.10	2.90	1.60	71.0	0	60.0	60.0
3 oz.	Tuna-canned in oil/drnd	85.0	51.9	165	24.0	0	0	7.00	1.40	1.90	3.10	55.0	0	23.0	23.0
3 oz.	Tuna-canned in water/drnd	85.0	53.6	135	30.0	0	0	1.00	0.300	0.200	0.300	48.0	0	32.0	32.0
1 cup	Tuna noodle casserole-hme	202	147	251	20.8	24.3	0.251	7.28	1.97	1.50	3.16	51.9	0	34.3	34.3
5 cup	Tuna salad	102	64.6	188	16.5	9.50	1.23	9.50	1.65	2.45	4.60	40.0	4.00	22.5	26.5
1 ea.	Tuna salad san/part WhlWt	116	54.4	303	13.6	31.2	3.73	14.3	2.42	4.22	6.65	25.4	2.00	19.6	21.6
1 ea.	Tuna salad san/firm white	126	58.1	335	13.8	37.2	2.40	14.6	2.75	4.26	6.71	25.4	2.00	19.6	21.6

B1 Mg	B2 Mg	B3 Mg	B6 Mg	B12 Mcg	Fol. Mcg	Panto Mg	Vit-C Mg	Vit-E Mg	Calc Mg	Cu Mg	Iron Mg	Mg Mg	Phos Mg	Potas Mg	Sel Mcg	Na Mg	Zinc Mg
0.128	0.119	2.47	0.221	1.19	4.25	0.510	0	0.850	40.0	0.051	1.62	36.6	196	183	29.8	52.7	0.435
0.094	0.085	1.62	0.492	3.06	8.50	0.498	0.009	0.850	24.7	0.081	0.595	38.3	244	357	25.5	86.8	0.833
0.094	0.094	1.53	0.468	2.98	6.80	0.430	0.009	0.850	29.8	0.081	0.765	38.3	219	309	25.5	267	0.808
0.064	0.066	2.55	0.336	1.70	9.36	0.213	0.001	0.885	20.4	0.106	0.510	22.1	187	316	30.9	191	0.638
0.017	0.017	1.53	0.078	0.723	2.38	0.040	0.001	1.96	68.0	0.106	0.425	20.4	170	315	18.1	85.0	0.850
0.068	0.072	1.62	0.349	1.70	8.50	0.213	0.009	1.28	21.3	0.106	0.680	22.1	212	335	30.9	92.7	0.638
0.077	0.077	2.55	0.315	2.55	10.2	0.170	0.001	0.459	12.8	0.119	0.425	17.9	204	306	32.7	85.0	0.638
0.051	0.051	1.02	0.043	0.850	6.80	0.213	0.017	0.850	59.5	0.115	0.850	15.3	93.6	221	12.8	425	0.340
0.322	0.266	3.30	0.098	0.840	23.8	0.476	2.80	2.22	132	0.098	1.85	29.4	223	274	35.0	667	0.952
0.030	0.050	0.600	0.059	0.560	5.05	0.094	0	0.089	11.0	0.021	0.300	8.00	58.0	94.0	4.50	53.0	0.201
0.050	0.080	1.60	0.284	1.27	10.0	0.429	1.00	1.61	14.0	0.076	0.300	18.7	187	273	72.0	151	0.723
0.128	0.111	2.13	0.219	0.680	9.78	0.213	1.70	1.37	68.9	0.096	0.546	19.6	179	225	73.0	197	0.344
0.050	0.080	1.70	0.285	1.28	10.2	0.430	0.001	1.37	24.7	0.076	0.430	18.7	213	238	72.3	102	0.723
0.060	0.100	2.90	0.130	0.791	13.6	0.213	0	1.02	34.0	0.026	1.00	29.5	183	270	30.0	123	0.600
0.060	0.060	0.936	0.238	1.70	2.55	0.111	0.001	0.374	49.3	0.119	0.850	21.3	213	247	28.9	1038	0.306
0.060	0.070	7.70	0.130	1.02	6.00	0.212	1.00	0.902	13.6	0.063	0.680	20.0	206	441	108	103	0.902
0.068	0.094	7.06	0.196	0.850	8.93	0.230	0.001	0.850	11.1	0.060	0.510	19.6	221	289	105	93.6	0.850
0.040	0.180	2.80	0.114	6.80	6.00	0.300	0	0.765	29.0	0.245	0.901	33.0	128	85.0	42.5	850	1.75
0.034	0.238	2.81	0.261	4.87	3.40	0.838	0	0.680	56.1	0.221	1.52	42.5	216	242	120	612	1.82
0.021	0.153	3.23	0.136	7.23	4.25	0.595	0.009	0.748	125	0.203	2.64	41.7	253	408	45.9	396	1.46
0.060	0.238	7.91	0.519	7.65	2.98	0.595	0	1.29	17.9	0.128	0.765	21.3	170	264	35.7	93.6	0.468
0.128	0.230	6.46	0.408	7.56	5.95	0.493	0	1.29	5.10	0.153	1.02	29.5	238	332	35.9	42.5	0.468
0.038	0.230	6.21	0.236	6.55	5.95	0.418	0	1.02	189	0.138	1.83	26.4	239	287	35.7	—	0.468
0.100	0.110	2.00	0.218	0.383	6.80	0.212	0	0.850	31.0	0.082	1.20	19.5	191	241	27.5	138	0.850
0.102	0.221	3.40	0.527	4.25	6.80	0.340	0.001	0.400	16.2	0.082	0.510	26.4	213	298	150	82.5	0.850
0.180	0.140	5.50	0.680	5.10	17.0	0.936	0	1.34	26.0	0.255	0.500	25.5	269	305	57.4	55.0	0.936
0.170	0.170	6.80	0.595	5.95	8.50	0.604	0	1.02	12.0	0.076	0.800	27.2	208	327	57.4	1701	0.340
0.026	0.153	5.53	0.282	3.83	14.0	0.468	0.009	1.28	79.1	0.068	0.544	25.5	204	255	59.5	485	0.765
0.030	0.150	6.80	0.383	5.86	17.0	0.480	0	1.28	167	0.060	0.700	23.0	243	307	60.0	443	0.765
0.034	0.145	6.23	0.282	3.83	16.8	0.447	0.009	1.28	133	0.078	0.663	25.0	243	255	59.5	329	0.765
0.010	0.057	1.53	0.094	5.74	4.27	0.198	0	0.085	124	0.022	0.867	14.7	141	116	7.07	142	0.737
0.006	0.045	1.25	0.094	4.68	4.39	0.191	0	0.312	100	0.030	0.992	12.2	123	159	5.67	145	0.822
0.003	0.085	2.10	0.071	3.18	4.54	0.142	0	0.085	85.9	0.011	0.992	8.50	128	79.4	7.09	184	0.737
0.003	0.077	1.53	0.062	3.18	4.25	0.142	0.003	0.085	127	0.011	0.680	8.50	136	90.7	5.67	113	0.737
0.003	0.085	2.10	0.079	3.52	4.25	0.142	0.000	0.085	85.9	0.011	0.936	8.50	100	73.7	5.67	215	0.822
0.054	0.064	2.89	0.233	1.36	7.65	0.202	0.001	0.706	18.2	0.041	0.255	28.7	91.0	414	147	44.2	0.340
0.077	0.077	3.06	0.284	0.850	11.1	0.264	0.009	0.332	17.9	0.102	0.442	17.0	213	238	57.8	102	0.850
0.034	0.043	8.76	1.53	1.28	8.50	1.53	0.009	0.902	23.0	0.063	1.11	20.4	234	425	28.9	114	0.902
0.070	0.070	2.30	0.415	2.38	5.95	1.17	1.00	0.128	26.0	0.221	1.00	29.8	259	297	59.5	122	0.221
0.040	0.090	10.1	0.466	2.72	12.8	0.315	0	0.455	7.00	0.090	1.60	27.0	199	298	73.0	303	0.871
0.030	0.100	13.2	0.425	2.89	13.6	0.315	0	0.453	17.0	0.090	0.600	26.0	202	255	73.0	468	0.871
0.144	0.169	8.59	0.243	1.78	12.8	0.473	0.725	0.108	36.6	0.225	1.94	30.8	182	224	62.3	—	—
0.030	0.070	6.65	0.243	1.79	20.5	0.321	3.00	11.2	15.5	0.163	1.25	21.3	140	265	56.0	438	0.580
0.275	0.217	5.85	0.186	0.897	35.7	0.422	1.50	9.14	79.6	0.241	2.63	36.6	176	215	—	—	—
0.327	0.243	5.81	0.146	0.897	33.7	0.468	1.5	9.06	92.8	0.199	2.56	24.7	144	210	—	—	—

SAUCES, SPREADS, GRAVIES

Qty	Name	Wgt G	Wtr G	Cal	Prot G	Carb G	Fiber G	F-Tot G	F-Sat G	Mono G	Poly G	Chol Mg	A-Car RE	A-Pre RE	A-Tot RE
1 Tbs	Barbecue sauce	15.6	12.7	10.0	0.237	1.50	0.094	0.375	0.037	0.137	0.131	0	14.0	0	14.0
1 Tbs	Bearnaise sauce	11.7	6.44	62.1	0.465	0.157	0.012	6.57	3.84	1.99	0.317	53.8	6.18	58.8	65.0
1 Tbs	Bechamel sauce	18.1	15.2	17.6	0.205	0.856	0.032	1.52	0.919	0.442	0.081	3.95	1.71	11.9	13.6
1 Tbs	Bordelaise sauce	29.1	25.1	24.6	0.334	1.13	0.084	1.50	0.919	0.431	0.061	3.92	2.88	11.9	14.7
1 Tbs	Catsup	17.1	11.8	18.1	0.313	4.31	0.085	0.069	0.012	0.012	0.025	0	23.9	0	23.9
1 Tbs	Cheese sauce	12.6	8.21	27.0	1.19	0.781	0.014	2.14	1.04	0.722	0.270	4.75	0.975	20.9	21.9
1 tsp	Hot chili sce-red pepper	5.17	4.85	1.000	0.046	0.200	0.061	0.031	0.003	0.002	0.018	0	49.0	0	49.0
1 tsp	Chili sauce-tomato based	5.69	3.87	5.92	0.142	1.41	0.040	0.017	0.002	0.002	0.006	0	7.96	0	7.96
1 Tbs	Chocolate syrup-thin	18.8	6.94	42.5	0.600	11.0	0.469	0.244	0.100	0.050	0.050	0	0.375	0	0.375
1 Tbs	Chocolate fudge topping	18.8	4.69	63.8	0.881	9.56	0.450	2.51	1.55	0.850	0.100	0	0	6.50	6.50
1 Tbs	Cranberry sauce-cnd/strnd	17.3	10.5	26.2	0.034	6.75	0.369	0.026	0.003	0.007	0.015	0	0.344	0	0.344
1 Tbs	Curry sauce	14.4	11.9	14.4	0.501	0.634	0.032	1.08	0.222	0.485	0.329	0.087	0.087	11.7	11.8
1 Tbs	Beef gravy-homemade	16.9	14.5	18.9	0.272	0.749	0.029	1.60	0.790	0.577	0.068	1.08	0	0	0
1 Tbs	Brown gravy fr/dry mix	16.3	15.0	5.00	0.188	0.875	0.015	0.125	0.056	0.050	0.006	0.125	0	0	0
1 Tbs	Chicken gravy-homemade	16.3	13.8	20.4	0.410	0.800	0.029	1.69	0.420	0.760	0.447	1.40	0	2.63	2.63
1 Tbs	Mushroom gravy-canned	14.9	13.2	7.50	0.188	0.813	0.019	0.375	0.063	0.175	0.150	0	0	0	0
1 Tbs	Onion gravy-dry-prepared	16.3	14.8	5.00	0.139	1.05	0.001	0.046	0.029	0.014	0.002	0.063	—	—	—
1 Tbs	Turkey gravy-dry-prepared	16.3	14.8	5.44	0.183	0.938	0.001	0.117	0.034	0.050	0.027	0.188	—	—	—
1 Tbs	Hollandaise sauce-recipe	10.0	3.40	54.2	0.750	0.140	0.003	5.66	1.27	2.63	1.37	65.5	0.019	76.5	76.6
1 Tbs	Horseradish-prepared	15.0	13.1	6.00	0.200	1.40	0.135	0.030	0.009	0.005	0.014	0	0	0	0
1 Tbs	Mayonnaise (soybean)	13.8	2.06	98.6	0.150	0.375	0	10.9	1.67	3.14	5.69	8.13	0	11.6	11.6
1 Tbs	Mayonnaise-imitation	15.0	9.45	35.0	0	2.00	0	3.00	0.500	0.700	1.60	4.00	0	0	0
1 Tbs	Mornay sauce	21.5	14.0	47.5	1.36	1.66	0.054	4.05	1.82	1.46	0.517	23.2	2.14	40.6	42.7
1 Tbs	Mushroom sauce-dry + milk	16.7	13.5	14.2	0.706	1.49	0.025	0.644	0.337	0.204	0.069	2.13	—	—	—
1 Tbs	Mustard-prepared	15.6	12.5	11.7	0.737	1.00	0.063	0.688	0.003	0.625	0.003	0	0	0	0
1 Tbs	Picante sauce-Tostitos	14.2	12.4	6.67	0.167	1.28	0.227	0.100	0.013	0.067	0.010	0.167	10.5	0	10.5
1 Tbs	Pickle relish	15.3	9.65	20.0	0.075	5.21	0.286	0.094	0.024	0.002	0.039	0	2.04	0	2.04
1 pce	Pickle slices-fresh pack	7.50	5.92	5.00	0.066	1.35	0.105	0.013	0.003	0.000	0.005	0	1.05	0	1.05
1 ea.	Dill pickle	65.0	60.4	5.00	0.500	1.40	0.910	0.100	0.026	0.002	0.042	0	7.00	0	7.00
1 ea.	Sweet pickle-small	15.0	9.15	20.0	0.090	5.50	0.210	0.045	0.013	0.001	0.021	0	1.00	0	1.00
1 Tbs	Salsa/Mex.sauce-hm-recipe	13.5	12.3	5.81	0.116	0.671	0.218	0.357	0.048	0.247	0.038	0	11.0	0	11.0
1 Tbs	Sour cream-mix-prep w/mlk	19.6	13.5	31.8	1.19	2.84	—	1.89	1.01	0.617	0.172	5.69	—	—	—
1 Tbs	Soy sauce	18.0	12.2	11.5	1.56	1.50	0	0	0	0	0	0	0	0	0
0.5 cup	Spaghetti sauce-homemade	110	82.5	89.5	3.00	11.4	1.33	4.85	0.695	2.47	1.32	0	117	0	117
0.5 cup	Spaghetti meat sauce-cnd	129	96.6	138	4.69	16.9	0.875	5.94	1.54	2.83	0.962	10.6	118	0	118
0.5 cup	Spag sce w/mushrooms-cnd	123	92.5	108	1.60	6.00	1.20	3.00	0.429	1.53	0.820	0	241	0	241
0.5 cup	Stroganoff sce + milk/water	148	116	135	5.85	16.9	0.300	5.35	3.38	1.50	0.175	19.0	—	—	—
.25 cup	Sweet & sour sce-prepared	78.2	59.5	73.5	0.190	18.2	0.002	0.020	0.002	0.005	0.010	0	—	—	—
1 Tbs	Tartar sauce	14.0	4.76	74.0	0.200	0.600	0.042	8.10	1.20	2.60	3.90	4.00	0	9.00	9.00
1 Tbs	Teriyaki sauce	18.0	15.1	15.0	1.07	2.87	0	0.057	0.009	0.014	0.034	0	0	0	0
0.5 cup	Tomato sauce-canned	122	109	37.0	1.63	8.80	1.60	0.205	0.029	0.030	0.082	0	120	0	120
0.5 cup	White sauce-homemade	125	91.2	197	5.00	12.0	0.215	15.0	4.55	5.95	3.60	16.0	3.50	166	170
0.5 cup	Sauerkraut-canned w/liqd	118	109	22.0	1.07	5.05	2.20	0.165	0.041	0.015	0.072	0	2.10	0	2.10

B1 Mg	B2 Mg	B3 Mg	B6 Mg	B12 Mcg	Fol. Mcg	Panto Mg	Vit-C Mg	Vit-E Mg	Calc Mg	Cu Mg	Iron Mg	Mg Mg	Phos Mg	Potas Mg	Sel Mcg	Na Mg	Zinc Mg
0.002	0.002	0.050	0.015	0	0.625	0.014	0.813	—	3.31	—	0.125	0.862	3.13	27.2	—	127	0.026
0.007	0.013	0.008	0.009	0.091	4.05	0.107	0.092	0.204	6.14	0.009	0.170	0.993	14.4	8.88	1.18	85.1	0.086
0.007	0.007	0.065	0.002	0	0.210	0.004	0.006	0.041	1.89	0.061	0.060	0.581	2.17	3.39	0.310	141	0.009
0.008	0.010	0.182	0.011	0.020	1.25	0.044	0.744	0.055	3.91	0.017	0.184	2.27	4.95	23.9	0.337	64.2	0.061
0.016	0.012	0.275	0.018	0	0.875	0.028	2.56	0.051	3.75	0.051	0.137	3.58	8.56	61.9	1.17	178	0.037
0.007	0.028	0.034	0.006	0.057	1.11	0.041	0.073	0.134	35.1	0.006	0.050	2.15	25.9	15.9	0.762	67.4	0.145
0.000	0.005	0.031	0.007	0	0.533	0.012	1.54	0.041	0.458	0.003	0.025	0.512	0.833	7.67	0.036	0.500	0.010
0.005	0.004	0.092	0.007	0	0.412	0.009	0.917	0.017	1.15	0.023	0.046	0.625	2.96	21.0	—	76.1	0.015
0.004	0.009	0.056	0.002	0	1.50	0.007	0	0.188	2.81	0.094	0.372	13.1	24.4	42.5	0.219	15.5	0.197
0.010	0.041	0.037	0.002	0	1.44	0.007	0	0.188	18.8	0.056	0.269	9.00	30.6	40.3	0.188	21.0	0.194
0.003	0.004	0.017	0.003	0	0.156	0.015	0.344	0.028	0.688	0.003	0.038	0.500	1.06	4.50	—	5.00	0.005
0.005	0.009	0.315	0.002	0.021	0.108	0.003	0.012	0.139	1.63	0.014	0.098	0.556	7.22	20.0	0.210	75.9	0.031
0.006	0.007	0.167	0.002	0.037	0.902	0.004	0	0.046	1.11	0.013	0.057	0.241	3.00	9.12	0.230	49.0	0.012
0.002	0.006	0.056	0.000	—	—	—	0	0.016	4.13	0.001	0.012	0.625	2.94	3.81	0	71.7	0.001
0.007	0.008	0.260	0.003	0.015	0.277	0.004	—	0.066	0.719	0.009	0.063	0.366	5.38	14.0	0.230	48.5	0.027
0.005	0.009	0.100	0.003	—	0	—	0	—	1.06	0.015	0.100	—	2.25	15.7	—	84.8	0.104
—	—	—	—	—	—	—	—	—	4.31	0.003	—	—	—	—	—	64.7	0.014
—	0.007	—	—	—	—	—	—	—	3.13	—	—	—	—	—	—	93.6	—
0.007	0.016	0.005	0.011	0.137	3.75	0.156	0.256	0.681	8.62	0.018	0.241	1.01	22.9	7.19	2.04	119	—
0.014	0.003	0.063	0.011	0	1.75	0.008	0.630	—	9.00	0.021	0.100	3.80	5.00	44.0	—	14.0	0.176
0.002	0.006	0.001	0.004	—	0.375	0.036	0	1.02	2.75	0.020	0.081	0.178	3.88	4.88	0.475	78.1	0.165
0	0	0	0	—	0.010	—	0	—	0	—	0	—	0	2.00	—	75.0	—
0.013	0.037	0.057	0.015	0.105	2.49	0.106	0.219	0.700	38.4	0.013	0.134	3.22	31.4	29.1	1.13	128	0.156
—	—	—	—	—	—	—	—	—	—	—	—	—	—	—	—	95.8	—
0.013	0.031	0.195	0.011	0	0	—	0	0.647	13.1	0.063	0.313	7.50	11.5	20.2	3.63	196	0.098
0.005	0.012	0.083	0.013	0	2.33	0.050	0.333	—	3.00	0.022	0.080	2.33	10.00	28.5	—	80.0	0.150
0.000	0.000	0.001	0.000	0	0	—	1.00	—	3.06	0.055	0.125	0.750	2.13	30.0	0.153	107	0.010
0	0.002	0.000	0.000	0	0	—	0.500	—	2.38	0.027	0.137	0.450	2.00	15.0	0.082	50.2	0
0.001	0.010	0.010	0.005	0	0.700	—	4.00	0	17.0	0.080	0.700	6.00	14.0	130	0.715	741	0.176
0.004	0.001	0.004	0.001	0	0	0.007	1.00	—	2.00	0.031	0.250	1.50	2.00	30.0	0.150	107	0.001
0.007	0.005	0.068	0.012	0	2.07	0.036	2.85	0.132	1.33	0.010	0.063	1.40	2.98	25.5	0.079	14.0	—
—	0.044	0.035	—	—	—	—	—	—	34.1	0.005	0.038	—	—	45.8	—	62.9	0.086
0.009	0.023	0.605	0.031	0	1.93	0.058	0	—	3.42	0.018	0.486	7.74	38.0	64.4	0.144	1029	0.036
0.101	0.064	1.50	0.197	0	11.5	0.271	10.0	1.65	26.0	0.475	1.47	18.5	43.0	457	1.50	450	0.289
0.125	0.100	2.12	0.166	1.10	8.13	0.217	1.25	1.000	22.5	0.182	1.75	9.25	66.2	277	2.69	653	0.656
0.080	0.080	0.933	0.159	0	12.5	0.426	9.33	1.93	14.7	0.393	1.000	14.7	30.0	333	2.21	496	0.340
0.429	0.385	0.379	—	—	—	—	—	—	260	0.043	0.665	—	151	336	—	914	0.550
—	0.024	—	—	—	—	—	—	—	10.2	0.007	0.405	—	—	16.5	—	195	0.023
0.001	0.004	0.001	0.005	0	0.600	0.036	0.001	4.00	3.00	0.038	0.100	0.448	4.00	11.0	0.825	182	0.020
0.005	0.013	0.229	0.018	0	3.60	0.036	0	—	4.00	0.018	0.310	11.0	28.0	41.0	—	690	0.018
0.081	0.071	1.41	0.166	0	19.4	0.378	16.0	0.600	17.0	0.240	0.940	23.0	39.0	454	0.725	740	0.300
0.075	0.215	0.400	0.058	0.413	7.40	0.403	1.00	5.10	146	0.025	0.450	15.2	119	190	2.50	444	0.585
0.025	0.026	0.168	0.153	0	2.00	0.109	17.4	—	36.0	0.113	1.73	15.5	23.0	200	—	780	0.220

SOUPS

Qty	Name	Wgt G	Wtr G	Cal	Prot G	Carb G	Fiber G	F-Tot G	F-Sat G	Mono G	Poly G	Chol Mg	A-Car RE	A-Pre RE	A-Tot RE
1 cup	Crm Asparagus soup+milk	248	213	161	6.31	16.4	0.750	8.18	3.33	2.07	2.24	22.0	49.0	34.0	83.0
1 cup	Bean w/bacon soup	253	213	173	7.89	22.8	2.55	5.94	1.53	2.18	1.82	3.00	89.0	0	89.0
1 cup	Beef soup-chunky-RTS	240	200	171	11.7	19.6	0.800	5.14	2.55	2.14	0.200	14.0	261	0	261
1 cup	Beef broth/bouillon f/cnd	240	235	16.0	2.74	0.100	0	0.530	0.260	0.220	0.020	0.600	0	0	0
1 cup	Beef/mushroom soup-cndnsd	251	238	106	11.5	2.00	0.020	6.02	3.01	2.51	0.250	13.0	0	0	0
1 cup	Beef noodle soup	244	224	84.0	4.83	8.97	0.240	3.08	1.15	1.24	0.490	5.00	63.0	0	63.0
1 cup	Black bean soup-prepared	247	216	116	5.64	19.8	2.00	1.51	0.400	0.540	0.470	0	49.0	0	49.0
1 cup	Cream/celery soup-w/milk	248	215	165	5.69	14.5	0.380	9.68	3.95	2.47	2.65	32.0	35.0	33.0	68.0
1 cup	Cheese soup prep w/milk	251	207	230	9.45	16.2	0.010	14.6	9.12	4.10	0.440	48.0	15.0	132	147
1 cup	Chicken soup-chunky-RTS	251	211	178	12.7	17.3	0.300	6.63	1.98	2.97	1.39	30.0	130	0	130
1 cup	Chicken broth from/canned	244	234	39.0	4.93	0.930	0	1.39	0.410	0.630	0.290	1.00	0	0	0
1 cup	Chicken+dumplings-prepard	241	221	97.0	5.61	6.04	0.020	5.52	1.31	2.53	1.30	34.0	52.0	0	52.0
1 cup	Crm.chicken soup w/milk	248	210	191	7.46	15.0	0.130	11.5	4.63	4.45	1.64	27.0	60.0	34.0	94.0
1 cup	Cream/chicken soup w/watr	244	221	115	3.43	9.26	0.610	7.36	2.08	3.28	1.49	10.0	56.0	0	56.0
1 cup	Chicken gumbo soup	244	229	56.0	2.64	8.37	0.150	1.43	0.330	0.650	0.350	5.00	13.6	0	13.6
1 cup	Chicken mushroom soup	244	220	67.0	4.39	2.00	0.050	9.16	2.39	4.03	2.32	10.0	112	0	112
1 cup	Chick-noodl soup-chnk-RTS	240	216	114	12.7	2.00	0.250	6.00	1.39	2.66	1.52	18.0	122	0	122
1 cup	Chicken noodle soup	241	222	75.0	4.04	9.35	0.240	2.45	0.650	1.11	0.550	7.00	71.0	0	71.0
1 cup	Chick-noodle+meatball-RTS	248	226	99.0	8.11	8.36	0.600	3.57	1.07	1.60	0.750	10.0	233	0	233
1 cup	Chicken rice-chunky-RTS	240	208	127	12.3	13.0	0.900	3.19	0.950	1.43	0.670	12.0	586	0	586
1 cup	Chicken rice soup	241	227	60.0	3.53	7.15	0.820	1.91	0.500	0.900	0.400	7.00	66.0	0	66.0
1 cup	Chicken/veg soup-prepared	241	223	74.0	3.61	8.58	0.300	2.84	0.850	1.27	0.600	—	266	0	266
1 cup	Chili con carne/beans-cnd	255	184	339	19.1	31.1	5.10	15.6	5.80	7.20	1.00	28.0	15.0	0	15.0
1 cup	Chili beef soup	250	212	169	6.69	21.5	1.45	6.61	3.34	2.80	0.270	12.0	0	503	503
1 cup	Clam chowder-New England	248	211	163	9.46	16.6	1.00	6.60	2.95	2.26	1.08	22.0	4.00	36.0	40.0
1 cup	Clam chowder-Manhatten	244	218	78.0	4.18	12.2	1.20	2.31	0.440	0.410	1.32	2.00	92.0	0	92.0
1 cup	Consomme with gelatin	241	232	29.0	5.35	1.76	0.010	0	0	0	0	0	0	0	0
1 cup	Gazpacho-ready to serve	244	229	57.0	8.70	0.780	0.640	2.24	0.290	0.540	1.32	0	0	20.0	20.0
1 cup	Leek soup-dry-prepared	254	236	71.0	2.11	11.4	0.300	2.05	1.02	0.860	0.080	3.00	—	—	—
1 cup	Minestrone	241	220	80.0	4.26	11.2	0.960	2.51	0.540	0.690	1.11	2.00	234	0	234
1 cup	Crm/mushroom soup-cnd-prp	248	210	205	6.05	15.0	0.250	13.6	5.12	2.98	4.61	20.0	4.00	34.0	38.0
1 cup	Crm mushroom soup-w/water	244	220	130	2.00	9.30	1.48	9.00	2.40	1.70	4.20	2.00	0	0	0
1 cup	Onion soup-canned	241	224	57.0	3.75	8.18	0.480	1.74	0.260	0.750	0.650	0	0	0	0
1 cup	Pea soup-prepared w/milk	254	198	239	12.6	32.2	0.600	7.03	4.00	2.18	0.520	18.0	24.0	34.0	58.0
1 cup	Cream of potato soup-cnd	248	215	148	5.78	17.2	0.340	6.45	3.76	1.73	0.560	22.0	33.0	34.0	67.0
1 cup	Split pea+ham soup-chkRTS	240	194	184	11.1	26.8	1.60	3.98	1.59	1.63	0.570	7.00	487	0	487
1 cup	Split pea soup w/ham-cnd	253	207	189	10.3	28.0	0.670	4.40	1.76	1.80	0.630	8.00	44.0	0	44.0
1 cup	Stock pot soup	248	225	100	4.86	11.5	0.500	3.90	0.860	1.02	1.76	5.00	398	0	398
1 cup	Tomato soup prep w/milk	248	211	160	6.00	22.3	0.500	6.01	2.90	1.60	1.10	17.0	73.0	36.0	109
1 cup	Tomato soup w/water-cnd	244	221	86.0	2.06	16.6	0.490	1.92	0.360	0.430	0.960	0	69.0	0	69.0
1 cup	Tomato soup-from dry	265	238	102	2.45	19.4	0.430	2.37	1.08	0.890	0.230	1.00	83.0	0	83.0
1 cup	Tomato beef noodle soup	244	212	140	4.45	21.2	0.200	4.29	1.59	1.73	0.680	5.00	53.3	0	53.3
1 cup	Tomato bisque prep w/milk	251	205	198	6.29	29.4	0.100	6.60	3.14	1.87	1.24	22.0	76.0	34.0	110
1 cup	Tomato rice soup	247	218	120	2.11	21.9	0.750	2.72	0.520	0.600	1.35	2.00	75.5	0	75.5
1 cup	Tomato-veg soup-from dry	253	237	55.0	2.00	10.2	0.530	0.870	0.400	0.330	0.080	0	19.0	0	19.0
1 cup	Turkey soup-chunky-RTS	236	204	136	10.2	14.1	1.00	4.41	2.75	1.78	1.08	9.00	1613	0	1613
1 cup	Turkey noodle soup	244	227	69.0	3.90	8.63	0.150	1.99	0.560	0.810	0.490	5.00	29.2	0	29.2
1 cup	Turkey vegetable soup	241	224	74.0	3.09	8.64	0.500	3.02	0.900	1.33	0.670	2.00	244	0	244
1 cup	Vegetable beef soup	244	224	79.0	5.58	10.2	0.810	1.90	0.850	0.800	0.110	5.00	189	0	189
1 cup	Vegetable soup+beef broth	241	221	81.0	2.96	13.1	0.650	1.91	0.440	0.550	0.780	2.00	209	0	209
1 cup	Vegetable soup-chunky-RTS	240	210	122	3.50	19.0	1.30	3.70	0.550	1.59	1.39	0	588	0	588
1 cup	Crm-vegetable soup Fr/dry	260	237	105	1.89	12.3	0.140	5.69	1.42	2.54	1.48	0	3.50	0	3.50
1 cup	Vegetarian vegetable soup	241	222	70.0	2.10	12.0	0.800	1.93	0.290	0.830	0.730	0	301	0	301

B1 Mg	B2 Mg	B3 Mg	B6 Mg	B12 Mcg	Fol. Mcg	Panto Mg	Vit-C Mg	Vit-E Mg	Calc Mg	Cu Mg	Iron	Mg Mg	Phos Mg	Potas Mg	Sel Mcg	Na Mg	Zinc Mg
0.102	0.275	0.880	0.064	—	—	—	3.90	—	175	0.139	0.870	20.0	153	359	—	1041	0.925
0.089	0.033	0.567	0.040	—	31.9	0.160	1.60	—	81.0	0.402	2.05	44.0	132	403	—	952	1.03
0.058	0.151	2.71	0.132	0.610	13.4	—	7.00	—	31.0	0.240	2.33	—	120	336	—	867	2.64
0.005	0.050	1.87	0.071	0.300	2.00	0.528	0	—	15.0	0.185	0.410	9.00	31.0	130	0	782	0.600
0.050	0.151	2.26	—	—	—	—	0	—	10.0	—	1.76	—	—	—	—	—	—
0.068	0.059	1.07	0.036	0.200	4.40	0.162	0.300	—	15.0	0.139	1.10	6.00	46.0	100	—	952	1.54
0.077	0.054	0.534	0.094	0.020	24.7	0.198	0.800	—	45.0	0.385	2.16	42.0	107	273	—	1198	1.41
0.074	0.248	0.436	0.064	—	8.50	—	1.40	—	186	0.154	0.690	22.0	151	309	8.49	1010	0.196
0.063	0.334	0.502	0.078	0.440	—	—	1.20	—	288	0.141	0.810	20.0	250	340	—	1020	0.688
0.085	0.173	4.42	0.050	0.250	4.60	—	1.30	—	24.0	0.251	1.73	—	113	176	—	887	1.00
0.010	0.071	3.35	0.024	0.240	—	—	0	—	9.00	0.124	0.510	2.00	73.0	210	—	776	0.249
0.017	0.072	1.75	0.036	0.160	—	—	0	—	15.0	0.123	0.620	4.00	61.0	116	—	861	0.366
0.074	0.258	0.923	0.067	0.450	7.70	0.400	1.30	0.111	180	0.139	0.670	18.0	152	273	8.49	1046	0.675
0.029	0.061	0.820	0.017	—	1.60	—	0.200	—	34.0	0.124	0.610	3.00	37.0	88.0	—	986	0.627
0.020	0.050	0.664	0.063	—	—	—	4.90	—	24.0	0.124	0.900	4.00	25.0	75.0	—	955	0.376
0.024	0.112	1.63	—	—	—	—	0	—	29.0	—	88.0	—	—	—	—	—	—
0.072	0.168	4.32	—	—	—	—	0	—	24.0	—	1.44	—	—	—	—	—	—
0.053	0.060	1.39	0.008	—	2.20	—	0.200	—	17.0	0.195	0.780	7.20	36.0	55.0	—	900	0.550
0.124	0.124	2.51	—	—	—	—	7.80	—	30.0	—	1.74	—	—	—	—	1039	—
0.024	0.098	4.10	—	—	3.80	—	3.80	—	35.0	—	1.87	—	—	—	—	888	—
0.017	0.024	1.13	0.024	—	1.10	—	0.100	—	17.0	0.118	0.750	1.00	22.0	101	3.13	815	0.263
0.043	0.055	1.23	0.048	—	—	—	1.00	—	18.0	0.123	0.870	6.00	41.0	154	—	944	0.366
0.080	0.180	3.30	0.268	0	41.0	0.357	8.00	1.40	82.0	0.395	4.30	60.0	321	594	2.60	1354	3.78
0.060	0.075	1.07	0.158	0.320	10.0	0.350	4.10	1.40	43.0	0.396	2.40	30.0	148	525	24.2	1035	1.40
0.067	0.236	1.03	0.126	10.3	12.0	0.400	3.50	0.111	187	0.139	1.48	23.0	157	300	—	992	1.30
0.063	0.049	1.34	0.083	2.19	9.50	0.122	3.20	—	34.0	0.148	1.89	10.0	58.0	261	—	1808	0.927
0.022	0.029	0.711	0.024	0	3.00	—	0.900	—	8.00	0.246	0.530	0	32.0	153	—	637	0.366
0.049	0.024	0.927	0.146	0	—	0.171	3.10	—	24.0	—	0.980	—	37.0	224	—	1183	—
—	—	—	—	—	—	—	—	—	—	0.036	—	—	—	—	—	966	0.236
0.053	0.043	0.942	0.099	0	16.1	—	1.00	—	34.0	0.123	0.920	7.00	56.0	312	—	911	0.735
0.077	0.280	0.813	0.064	0.444	15.0	0.683	2.30	—	178	0.139	0.590	20.0	156	270	8.49	1076	0.640
0.050	0.090	0.700	0.015	—	3.00	—	1.00	—	46.0	—	0.500	4.90	49.0	100	7.30	1032	0.593
0.034	0.024	0.600	0.048	0	15.2	—	1.20	—	26.0	0.123	0.670	2.00	11.0	69.0	—	1053	0.612
0.155	0.267	1.34	0.104	0.440	7.90	—	2.90	—	173	0.391	2.01	55.0	238	377	—	1048	1.76
0.082	0.236	0.642	0.089	0	9.20	0.838	1.10	—	166	0.263	0.540	17.0	160	323	—	1060	0.675
0.115	0.094	2.52	—	—	4.70	—	7.00	—	33.0	—	2.14	—	—	—	—	965	—
0.147	0.076	1.48	0.068	—	2.50	—	1.40	—	22.0	0.369	2.28	48.0	213	399	—	1008	1.32
0.044	0.052	1.22	0.089	0	—	—	2.10	—	22.0	0.128	0.870	4.00	54.0	238	—	1048	1.16
0.134	0.248	1.52	0.164	0.440	20.9	0.109	68.0	0.111	159	0.268	1.82	23.0	148	450	8.49	932	0.290
0.088	0.051	1.42	0.112	0	14.7	0.109	66.5	—	13.0	0.260	1.76	8.00	34.0	263	1.22	872	0.244
0.061	0.048	0.782	0.098	—	6.70	—	4.60	—	54.0	0.093	0.420	15.0	66.0	295	—	943	0.209
0.083	0.090	1.87	0.088	0.190	—	—	0	—	18.0	0.124	1.12	8.00	56.0	221	—	917	0.752
0.113	0.269	1.25	0.141	0.440	—	—	7.10	—	186	0.141	0.880	25.0	174	604	—	1108	0.633
0.062	0.049	1.06	0.077	0	—	—	14.8	—	23.0	0.128	0.790	5.00	33.0	330	—	815	0.514
0.058	0.046	0.789	0.094	—	3.00	0.144	6.00	—	8.00	0.033	0.630	20.0	29.0	103	—	1146	0.167
0.080	0.239	8.89	0.692	4.79	25.0	—	14.4	—	50.0	0.532	1.91	—	234	814	—	2082	4.79
0.073	0.063	1.40	0.037	—	—	—	0.200	—	12.0	0.124	0.940	5.00	48.0	75.0	—	815	0.583
0.029	0.039	1.01	0.048	0.170	—	—	0	—	17.0	0.123	0.760	4.00	40.0	175	—	905	0.612
0.037	0.049	1.03	0.076	0.310	10.6	0.337	2.40	—	17.0	0.140	1.11	6.00	41.0	173	—	956	2.00
0.051	0.046	0.966	0.055	0	—	—	2.40	—	18.0	0.154	0.970	7.00	39.0	192	—	810	0.795
0.072	0.065	1.20	0.192	0	16.5	—	6.00	—	56.0	0.240	1.63	—	72.0	396	—	1010	3.12
1.22	0.107	0.520	0.052	—	—	—	3.90	—	—	—	—	—	54.0	96.0	—	1171	—
0.053	0.046	0.916	0.055	0	10.6	0.337	1.00	—	21.0	0.220	1.08	7.00	35.0	209	—	823	0.460

SWEETS, DESSERTS

Qty	Name	Wgt G	Wtr G	Cal	Prot G	Carb G	Fiber G	F-Tot G	F-Sat G	Mono G	Poly G	Chol Mg	A-Car RE	A-Pre RE	A-Tot RE
1 ea.	Brownies w/nuts-homemade	20.0	2.00	95.0	1.30	11.0	0.200	6.30	1.40	2.80	1.20	18.0	0	6.00	6.00
1 ea.	Brownies w/nuts/frst/comm	25.0	3.27	100	1.18	15.9	0.220	4.40	1.60	2.00	0.800	14.0	1.50	16.5	18.0
1 pce	Angel food cake (1/12th)	53.0	20.0	125	3.20	28.5	0.250	0.167	0.033	0.017	0.083	0	0	0	0
1 pce	Boston cream pie-1/8 cake	120	42.0	260	2.50	44.0	0.375	8.00	2.75	3.05	1.50	20.0	3.00	67.0	70.0
1 pce	Carrot cake/crmchz 2x3 in	96.0	22.1	385	4.20	48.0	0.690	21.0	4.10	8.40	6.80	74.0	13.0	2.00	15.0
1 pce	Cheesecake 1/12 of cake	92.0	42.2	278	4.99	26.3	0.414	17.7	9.94	5.43	1.19	170	0.600	68.4	69.0
1 ea.	Choc cupcake/choc frostng	42.0	10.1	143	1.83	24.5	0.450	4.87	2.13	1.95	0.730	22.5	0	18.9	18.9
1 pce	Choc cake + icng-mix-1/16ck	69.0	16.6	235	3.00	40.2	0.740	8.00	3.50	3.20	1.20	37.0	0	31.0	31.0
1 pce	White cake/coconut-comm	70.0	16.8	270	3.20	42.0	1.30	10.0	3.89	3.93	2.65	3.00	0	12.0	12.0
1 pce	Coffee cake f/mix (1/6th)	72.0	21.6	230	4.52	37.7	0.540	6.87	1.98	2.80	1.61	47.0	2.00	30.0	32.0
1 pce	Dark fruitcake 2/3in arc	43.0	7.74	165	2.00	25.0	1.20	7.00	1.50	3.60	1.60	20.0	1.00	12.0	13.0
1 pce	Gingerbread cake-homemade	110	41.8	351	4.46	59.0	1.08	11.1	2.24	4.79	3.44	30.4	0.400	134	134
1 pce	Pound cake-1/2in slc-mix	30.0	6.60	120	2.00	15.0	0.220	5.00	1.20	2.40	1.60	32.0	0	60.0	60.0
1 pce	Sheet cake-wht frstg-pce	121	25.4	445	4.00	77.0	0.340	14.0	4.60	5.60	2.90	70.0	0.600	70.4	71.0
1 ea.	Snack cake/choc w/filling	28.0	5.60	105	1.00	17.0	0.080	4.00	1.70	1.50	0.600	15.0	1.00	3.00	4.00
1 ea.	Sponge snack cake w/fill	42.0	7.98	155	1.00	27.0	0.100	5.00	2.30	2.10	0.500	7.00	0	9.00	9.00
1 pce	Sponge cake-1/12th tube	66.0	21.1	194	4.68	37.3	0.443	2.95	0.860	1.13	0.430	137	0.020	39.0	39.0
1 pce	White cake/coconut-comm	70.0	16.8	270	3.20	42.0	1.30	10.0	3.89	3.93	2.65	3.00	0	12.0	12.0
1 pce	White cake/choc icng-mix	77.0	17.7	291	3.74	43.6	0.656	12.2	4.00	4.79	2.74	3.00	0.200	12.0	12.2
1 pce	Yellow cake/choc-pce-f/mx	69.0	17.9	235	2.80	40.0	0.312	7.78	2.99	3.05	1.36	36.0	0.500	28.5	29.0
1 cup	Cake icing-canned avg all	250	—	1024	0	154	0	0	10.6	18.8	11.0	0	0	0	0
1 cup	Cake icing prep from mix	250	—	1069	0	180	0	39.7	—	—	—	0	0	0	0
1 oz.	Almond Joy candy bar	28.3	—	153	1.71	18.7	0.395	7.93	6.74	0.639	0.117	0	0	0	0
1 oz.	Sugar coated almonds	28.3	—	148	3.15	14.8	2.46	9.25	—	—	—	0	0	0	0
1 oz.	Bittersweet chocolate	28.3	0.283	143	1.92	15.9	0.901	9.87	5.97	3.34	0.304	0	1.01	0	1.01
1 oz.	Caramel-plain or choc.	28.3	2.27	116	1.01	22.3	0.057	3.04	2.23	0.304	0.101	1.01	0	0.304	0.304
1 oz.	Chocolate coated almonds	28.3	0.850	161	3.92	7.99	3.01	12.7	2.75	7.73	2.23	0	0.447	0	0.447
1 oz.	Choc-covrd coconut candy	28.3	—	135	0.918	17.7	2.44	7.21	—	—	—	0	0.911	0	0.911
1 oz.	Chocolate covered mints	28.3	0.850	117	0.506	23.3	0.028	3.04	1.82	0.992	0.091	0	0.101	0	0.101
1 oz.	Chocolate coated peanuts	28.3	0.850	159	5.00	9.76	1.83	11.7	2.68	5.02	2.77	0	1.07	0	1.07
1 oz.	Chocolate covered raisins	28.3	3.69	111	1.06	20.6	1.61	2.71	1.41	0.763	0.103	0	0.667	0	0.667
1 oz.	Chocolate fudge	28.3	2.27	116	0.572	21.3	0.063	2.81	2.13	1.01	0.101	1.01	2.02	14.2	16.2
1 oz.	Chocolate fudge with nuts	28.3	2.24	115	1.07	19.0	0.238	5.06	2.28	1.44	1.32	7.45	1.01	13.2	14.2
1 ea.	REESE's peanut butter cup	22.5	—	120	2.90	11.0	0.845	7.20	—	—	—	1.28	—	—	4.00
1 oz.	Divinity w/nuts candy	28.3	—	113	0.868	22.7	0.221	2.72	—	—	—	0	0.142	0	0.142
1 oz.	English toffee candy bar	28.3	—	195	0.886	9.83	0.089	16.9	—	—	—	0	—	—	4.43
1 oz.	Fondant candy-candy corn	28.3	0.850	106	0	27.3	0	0	0	0	0	0	0	0	0
1 oz.	Hard candy-all flavors	28.3	0.283	110	0	27.9	0	0	0	0	0	0	0	0	0
1 oz.	Jelly beans	28.3	1.70	105	0	26.7	0	0.101	0	0	0.101	0	0	0	0
1 oz.	Gum drops	28.3	3.40	99.2	0	25.1	0	0.202	0	0	0.101	0	0	0	0
1 oz.	Chocolate candy kisses	28.3	—	156	2.13	16.1	0.304	9.11	—	—	—	—	0	5.06	5.06
1 oz.	Kit Kat candy bar	28.3	—	138	1.98	16.5	0.066	7.25	—	—	—	—	0	5.93	5.93
1 oz.	Krackle candy bar	28.3	—	149	2.00	16.9	0.167	8.09	—	—	—	—	0	6.00	6.00
1 oz.	Malted milk balls	28.3	—	137	2.33	18.0	0.101	7.09	—	—	—	—	—	—	—
1 oz.	M&M's Plain choc. candies	28.3	—	140	1.95	19.5	0.142	6.08	—	—	—	0	0	7.68	7.68
1 oz.	M&M's Peanut choc candies	28.3	—	144	3.23	16.5	0.809	7.25	—	—	—	0	—	—	0.060
1 oz.	MARS bar	28.3	—	136	2.27	17.0	0.493	6.24	2.72	2.49	0.454	0	—	—	0.057
1 oz.	Milk chocolate-plain	28.3	0.283	147	2.02	16.2	0.312	9.11	5.47	3.04	0.304	6.07	0	10.1	10.1
1 oz.	Milk chocolate w/almonds	28.3	0.567	152	2.95	15.2	0.996	10.5	4.45	4.71	1.01	4.56	0	8.10	8.10
1 oz.	Milk chocolate w/peanuts	28.3	0.283	157	4.96	10.1	1.61	11.8	3.54	5.26	2.73	3.04	0	8.10	8.10
1 oz.	MILKY WAY candy bar	28.3	—	123	1.53	20.3	0.033	4.25	2.55	1.42	0.142	6.61	—	—	11.8
1 oz.	Mr. Goodbar candy bar	28.3	—	151	3.62	13.9	0.302	9.05	4.70	—	1.57	4.22	0	3.26	3.26
1 oz.	SNICKERS candy bar	28.3	—	134	3.08	17.0	0.709	6.62	—	—	—	0	—	—	2.32
1 oz.	Vanilla fudge	28.3	—	119	0.709	22.3	0	3.20	—	—	—	10.1	12.1	0	12.1
1 oz.	Vanilla fudge with nuts	28.3	—	124	1.01	18.5	0.202	5.08	—	—	—	8.66	12.1	0	12.1
1 oz.	Chocolate fudge	28.3	2.27	116	0.572	21.3	0.063	2.81	2.13	1.01	0.101	1.01	2.02	14.2	16.2
1 oz.	Chocolate fudge with nuts	28.3	2.24	115	1.07	19.0	0.238	5.06	2.28	1.44	1.32	7.45	1.01	13.2	14.2
1 cup	Chocolate milk-whole	250	206	210	7.92	25.9	0.150	8.48	5.26	2.48	0.310	31.0	8.80	64.2	73.0
1 cup	Chocolate milkshake	226	162	288	7.68	46.3	0.232	8.40	5.24	2.43	0.317	29.6	5.60	45.6	51.2

B1 Mg	B2 Mg	B3 Mg	B6 Mg	B12 Mcg	Fol. Mcg	Panto Mg	Vit-C Mg	Vit-E Mg	Calc Mg	Cu Mg	Iron Mg	Mg Mg	Phos Mg	Potas Mg	Sel Mcg	Na Mg	Zinc Mg
0.050	0.050	0.300	0.035	0.044	4.00	0.100	0.010	0.500	9.00	0.091	0.400	11.2	26.0	35.0	3.00	51.0	0.310
0.080	0.065	0.325	0.043	0.052	5.00	0.124	0.012	0.440	13.0	0.114	0.605	14.0	26.0	50.0	3.20	59.0	0.360
0.027	0.106	0.134	0.007	0	4.00	0.115	0	0.010	44.0	0.032	0.230	4.30	91.0	71.0	3.10	269	0.068
0.010	0.180	0.700	0.050	0.320	7.00	0.320	0	2.00	26.0	0.093	0.600	11.0	70.0	40.0	3.07	225	0.230
0.110	0.120	0.900	0.864	0.152	15.2	0.303	1.00	95.2	44.0	0.146	1.30	12.3	62.0	108	4.36	279	0.510
0.028	0.119	0.423	0.058	0.455	16.6	0.527	4.64	2.50	51.6	0.055	0.441	9.19	80.9	90.2	6.20	204	—
0.043	0.061	0.365	0.012	0.060	2.52	0.084	0.061	0.956	25.0	0.021	0.852	5.48	43.8	54.8	2.47	—	—
0.070	0.100	0.600	0.020	0.098	4.14	0.138	0.100	1.57	41.0	0.090	1.40	21.7	72.0	90.0	1.70	181	0.530
0.102	0.131	1.72	0.010	0.040	4.00	0.210	0	0.273	33.9	0.050	1.12	6.89	106	72.7	3.18	177	0.212
0.137	0.151	1.29	0.020	0.107	5.00	0.150	0.170	2.16	44.0	0.034	1.22	4.50	125	78.0	2.53	310	0.619
0.080	0.080	0.500	0.054	0.049	1.70	0.086	16.0	0.602	41.0	0.072	1.20	10.7	50.0	194	0.029	67.0	0.215
0.164	0.148	1.78	0.058	0.085	8.20	0.305	0.050	1.97	47.3	0.329	2.74	17.2	51.9	214	14.1	—	—
0.050	0.060	0.500	0.023	0.134	3.20	0.131	0.221	0.265	20.0	0.020	0.500	3.00	28.0	28.0	3.12	98.0	0.158
0.130	0.160	1.10	0.030	0.071	12.0	0.231	0.221	0.278	61.0	0.036	1.20	12.0	91.0	74.0	7.00	275	0.322
0.060	0.090	0.700	0.013	0.096	3.00	0.119	0	0.300	21.0	0.018	1.00	2.50	26.0	34.0	1.30	105	0.172
0.070	0.060	0.600	0.016	0.120	4.00	0.099	0	0.700	14.0	0.023	0.600	3.00	44.0	37.0	1.20	155	0.210
0.100	0.107	0.802	0.028	0.328	11.2	0.401	0.223	0.401	25.1	0.049	1.22	6.59	69.8	50.2	11.0	210	—
0.102	0.131	1.72	0.010	0.040	4.00	0.210	0	0.273	33.9	0.050	1.12	6.89	106	72.7	3.18	177	0.212
0.203	0.151	1.78	0.012	0.040	7.80	0.221	0	0.600	38.0	0.149	1.40	21.0	122	102	3.41	176	0.323
0.076	0.103	0.691	0.028	0.098	5.00	0.200	0.062	2.07	63.0	0.034	0.965	4.50	126	75.0	2.90	157	0.206
—	—	—	—	0	—	—	—	—	—	—	—	—	—	—	—	538	—
—	—	—	—	0	—	—	—	—	—	—	—	—	—	—	—	582	—
—	—	—	—	0	—	—	—	0.101	2.02	—	0.789	—	—	—	—	—	—
0.043	0.158	0.605	0.017	0	16.4	0.094	0	3.96	40.2	0.128	0.786	46.4	87.1	134	0.723	1.01	0.533
0.015	0.051	0.322	0.010	0	14.2	0.051	0	1.70	13.2	0.253	1.05	28.3	60.7	131	—	2.02	1.14
0.010	0.051	0.101	0.003	0.020	0	0.034	0.001	0.075	42.5	0.025	0.405	5.77	35.4	54.7	1.01	64.8	0.155
0.052	0.186	0.716	0.022	0	22.0	0.116	0	4.93	47.8	0.235	1.09	62.5	108	174	0.780	2.06	0.723
0.008	0.016	0.152	0.101	0	5.49	0.026	0	0.519	8.49	0.132	0.623	16.6	29.4	75.9	1.81	7.09	0.409
0.010	0.020	0.132	—	0	—	—	—	—	16.2	0.081	0.304	16.2	15.2	26.3	0.010	52.6	0.223
0.086	0.043	2.67	0.070	0	28.5	0.415	—	2.75	32.9	0.215	0.689	47.0	84.5	143	7.32	17.0	0.744
0.034	0.025	0.196	0.052	0	2.61	0.018	0.652	0.529	12.2	0.170	0.663	18.0	29.9	175	2.06	3.94	0.190
0.010	0.030	0.101	0.004	0.037	2.05	0.053	0.001	0.068	22.3	0.052	0.304	14.2	24.3	42.5	1.07	54.7	0.157
0.016	0.030	0.111	0.032	0.037	3.68	0.065	0.117	0.729	22.3	0.083	0.304	15.2	31.4	46.6	0.871	48.6	0.248
0.016	0.025	1.06	0.029	0	8.30	0.249	—	2.20	17.2	0.128	0.341	23.5	43.5	84.0	0.585	46.0	0.346
0.014	0.011	0.048	0.035	0	3.61	0.045	0.081	0.832	7.30	0.045	0.173	6.00	17.0	22.7	1.69	26.9	0.125
0.470	0.044	0.089	0.035	0	—	—	0	—	0	—	0.177	—	0	44.3	—	79.7	—
0.001	0.001	0.010	0.001	0	0	—	0	0	2.02	—	0.101	—	2.02	1.01	1.09	57.7	0.101
0	0	0	0	0	0	0	0	0	6.07	0.025	0.101	0.405	2.02	1.01	0.081	7.09	0
0	0.001	0.010	—	0	0	0	0	—	1.01	—	0.304	—	1.01	11.1	0.081	7.09	0
0	0.001	0.010	0	0	0	0	0	—	2.02	—	0.101	—	—	1.01	0.081	10.1	0
0.020	0.081	0.101	—	—	—	—	—	—	53.7	0.111	0.506	18.2	88.1	116	—	25.3	0.364
0.020	0.073	0.066	—	—	—	—	—	—	42.9	0.053	0.369	12.5	51.4	85.0	—	25.1	0.283
0.017	0.075	0.083	—	—	—	—	—	—	50.0	0.117	0.400	16.7	68.4	96.7	—	40.9	0.309
—	—	—	—	—	—	—	—	—	63.8	—	—	—	87.1	114	—	28.3	—
0.015	0.073	0.159	0.006	0	2.84	0.171	—	—	46.7	0.089	0.449	17.7	38.4	101	—	24.2	0.337
0.016	0.056	0.887	0.020	0	2.83	0.170	—	—	35.4	0.102	0.402	22.7	38.4	97.1	—	17.4	0.396
0.014	0.093	0.272	0.006	0	3.01	0.180	—	—	48.2	0.074	0.312	21.0	35.7	99.8	—	48.2	0.332
0.020	0.101	0.101	0.016	0	0.283	0.200	0.001	1.42	50.6	0.112	0.405	16.4	61.8	97.2	1.11	23.3	0.372
0.030	0.132	0.317	0.020	0	4.45	0.184	0.101	2.78	61.8	0.152	0.567	33.4	78.0	127	1.21	23.3	0.488
0.113	0.066	2.23	0.054	0	16.2	0.506	0.001	2.08	32.4	0.202	0.688	35.4	88.1	157	1.69	19.2	0.684
0.013	0.070	0.094	0.006	0	3.09	0.186	0.282	—	40.6	0.043	0.232	10.3	37.8	78.9	—	66.1	0.211
0.030	0.072	1.27	—	—	—	—	—	—	39.2	0.145	0.567	27.1	79.6	128	—	12.7	0.513
0.013	0.050	0.852	0.009	0	2.89	0.173	—	—	32.4	0.065	0.227	18.1	34.7	96.8	0.269	78.7	0.319
0.006	0.025	0.013	0.004	0.055	0.848	0.045	0.078	0.060	30.4	0.012	0.030	1.73	24.3	36.4	0.337	50.6	0.097
0.017	0.026	0.048	0.036	0.044	3.74	0.072	0.137	0.815	25.3	0.046	0.161	6.53	26.3	38.5	1.01	36.4	0.181
0.010	0.030	0.101	0.004	0.037	2.05	0.053	0.001	0.068	22.3	0.052	0.304	14.2	24.3	42.5	1.07	54.7	0.157
0.016	0.030	0.111	0.032	0.037	3.68	0.065	0.117	0.729	22.3	0.083	0.304	15.2	31.4	46.6	0.871	48.6	0.248
0.092	0.405	0.313	0.100	0.835	12.0	0.738	2.28	0.222	280	0.085	0.600	33.0	251	417	3.05	149	1.02
0.131	0.554	0.365	0.114	0.776	7.92	0.880	1.04	0.560	255	0.147	0.704	37.6	230	454	—	218	0.920

Qty	Name	Wgt G	Wtr G	Cal	Prot G	Carb G	Fiber G	F-Tot G	F-Sat G	Mono G	Poly G	Chol Mg	A-Car RE	A-Pre RE	A-Tot RE
1 cup	Chocolate pudding-Recipe	260	172	385	8.10	66.8	0.520	11.5	7.08	3.24	0.300	39.0	8.00	93.0	101
1 Tbs	Chocolate syrup-thin	18.8	6.94	42.5	0.600	11.0	0.469	0.244	0.100	0.050	0.050	0	0.375	0	0.375
5 ea.	Animal cookies	5.19	0.156	22.2	0.352	4.07	0.019	0.537	0.138	0.230	0.138	0.019	0	0	0
3 ea.	Butter cookies	15.0	0.600	69.0	0.930	10.7	0.015	2.55	1.58	0.732	0.942	2.16	2.70	21.9	24.6
3 ea.	Choc chip cookies-comm	31.5	1.20	135	1.71	21.0	0.337	6.60	2.17	2.32	1.95	3.75	0	11.3	11.3
3 ea.	Choc chip cookies-home	30.0	0.900	139	1.50	19.2	0.720	8.02	2.92	3.22	1.50	13.5	0	3.75	3.75
3 ea.	Fig bars	42.0	5.17	157	1.51	31.7	0.600	2.86	0.750	1.13	0.750	20.2	4.72	0	4.72
3 ea.	Lady fingers	33.0	6.34	118	2.55	21.3	0.033	2.55	0.945	1.22	0.390	118	0	56.3	56.3
3 ea.	Oatmeal raisin cookies	39.0	1.56	184	2.25	27.0	0.600	7.50	1.88	3.38	2.10	1.50	0	9.00	9.00
3 ea.	Peanut butter cookies-hme	36.0	1.08	184	3.00	21.0	0.750	10.5	3.00	4.35	2.10	16.5	3.75	3.38	3.75
3 ea.	Sandwich type cookies-all	30.0	0.600	146	1.50	21.7	0.030	6.00	1.50	2.70	1.65	0	0	0	0
3 ea.	Snickerdoodle cookies	60.0	4.80	330	3.81	48.0	1.16	14.3	8.76	4.05	0.648	37.8	14.5	115	130
3 ea.	Shortbread cookies-comm	24.0	1.44	116	1.50	15.0	0.048	6.00	2.17	2.25	0.825	20.2	0.375	5.63	6.00
3 ea.	Shortbread cookies-lrg-hm	42.0	1.26	217	2.47	25.8	0.067	12.4	1.95	4.05	5.10	0	0	133	133
3 ea.	Sugar cookies f/refrig do	36.0	1.44	176	1.50	23.2	0.036	9.00	1.72	3.75	2.70	21.7	0	8.25	8.25
3 ea.	Vanilla wafers	12.0	0.480	55.5	0.600	8.70	0.012	2.10	0.540	0.900	0.540	7.50	0.150	4.05	4.20
1 Tbs	Corn syrup-dark	20.5	5.13	59.0	0	15.4	0	0	0	0	0	0	0	0	0
1 Tbs	Whipped cream	7.44	4.29	25.7	0.152	0.207	0	2.75	1.71	0.794	0.102	10.2	0.750	30.6	31.3
1 Tbs	Dessert top-fzn/non-dairy	4.69	2.35	14.9	0.059	1.08	0	1.19	1.02	0.076	0.024	0	4.06	0	4.06
1 cup	Apple brown betty	207	137	316	2.21	54.0	4.85	11.7	6.80	3.25	0.741	27.6	16.4	84.8	101
1 pce	Apple cobbler pce=3x3in	104	58.2	201	1.93	35.1	2.01	6.40	1.39	2.66	1.94	1.38	2.65	73.2	75.9
1 pce	Apple crisp-3x3 in piece	78.0	45.2	146	0.901	25.0	1.78	5.32	1.04	2.27	1.69	0	2.74	62.6	65.3
1 ea.	Apple dumpling	151	87.6	295	1.72	46.0	3.77	12.6	2.78	5.44	3.67	0	5.70	70.4	76.1
1 cup	Bread + raisin pudding	165	96.7	349	7.24	49.7	2.06	14.4	4.52	6.04	2.82	142	3.00	164	167
1 pce	Cheesecake 1/12 of cake	92.0	42.2	278	4.99	26.3	0.414	17.7	9.94	5.43	1.19	170	0.600	68.4	69.0
1 pce	Cherry cobbler-pce=3x3 in	129	83.8	199	2.39	34.2	1.31	6.24	1.37	2.67	1.90	1.38	61.7	73.2	135
1 pce	Cherry & cream cheese torte	161	71.6	451	7.28	57.2	2.32	22.5	8.04	3.59	0.494	63.5	35.0	143	178
1 pce	Cherry crisp-3x3 in piece	138	101	157	1.64	27.2	1.46	5.25	1.03	2.29	1.67	0	81.9	62.6	144
1 cup	Chocolate mousse	237	167	460	11.1	18.3	0.600	39.9	22.9	12.3	1.89	349	10.7	371	381
1 ea.	Cream puff w/custard fill	110	52.8	280	4.83	26.5	0.241	17.6	9.69	5.80	0.754	228	9.00	193	202
1 ea.	Choc eclair w/custard fil	94.0	45.1	262	4.00	29.7	0.247	14.7	7.89	4.92	0.829	167	6.90	154	161
1 cup	Gelatin salad/dessert	240	202	140	3.60	33.8	0.200	0	0	0	0	0	0	0	0
1 pce	Peach cobbler-3x3in piece	130	83.2	130	2.29	36.5	1.78	6.19	1.36	2.66	1.88	1.38	31.7	73.2	105
1 pce	Peach crisp-3x3in piece	139	100	166	1.51	30.3	2.09	5.18	1.01	2.28	1.65	0	41.9	62.6	104
1 ea.	Doughnut-cake type-medium	50.0	10.4	210	2.35	24.5	0.500	11.9	3.40	5.80	2.00	20.0	0.500	4.50	5.00
1 ea.	Doughnut-jelly filled	65.0	18.2	226	3.40	30.0	0.500	8.80	3.52	3.72	0.610	0	12.0	0	12.0
1 ea.	Doughnut-yeast raised	60.0	16.0	235	4.00	26.0	0.480	13.3	5.20	5.50	0.900	21.0	0	0.300	0.300
1 pce	Gingerbread cake-homemade	110	41.8	351	4.46	59.0	1.08	11.1	2.24	4.79	3.44	30.4	0.400	134	134
1 Tbs	Honey	21.2	3.60	64.4	0.063	17.4	0	0	0	0	0	0	0	0	0
1 cup	Ice cream-regular-vanilla	133	80.9	269	4.80	31.7	0	14.3	8.29	4.14	0.530	59.0	15.0	118	133
1 cup	Ice cream-rich-vanilla	148	87.2	349	4.13	32.0	0	23.7	14.7	6.84	0.880	88.0	25.0	194	219
1 cup	Ice cream-soft serve	173	103	377	7.04	38.3	0	22.5	13.5	6.68	0.980	153	20.0	179	199
1 ea.	Soft ice cream cone-small	115	74.3	189	4.30	31.2	0.115	5.20	2.24	1.29	0.250	23.5	5.00	50.0	55.0
1 ea.	Hot fudge sundae-small	164	97.9	357	7.00	58.0	0.164	10.8	5.42	2.88	1.00	26.6	5.50	53.5	58.0
1 ea.	Strawberry sundae-small	164	101	320	6.00	54.0	0.164	8.70	3.18	2.81	1.11	25.0	5.50	53.5	58.0
1 ea.	Caramel sundae-small	165	93.2	361	7.20	60.8	0.165	10.0	3.47	2.71	0.910	31.4	6.60	63.4	70.0
1 cup	Ice milk	131	89.9	184	5.16	29.0	0	5.63	3.51	1.63	0.210	18.0	6.00	46.0	52.0
1 cup	Ice milk-soft serve-3%fat	175	122	223	8.03	38.4	0	4.62	2.88	1.33	0.170	13.0	4.30	39.7	44.0
1 cup	Ice slushy	193	154	247	0	62.7	0	0	0	0	0	0	0	0	0
1 cup	Gelatin salad/dessert	240	202	140	3.60	33.8	0.200	0	0	0	0	0	0	0	0
1 cup	Malt powder-choc flavored	336	4.37	1264	17.6	294	6.40	12.8	7.25	3.50	1.20	16.0	16.0	48.0	64.0
1 cup	Malted milk powder/natrl	336	6.72	1392	37.0	254	4.80	27.2	14.1	6.86	4.05	64.0	0	304	304
1 cup	Chocolate milkshake	226	162	288	7.68	46.3	0.232	8.40	5.24	2.43	0.317	29.6	5.60	45.6	51.2
1 cup	Strawberry milkshake	226	168	255	7.60	42.7	0.192	6.40	4.01	1.86	0.240	24.8	7.60	58.8	66.4
1 cup	Vanilla milkshake	226	169	251	7.84	40.6	0.152	6.72	4.21	1.95	0.251	25.6	8.00	64.0	72.0
1 Tbs	Molasses-blackstrap	20.0	4.80	42.5	0	11.0	0	0	0	0	0	0	0	0	0
1 Tbs	Pancake syrup	21.0	5.25	61.0	0	16.0	0	0	0	0	0	0	0	0	0
1 pce	Apple pie 1/6th pie	158	75.8	405	3.67	59.5	3.13	17.5	4.12	7.62	4.85	0	5.00	0	5.00
1 ea.	Apple pie-fried	85.0	36.5	255	2.20	32.0	1.70	14.0	5.80	6.60	0.600	14.0	3.00	0	3.00

B1 Mg	B2 Mg	B3 Mg	B6 Mg	B12 Mcg	Fol. Mcg	Panto Mg	Vit-C Mg	Vit-E Mg	Calc Mg	Cu Mg	Iron Mg	Mg Mg	Phos Mg	Potas Mg	Sel Mcg	Na Mg	Zinc Mg
0.050	0.360	0.300	0.128	0.481	10.0	0.780	1.00	0.255	250	0.077	1.30	48.4	255	445	4.00	146	1.53
0.004	0.009	0.056	0.002	0	1.50	0.007	0	0.188	2.81	0.094	0.372	13.1	24.4	42.5	0.219	15.5	0.197
0.015	0.024	0.204	0.002	0.002	0.741	0.011	0	—	0.556	0.004	0.170	0.556	3.15	4.81	—	20.9	0.026
0.006	0.009	0.060	0.012	0.007	1.29	0.022	0	0.450	19.2	0.007	0.090	4.50	14.4	9.00	1.02	63.0	0.072
0.075	0.172	0.675	0.015	0.015	2.85	0.405	0.001	1.24	12.3	0.060	0.600	7.50	30.7	42.0	0.300	105	0.228
0.045	0.045	0.438	0.022	0.030	2.70	0.080	0	0.900	9.75	0.097	0.750	10.5	25.5	61.5	0.300	61.5	0.165
0.058	0.055	0.546	0.052	0.001	2.63	0.150	0.001	—	30.0	0.120	1.02	10.9	25.5	121	1.13	135	0.268
0.022	0.045	0.075	0.034	0.394	15.0	0.518	0	—	13.5	—	0.600	3.60	54.0	39.0	2.85	37.5	0.432
0.067	0.060	0.750	0.021	0.022	4.80	0.052	0	1.80	13.5	0.046	0.825	19.8	43.5	67.5	3.51	111	0.397
0.052	0.052	1.42	0.029	0.014	8.62	0.050	0	4.57	15.7	0.056	0.825	14.2	45.0	82.5	2.25	106	0.270
0.067	0.052	0.600	0.009	0.011	0.900	0.033	0	1.24	9.00	0.022	1.05	11.3	30.0	49.5	0.300	142	0.160
0.120	0.141	1.52	0.027	0.021	6.03	0.150	0.480	1.35	34.5	0.054	1.87	8.28	34.2	53.4	9.69	278	—
0.075	0.067	0.675	0.009	0	1.95	0.036	0	0.698	9.75	0.015	0.600	3.30	29.2	28.5	1.44	92.2	0.110
0.115	0.090	1.06	0.013	0.012	3.45	0.115	0.001	1.24	9.00	0.024	0.825	6.00	46.5	27.0	2.88	188	0.192
0.067	0.045	0.825	0.015	0.018	3.22	0.054	0	1.05	37.5	0.047	0.675	5.77	68.2	24.7	1.26	196	0.180
0.021	0.030	0.300	0.004	0.006	1.05	0.018	0	0.330	4.80	0.009	0.240	1.80	10.8	15.0	0.864	45.0	0.036
0	0	0	—	0	1.00	—	0	—	9.44	0.007	0.205	0.688	3.25	0.813	2.00	13.9	0
0.002	0.008	0.003	0.002	0.013	0.313	0.019	0.043	0.047	4.81	0.008	0.002	0.531	4.66	5.59	0.044	2.78	0.017
0	0	0	0	0	0	0	0	0.003	0.313	—	0.006	0.063	0.375	0.875	—	1.19	0.002
0.117	0.084	0.853	0.079	0	8.20	0.156	0.516	0.751	39.1	0.108	0.949	10.2	37.3	169	6.88	208	—
0.083	0.070	0.701	0.036	0.043	2.76	0.106	0.327	1.12	32.4	0.062	0.756	6.57	42.0	86.2	4.49	—	—
0.049	0.037	0.409	0.030	0.006	2.79	0.061	3.68	1.08	20.4	0.084	0.765	11.8	14.6	112	2.57	—	—
0.065	0.070	0.679	0.060	0.007	6.00	0.112	3.00	1.57	38.0	0.152	1.35	20.6	37.6	209	4.10	260	0.147
0.176	0.280	1.36	0.115	0.574	21.0	0.750	1.00	1.54	161	0.165	1.77	25.6	172	306	15.2	379	0.863
0.028	0.119	0.423	0.058	0.455	16.6	0.527	4.64	2.50	51.6	0.055	0.441	9.19	80.9	90.2	6.20	204	—
0.085	0.097	0.811	0.046	0.043	8.99	0.166	1.86	0.964	38.7	0.093	1.78	9.57	45.7	113	4.23	—	—
0.083	0.297	1.07	0.071	0.304	15.2	0.554	4.25	0.403	162	0.181	1.51	25.2	174	298	3.69	—	—
0.059	0.075	0.563	0.054	0.006	10.1	0.145	3.20	0.787	28.9	0.140	2.16	16.2	22.2	163	2.35	—	—
0.107	0.397	0.244	0.121	1.19	39.5	1.30	1.40	2.20	203	0.397	1.64	50.3	243	337	13.5	143	1.37
0.060	0.158	0.436	0.054	0.529	18.0	0.698	0.150	0.628	63.8	0.072	1.07	9.42	104	85.0	9.60	122	—
0.062	0.137	0.321	0.044	0.425	14.0	0.544	0.360	0.650	61.7	0.086	0.856	12.2	91.6	90.3	7.00	101	—
0.020	0.020	0.400	0.002	0	0	—	0	0	4.00	0.150	0.200	0.940	46.0	182	4.00	110	0.060
0.082	0.077	1.15	0.026	0.043	5.19	0.497	3.09	2.60	34.7	0.077	0.903	10.6	51.7	139	4.48	—	—
0.050	0.049	1.01	0.027	0.006	5.06	0.587	4.84	2.97	23.5	0.119	0.997	17.6	30.2	197	2.69	—	—
0.120	0.120	1.10	0.020	0	4.00	0.194	0.001	2.02	23.0	0.065	0.800	11.5	111	58.0	4.50	192	0.250
0.120	0.100	0.900	0.300	0	6.00	0.160	0.200	1.70	28.0	0.016	0.800	16.0	42.0	30.0	4.00	40.0	0.200
0.280	0.120	1.80	0.277	0	12.8	0.231	0	2.43	17.0	0.084	1.40	13.0	55.0	64.0	5.40	222	0.300
0.164	0.148	1.78	0.058	0.085	8.20	0.305	0.050	1.97	47.3	0.329	2.74	17.2	51.9	214	14.1	—	—
0.001	0.009	0.063	0.004	0	2.13	0.042	0.188	0	1.06	0.007	0.106	0.438	1.25	10.8	0.169	1.06	0.025
0.052	0.329	0.134	0.061	0.625	3.00	0.654	0.700	0.492	176	0.027	0.120	18.0	134	257	9.31	116	1.41
0.044	0.283	0.115	0.053	0.537	2.00	0.562	0.610	0.518	151	0.030	0.100	16.0	115	221	8.01	108	1.21
0.080	0.448	0.178	0.095	0.996	9.00	1.07	0.920	0.605	236	0.035	0.430	25.0	199	338	12.6	153	1.99
0.056	0.356	0.437	0.061	0.031	3.00	0.138	1.15	0.193	183	0.003	0.115	17.1	160	182	7.40	109	0.644
0.066	0.312	1.12	0.134	0.672	11.0	0.344	2.46	0.230	215	0.134	0.607	35.1	236	410	9.00	170	0.984
0.066	0.295	1.03	0.054	0.607	20.0	0.410	2.79	0.280	174	0.107	0.377	28.2	180	290	8.60	90.0	0.804
0.066	0.312	1.01	0.051	0.640	13.0	0.394	3.61	0.317	200	0.087	0.230	29.5	230	338	8.60	145	0.869
0.076	0.347	0.118	0.085	0.875	3.00	0.662	0.760	0.458	176	0.079	0.180	19.0	129	265	5.00	105	0.550
0.117	0.541	0.184	0.133	1.36	5.00	1.03	1.17	0.612	274	0.105	0.280	29.0	202	412	13.0	163	0.860
0	0	0	0	0	0	0	2.00	0	0	—	—	0	6.00	—	—	—	0
0.020	0.020	0.400	0.002	0	0	—	0	0	4.00	0.150	0.200	0.940	46.0	182	4.00	110	0.060
0.576	0.672	6.74	0.528	0.688	67.2	—	4.80	—	208	0.672	7.68	240	592	2080	—	848	2.72
1.70	3.09	17.6	1.38	2.56	155	—	9.60	—	1008	0.672	2.48	320	1200	2544	—	1648	3.36
0.131	0.554	0.365	0.114	0.776	7.92	0.880	1.04	0.560	255	0.147	0.704	37.6	230	454	—	218	0.920
0.102	0.442	0.396	0.100	0.704	6.80	1.11	1.68	0.560	256	0.050	0.240	28.8	226	413	—	187	0.800
0.102	0.412	0.419	0.118	0.808	7.36	0.944	1.76	0.560	275	0.115	0.208	28.0	231	394	—	186	0.808
0.020	0.040	0.400	0.054	0	2.90	0.100	0	0.082	137	0.284	5.05	51.5	17.0	585	12.1	19.0	0
0	0	0	0	0	0.002	0	0	—	0.500	0.001	0.015	0.600	2.00	3.50	0.600	9.50	0.020
0.175	0.128	1.60	0.083	0.003	8.00	0.172	0.333	1.08	28.0	0.100	1.67	11.5	50.0	100	9.20	476	0.267
0.090	0.060	1.00	0.030	0.001	4.00	0.093	1.00	0.640	12.0	0.050	0.935	6.35	34.0	42.0	5.00	326	0.144

Qty	Name	Wgt G	Wtr G	Cal	Prot G	Carb G	Fiber G	F-Tot G	F-Sat G	Mono G	Poly G	Chol Mg	A-Car RE	A-Pre RE	A-Tot RE
1 pce	Banana cream pie-1/6 pie	198	130	319	6.31	47.1	1.69	12.9	4.50	4.87	2.48	15.0	7.10	30.0	37.1
1 pce	Blueberry pie-1/6th pie	158	80.6	380	4.00	55.0	3.72	17.0	4.01	7.47	4.73	0	14.0	0	14.0
1 pce	Boston cream pie-1/8 cake	120	42.0	260	2.50	44.0	0.375	8.00	2.75	3.05	1.50	20.0	3.00	67.0	70.0
1 pce	Cherry pie 1/6th pie	158	74.3	410	4.30	60.5	2.43	17.8	4.21	7.83	4.93	0	70.0	0	70.0
1 ea.	Cherry pie fried	85.0	36.5	250	2.04	32.2	1.31	14.2	5.80	6.70	0.600	13.0	19.0	0	19.0
1 pce	Chocolate cream pie 1/6	175	110	311	7.43	42.4	0.730	12.6	4.53	4.95	2.45	15.0	4.00	30.0	34.0
1 pce	Coconut cream pie 1/6	172	104	343	6.25	43.8	3.35	16.9	8.08	5.02	2.48	15.0	4.00	30.0	34.0
1 pce	Coconut custard pie	165	95.7	384	9.84	36.4	3.38	22.4	6.19	6.37	3.06	183	4.50	91.5	96.0
1 pce	Cream pie commercial	152	65.4	455	3.00	59.0	0.600	23.0	15.0	4.00	1.10	8.00	0	65.0	65.0
1 pce	Custard pie 1/6th pie	152	88.2	293	7.67	34.0	0.600	14.2	0.933	5.75	2.80	148	4.50	91.5	96.0
1 pce	Lemon meringue pie-1/6th	140	65.8	355	4.70	53.0	0.792	14.3	3.50	6.20	3.67	137	3.00	63.0	66.0
1 pce	Mincemeat pie	160	68.8	395	3.69	72.5	4.70	12.0	2.93	5.15	3.24	0	3.40	0	3.40
1 pce	Peach pie 1/6th pie	158	75.8	405	3.50	60.7	2.83	17.5	4.13	7.72	4.83	0	115	0	115
1 pce	Pecan pie 1/6th pie	138	27.6	583	6.33	91.8	1.68	23.7	3.93	12.6	5.72	137	2.30	39.0	41.3
1 pce	Pumpkin pie 1/6th pie	200	118	367	9.00	51.3	2.52	15.7	5.70	6.08	2.75	109	1805	56.0	1861
1 pce	Strawberry chiffon pie	162	90.7	372	4.84	45.7	2.55	19.8	8.99	7.04	2.80	40.7	6.30	122	129
1 ea.	Toaster pastry-fortified	54.0	6.97	210	2.08	38.0	0.600	6.00	1.70	3.60	0.400	0	0	150	150
1 cup	Bread + raisin pudding	165	96.7	349	7.24	49.7	2.06	14.4	4.52	6.04	2.82	142	3.00	164	167
1 cup	Chocolate pudding-Recipe	260	172	385	8.10	66.8	0.520	11.5	7.08	3.24	0.300	39.0	8.00	93.0	101
1 cup	Tapioca pudding-homemade	165	118	220	8.30	28.2	0	8.39	5.16	2.37	0.215	159	8.00	120	128
1 cup	Vanilla pudding-homemade	255	194	285	8.89	40.5	0.010	9.89	6.09	2.80	0.254	37.0	8.00	99.0	107
1 cup	Fruit flavored soda pop	248	221	113	0	28.0	0	0	0	0	0	0	0	0	0
1 cup	Cola beverage-regular	247	221	101	0	25.7	0	0	0	0	0	0	0	0	0
1 cup	Cream soda	247	214	127	0	32.9	0	0	0	0	0	0	0	0	0
1 cup	Ginger ale	244	223	82.7	0.067	21.3	0	0	0	0	0	0	0	0	0
1 cup	Grape soda carbonated	248	220	107	0	27.8	0	0	0	0	0	0	0	0	0
1 cup	Lemon-lime soda	245	220	99.3	0	25.6	0	0	0	0	0	0	0	0	0
1 cup	Orange drink/carbonated	248	217	118	0	30.5	0	0	0	0	0	0	0	0	0
1 cup	Pepper type soda	245	219	101	0	25.5	0	0	0	0	0	0	0	0	0
1 cup	Root beer	247	220	101	0.067	26.1	0	0	0	0	0	0	0	0	0
1 Tbs	Brown sugar	13.8	0.275	51.3	0	13.2	0	0	0	0	0	0	0	0	0
1 Tbs	White sugar	12.5	0.125	48.1	0	12.4	0	0	0	0	0	0	0	0	0
1 Tbs	Maple syrup	20.0	4.80	50.0	0	12.8	0	0	0	0	0	0	0	0	0

VEGETABLES

Qty	Name	Wgt G	Wtr G	Cal	Prot G	Carb G	Fiber G	F-Tot G	F-Sat G	Mono G	Poly G	Chol Mg	A-Car RE	A-Pre RE	A-Tot RE
1 cup	Acorn Squash-baked cubes	205	170	115	2.29	29.9	5.71	0.287	0.059	0.021	0.121	0	88.0	0	88.0
1 oz.	Seaweed (agar) dried	28.3	2.46	86.8	1.76	22.9	1.50	0.085	0.017	0.008	0.029	0	0	0	0
1 cup	Alfalfa sprouts	33.0	30.1	10.0	1.32	1.25	1.20	0.228	0.023	0.019	0.135	0	5.10	0	5.10
1 cup	Amaranth-chopped leaves	28.0	25.7	7.40	0.697	1.14	0.375	0.094	0.026	0.022	0.042	0	83.0	0	83.0
1 cup	Artichoke hearts-raw	168	145	74.0	3.86	17.3	5.60	0.286	0.068	0.008	0.120	0	24.2	0	24.2
1 ea.	Artichoke-globe-cooked	120	104	53.0	2.76	12.4	3.96	0.204	0.048	0.006	0.086	0	17.2	0	17.2
1 cup	Jerusalem artichoke-raw	150	117	114	3.00	26.2	1.95	0.020	0	0.006	0.002	0	3.00	0	3.00
1 cup	Asparagus-raw pieces	134	124	30.0	4.10	4.94	2.04	0.294	0.068	0.010	0.128	0	120	0	120
4 ea.	Asparagus-raw spears	58.0	53.5	13.0	1.77	2.14	0.808	0.128	0.029	0.004	0.056	0	52.0	0	52.0
1 cup	Asparagus-ckd-pieces	180	166	45.0	4.66	7.92	3.00	0.558	0.128	0.018	0.246	0	149	0	149
4 ea.	Asparagus-ckd-spears	60.0	55.2	15.0	1.55	2.64	1.00	0.186	0.043	0.006	0.082	0	49.8	0	49.8
4 ea.	Asparagus-canned-spears	80.0	76.0	15.2	1.71	1.98	1.28	0.520	0.118	0.017	0.227	0	38.0	0	38.0
1 cup	Bamboo shoots-sliced-raw	151	137	41.0	3.93	7.85	3.93	0.470	0.104	0.011	0.202	0	3.00	0	3.00
1 cup	Green beans-raw/uncooked	110	99.3	34.0	2.00	7.85	4.90	0.130	0.029	0.006	0.065	0	73.5	0	73.5
1 cup	Green beans-fresh-cooked	125	111	44.0	2.36	9.86	3.25	0.360	0.080	0.014	0.181	0	83.3	0	83.3
1 cup	Green beans-frzn-cooked	135	124	36.0	1.84	8.26	3.38	0.180	0.041	0.007	0.093	0	71.3	0	71.3
1 cup	Green beans-canned/draind	135	126	26.0	1.55	6.08	2.03	0.135	0.030	0.006	0.070	0	47.1	0	47.1
1 cup	Lima beans-raw	156	110	176	10.7	31.5	7.64	1.34	0.309	0.078	0.654	0	47.3	0	47.3
1 cup	Lima beans-baby-frzn-ckd	180	130	188	12.0	35.0	9.72	0.540	0.122	0.030	0.260	0	30.0	0	30.0

B1 Mg	B2 Mg	B3 Mg	B6 Mg	B12 Mcg	Fol. Mcg	Panto Mg	Vit-C Mg	Vit-E Mg	Calc Mg	Cu Mg	Iron Mg	Mg Mg	Phos Mg	Potas Mg	Sel Mcg	Na Mg	Zinc Mg
0.157	0.292	1.23	0.296	0.400	19.3	0.521	4.43	0.498	147	0.111	1.09	30.9	135	333	6.34	422	—
0.173	0.142	1.73	0.072	0.003	14.0	0.154	6.00	0.883	26.0	0.088	2.10	10.0	46.0	126	8.33	423	0.280
0.010	0.180	0.700	0.050	0.320	7.00	0.320	0	2.00	26.0	0.093	0.600	11.0	70.0	40.0	3.07	225	0.230
0.188	0.142	1.58	0.083	0.002	15.5	0.187	0.830	0.850	37.0	0.154	3.17	15.2	58.0	153	8.22	480	0.312
0.060	0.060	0.600	0.040	0.001	8.00	0.101	1.00	0.640	11.0	0.060	0.700	6.51	41.0	61.0	4.00	371	0.150
0.151	0.300	1.06	0.089	0.107	11.0	0.457	0.500	0.385	160	0.101	1.08	29.3	147	222	8.82	427	0.743
0.130	0.257	1.08	1.01	0.400	11.2	0.517	0.550	0.490	146	0.108	1.20	26.0	140	222	7.48	452	0.823
0.166	0.318	1.10	0.236	0.762	25.0	0.949	0.690	0.729	146	0.164	1.77	32.2	195	289	11.6	430	1.21
0.060	0.150	1.10	0.065	—	18.0	—	0	—	46.0	—	1.10	19.0	154	133	—	369	0.785
0.137	0.267	0.917	0.084	0.617	15.0	0.683	0.170	0.560	124	0.086	1.44	18.0	147	173	11.8	333	0.792
0.100	0.140	0.833	0.050	0.328	13.0	0.420	4.20	0.970	25.0	0.077	1.40	9.00	70.0	70.0	9.00	395	0.510
0.157	0.136	1.57	0.147	0	8.65	0.126	3.00	2.45	38.9	0.164	2.03	18.7	69.7	349	8.10	330	0.293
0.175	0.155	2.30	0.065	0.003	12.0	0.567	4.67	0.900	27.0	0.122	1.90	16.3	55.0	235	9.00	423	0.352
0.217	0.165	1.10	0.080	0.307	18.3	0.773	0	1.02	35.0	0.287	1.85	32.0	130	130	18.5	304	1.47
0.137	0.293	1.22	0.107	0.322	20.0	0.850	1.00	1.23	212	0.221	2.63	40.0	211	400	9.62	338	0.993
0.123	0.134	1.28	0.055	0.053	20.5	0.211	31.0	0.604	43.7	0.115	1.45	15.0	54.1	151	5.43	259	—
0.173	0.184	2.27	0.205	0	43.0	0.118	4.00	10.5	104	0.081	2.16	9.72	104	91.0	0.015	248	0.313
0.176	0.280	1.36	0.115	0.574	21.0	0.750	1.00	1.54	161	0.165	1.77	25.6	172	306	15.2	379	0.863
0.050	0.360	0.300	0.128	0.481	10.0	0.780	1.00	0.255	250	0.077	1.30	48.4	255	445	4.00	146	1.53
0.070	0.300	0.200	0.083	0.481	9.50	0.495	2.00	0.165	173	0.080	0.700	13.2	180	223	9.57	257	0.832
0.080	0.410	0.300	0.109	0.481	14.0	0.765	2.00	0.255	298	0.102	0.800	20.4	232	352	5.66	166	1.18
0	0	0.013	0	0	0	0	0	0	10.00	0.041	0.174	2.67	1.33	13.3	0	32.0	0.181
0	0	0	0	0	0	0	0	0	6.00	0.027	0.080	2.00	30.7	2.67	0	10.00	0.033
0	0	0	0	0	0	0	0	0	12.7	0.020	0.127	2.00	0	2.67	—	28.7	0.160
0	0	0	0	0	0	0	0	0	8.00	0.044	0.440	2.00	0.667	3.33	—	16.7	0.122
0	0	0	0	0	0	0	0	0	8.00	0.055	0.207	2.67	0	2.00	—	38.0	0.173
0	0	0.037	0	0	0	0	0	0	6.00	0.029	0.167	1.33	0.667	2.67	0	27.3	0.120
0	0	0	0	0	0	0	0	0	12.7	0.037	0.153	2.67	2.67	6.00	—	30.7	0.253
0	0	0	0	0	0	0	0	0	8.00	0.015	0.093	0.667	27.3	1.33	—	25.3	0.100
0	0	0	0	0	0	0	0	0	12.7	0.017	0.123	2.67	1.33	2.00	—	32.7	0.173
0.001	0.004	0.012	0	0	0	—	0	0	11.7	0.048	0.300	8.44	3.50	47.3	0.151	6.06	0.005
0	0	0	0	0	0	0	0	0	0.188	0.002	0.006	0.012	0.006	0.438	0.037	0.313	0.002
—	—	—	—	0	—	0	0	—	33.0	0.090	0.240	4.70	3.00	26.0	—	3.00	0.010

B1 Mg	B2 Mg	B3 Mg	B6 Mg	B12 Mcg	Fol. Mcg	Panto Mg	Vit-C Mg	Vit-E Mg	Calc Mg	Cu Mg	Iron Mg	Mg Mg	Phos Mg	Potas Mg	Sel Mcg	Na Mg	Zinc Mg
0.342	0.027	1.81	0.398	0	38.4	1.03	22.1	1.35	90.0	0.176	1.91	87.0	93.0	896	2.64	9.00	0.349
0.003	0.063	0.057	—	0	—	—	0	—	177	—	6.06	218	1.50	318	—	28.9	—
0.025	0.042	0.159	0.011	0	12.2	0.186	2.70	—	11.0	0.052	0.317	9.00	23.0	26.0	—	2.00	0.304
0.008	0.045	0.187	—	0	24.2	—	12.3	—	61.0	0.046	0.658	15.6	14.0	173	—	6.00	0.255
0.096	0.082	0.992	0.146	0	74.8	0.336	12.4	0.026	66.0	0.102	2.26	66.0	100	442	—	110	0.504
0.068	0.059	0.709	0.104	0	53.4	0.240	8.90	0.018	47.0	0.073	1.62	47.0	72.0	316	—	79.0	0.432
0.300	0.090	1.95	0.107	0	15.0	0.405	6.00	0.270	21.0	0.189	5.10	26.0	117	644	—	6.00	0.105
0.152	0.166	1.52	0.206	0	140	66.0	44.2	2.66	30.0	0.206	0.912	24.0	70.0	404	10.7	2.00	0.938
0.066	0.072	0.660	0.089	0	61.0	0.101	19.1	1.15	13.0	0.089	0.394	10.0	30.0	175	4.63	1.00	0.406
0.178	0.218	1.89	0.254	0	176	0.580	49.0	4.90	44.0	0.180	1.19	34.0	110	558	4.50	8.00	0.864
0.059	0.073	0.631	0.085	0	58.8	0.193	16.0	1.63	14.4	0.060	0.396	11.4	37.0	186	1.50	2.00	0.288
0.047	0.070	0.700	0.040	0	69.0	0.093	13.0	0.728	11.0	0.076	0.500	7.90	30.0	122	1.75	278	0.320
0.227	0.106	0.906	0.085	0	49.0	—	6.00	—	20.0	—	0.760	4.00	89.0	805	—	7.00	0.369
0.092	0.116	0.827	0.081	0	40.1	0.200	17.9	0.121	41.0	0.076	1.41	27.0	42.0	230	0.660	6.00	0.260
0.093	0.121	0.768	0.070	0	41.6	0.240	12.1	0.165	58.0	0.129	1.60	32.0	48.0	373	1.00	4.00	0.450
0.065	0.100	0.563	0.076	0	42.0	0.180	11.1	0.126	61.0	0.090	1.11	29.0	33.0	151	1.08	17.0	0.840
0.020	0.076	0.272	0.050	0	43.0	0.140	6.40	0.050	36.0	0.052	1.22	18.0	26.0	147	0.750	339	0.392
0.339	0.161	2.30	0.318	0	171	0.385	36.6	4.90	54.0	0.496	4.89	90.0	213	729	3.05	13.0	1.21
0.126	0.100	1.39	0.208	0	116	0.318	10.4	3.14	50.0	0.354	3.52	100	202	740	3.40	52.0	1.00

Qty	Name	Wgt G	Wtr G	Cal	Prot G	Carb G	Fiber G	F-Tot G	F-Sat G	Mono G	Poly G	Chol Mg	A-Car RE	A-Pre RE	A-Tot RE
1 cup	Lima beans-lrge-frzn-ckd	170	125	170	10.3	32.0	9.20	0.580	0.130	0.034	0.278	0	32.0	0	32.0
1 cup	Lima beans-canned/drained	170	114	164	9.20	31.2	9.20	0.600	0.186	0.078	0.390	0	32.2	0	32.2
1 cup	Yellow wax beans-raw	110	99.3	34.0	2.00	7.85	4.90	0.130	0.029	0.006	0.065	0	11.9	0	11.9
1 cup	Yellow wax beans-raw-ckd	125	111	44.0	2.36	9.86	3.20	0.360	0.080	0.014	0.181	0	10.1	0	10.1
1 cup	Yellow wax beans-frzn-ckd	135	124	36.0	1.84	8.26	3.38	0.180	0.041	0.007	0.093	0	15.1	0	15.1
1 cup	Yellow wax beans-cnd/drnd	135	126	26.0	1.55	6.08	2.03	0.135	0.030	0.006	0.070	0	14.3	0	14.3
1 cup	Beet greens-raw-ckd-drnd	144	128	40.0	3.70	7.87	2.97	0.290	0.045	0.055	0.101	0	734	0	734
1 cup	Beets-raw-cooked-diced	170	155	52.0	1.80	11.4	3.92	0.080	0.014	0.018	0.030	0	2.20	0	2.20
1 ea.	Beets-raw-cooked-whole	50.0	45.4	15.5	0.530	3.34	1.15	0.025	0.004	0.005	0.009	0	0.650	0	0.650
1 cup	Beets-canned/draind-diced	170	155	54.0	1.56	12.2	4.26	0.240	0.040	0.048	0.086	0	2.00	0	2.00
1 cup	Black-eyed peas-raw-ckd	165	118	179	13.4	29.9	7.13	1.32	0.345	0.117	0.558	0	105	0	105
1 cup	Black-eyed peas-frzn-ckd	170	112	224	14.4	40.4	7.34	1.13	0.298	0.102	0.476	0	12.8	0	12.8
1 cup	Broccoli-raw-chopped	88.0	79.8	24.0	2.62	4.62	3.34	0.300	0.048	0.022	0.148	0	136	0	136
1 ea.	Broccoli-raw-spears	151	137	42.0	4.50	7.91	5.74	0.520	0.082	0.036	0.252	0	233	0	233
1 cup	Broccoli-raw-ckd-chopped	156	141	46.0	4.64	8.68	5.40	0.440	0.067	0.031	0.209	0	220	0	220
1 ea.	Broccoli-raw-ckd-spear	180	162	53.0	5.35	10.0	6.19	0.500	0.077	0.036	0.241	0	254	0	254
1 cup	Broccoli-frzn-ckd-chopped	184	167	51.0	5.71	9.84	5.58	0.221	0.033	0.015	0.101	0	348	0	348
1 pce	Broccoli-frzn-ckd-spears	30.0	27.3	8.40	0.930	1.60	0.900	0.036	0.005	0.002	0.016	0	56.8	0	56.8
1 cup	Brussels sprouts-raw	88.0	75.7	38.0	2.98	7.88	3.31	0.260	0.055	0.020	0.135	0	77.0	0	77.0
1 cup	Brussels sprouts-raw-ckd	156	136	60.0	5.98	13.5	5.15	0.796	0.164	0.061	0.406	0	112	0	112
1 cup	Brussels sprouts-frzn-ckd	155	135	65.0	5.64	12.9	4.54	0.610	0.126	0.047	0.310	0	91.2	0	91.2
1 cup	Butternut squash-bkd-mshd	245	215	99.0	2.20	25.7	5.88	0.221	0.047	0.017	0.093	0	1715	0	1715
1 cup	Butternut squash-bkd-cube	205	180	83.0	1.85	21.5	4.92	0.185	0.039	0.014	0.078	0	1435	0	1435
1 cup	Cabbage raw-shredded	70.0	64.7	16.0	0.840	3.76	1.40	0.120	0.016	0.010	0.060	0	8.80	0	8.80
1 cup	Cabbage-cooked	150	140	32.0	1.44	7.16	3.30	0.375	0.048	0.027	0.179	0	13.0	0	13.0
1 cup	Bok-choy cabbage-raw-shrd	70.0	66.7	9.00	1.05	1.53	1.70	0.140	0.018	0.011	0.067	0	210	0	210
1 cup	Pe-tsai cabbage-raw-chpd	76.0	71.7	11.0	0.910	2.46	1.67	0.150	0.033	0.017	0.055	0	91.0	0	91.0
1 cup	Red cabbage raw	70.0	64.1	19.0	0.970	4.30	1.82	0.180	0.024	0.013	0.088	0	3.00	0	3.00
1 cup	Savoy cabbage raw	70.0	63.7	20.0	1.40	4.27	1.62	0.070	0.009	0.005	0.034	0	70.0	0	70.0
1 cup	Carrot juice	246	219	98.0	2.32	22.8	3.34	0.360	0.066	0.018	0.174	0	6318	0	6318
1 ea.	Carrot-whole-fresh	72.0	63.2	31.0	0.740	7.30	2.03	0.140	0.022	0.006	0.055	0	2025	0	2025
1 cup	Carrots-grated-fresh	110	96.6	48.0	1.12	11.2	3.10	0.200	0.034	0.008	0.084	0	3094	0	3094
1 cup	Carrots-sliced-ckd	156	136	70.0	1.70	16.4	5.22	0.280	0.054	0.014	0.138	0	3830	0	3830
1 cup	Carrots-sliced-frzn-ckd	146	131	52.0	1.74	12.0	4.88	0.160	0.030	0.008	0.078	0	2584	0	2584
1 cup	Carrots-canned/drained	146	136	34.0	0.940	8.08	3.80	0.278	0.052	0.014	0.134	0	2012	0	2012
1 cup	Cauliflower raw	100	92.3	24.0	1.98	4.92	2.68	0.180	0.028	0.012	0.084	0	1.60	0	1.60
1 cup	Cauliflower-raw-cooked	124	115	30.0	2.32	5.74	2.70	0.220	0.046	0.022	0.144	0	1.80	0	1.80
1 cup	Cauliflower-frzn-cooked	180	169	34.0	2.90	6.75	3.17	0.390	0.059	0.027	0.185	0	4.00	0	4.00
1 cup	Celery-raw-chopped	120	114	19.2	0.800	4.36	2.00	0.140	0.038	0.028	0.072	0	15.2	0	15.2
1 ea.	Celery-raw-lg outer stalk	40.0	37.9	6.40	0.260	1.45	0.670	0.048	0.013	0.010	0.024	0	5.00	0	5.00
1 cup	Celery diced-cooked	150	142	22.0	0.760	5.29	2.44	0.170	0.042	0.032	0.080	0	16.2	0	16.2
1 cup	Swiss chard-raw	36.0	33.4	6.84	0.648	1.35	0.650	0.072	0.016	0.003	0.041	0	119	0	119
1 cup	Swiss chard-cooked	175	162	35.0	3.29	7.24	3.80	0.140	0.031	0.006	0.080	0	549	0	549
1 Tbs	Chives-fresh	3.00	2.76	1.00	0.040	0.130	0.020	0.010	0.003	0.003	0.007	0	14.0	0	14.0
1 cup	Collards-fresh	36.0	33.8	6.84	0.565	1.36	0.750	0.079	0.011	0.011	0.046	0	120	0	120
1 cup	Collards-fresh-cooked	145	139	20.3	1.60	3.83	4.08	0.218	0.062	0.031	0.125	0	322	0	322
1 cup	Collards-frozen-cooked	170	150	61.0	5.04	12.1	4.76	0.690	0.100	0.100	0.400	0	1017	0	1017
1 cup	Corn-raw-kernels	154	117	132	4.96	29.2	8.32	1.82	0.280	0.534	0.860	0	43.2	0	43.2
1 ea.	Corn on cob-5 inch-cooked	77.0	53.6	83.0	2.56	19.4	3.62	0.986	0.152	0.288	0.464	0	16.7	0	16.7
1 ea.	Corn on cob-3.5in/frn/ckd	63.0	46.1	59.0	1.96	14.1	2.96	0.466	0.072	0.136	0.219	0	13.3	0	13.3
1 cup	Corn-cooked from raw	164	114	178	5.44	41.2	11.3	2.10	0.324	0.614	0.988	0	35.6	0	35.6
1 cup	Corn-frozen/cooked	164	124	134	4.96	33.6	7.70	0.114	0.018	0.034	0.056	0	40.8	0	40.8
1 cup	Corn-canned/drained	164	126	132	4.30	30.4	5.00	1.64	0.252	0.478	0.772	0	25.6	0	25.6
1 cup	Corn-canned/drained-diet	164	126	132	4.30	30.4	5.00	1.64	0.252	0.478	0.772	0	25.6	0	25.6
1 cup	Corn-cream style-canned	256	201	186	4.46	46.4	9.00	1.08	0.166	0.314	0.506	0	24.8	0	24.8
1 cup	Corn-canned w/liquid	256	210	158	4.96	38.0	7.20	1.14	0.176	0.332	0.538	0	30.6	0	30.6
1 cup	Corn-white kernal-fzn/ckd	164	124	134	4.96	33.6	5.00	0.114	0.018	0.034	0.056	0	0.200	0	0.200
1 cup	Garden cress-raw	50.0	44.7	16.0	1.30	2.76	0.560	0.360	0.012	0.120	0.114	0	44.6	0	44.6
1 cup	Crookneck squash-raw	130	122	24.0	1.22	5.26	2.21	0.310	0.064	0.023	0.130	0	44.0	0	44.0

B1 Mg	B2 Mg	B3 Mg	B6 Mg	B12 Mcg	Fol. Mcg	Panto Mg	Vit-C Mg	Vit-E Mg	Calc Mg	Cu Mg	Iron Mg	Mg Mg	Phos Mg	Potas Mg	Sel Mcg	Na Mg	Zinc Mg
0.126	0.104	1.82	0.208	0	130	0.278	22.0	3.00	38.0	0.094	2.32	58.0	107	694	0.010	90.0	0.740
0.060	0.080	0.800	0.039	0	40.0	0.129	10.0	3.00	48.0	0.360	2.92	70.0	120	378	—	402	1.60
0.092	0.116	0.827	0.081	0	40.1	0.200	17.9	0.121	41.0	0.076	1.14	27.0	42.0	230	0.660	6.00	0.260
0.093	0.121	0.768	0.070	0	41.6	0.240	12.1	0.165	58.0	0.129	1.60	32.0	48.0	373	0.750	4.00	0.450
0.065	0.100	0.563	0.076	0	42.0	0.180	11.1	0.176	61.0	0.090	1.11	29.0	33.0	151	121	17.0	0.840
0.020	0.076	0.272	0.050	0	43.0	0.140	6.40	0.050	36.0	0.052	1.22	18.0	26.0	147	0.750	339	0.392
0.168	0.416	0.719	0.190	0	47.0	0.474	35.9	2.39	165	0.361	2.74	97.0	58.0	1308	1.70	346	0.720
0.052	0.024	0.464	0.052	0	98.0	0.164	9.40	0.050	18.0	0.096	1.05	62.0	52.0	532	0.680	84.0	0.426
0.015	0.007	0.136	0.015	0	43.0	0.048	2.75	0.014	5.50	0.028	0.310	18.5	15.5	156	0.200	24.5	0.125
0.020	0.070	0.300	0.090	0	44.0	0.166	7.00	0.052	26.0	0.100	3.10	26.0	30.0	252	0.450	466	0.360
0.112	0.177	1.77	0.083	0	173	0.195	2.60	—	46.0	0.167	2.36	83.0	197	693	31.0	7.00	1.30
0.422	0.109	1.24	0.162	0	240	0.362	4.50	—	40.0	0.313	3.60	85.0	208	638	31.9	9.00	2.42
0.058	0.104	0.562	0.140	0	62.4	0.470	82.0	0.603	42.0	0.040	0.780	22.0	58.0	286	0.176	24.0	0.360
0.098	0.180	0.963	0.240	0	107	0.808	141	0.154	72.0	0.068	1.33	38.0	99.0	490	0.302	41.0	0.600
0.128	0.322	1.18	0.308	0	107	0.450	98.0	1.80	178	0.108	1.78	94.0	74.0	254	0.312	16.0	0.234
0.148	0.373	1.36	0.356	0	123	0.518	113	2.08	205	0.124	2.06	108	86.0	293	0.360	20.0	0.270
0.101	0.149	0.843	0.239	0	104	0.504	73.7	1.97	94.0	0.079	1.13	37.0	101	331	0.368	44.0	0.560
0.016	0.024	0.137	0.039	0	25.8	0.082	12.0	0.330	15.3	0.013	0.183	6.03	16.4	54.0	0.060	7.20	0.090
0.122	0.080	0.656	0.192	0	53.8	0.272	74.8	0.774	36.0	0.062	1.23	20.0	60.0	342	8.10	22.0	0.370
0.166	0.124	0.946	0.310	0	93.6	0.560	96.8	1.33	56.0	0.130	1.88	32.0	87.0	491	10.7	17.0	0.500
0.160	0.175	0.832	0.271	0	157	0.530	70.8	1.00	38.0	0.109	1.15	37.0	84.0	504	9.90	36.0	0.550
0.177	0.042	2.38	0.303	0	47.0	0.880	36.9	1.61	100	0.159	1.47	70.5	66.0	697	3.16	8.40	0.319
0.148	0.035	1.99	0.254	0	39.3	0.736	30.9	1.35	84.0	0.133	1.23	59.0	55.0	582	2.64	7.00	0.267
0.036	0.022	0.210	0.066	0	39.6	0.098	33.0	0.041	32.0	0.016	0.400	10.0	16.0	172	1.57	12.0	0.120
0.086	0.083	0.345	0.096	0	31.0	0.095	36.4	0.043	50.0	0.042	0.585	22.5	38.0	308	2.56	29.0	0.240
0.028	0.049	0.350	0.066	0	57.0	0.100	31.5	0.091	74.0	0.038	0.560	13.0	26.0	176	—	0.450	0.288
0.030	0.038	0.304	0.176	0	60.0	0.080	20.5	0.099	59.0	0.027	0.230	10.0	22.0	181	—	7.00	0.170
0.045	0.021	0.210	0.147	0	19.0	0.227	39.9	0.140	36.0	0.068	0.350	11.0	29.0	144	5.20	8.00	0.150
0.049	0.021	0.210	0.133	0	32.0	0.100	21.7	0.140	25.0	0.049	0.280	20.0	29.0	161	2.60	20.0	0.255
0.226	0.134	0.946	0.532	0	9.40	0.560	21.0	—	58.0	0.114	1.13	34.6	102	716	0.666	72.0	0.442
0.070	0.042	0.668	0.106	0	10.1	0.142	6.70	0.294	19.0	0.034	0.360	11.0	32.0	233	0.816	25.0	0.144
0.106	0.064	1.02	0.162	0	15.4	0.216	10.2	0.448	30.0	0.052	0.550	16.0	48.0	356	1.25	38.0	0.220
0.054	0.888	0.790	0.384	0	21.6	0.474	4.00	1.42	48.0	0.210	0.968	20.0	48.0	354	1.77	104	0.468
0.040	0.054	0.640	0.188	0	15.8	0.236	4.00	1.33	42.0	0.106	0.700	14.0	38.0	230	1.78	86.0	0.350
0.026	0.044	0.806	0.164	0	13.4	0.198	4.00	1.32	38.0	0.152	0.934	12.0	34.0	262	1.65	352	0.380
0.076	0.058	0.634	0.232	0	66.2	0.142	71.6	0.260	28.0	0.032	0.580	14.0	46.0	356	0.650	14.0	0.180
0.078	0.080	0.684	0.250	0	63.4	0.152	68.6	0.200	34.0	0.112	0.520	14.0	44.0	400	0.812	8.00	0.298
0.067	0.095	0.558	0.158	0	73.7	0.176	56.3	0.200	31.0	0.043	0.738	16.0	43.0	250	1.17	33.0	0.234
0.036	0.036	0.360	0.036	0	10.6	0.202	7.60	0.660	44.0	0.042	0.580	14.0	32.0	340	2.64	106	0.204
0.012	0.012	0.120	0.012	0	3.60	0.068	2.50	0.220	14.4	0.014	0.192	4.80	10.0	114	0.880	35.0	0.068
0.039	0.045	0.375	0.045	0	10.1	0.215	7.10	0.200	53.0	0.047	0.200	18.0	36.0	531	1.65	97.0	0.230
0.014	0.032	0.144	0.032	0	19.5	0.062	10.8	0.540	18.4	0.392	0.648	29.2	16.6	136	—	76.7	0.163
0.060	0.150	0.630	0.117	0	57.0	0.285	31.5	3.00	102	0.172	3.96	150	58.0	961	—	313	0.589
0.002	0.003	0.012	0.005	0	—	—	1.30	—	2.00	—	0.040	—	1.00	6.00	—	—	—
0.011	0.023	0.135	0.025	0	40.0	0.023	8.40	—	42.0	0.094	0.380	6.10	6.00	53.0	—	10.0	0.346
0.025	0.062	0.342	0.061	0	55.0	0.061	14.2	—	113	0.218	0.595	16.0	15.0	135	—	27.0	0.928
0.080	0.196	1.08	0.194	0	129	0.196	45.0	—	357	0.094	1.90	52.0	46.0	427	—	85.0	0.460
0.308	0.092	2.62	0.084	0	70.6	1.17	10.6	1.02	3.08	0.084	0.800	57.0	138	416	0.620	23.4	0.694
0.166	0.055	1.24	0.184	0	35.7	0.676	4.80	0.377	1.54	0.041	0.470	24.6	79.0	192	0.385	13.0	0.370
0.110	0.043	0.956	0.141	0	19.2	0.158	3.00	0.190	2.00	0.029	0.384	21.0	47.0	158	0.315	2.50	0.400
0.352	0.118	2.64	0.276	0	76.2	1.44	10.2	0.804	3.28	0.086	1.00	52.4	170	408	0.660	28.0	0.788
0.114	0.120	2.10	0.356	0	37.4	0.356	4.20	0.444	3.28	0.054	0.492	29.6	78.0	228	0.820	8.00	0.574
0.050	0.082	1.44	0.080	0	60.0	0.412	6.76	0.108	8.00	0.096	0.820	30.8	130	252	0.600	380	0.762
0.050	0.082	1.44	0.080	0	60.0	0.412	6.76	0.108	8.00	0.096	0.820	30.8	130	252	0.600	7.60	0.762
0.064	0.136	2.46	0.162	0	115	0.460	11.8	1.28	8.00	0.104	0.972	43.6	130	344	1.28	730	1.36
0.066	0.156	2.40	0.512	0	97.6	1.34	17.0	0.108	10.0	0.144	0.880	40.0	130	392	0.696	648	0.920
0.114	0.120	2.10	0.356	0	37.4	0.356	4.20	0.644	3.28	0.054	0.492	29.6	78.0	228	0.820	8.00	0.574
0.040	0.130	0.500	0.124	0	—	—	34.6	0.360	40.0	—	0.660	—	38.0	304	—	8.00	2.40
0.068	0.056	0.590	0.142	0	29.7	0.133	10.9	0.400	28.0	0.133	0.620	27.0	42.0	276	1.95	2.00	0.380

Qty	Name	Wgt G	Wtr G	Cal	Prot G	Carb G	Fiber G	F-Tot G	F-Sat G	Mono G	Poly G	Chol Mg	A-Car RE	A-Pre RE	A-Tot RE
1 cup	Crookneck squash-cooked	180	169	36.0	1.63	7.76	3.24	0.560	0.115	0.041	0.236	0	51.7	0	51.7
1 ea.	Cucumber slices with peel	104	99.9	14.0	0.560	3.02	1.20	0.140	0.034	0.004	0.054	0	4.60	0	4.60
1 ea.	Cucumber-whole-8 x 2+ in	301	289	39.0	1.63	8.76	3.50	0.390	0.099	0.009	0.153	0	13.5	0	13.5
1 cup	Dandelion greens-fresh	55.0	47.1	25.0	1.49	5.06	0.940	0.390	0.050	0.040	0.230	0	770	0	770
1 cup	Dandelion greens-cooked	105	94.3	35.0	2.10	6.72	1.27	0.630	0.082	0.071	0.367	0	1229	0	1229
1 cup	Dock/sorrel greens-raw	133	124	29.0	2.66	4.26	1.06	0.930	—	—	—	0	532	0	532
1 cup	Eggplant cooked	160	147	44.8	1.33	10.6	6.00	0.370	0.070	0.032	0.149	0	10.2	0	10.2
1 cup	Endive-raw-chopped	50.0	46.9	8.00	0.620	1.68	0.460	0.100	0.024	0.002	0.044	0	103	0	103
10 ea.	French fries-frzn-veg oil	50.0	19.0	158	2.01	19.8	1.11	8.28	2.50	1.64	3.78	0	0	0	0
10 ea.	French fries-veg/aml oil	50.0	19.0	158	2.01	19.8	1.11	8.28	3.40	4.00	0.521	0	0	0	0
10 pce	French fries-oven heated	50.0	26.4	111	1.73	17.0	1.11	4.38	2.08	1.78	0.329	0	0	0	0
1 ea.	Garlic cloves	3.00	1.76	4.47	0.191	0.992	0.050	0.015	0.003	0.000	0.007	0	0	0	0
1 tsp	Garlic powder	2.80	0.182	9.33	0.470	2.04	0.053	0.020	0.007	0.001	0.010	0	0	0	0
1 cup	Kale-fresh-chopped	67.0	37.9	33.0	2.21	6.71	3.89	0.469	0.061	0.035	0.226	0	596	0	596
1 cup	Kale-fresh-chopped-cooked	130	119	41.6	3.47	7.32	3.55	0.520	0.068	0.039	0.251	0	962	0	962
1 cup	Kale-frzn-chopped-cooked	130	118	39.0	3.69	6.81	3.24	0.637	0.082	0.047	0.306	0	826	0	826
1 oz.	Seaweed (kelp) raw	28.3	23.1	12.2	0.477	2.71	0.401	0.159	0.070	0.028	0.013	0	3.31	0	3.31
1 cup	Kohlrabi-raw slices	140	127	38.0	2.38	8.68	2.00	0.140	0.018	0.010	0.067	0	5.00	0	5.00
1 cup	Kohlrabi-raw-cooked	165	149	48.0	2.97	11.4	2.30	0.180	0.023	0.013	0.087	0	5.80	0	5.80
1 cup	Leeks-chopped-cooked	104	94.4	32.2	0.842	7.92	3.40	0.208	0.028	0.004	0.116	0	4.80	0	4.80
1 cup	Lentils sprouted-raw	77.0	51.8	81.0	6.90	17.1	3.12	0.423	0.044	0.080	0.169	0	3.50	0	3.50
1 cup	Butterhead lettuce-chpd	56.0	53.5	7.28	0.722	1.30	0.840	0.123	0.016	0.005	0.066	0	54.3	0	54.3
1 cup	Iceberg lettuce-chopped	56.0	53.7	7.28	0.566	1.17	0.840	0.106	0.014	0.004	0.056	0	18.5	0	18.5
2 ea.	Iceberg lettuce leaf	40.0	38.4	5.20	0.404	0.836	0.540	0.076	0.010	0.002	0.040	0	13.2	0	13.2
1 cup	Loose leaf lettuce-chpd	56.0	52.6	10.1	0.728	1.96	0.930	0.168	0.022	0.007	0.089	0	106	0	106
1 cup	Romaine lettuce-chopped	56.0	53.1	8.96	0.907	1.33	0.930	0.112	0.015	0.005	0.059	0	146	0	146
1 cup	Mushrooms-raw sliced	70.0	64.3	17.5	1.46	3.26	1.75	0.294	0.040	0.006	0.120	0	0	0	0
5 ea.	Mushroom-raw-18grams each	90.0	82.6	22.5	1.88	419	2.25	0.380	0.050	0.005	0.155	0	0	0	0
1 cup	Mustard greens-fresh	56.0	50.8	14.6	1.51	2.75	1.51	0.112	0.006	0.052	0.021	0	297	0	297
10 oz.	Okra pods-fresh-cooked	283	255	90.7	5.30	20.4	6.24	0.484	0.127	0.080	0.130	0	163	0	163
10 ea.	Green olives-wo/pits	39.0	30.4	45.0	0.500	0.500	1.72	6.00	0.600	3.60	0.300	0	12.0	0	12.0
10 ea.	Ripe olives-large∅pits	47.0	34.3	78.0	0.500	1.20	2.08	10.4	1.57	6.80	1.04	0	5.20	0	5.20
1 tsp	Onion powder	2.17	0.108	5.00	0.220	1.75	0.123	0.023	0.005	0.004	0.010	0	0	0	0
1 cup	Onions-chopped-raw	160	145	54.0	1.89	11.7	2.36	0.416	0.070	0.059	0.163	0	0	0	0
1 cup	Onion slices-raw	115	104	39.0	1.36	8.42	1.70	0.299	0.051	0.043	0.117	0	0	0	0
1 cup	Onions-chopped-raw-cooked	210	194	58.0	1.90	13.2	3.06	0.340	0.056	0.048	0.132	0	0	0	0
1 cup	Onions-chopped-frzn-ckd	210	194	60.0	1.60	13.9	3.06	0.200	0.034	0.028	0.080	0	7.20	0	7.20
1 cup	Green onion-all-chopped	100	91.9	26.0	1.74	5.56	2.64	0.140	0.024	0.020	0.054	0	500	0	500
1 tsp	Parsley-freeze dried	0.117	0.002	0.333	0.037	0.049	0.047	0.006	0.001	0.000	0.003	0	7.42	0	7.42
1 Tbs	Parsley-fresh-chopped	3.75	3.31	1.25	0.082	0.259	0.244	0.011	0.001	0.001	0.005	0	19.5	0	19.5
1 cup	Parsnips-sliced-cooked	156	121	125	2.06	30.4	5.46	1.40	0.100	0.200	0.100	0	0	0	0
1 cup	Peas-fresh/raw	146	115	118	7.90	21.1	7.10	0.580	0.104	0.051	0.273	0	93.4	0	93.4
1 cup	Peas-fresh-cooked	160	125	134	8.57	25.0	7.68	0.340	0.062	0.030	0.163	0	95.5	0	95.5
1 cup	Peas-frozen-cooked	160	127	126	8.24	22.8	7.22	0.440	0.078	0.038	0.206	0	107	0	107
1 cup	Peas-canned/drained	170	139	118	7.52	21.4	10.1	0.580	0.106	0.052	0.278	0	130	0	130
1 cup	Peas-canned/drained-diet	170	139	118	7.52	21.4	10.1	0.580	0.106	0.052	0.278	0	130	0	130
1 cup	Peas + carrots-frzn-cooked	160	137	76.0	4.94	16.2	6.60	0.680	0.124	0.056	0.322	0	1242	0	1242
1 cup	Peas + carrots-cnd + liq	256	226	96.0	5.54	21.8	8.28	0.700	0.126	0.058	0.330	0	1478	0	1478
1 cup	Peas/carrots/onions-frzn	182	154	108	6.20	20.2	—	0.600	—	—	0.200	0	1272	0	1272
1 cup	Peas & mushrooms-frozen	190	151	146	10.0	26.2	—	0.800	0.200	—	0.400	0	149	0	149
1 cup	Peas & onions-frzn	190	151	142	9.20	27.0	—	0.400	—	—	0.200	0	127	0	127
1 cup	Peas-edible pods-fresh	145	129	61.0	4.06	11.0	4.35	0.290	0.057	0.030	0.129	0	21.1	0	21.1
1 cup	Peas-edible pods-cooked	160	142	67.0	5.24	11.3	4.47	0.360	0.070	0.037	0.160	0	21.0	0	21.0
1 cup	Sprouted peas-mature-raw	120	74.8	154	10.6	33.9	4.34	0.820	0.149	0.073	0.391	0	20.0	0	20.0
1 Tbs	Hot green pepper-canned	8.50	7.86	2.13	0.076	0.519	0.135	0.009	0.001	0.000	0.005	0	5.25	0	5.25
1 Tbs	Grn chili pepper-raw-chpd	9.38	8.22	3.75	0.188	0.887	0.150	0.019	0.002	0.001	0.010	0	7.22	0	7.22
1 ea.	Green chili pepper-raw-ea	45.0	39.5	18.0	0.900	4.26	0.800	0.090	0.009	0.005	0.049	0	35.0	0	35.0
1 ea.	Red chili pepper-raw-whl	45.0	39.5	18.0	0.900	4.26	0.810	0.090	0.009	0.005	0.049	0	484	0	484
1 Tbs	Red chili peppers raw/chp	9.38	8.22	3.75	0.188	0.887	0.150	0.019	0.002	0.001	0.010	0	101	0	101

B1 Mg	B2 Mg	B3 Mg	B6 Mg	B12 Mcg	Fol. Mcg	Panto Mg	Vit-C Mg	Vit-E Mg	Calc Mg	Cu Mg	Iron Mg	Mg Mg	Phos Mg	Potas Mg	Sel Mcg	Na Mg	Zinc Mg
0.088	0.088	0.923	0.169	0	36.2	0.247	10.0	0.252	48.0	0.185	0.640	44.0	69.0	346	2.50	2.00	0.710
0.032	0.020	0.312	0.054	0	14.4	0.260	4.80	0.156	14.0	0.042	0.280	12.0	18.0	156	12.4	2.00	0.240
0.090	0.060	0.903	0.156	0	41.8	0.752	14.2	0.452	42.0	0.120	0.840	33.0	51.0	448	35.0	6.00	0.690
0.105	0.143	0.390	0.037	0	64.0	0.035	19.3	1.38	103	0.082	1.71	20.0	36.0	218	—	42.0	0.620
0.137	0.184	0.500	0.044	0	82.0	0.044	18.9	2.35	147	0.116	1.89	26.0	44.0	244	—	46.0	0.800
0.053	0.133	0.665	—	0	—	—	63.8	—	59.0	—	3.19	137	84.0	519	—	5.00	—
0.122	0.032	0.960	0.138	0	23.0	0.120	2.08	0.051	9.60	0.173	0.560	21.0	35.0	397	—	4.80	0.240
0.040	0.038	0.200	0.010	0	71.0	0.450	3.20	—	26.0	0.050	0.420	8.00	14.0	158	—	12.0	0.400
0.089	0.014	1.63	0.118	0	14.5	0.328	5.20	0.291	10.0	0.069	0.380	17.0	47.0	366	0.450	108	0.190
0.089	0.014	1.63	0.118	0	14.5	0.328	5.20	0.291	10.0	0.069	0.380	17.0	47.0	366	0.450	108	0.190
0.061	0.015	1.15	0.116	0	8.30	0.329	5.50	0.291	4.00	0.082	0.670	11.0	43.0	229	0.450	15.0	0.210
0.006	0.003	0.021	0.100	0	0.092	—	0.935	0.000	5.42	0.008	0.051	0.750	4.60	12.0	0.747	0.510	0.265
0.013	0.004	0.019	0.567	0	1.67	—	0.003	0.001	2.33	0.021	0.077	1.67	11.7	31.0	1.77	0.667	0.074
0.074	0.087	0.670	0.182	0	19.6	0.061	80.4	5.36	90.0	0.194	1.14	23.0	38.0	299	0.124	29.0	0.295
0.069	0.090	0.700	0.179	0	30.0	0.064	53.3	7.41	94.0	0.203	1.17	23.0	36.0	296	0.240	30.0	0.312
0.056	0.148	0.874	0.112	0	31.0	0.069	32.8	6.13	179	0.061	1.22	23.0	36.0	417	0.290	20.0	0.234
0.014	0.043	0.133	—	0	51.1	—	—	0.247	47.7	0.037	0.809	34.4	11.9	25.2	—	66.1	0.350
0.070	0.028	0.560	0.210	0	14.1	0.231	86.8	—	34.0	0.196	0.560	27.0	64.0	490	11.2	28.0	0.322
0.066	0.033	0.644	0.139	0	13.3	0.168	89.1	—	41.0	0.196	0.660	31.0	74.0	561	13.2	34.0	0.322
0.026	0.022	0.208	0.150	0	32.0	0.100	4.40	0.900	31.2	0.090	1.14	14.6	17.6	90.4	5.10	10.4	0.240
0.176	0.099	0.869	0.146	0	76.9	0.445	12.7	—	19.0	0.271	2.47	28.0	133	248	—	8.00	1.16
0.034	0.034	0.168	0.037	0	41.0	0.176	4.50	0.576	18.7	0.013	0.168	6.20	13.0	144	0.450	2.80	0.144
0.026	0.017	0.105	0.022	0	31.4	0.026	2.18	0.060	10.6	0.016	0.280	5.04	11.2	88.5	0.224	5.04	—
0.018	0.012	0.074	0.016	0	22.4	0.018	1.56	0.042	7.60	0.012	0.200	3.60	8.00	63.2	1.43	3.60	0.088
0.028	0.045	0.224	0.031	0	60.0	0.112	10.1	0.224	38.0	0.015	0.784	6.20	14.0	148	0.224	5.00	0.185
0.056	0.056	0.280	0.034	0	76.0	0.112	13.4	0.224	20.2	0.015	0.616	3.40	25.0	162	0.224	4.48	0.185
0.072	0.314	2.88	0.068	0	14.8	1.54	2.46	0.056	3.50	0.344	0.868	7.00	72.8	260	7.80	2.80	0.600
0.900	0.405	3.71	0.090	0	20.7	1.98	3.15	—	4.50	0.445	1.12	9.00	93.5	335	—	3.50	0.655
0.045	0.062	0.448	0.096	0	33.0	0.118	39.2	1.13	58.0	0.066	0.818	18.0	24.0	198	—	14.0	0.144
0.374	0.157	2.47	0.530	0	129	0.604	46.4	—	179	0.243	1.28	160	160	914	—	13.3	1.56
0.001	0.001	0.010	0.006	0	0.340	0.007	0.001	0.620	24.0	0.133	0.600	8.58	6.00	21.0	—	936	0.027
0.001	0.002	0.010	0.007	0	0.343	0.008	0.001	1.20	52.0	0.109	1.04	10.0	10.0	10.0	—	355	0.142
0.009	0.001	0.014	0.033	0	3.00	0.032	0.317	—	8.00	0.067	0.057	2.67	7.00	20.0	—	1.000	0.050
0.096	0.016	0.160	0.251	0	31.8	0.211	13.4	0.496	40.0	0.064	0.592	16.0	46.0	248	2.56	3.20	0.288
0.069	0.012	0.115	0.181	0	22.9	0.152	9.66	0.357	29.0	0.046	0.426	11.5	33.0	178	1.84	2.30	0.207
0.088	0.016	0.168	0.378	0	26.6	0.266	12.0	0.620	58.0	0.084	0.420	22.0	48.0	318	2.90	16.0	0.380
0.048	0.052	0.292	0.144	0	28.0	0.208	5.40	0.360	34.0	0.040	0.630	14.0	40.0	228	2.70	26.0	0.148
0.070	0.140	0.200	0.050	0	16.0	0.144	45.0	0.300	60.0	0.060	1.88	20.0	32.0	256	1.20	4.00	0.440
0.001	0.003	0.012	0.002	0	1.79	0.003	0.175	0.017	0.167	0.000	0.062	0.417	0.667	7.33	0.007	0.417	0.007
0.003	0.004	0.026	0.006	0	6.86	0.011	3.38	0.063	4.88	0.002	0.232	1.63	1.50	20.1	0.019	1.50	0.027
0.130	0.080	1.10	0.146	0	91.0	0.918	20.2	1.20	58.0	0.216	0.900	46.0	108	573	3.62	16.0	0.400
0.387	0.193	3.05	0.247	0	95.3	0.152	58.4	2.03	36.0	0.257	2.14	48.0	157	357	7.97	7.00	1.81
0.414	0.238	3.23	0.250	0	101	0.245	22.8	3.40	44.0	0.277	2.47	63.0	187	434	8.80	4.00	1.90
0.452	0.280	2.36	0.180	0	93.8	0.228	15.8	0.800	38.0	0.222	2.50	46.0	144	268	6.40	140	1.50
0.206	0.132	1.24	0.108	0	75.4	0.218	16.2	1.52	34.0	0.140	1.62	30.0	114	294	6.80	372	1.20
0.206	0.132	1.24	0.108	0	75.4	0.218	16.2	1.52	34.0	0.140	1.62	30.0	114	294	6.80	3.40	1.20
0.360	0.112	1.85	0.140	0	41.6	0.260	13.0	1.79	36.0	0.122	1.50	26.0	78.0	254	4.46	110	0.720
0.190	0.136	1.49	0.226	0	47.0	0.308	16.8	1.45	58.0	0.264	1.94	0.360	116	256	5.18	664	1.48
0.340	0.140	2.60	0.180	0	112	0.440	24.0	—	52.0	0.164	2.06	34.0	112	316	—	120	1.02
0.500	0.220	4.20	0.260	0	162	0.220	40.0	—	26.0	0.196	1.86	38.0	140	352	—	430	1.10
0.480	0.160	3.60	0.260	0	146	0.340	38.0	—	30.0	0.166	1.70	36.0	118	344	—	624	0.970
0.218	0.116	0.870	0.232	0	43.5	1.09	87.0	3.90	62.0	0.120	3.01	35.0	77.0	290	4.60	6.00	0.590
0.205	0.122	0.862	0.230	0	48.0	1.08	76.6	4.70	67.0	0.123	3.15	42.0	89.0	383	3.50	6.00	0.600
0.270	0.186	3.71	0.318	0	173	1.24	12.5	—	43.0	0.326	2.71	67.0	198	457	8.80	24.0	1.26
0.002	0.004	0.068	0.010	0	4.38	0.058	5.77	0.030	0.625	0.009	0.042	1.02	1.50	17.9	—	1.19	0.002
0.008	0.008	0.089	0.026	0	2.19	0.006	22.7	0.063	1.63	0.016	0.112	2.38	4.25	31.9	0.075	0.625	0.028
0.041	0.041	0.428	0.125	0	10.5	0.027	109	0.300	8.00	0.078	0.540	11.0	21.0	153	—	3.00	0.135
0.041	0.041	0.428	0.125	0	10.5	0.027	109	0.300	8.00	0.078	0.540	11.0	21.0	153	0.360	3.00	0.135
0.008	0.008	0.089	0.026	0	2.19	0.006	22.7	0.063	1.63	0.016	0.112	2.38	4.25	31.9	0.075	0.625	0.028

Qty	Name	Wgt G	Wtr G	Cal	Prot G	Carb G	Fiber G	F-Tot G	F-Sat G	Mono G	Poly G	Chol Mg	A-Car RE	A-Pre RE	A-Tot RE
1 Tbs	Jalapeno peppers cnd/chpd	8.50	7.64	2.13	0.067	0.416	0.255	0.051	0.052	0.003	0.028	0	14.5	0	14.5
1 cup	Pepper-swt green-raw-chpd	100	92.8	24.0	0.860	5.32	1.50	0.460	0.068	0.030	0.242	0	53.0	0	53.0
1 ea.	Pepper-swt green-raw-pod	74.0	68.7	18.0	0.630	3.93	1.11	0.330	0.050	0.022	0.178	0	39.2	0	39.2
1 cup	Pepper-swt green-ckd-chpd	136	129	24.0	0.840	5.30	1.50	0.440	0.066	0.030	0.240	0	52.8	0	52.8
1 ea.	Pepper-swt green-ckd-pod	73.0	69.1	13.0	0.453	2.84	0.800	0.241	0.036	0.016	0.129	0	28.3	0	28.3
1 cup	Pepper-swt green-fzn/ckd	136	129	24.4	1.29	5.30	1.62	0.244	0.036	0.016	0.134	0	39.4	0	39.4
1 cup	Sweet red pepper-raw-chpd	100	92.8	24.0	0.860	5.32	1.50	0.460	0.068	0.030	0.242	0	570	0	570
1 cup	Sweet red pepper-ckd-chpd	136	129	24.0	0.840	5.30	1.50	0.440	0.066	0.030	0.240	0	512	0	512
1 cup	Sweet red repper ckd/frzn	136	129	24.4	1.29	5.30	1.62	0.244	0.036	0.016	0.134	0	454	0	454
1 Tbs	Pepper-sweet red-frzdried	0.400	0.008	1.25	0.072	0.275	0.077	0.012	0.002	0.001	0.006	0	31.0	0	31.0
1 ea.	Baked potato with skin	202	144	220	4.65	51.0	3.90	0.200	0.052	0.004	0.087	0	0	0	0
1 ea.	Baked potato-flesh only	156	118	145	3.06	33.6	2.70	0.160	0.041	0.003	0.067	0	0	0	0
1 ea.	Potato skin-oven baked	58.0	27.4	115	2.49	27.0	1.54	0.060	0.015	0.001	0.025	0	0	0	0
1 ea.	Potato + peel-microwaved	202	145	212	4.93	48.7	3.90	0.200	0.052	0.004	0.087	0	0	0	0
1 ea.	Potato-boiled-peeled aftr	136	105	119	2.54	27.4	2.20	0.140	0.035	0.003	0.058	0	0	0	0
1 ea.	Peeled potato-boiled	135	105	116	2.31	27.0	1.11	0.140	0.035	0.003	0.058	0	0	0	0
1 ea.	Potato-ckd f/frzn-small	70.0	58.0	46.0	1.39	10.2	0.500	0.091	0.024	0.002	0.039	0	0	0	0
2 ea.	Potatoes-canned-1 in diam	70.0	59.0	42.0	0.980	9.52	0.560	0.140	0.038	0.004	0.062	0	0	0	0
10 pce	French fries-oven heated	50.0	26.4	111	1.73	17.0	1.11	4.38	2.08	1.78	0.329	0	0	0	0
10 ea.	French fries-frzn-veg oil	50.0	19.0	158	2.01	19.8	1.11	8.28	2.50	1.64	3.78	0	0	0	0
1 ea.	Cottage frd potatoes f/Fz	5.00	2.64	10.9	0.172	1.70	0.111	0.410	0.195	0.166	0.031	0	0	0	0
1 cup	Hash brown potatoes f/fzn	156	87.5	340	4.93	44.0	1.11	18.0	7.01	8.01	2.07	0	0	0	0
1 cup	Mashed potatoes prep/milk	210	165	162	4.06	36.9	1.23	1.23	0.699	0.307	0.116	4.00	0	12.0	12.0
1 cup	Mashed potatoes-mlk&marg	210	160	222	3.95	35.1	1.23	8.87	2.17	3.72	2.54	4.00	33.0	8.00	41.0
1 cup	Mashed potatoes-prep inst	210	160	237	4.00	31.5	1.20	11.8	7.21	3.32	0.521	4.00	34.0	10.0	44.0
1 cup	Mashed potatoes-prep inst	210	160	237	4.00	31.5	1.20	11.8	7.21	3.32	0.521	4.00	34.0	10.0	44.0
10 ea.	Potato chips	20.3	0.507	106	1.14	10.5	0.207	7.21	1.84	1.26	3.69	0	0	0	0
1 cup	Pumpkin-canned	246	221	84.0	2.70	19.8	4.50	0.690	0.358	0.090	0.038	0	5404	0	5404
1 cup	Pumpkin-ckd fr/raw/mashed	245	230	50.0	2.00	11.9	4.30	0.172	0.091	0.022	0.010	0	265	0	265
1 cup	Purslane raw	43.0	40.4	7.00	0.560	1.47	0.340	0.040	—	—	—	0	56.8	0	56.8
4 ea.	Radishes-red	18.0	17.1	2.80	0.108	0.644	0.396	0.096	0.006	0.003	0.008	0	0.120	0	0.120
1 cup	Radishes-daikon	88.0	83.2	16.0	0.520	3.62	2.00	0.080	0.026	0.014	0.040	0	0	0	0
1 cup	Radish seeds-sprouted	38.0	34.2	15.6	1.45	1.16	0.990	0.961	0.291	0.159	0.434	0	15.0	0	15.0
1 cup	Sauerkraut-canned w/liqd	236	218	44.0	2.15	10.1	4.40	0.330	0.083	0.031	0.144	0	4.20	0	4.20
1 cup	Soybeans-sprouted-raw	70.0	48.4	90.0	9.16	7.82	1.62	4.68	0.508	0.526	2.60	0	0.800	0	0.800
1 cup	Bean sprouts-fresh/raw	104	94.0	31.2	3.16	6.16	2.70	0.187	0.048	0.023	0.060	0	2.20	0	2.20
1 cup	Spinach-fresh-chopped	56.0	51.3	12.3	1.60	1.96	2.28	0.196	0.031	0.006	0.082	0	376	0	376
1 cup	Spinach-fresh-cooked	180	164	41.0	5.35	6.75	4.95	0.470	0.076	0.013	0.194	0	1474	0	1474
1 cup	Spinach-leaf-frzn-cooked	190	171	53.2	5.97	10.2	6.27	0.399	0.063	0.012	0.164	0	1479	0	1479
1 cup	Spinach-canned/drained	214	196	50.0	6.02	7.28	7.70	1.07	0.173	0.030	0.447	0	1878	0	1878
1 cup	Summer squash-slices-raw	130	122	26.0	1.53	5.65	2.34	0.280	0.057	0.021	0.116	0	25.5	0	25.5
1 cup	Summer squash-all-cooked	180	169	36.0	1.63	7.76	3.00	0.560	0.115	0.041	0.236	0	51.7	0	51.7
1 cup	Zucchini squash-raw	130	124	19.0	1.50	3.78	1.60	0.180	0.038	0.014	0.078	0	44.2	0	44.2
1 cup	Zucchini squash-cooked	180	170	29.0	1.15	7.07	3.60	0.090	0.018	0.007	0.038	0	43.2	0	43.2
1 cup	Winter squash-avg-bkd-msh	245	218	96.0	2.20	21.4	5.88	1.54	0.320	0.115	0.650	0	872	0	872
1 cup	Winter squash-avg-bkd-cbs	205	182	79.0	1.81	17.9	4.92	1.29	0.267	0.096	0.543	0	730	0	730
1 cup	Winter squash-avg-frz-ckd	240	211	95.0	2.95	24.1	6.68	0.168	0.034	0.012	0.070	0	801	0	801
1 cup	Succotash-frozen-cooked	170	126	158	7.32	33.9	8.80	1.52	0.282	0.294	0.726	0	39.3	0	39.3
1 ea.	Sweet potato-bkd in skin	114	83.1	118	1.96	27.7	2.84	0.130	0.027	0.005	0.056	0	2488	0	2488

B1 Mg	B2 Mg	B3 Mg	B6 Mg	B12 Mcg	Fol. Mcg	Panto Mg	Vit-C Mg	Vit-E Mg	Calc Mg	Cu Mg	Iron Mg	Mg Mg	Phos Mg	Potas Mg	Sel Mcg	Na Mg	Zinc Mg
0.002	0.004	0.042	0.010	0	4.38	0.092	1.10	0.057	2.25	0.012	0.237	1.00	1.50	11.5	0.067	124	0.016
0.086	0.050	0.550	0.164	0	17.8	0.036	128	0.620	6.00	0.104	1.26	14.0	22.0	196	1.06	4.00	0.180
0.063	0.037	0.407	0.121	0	12.5	0.027	94.7	0.459	4.00	0.076	0.940	10.0	16.0	144	0.592	2.00	0.133
0.072	0.048	0.494	0.146	0	19.8	0.032	152	0.488	6.00	0.096	1.20	14.0	20.0	176	1.09	2.00	0.164
0.039	0.026	0.265	0.079	0	72.0	0.017	81.3	0.361	3.00	0.052	0.642	7.30	15.0	94.0	0.584	2.00	0.088
0.070	0.042	1.47	0.146	0	13.4	0.032	56.0	0.814	10.9	0.060	0.708	9.52	17.6	98.0	1.09	6.00	0.068
0.086	0.050	0.550	0.164	0	17.8	0.036	190	0.740	6.00	0.104	1.26	14.0	22.0	196	1.06	4.00	0.180
0.072	0.048	0.494	0.146	0	19.8	0.032	226	1.09	6.00	0.096	1.20	14.0	20.0	176	0.950	2.00	0.160
0.070	0.042	1.47	0.146	0	13.4	0.032	112	0.800	10.9	0.060	0.708	9.52	17.6	98.0	1.09	6.00	0.680
0.005	0.005	0.029	0.009	0	0.925	0.002	7.60	0.022	0.500	0.005	0.041	0.750	1.25	12.7	0.029	0.750	0.010
0.216	0.067	3.32	0.701	0	22.2	1.12	26.1	0.100	20.0	0.616	2.75	55.0	115	844	1.80	16.0	0.650
0.164	0.033	2.18	0.470	0	14.2	0.866	20.0	0.090	8.00	0.335	0.550	39.0	78.0	610	1.41	8.00	0.450
0.071	0.069	1.78	0.352	0	12.5	0.256	7.80	0.010	20.0	0.474	2.20	25.0	59.0	332	—	12.0	0.280
0.242	0.065	3.46	0.695	0	24.2	1.12	30.5	0.100	22.0	0.675	2.50	54.0	212	903	1.80	16.0	0.730
0.144	0.027	1.96	0.407	0	13.6	0.707	17.6	0.070	7.00	0.256	0.420	30.0	60.0	515	1.23	6.00	0.410
0.132	0.026	0.177	0.363	0	11.9	0.687	10.0	0.070	10.0	0.225	0.420	26.0	54.0	443	1.21	7.00	0.370
0.071	0.018	0.928	0.141	0	5.88	0.196	6.58	0.038	4.90	0.055	0.588	7.70	18.0	201	0.584	14.0	0.175
48.0	0.010	0.640	0.132	0	4.40	0.248	3.60	0.030	4.00	0.040	0.880	10.0	20.0	160	0.600	—	0.200
0.061	0.015	1.15	0.116	0	8.30	0.329	5.50	0.291	4.00	0.082	0.670	11.0	43.0	229	0.450	15.0	0.210
0.089	0.014	1.63	0.118	0	14.5	0.328	5.20	0.291	10.0	0.069	0.380	17.0	47.0	366	0.450	108	0.190
0.006	0.002	0.121	0.012	0	0.830	0.034	0.480	0.029	0.500	0.010	0.075	1.10	3.30	24.0	0.045	2.30	0.021
0.173	0.031	3.78	0.197	0	26.0	0.696	9.83	0.100	24.0	0.237	2.36	26.5	112	680	1.39	53.0	0.500
0.185	0.084	2.35	0.489	0.113	17.2	1.00	14.0	0.210	55.0	0.294	0.570	39.0	100	628	1.89	636	0.600
0.176	0.106	2.27	0.470	0.107	16.7	1.20	12.9	0.210	54.0	0.288	0.550	37.0	97.0	607	1.89	619	0.580
0.233	0.080	1.41	0.019	0.164	9.40	0.252	20.4	0.044	103	0.034	0.460	37.0	118	490	1.95	697	0.370
0.233	0.080	1.41	0.019	0.164	9.40	0.252	20.4	0.044	103	0.034	0.460	37.0	118	490	1.95	697	0.370
0.029	0.004	0.850	0.103	0	9.14	0.081	8.43	1.34	5.00	0.041	0.243	12.1	30.7	264	1.54	95.0	0.214
0.060	0.132	0.900	0.138	0	30.0	0.980	10.2	2.20	64.0	0.262	3.42	56.0	86.0	504	—	12.0	0.418
0.076	0.191	1.01	0.157	0	33.0	0.726	11.5	1.63	37.0	0.194	1.40	22.0	74.0	564	—	3.00	0.450
0.020	0.048	0.206	—	0	—	—	9.00	—	28.0	—	0.860	29.0	19.0	213	—	20.0	—
0.001	0.008	0.054	0.013	0	4.88	0.016	4.12	0	3.60	0.007	0.052	1.60	3.20	41.6	0.560	4.40	0.052
0.018	0.018	0.176	0.306	0	19.2	0.190	19.4	0	24.0	0.122	0.360	14.0	20.0	200	2.44	18.0	0.140
0.039	0.039	1.08	0.108	0	36.0	0.279	11.0	—	19.4	0.046	0.327	16.7	43.0	33.0	—	2.00	0.213
0.050	0.052	0.337	0.307	0	4.00	0.219	34.8	—	72.0	0.227	3.47	31.0	46.0	401	—	1561	0.440
0.238	0.082	0.804	0.124	0	120	0.650	10.8	—	48.0	0.300	1.48	50.0	114	338	—	10.0	0.820
0.087	0.129	0.779	0.092	0	63.2	0.396	13.7	0.210	14.0	0.171	0.946	22.0	56.0	154	—	6.00	0.426
0.044	0.106	0.405	0.109	0	109	0.036	15.7	1.50	55.4	0.073	1.52	44.2	27.4	312	0.816	44.0	0.297
0.171	0.425	0.882	0.436	0	262	0.261	40.0	4.00	244	0.313	6.42	157	100	838	2.70	126	1.37
0.114	0.319	0.796	0.278	0	204	0.158	23.4	3.50	277	0.268	2.89	131	91.2	566	2.96	163	—
0.034	0.295	0.830	0.214	0	209	0.101	31.0	0.500	271	0.385	4.92	162	94.0	740	1.50	683	0.990
0.083	0.048	0.716	0.142	0	33.3	0.133	19.2	0.330	26.0	0.099	0.600	30.0	46.0	253	4.10	3.00	0.330
0.079	0.074	0.923	0.117	0	36.2	0.247	9.20	0.252	48.0	0.185	0.640	44.0	69.0	346	4.16	2.00	0.710
0.091	0.039	0.520	0.116	0	28.8	0.108	11.7	0.507	20.0	0.074	0.550	28.0	42.0	322	1.95	3.00	0.260
0.074	0.074	0.770	0.140	0	30.2	0.205	8.30	0.252	23.0	0.155	0.630	40.0	72.0	455	1.50	5.40	0.324
0.208	0.059	1.72	0.176	0	69.0	0.086	23.5	0.294	34.3	0.232	0.810	19.6	49.0	1071	3.15	2.45	0.637
0.174	0.049	1.43	0.148	0	57.4	0.718	19.7	0.246	28.0	0.195	0.670	16.0	41.0	895	2.63	3.00	0.540
0.120	0.060	1.11	0.218	0	38.0	0.370	8.30	1.20	46.0	0.086	1.39	22.0	34.0	319	2.50	4.80	0.288
0.126	0.116	2.22	0.162	0	56.5	0.394	10.1	1.74	25.0	0.102	1.51	39.0	119	451	0.850	77.0	0.760
0.083	0.145	0.700	0.275	0	25.7	0.736	28.1	5.20	32.0	0.237	0.520	23.0	63.0	397	0.704	12.0	0.330

VEGETABLES (continued)

Qty	Name	Wgt G	Wtr G	Cal	Prot G	Carb G	Fiber G	F-Tot G	F-Sat G	Mono G	Poly G	Chol Mg	A-Car RE	A-Pre RE	A-Tot RE
1 ea.	Sweet potato-peeled-bld	151	110	160	2.00	37.0	3.68	0.453	0.097	0.017	0.200	0	2575	0	2575
1 pce	Candied sweet potatoes	105	70.3	144	0.910	29.3	2.15	3.41	1.42	0.658	0.154	0	440	0	440
1 cup	Sweet potatoes-cnd-mshd	256	189	258	5.04	59.2	6.40	0.510	0.110	0.020	0.228	0	3858	0	3858
1 cup	Tomato juice-canned	244	229	41.5	1.85	10.3	1.70	0.146	0.020	0.022	0.059	0	136	0	136
1 cup	Tomato juice-cnd-unsalted	244	229	41.5	1.85	10.3	1.70	0.146	0.020	0.022	0.059	0	136	0	136
1 cup	Tomato paste-canned	262	194	220	9.90	49.3	6.20	2.30	0.333	0.351	0.948	0	647	0	647
1 cup	Tomato sauce-canned	245	218	74.0	3.25	17.6	3.20	0.410	0.059	0.061	0.164	0	240	0	240
1 cup	Tomato puree-canned	250	218	102	4.18	25.1	4.20	0.290	0.040	0.043	0.118	0	340	0	340
1 ea.	Tomato-fresh-whole	123	116	24.0	1.09	5.34	2.00	0.260	0.037	0.039	0.107	0	139	0	139
1 cup	Tomatoes-fresh-chopped	180	169	35.0	1.60	7.81	2.93	0.390	0.054	0.058	0.157	0	204	0	204
1 cup	Tomatoes-cooked fr/fresh	240	222	60.0	2.68	13.5	5.00	0.650	0.091	0.096	0.262	0	325	0	325
1 cup	Tomatoes-whole-canned	240	225	47.0	2.24	10.3	2.16	0.590	0.084	0.089	0.238	0	145	0	145
1 Tbs	Catsup	17.1	11.8	18.1	0.313	4.31	0.085	0.069	0.012	0.012	0.025	0	23.9	0	23.9
1 cup	Turnip cubes-raw	130	119	35.0	1.17	8.09	3.03	0.130	0.014	0.008	0.069	0	0	0	0
1 cup	Turnip cubes-ckd from raw	156	146	28.0	1.10	7.66	3.44	0.120	0.012	0.008	0.066	0	0	0	0
1 cup	Turnip greens-fresh-ckd	144	135	29.0	1.64	6.28	3.60	0.330	0.076	0.022	0.131	0	792	0	792
1 cup	Mixed vegetables-frzn-ckd	182	151	107	5.21	23.8	7.50	0.273	0.056	0.016	0.120	0	779	0	779
1 cup	Mixed vegetables-cnd-drnd	163	142	77.0	4.22	15.1	6.60	0.410	0.083	0.026	0.194	0	1899	0	1899
1 cup	Watercress-fresh	34.0	32.3	4.00	0.780	0.440	0.940	0.040	0.010	0.002	0.012	0	160	0	160
1 cup	Hawaii mtn yam/ckd-steamd	145	112	119	2.51	29.0	0.812	0.116	0.026	0.004	0.052	0	0	0	0
1 cup	Yams-white-cooked cubes	136	95.3	158	2.02	37.5	3.90	0.190	0.039	0.007	0.082	0	0	0	0
1 cup	Yardlong beans-boild slcs	104	91.0	49.0	2.63	9.54	1.57	0.100	0.027	0.009	0.044	0	46.8	0	46.8

B1 Mg	B2 Mg	B3 Mg	B6 Mg	B12 Mcg	Fol. Mcg	Panto Mg	Vit-C Mg	Vit-E Mg	Calc Mg	Cu Mg	Iron Mg	Mg Mg	Phos Mg	Potas Mg	Sel Mcg	Na Mg	Zinc Mg
0.080	0.210	1.00	0.360	0	22.0	0.803	26.0	6.04	32.0	0.243	0.800	15.0	41.0	278	0.700	20.0	0.400
0.019	0.044	0.414	0.165	0	12.0	0.450	7.00	0.780	27.0	0.107	1.20	12.0	27.0	198	0.679	73.0	0.160
0.068	0.230	2.40	0.486	0	42.4	1.33	13.0	9.00	77.0	0.710	3.40	60.0	134	536	1.49	190	0.540
0.115	0.076	1.64	0.271	0	48.6	0.610	44.7	0.537	22.0	0.246	1.41	26.8	46.4	537	0.488	881	0.342
0.115	0.076	1.64	0.271	0	48.6	0.610	44.7	0.537	22.0	0.246	1.41	26.8	46.4	537	0.488	24.0	0.342
0.406	0.498	8.44	0.996	0	40.0	1.97	111	3.52	91.7	1.55	7.84	134	207	2442	1.40	170	2.10
0.162	0.142	2.82	0.333	0	38.8	0.757	32.1	1.20	34.0	0.480	1.88	46.0	78.0	908	1.45	1481	0.600
0.178	0.135	4.29	0.380	0	38.8	1.10	88.2	0.600	37.0	0.408	2.32	60.0	99.0	1051	2.00	49.0	0.540
0.074	0.062	0.738	0.094	0	11.5	0.304	21.6	0.860	9.00	0.095	0.590	14.0	28.0	255	0.615	10.0	0.130
0.108	0.090	1.08	0.138	0	16.8	0.445	31.6	1.26	12.0	0.139	0.860	20.0	42.0	372	0.900	15.0	0.190
0.170	0.144	1.72	0.151	0	22.6	0.706	50.3	1.60	20.0	0.233	1.44	33.0	70.0	624	1.40	25.0	0.320
0.108	0.074	1.76	0.216	0	35.3	0.401	36.3	0.890	63.0	0.264	1.45	29.0	46.0	529	1.10	390	0.380
0.016	0.012	0.275	0.018	0	0.875	0.028	2.56	0.051	3.75	0.051	0.137	3.58	8.56	61.9	1.17	178	0.037
0.052	0.039	0.520	0.117	0	18.9	0.260	27.3	0.032	39.0	0.078	0.390	14.0	35.0	248	0.910	88.0	0.156
0.042	0.036	0.466	0.104	0	14.2	0.222	18.0	0.024	36.0	0.062	0.340	12.0	30.0	212	1.08	78.0	0.166
0.065	0.104	0.592	0.259	0	171	0.395	39.5	2.46	198	0.364	1.15	32.0	41.0	293	1.30	41.0	0.290
0.129	0.218	1.55	0.135	0	34.6	0.275	5.80	0.756	46.0	0.151	1.49	40.0	93.0	308	3.68	64.0	0.892
0.075	0.078	0.941	0.129	0	38.5	0.233	8.20	0.680	44.0	0.119	1.71	26.0	68.0	474	3.30	243	0.668
0.030	0.040	0.068	0.044	0	68.0	0.106	14.6	0.340	40.0	0.030	0.060	8.00	20.0	112	—	14.0	0.060
0.125	0.020	0.189	—	0	—	—	0	—	11.6	—	0.624	14.5	58.0	718	—	17.4	—
0.129	0.038	0.751	0.310	0	21.8	0.423	16.5	—	19.0	0.207	0.707	25.0	67.0	911	—	11.0	0.272
0.088	0.103	0.655	—	0	—	—	16.8	—	46.0	—	1.02	43.0	59.0	302	—	4.00	—

C

The Human Digestive System

Humans and other animals must ingest food into the body from the environment to live. Figure C.1 illustrates the entire digestive system that functions primarily to organize this important process. This amazing tract from the mouth to the anus allows us to ingest, chew, and swallow food, then break it down into absorbable molecules, and finally discharge food waste from the body.

Food is composed of water, dietary fiber, vitamins, minerals, carbohydrate, protein, and fat. The latter three are needed for their energy value and for making body tissue. Within the stomach and intestines, the large molecules of carbohydrate, protein, and fat are digested by the process of hydrolysis into their very smallest units, or monomers (glucose and other mono-saccharides, amino acids, and fatty acids and glycerol) (see figure C.2). These monomers are then transported across the wall of the intestine into the blood and lymph. This process is called absorption. Enzymes facilitate the process of digestion and absorption.

The stomach receives the food in bolus form from the esophagus. The food has already been broken down somewhat from the chewing action of the mouth, and mixed with saliva. Saliva contains enzymes that begin the process of starch digestion. In the stomach, hydrochloric acid and an enzyme called pepsinogen are secreted, both of which help to begin the digestion of protein. Carbohydrates are not digested at all in the stomach, and fats are digested only in small part due to the action of an enzyme secreted with the saliva. The complete digestion of food molecules occurs later, when the contents of the stomach enter the small intestine. No food is absorbed through the stomach wall. Only alcohol can be absorbed across the stomach wall.

The small intestine is that portion of the digestive tract between the stomach and the large intestine. The small intestine is twelve feet long and one inch wide. The small intestine serves as the major site of digestion and absorption in the digestive tract.

The small intestine is divided into three regions—duodenum, jejunum, and ileum. The duodenum is a C-shaped, ten-inch-long tube. It receives secretions from both the liver and the pancreas. The jejunum is approximately three feet long and extends from the duodenum to the ileum. The ileum makes up the remaining six to seven feet of the small intestine.

Enzymes from the pancreas and the small intestine digest the starches, proteins, and fats into their final monomer units (see table C.1). Although the digestion of starch begins in the mouth with the action of the enzyme called salivary amylase (also called ptyalin), most of the action takes place in the duodenum as a result of the enzyme called pancreatic amylase. This enzyme cleaves the straight chains of starch to smaller particles, which are finally broken down to glucose by the action of enzymes on the brush border of the intestinal wall. Sucrose and lactose (disaccharides) are also hydrolyzed to their monosaccharides by enzymes located on the wall of the small intestine (see chapter 4).

The digestive system, including the alimentary canal and the accessory digestive organs.

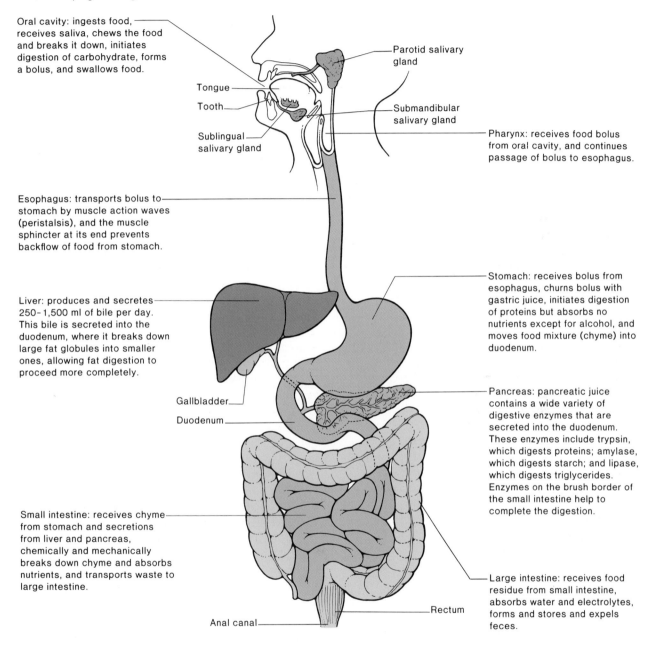

Oral cavity: ingests food, receives saliva, chews the food and breaks it down, initiates digestion of carbohydrate, forms a bolus, and swallows food.

Tongue

Tooth

Sublingual salivary gland

Parotid salivary gland

Submandibular salivary gland

Pharynx: receives food bolus from oral cavity, and continues passage of bolus to esophagus.

Esophagus: transports bolus to stomach by muscle action waves (peristalsis), and the muscle sphincter at its end prevents backflow of food from stomach.

Stomach: receives bolus from esophagus, churns bolus with gastric juice, initiates digestion of proteins but absorbs no nutrients except for alcohol, and moves food mixture (chyme) into duodenum.

Liver: produces and secretes 250-1,500 ml of bile per day. This bile is secreted into the duodenum, where it breaks down large fat globules into smaller ones, allowing fat digestion to proceed more completely.

Gallbladder

Duodenum

Pancreas: pancreatic juice contains a wide variety of digestive enzymes that are secreted into the duodenum. These enzymes include trypsin, which digests proteins; amylase, which digests starch; and lipase, which digests triglycerides. Enzymes on the brush border of the small intestine help to complete the digestion.

Small intestine: receives chyme from stomach and secretions from liver and pancreas, chemically and mechanically breaks down chyme and absorbs nutrients, and transports waste to large intestine.

Large intestine: receives food residue from small intestine, absorbs water and electrolytes, forms and stores and expels feces.

Anal canal

Rectum

*F*IGURE C.2

The digestion of food molecules occurs by means of hydrolysis reactions.

Maltose   +   Water   ⟶   Glucose   +   Glucose

Disaccharide   **Monosaccharides**

Peptide (portion of protein molecule)   +   Water   ⟶   Amino acid   +   Amino acid

Fat   +   Water   ⟶   Fatty acids   +   Glycerol

TABLE C.1
Summary of the sources and activities of the major digestive enzymes

Region or source					
Organ	Source	Substrate	Enzymes	Optimum pH	Products
Mouth	Saliva	Starch	Salivary amylase	6.7	Maltose
Stomach	Gastric glands	Protein	Pepsin	1.6–2.4	Shorter polypeptides
Duodenum	Pancreatic juice	Starch	Pancreatic amylase	6.7–7.0	Maltose, maltriose, and oligosaccharides
		Polypeptides	Trypsin, chymotrypsin, carboxypeptidase	8.0	Amino acids, dipeptides, and tripeptides
		Triglycerides	Pancreatic lipase	8.0	Fatty acids and monoglycerides
	Epithelial membranes	Maltose	Maltase	5.0–7.0	Glucose
		Sucrose	Sucrase	5.0–7.0	Glucose + fructose
		Lactose	Lactase	5.8–6.2	Glucose + galactose
		Polypeptides	Aminopeptidase	8.0	Amino acids, dipeptides, tripeptides

Source: Fox, Stuart Ira, *Human Physiology.* © 1984 Wm. C. Brown Publishers, Dubuque, Iowa. All Rights Reserved. Reprinted by permission.

Protein digestion begins in the stomach with the action of pepsin. Most of the protein digestion, however, occurs in the duodenum and jejunum. The pancreatic enzymes trypsin, chymotrypsin, and elastase cleave peptide bonds (see chapter 6). Other enzymes called carboxypeptidase and the brush border enzyme aminopeptidase also help digest proteins down to their final amino acids.

Most of the ingested fat enters the duodenum undigested in the form of fat globules. Bile salts from the liver break up these droplets into much finer droplets. An enzyme from the pancreas, pancreatic lipase, breaks down the fats into fatty acids and monoglycerides (see chapter 5).

The large intestine is about five feet long and two and one-half inches in diameter. The large intestine has little or no digestive function, but it does absorb water and electrolytes from the remaining food residue. In addition, the large intestine functions to form, store, and expel feces from the body.

A P P E N D I X

Weights, Measures, and Conversions

Arabic numbers are used with weights and measures, as 10 gm., or 3 ml., etc. Portions of weights and measures are usually expressed decimally. For practical purposes, 1 cc. is equivalent to 1 ml. and 1 drop (gtt) of water is equivalent to a minim (m).

Household Measures* and Weights

Approximate Equivalents: 60 gtt = 1 teaspoonful = 5 ml = 60 minims = 60 grains = 1 dram = ⅛ ounce.

1 teaspoon = ⅛ fl oz; 1 dram
3 teaspoons = 1 tablespoon
1 tablespoon = ½ fl oz; 4 drams
16 tablespoons (liquid) = 1 cup
12 tablespoons (dry) = 1 cup

1 cup = 8 fl oz
1 tumbler or glass = 8 fl oz; ½ pint

*Household measures are not precise. For instance, household tsp will hold from 3 to 5 ml of liquid substances. Therefore, do not substitute household equivalents for medication prescribed by the physician.

To Convert Centigrade or Celsius Degrees to Fahrenheit Degrees

Multiply the number of Centigrade degrees by 9/5 and add 32 to the result.

Example: 55° C × 9/5 = 99 + 32 = 131° F.

To convert Fahrenheit degrees to Centigrade degrees: Subtract 32 from the number of Fahrenheit degrees and multiply the difference by 5/9.

Example: 243° F − 32 = 211 × 5/9 = 117.2° C.

Metric system (weights)						
Scale		**Table**		**Grams**		**Grains**
Kilo	1	Kilomgram	=	1000.0	=	15,432.35
Hecto	1	Hectogram	=	100.0	=	1,543.23
Deca	1	Decagram	=	10.0	=	154.323
Unit	1	Gram	=	1.0	=	15.432
Deci	1	Decigram	=	0.1	=	1.5432
Centi	1	Centigram	=	0.01	=	0.15432
Milli	1	Milligram	=	0.001	=	0.01543
Micro	1	Microgram	=	10^{-6}	=	15.432×10^{-6}
Nano	1	Nanogram	=	10^{-9}	=	15.432×10^{-9}
Pico	1	Picogram	=	10^{-12}	=	15.432×10^{-12}
Femto	1	Femtogram	=	10^{-15}	=	15.432×10^{-15}
Atto	1	Attogram	=	10^{-18}	=	15.432×10^{-18}

Units of length

Millimeters	Centimeters	Inches	Feet	Yards	Meters
1 mm = 1.0	0.1	0.03937	0.00328	0.0011	0.001
1 cm = 10.0	1.0	0.3937	0.03281	0.0109	0.01
1 in = 25.4	2.54	1.0	0.0833	0.0278	0.0254
1 ft = 304.8	30.48	12.0	1.0	0.333	0.3048
1 yd = 914.40	91.44	36.0	3.0	1.0	0.9144
1 m = 1000.0	100.0	39.37	3.2808	1.0936	1.0

$1\ \mu$ = 1 mu = 1 micrometer = 0.001 millimeter. 1 mm = 1000 μ.
1 km = 1 kilometer = 1000 meters = 0.6215 mile.
1 mile = 5280 feet = 1.609 kilometers.

Units of volume (fluid or liquid)

Milliliters	U.S. Fluid Drams	Cubic Inches	U.S. Fluid Ounces	U.S. Fluid Quarts	Liters
1 ml = 1.0	0.2705	0.061	0.03381	0.00106	0.001
1 fl ʒ = 3.697	1.0	0.226	0.125	0.00391	0.00369
1 cu in = 16.3866	4.4329	1.0	0.5541	0.0173	0.01639
1 fl ʒ = 29.573	8.0	1.8047	1.0	0.03125	0.02957
1 qt = 946.332	256.0	57.75	32.0	1.0	0.9463
1 L = 1000.0	270.52	61.025	33.815	1.0567	1.0

1 gallon = 4 quarts = 8 pints = 3.785 liters.
1 pint = 473.16 ml

Units of weight

Grains	Grams	Apothecaries Ounces	Avoirdupois Pounds	Kilograms
1 gr = 1.0	0.0648	0.00208	0.0001429	0.000065
1 gm = 15.432	1.0	0.03215	0.002205	0.001
1 ʒ = 480.0	31.1	1.0	0.06855	0.0311
1 lb = 7000.0	453.5924	14.583	1.0	0.45354
1 kg = 15432.358	1000.0	32.15	2.2046	1.0

$1\ \gamma$ = 1 gamma = 1 microgram = 0.001 milligram; 1000 γ = 1 mg
1 mg = 1 milligram = 0.001 gm; 1000 mg = 1 gm
1 grain = 64.8 mg; 1 mg = 0.0154 grain.

A P P E N D I X

E

Nutrition Resource Organizations

The following organizations are excellent resources for nutrition information. Most of these are nonprofit and may request a small charge for their pamphlets.

American Cancer Society
National Headquarters
90 Park Avenue
New York, NY 10016

American Diabetes Association
1660 Duke Street
Alexandria, VA 22314

American Dietetic Association
216 West Jackson Blvd.
Chicago, IL 60606–9715

American Health Foundation
1370 Avenue of the Americas
New York, NY 10019

American Heart Association
7320 Greenville Avenue
Dallas, TX 75231
(Also see your local association)

Center for Science in the Public Interest
1501 16th St., NW
Washington, D.C. 20036

Consumer Information Center
Dept. 88
Pueblo, CO 81009

Cooperative Extensive Service
(see your local listings)

Current Diet Review
P.O. Box 1914
Rialto, CA 92376

Food and Drug Administration
5600 Fishers Lane
Rockville, MD 20852

High Blood Pressure Information Center
120/80 National Institutes of Health
Bethesda, MD 20205

The National Council Against Health Fraud
Resource Center
2800 Main St.
Trinity Lutheran Hospital
Kansas City, MO 64108

National Institutes of Health
Office of Information, OD
RM 2310, Bldg 31
9000 Rockville Pike
Bethesda, MD 20014

U.S. Department of Agriculture
Office of Governmental and Public Affairs
Washington, D.C. 20250

A P P E N D I X

Eating for Health: Recommended Cookbooks and Magazines

1. American Harvest: *Regional Recipes for the Vegetarian Kitchen,* by Nava Atlas. Ballantine Books, NY, 1987.
2. *American Wholefoods Cuisine,* by Nicki and David Goldbeck.
3. *Choices for a Healthy Heart,* by Joseph and Bernice Piscatella. Workman Publishing, NY, 1987.
4. *Controlling Cholesterol,* by Kenneth Cooper. Bantam Books, NY, 1988.
5. *Cooking Light—Cooking Guide/Menus/Recipes,* by Susan McIntosh. Southern Living, Oxmoor House, Inc., Birmingham, Alabama, 1983.
6. *Cooking Light: The Magazine of Food and Fitness.* P.O. Box C–549, Birmingham, Alabama 35201.
7. *Deliciously Low—The Gourmet Guide to Low-Sodium, Low-Fat, Low-Cholesterol, Low-Sugar Cooking,* by Harriet Roth. The New American Library, NY, 1983.
8. *Dietitian's Food Favorites—A Cookbook from the American Dietetic Association Foundation,* featuring recipes for health and good taste. Cahners Publishing Co., Des Plaines, IL, 1985.
9. *Fit or Fat Target Recipes,* by Covert Bailey and Lea Bishop. Houghton Mifflin Co., Boston, MA, 1985.
10. *Good Food Book, Living the High Carbohydrate Way,* by Jane Brody. Bantam Books, NY, 1987.
11. *Heart Smart, A Plan for Low-Cholesterol Living,* by Gail Becker. Simon and Schuster, Inc., NY, 1987.
12. *Opening the Door to Good Nutrition, Tips for Health Eating, Grocery Shopping, Cooking, and Putting It All Together!,* by Marion Franz, Betsy Hedding, and Gayle Leitch. International Diabetes Center, Park Nicollet Medical Foundation, Minneapolis, MN, 1985.
13. *The Dieter's Cookbook.* Better Homes and Gardens, Meredith Corporation, Des Moines, Iowa, 1982.
14. *The Fit or Fat Target Diet,* by Covert Bailey. Houghton Mifflin Co., Boston, 1984.
15. *The Greens Cook Book,* by Deborah Madison with Edward Espe Brown. Bantam Books, New York, NY, 1987.
16. *The Laurel's Kitchen Bread Book,* by Laurel Robertson, Carol Flinders, Bronwen Godfrey. Random House, New York, NY, 1984.
17. *The New American Diet,* by Sonja and William Connor. Simon and Schuster, New York, NY, 1986.
18. *The New Laurel's Kitchen,* by Laurel Robertson, Carol Flinders, Brian Ruppenthal. Ten Speed Press, Berkeley, CA, 1986.
19. *Tofu Cookery,* by Louise Hagler. The Book Publishing Co., Summertown, TN, 1982.
20. *Vegetarian Soup Cookbook,* by Janice Migliaccio. Woodbridge Press, Santa Barbara, CA, 1983.
21. *Whole Grains—Grow, Harvest, and Cook Your Own,* by Sara Pitzer. Garden Way Publishing, Charlotte, VT, 1981.
22. The following books can be ordered from: Center for Science in the Public Interest 1501 6th St., NW Washington, D.C. 20036
   A. *Creative Food Experiences for Children,* by Mary Goodwin and Gerry Pollen.
   B. *Eater's Choice: A Food Lover's Guide to Lower Cholesterol,* by Ron and Nancy Goor.
   C. *Fast-Food: An Eater's Guide,* by Michael Jacobson and Sara Fritschner.
   D. *Fast Vegetarian Feasts,* by Martha Rose Shulman.
   E. *Salt: The Brand Name Guide to Sodium Content,* by Michael Jacobson, Bonnie Liebman, and Greg Moyer.
   F. *The Complete Eater's Digest and Nutrition Scoreboard,* by Michael Jacobson.

A P P E N D I X

G

Dietary Guidelines for Americans

What should Americans eat to stay healthy?

These guidelines help answer this question. They are advice for healthy Americans ages 2 years and over—not for younger children and infants, whose dietary needs differ. The guidelines reflect recommendations of nutrition authorities who agree that enough is known about diet's effect on health to encourage certain dietary practices by Americans (see page 499).

Many American diets have too many calories and too much fat (especially saturated fat), cholesterol, and sodium. They also have too little complex carbohydrates and fiber. Such diets are one cause of America's high rates of obesity and of certain diseases—heart disease, high blood pressure, stroke, diabetes, and some forms of cancer. The exact role of diet in some of these is still being studied.

Diseases caused by vitamin and mineral deficiencies are rare in this country. But some people do not get recommended amounts of a few nutrients, especially calcium and iron.

Food alone cannot make you healthy. Good health also depends on your heredity, your environment, and the health care you get. Your lifestyle is also important to your health—how much you exercise and whether you smoke, drink alcoholic beverages to excess, or abuse drugs, for example. But a diet based on these guidelines can help you keep healthy and may improve your health.

The first two guidelines form the framework for the diet: "Eat a variety of foods" for the nutrients you need and for energy (calories) to "Maintain healthy weight." The next two guidelines stress the need for many Americans to change their diets to be lower in fat, especially saturated fat, and higher in complex carbohydrates and fiber. Other guidelines suggest only moderate use of sugars, salt, and, if used at all, alcoholic beverages.

These guidelines call for moderation—avoiding extremes in diet. Both eating too much and eating too little can be harmful. Also, be cautious of diets based on the belief that a food or supplement alone can cure or prevent disease.

Your good health may depend on your learning more about yourself. Are you at your healthy weight? Are your blood pressure and your blood cholesterol levels too high? If so, diet or medicine your doctor prescribes may help reduce them. Generally, the sooner a problem is found, the easier it is to treat.

The foods Americans have to choose from are varied, plentiful, and safe to eat. These guidelines can help you choose a diet that is both healthful and enjoyable.

Read on for more about each guideline—what it means, how it is important to health, brief "advice for today," and some tips on using the guideline. See page 500 for how to get more help.

Eat a Variety of Foods

You need more than 40 different nutrients for good health. Essential nutrients include vitamins, minerals, amino acids from protein, certain fatty acids from fat, and sources of calories (protein, carbohydrates, and fat).

These nutrients should come from a variety of foods, not from a few highly fortified foods or supplements. Any food that supplies

Source: USDA's Food Guide (see pages 496–97).

calories and nutrients can be part of a nutritious diet. The content of the total diet over a day or more is what counts.

Many foods are good sources of several nutrients. For example, vegetables and fruits are important for vitamins A and C, folic acid, minerals, and fiber. Breads and cereals supply B vitamins, iron, and protein; whole-grain types are also good sources of fiber. Milk provides protein, B vitamins, vitamins A and D, calcium, and phosphorus. Meat, poultry, and fish provide protein, B vitamins, iron, and zinc.

No single food can supply all nutrients in the amounts you need. For example, milk supplies calcium but little iron; meat supplies iron but little calcium. To have a nutritious diet, you must eat a variety of foods.

One way to assure variety—and with it, an enjoyable and nutritious diet—is to choose foods each day from five major food groups (see box). Individuals who do not eat foods from one or more of the food groups may want to contact a dietitian for help in planning how to meet nutritional needs.

People who are inactive or are trying to lose weight may eat little food. They need to take special care to choose lower calorie, nutrient-rich foods from the five major food groups. They also need to eat less of foods high in calories and low in essential nutrients, such as fats and oils, sugars, and alcoholic beverages.

Diets of some groups of people are notably low in some nutrients. Many women and adolescent girls need to eat more calcium-rich foods, such as milk and milk products, to get the calcium they need for healthy bones throughout life. Young children, teenage girls, and women of childbearing age must take care to eat enough iron-rich foods such as lean meats; dry beans; and whole-grain and iron-enriched breads, cereals, and other grain products.

Supplements of some nutrients taken regularly in large amounts can be harmful. Vitamin and mineral supplements at or below the Recommended Dietary Allowances (RDA) are safe, but are rarely needed if you eat a variety of foods. Here are exceptions in which your doctor may recommend a supplement:

Pregnant women often need an iron supplement. Some other women in their childbearing years may also need an iron supplement to help replace iron lost in menstrual bleeding.

Certain women who are pregnant or breastfeeding may need a supplement to meet their increased requirements for some nutrients.

People who are unable to be active and eat little food may need supplements.

People, especially older people, who take medicines that interact with nutrients may need supplements.

Advice for today: Get the many nutrients your body needs by choosing different foods you enjoy eating from these five groups daily: vegetables, fruits, grain products, milk and milk products, and meats and meat alternatives.

Maintain Healthy Weight

If you are too fat or too thin, your chances of developing health problems are increased.

Being too fat is common in the United States. It is linked with high blood pressure, heart disease, stroke, the most common type of diabetes, certain cancers, and other types of illness.

Being too thin is a less common problem. It occurs with anorexia nervosa and is linked with osteoporosis in women and greater risk of early death in both women and men.

Whether your weight is "healthy" depends on how much of your weight is fat, where in your body the fat is located, and whether you have weight-related medical problems, such as high blood pressure, or a family history of such problems.

What is a healthy weight for you? There is no exact answer right now. Researchers are trying to develop more precise ways to describe healthy weight. In the meantime, you can use the guidelines suggested below to help judge if your weight is healthy.

See if your weight is within the range suggested in the table for persons of your age and height. The table shows higher weights for people 35 years and above than for younger adults. This is because recent research suggests that people can be a little heavier as they grow older without added risk to health. Just how much heavier is not yet clear. The weight ranges given in the table are likely to change based on research under way.

Ranges of weights are given in the table because people of the same height may have equal amounts of body fat but differ in muscle and bone. The higher weights in the ranges are suggested for people with more muscle and bone.

Weights above the range are believed to be unhealthy for most people. Weights slightly below the range may be healthy for some small-boned people but are sometimes linked to health problems, especially if sudden weight loss has occurred.

Research also suggests that, for adults, body shape as well as weight is important to health. Excess fat in the abdomen is believed to be of greater health risk than that in the hips and thighs. There are several ways to check body shape. Some require the help of a doctor; others you can do yourself.

TABLE
Suggested Weights for Adults

Height[1]	Weight in pounds[2]	
	19 to 34 years	35 years and over
5'0"	[3]97–128	108–138
5'1"	101–132	111–143
5'2"	104–137	115–148
5'3"	107–141	119–152
5'4"	111–146	122–157
5'5"	114–150	126–162
5'6"	118–155	130–167
5'7"	121–160	134–172
5'8"	125–164	138–178
5'9"	129–169	142–183
5'10"	132–174	146–188
5'11"	136–179	151–194
6'0"	140–184	155–199
6'1"	144–189	159–205
6'2"	148–195	164–210
6'3"	152–200	168–216
6'4"	156–205	173–222
6'5"	160–211	177–228
6'6"	164–216	182–234

[1]Without shoes.
[2]Without clothes.
[3]The higher weights in the ranges generally apply to men, who tend to have more muscle and bone; the lower weights more often apply to women, who have less muscle and bone.

Source: Derived from National Research Council, 1989 (see page 499).

A look at your profile in the mirror may be enough to make it clear that you have too much fat in the abdomen. Or you can check your body shape this way:

Measure around your waist near your navel while you stand relaxed, not pulling in your stomach.

Measure around your hips, over the buttocks, where they are largest.

Divide the waist measure by the hips measure to get your waist-to-hip ratio. Research in adults suggests that ratios close to or above one are linked with greater risk for several diseases. However, ratios have not been defined for all populations or age groups.

If your weight is within the range in the table, if your waist-to-hip ratio does not place you at risk, and if you have no medical problem for which your doctor advises you to gain or lose

To Increase Calorie Expenditure—be more physically active.		
Activity	**Calories expended per hour[1]**	
	Man[2]	**Woman[2]**
Sitting quietly	100	80
Standing quietly	120	95
Light activity:	300	240
Cleaning house		
Office work		
Playing baseball		
Playing golf		
Moderate activity:	460	370
Walking briskly (3.5 mph)		
Gardening		
Cycling (5.5 mph)		
Dancing		
Playing basketball		
Strenuous activity:	730	580
Jogging (9 min./mile)		
Playing football		
Swimming		
Very strenuous activity:	920	740
Running (7 min./mile)		
Racquetball		
Skiing		

[1]May vary depending on environmental conditions.
[2]Healthy man, 175 lbs; healthy woman, 140 lbs

Source: Derived from McArdle, et al., **Exercise Physiology,** 1986.

To Decrease Calorie Intake—

Eat a variety of foods that is low in calories and high in nutrients:

- Eat less fat and fatty foods.
- Eat more fruits, vegetables, and breads and cereals—without fats and sugars added in preparation and at the table.
- Eat less sugars and sweets.
- Drink little or no alcoholic beverages.

Eat smaller portions; limit second helpings.

weight, there appears to be no health advantage to changing your weight. If you do not meet all of these conditions, or if you are not sure, you may want to talk to your doctor about how your weight might affect your health and what you should do about it.

Heredity plays a role in body size and shape as do exercise and what you eat. Some people seem to be able to eat more than others and still maintain a good body size and shape.

No one plan for losing weight is best for everyone. If you are not physically active, regular exercise may help you lose weight and keep if off. See the table above for the calories expended in some activities. If you eat too much, decreasing your calorie intake as advised in the following box may help. However, getting enough of some nutrients is difficult in diets of 1,200 calories or less. Long-term success usually depends upon new and better lifelong habits of both exercise and eating.

Do not try to lose weight too fast. A steady loss of ½ to 1 pound a week until you reach your goal is generally safe. Avoid crash weight-loss diets that severely restrict the variety of foods or the calories you can have.

Avoid other extreme approaches to losing weight. These include inducing vomiting and using medications such as laxatives, amphetamines, and diuretics. Such approaches are not appropriate for losing weight and can be dangerous.

You probably do not need to try to lose weight if your weight is already below the suggested range in the table and if you are otherwise healthy. If you lose weight suddenly or for unknown reasons, see a doctor. Unexplained weight loss may be an early clue to a health problem.

Children need calories to grow and develop normally; weight-reducing diets are usually not recommended for them. Overweight children may need special help in choosing physical activities they enjoy and nutritious diets with adequate but not excessive calories.

Advice for today: Check to see if you are at a healthy weight. If not, set reasonable weight goals and try for long-term success through better habits of eating and exercise. Have children's heights and weights checked regularly by a doctor.

Choose a Diet Low in Fat, Saturated Fat, and Cholesterol

Most health authorities recommend an American diet with less fat, saturated fat, and cholesterol. Populations like ours with diets high in fat have more obesity and certain types of cancer.

The higher levels of saturated fat and cholesterol in our diets are linked to our increased risk for heart disease.

A diet low in fat makes it easier for you to include the variety of foods you need for nutrients without exceeding your calorie needs because fat contains over twice the calories of an equal amount of carbohydrates or protein.

A diet low in saturated fat and cholesterol can help maintain a desirable level of blood cholesterol. For adults this level is below 200 mg/dl. As blood cholesterol increases above this level, greater risk for heart disease occurs. Risk can also be increased by high blood pressure, cigarette smoking, diabetes, a family history of premature heart disease, obesity, and being a male.

The way diet affects blood cholesterol varies among individuals. However, blood cholesterol does increase in most people when they eat a diet high in saturated fat and cholesterol and excessive in calories. Of these, dietary saturated fat has the greatest effect; dietary cholesterol has less.

Suggested goals for fats in American diets are as follows:

Total fat. An amount that provides 30 percent or less of calories is suggested. Thus, the upper limit on the grams of fat in your diet depends on the calories you need. For example, at 2,000 calories per day, your suggested upper limit is 600 calories from fat (2,000 × .30). This is equal to 67 grams of fat (600 ÷ 9, the number of calories each gram of fat provides). The grams of fat in some foods are shown in the box.

Saturated fat. An amount that provides less than 10 percent of calories (less than 22 grams at 2,000 calories per day) is suggested. All fats contain both saturated and unsaturated fat (fatty acids). The fats in animal products are the main sources of saturated fat in most diets, with tropical oils (coconut, palm kernel, and palm oils) and hydrogenated fats providing smaller amounts.

Cholesterol. Animal products are the source of all dietary cholesterol. Eating less fat from animal sources will help lower cholesterol as well as total fat and saturated fat in your diet.

These goals for fats are not for children under 2 years, who have special dietary needs. As children begin to eat with the family, usually at about 2 years of age or older, they should be

---

For a Diet Low in Fat, Saturated Fat, and Cholesterol

Fats and Oils
- Use fats and oils sparingly in cooking.
- Use small amounts of salad dressings and spreads, such as butter, margarine, and mayonnaise. One tablespoon of most of these spreads provides 10 to 11 grams of fat.
- Choose liquid vegetable oils most often because they are lower in saturated fat.
- Check labels on foods to see how much fat and saturated fat are in a serving.

Meat, Poultry, Fish, Dry Beans, and Eggs
- Have two or three servings, with a daily total of about 6 ounces. Three ounces of cooked lean beef or chicken without skin—the size of a deck of cards—provides about 6 grams of fat
- Trim fat from meat; take skin off poultry.
- Have cooked dry beans and peas instead of meat occasionally.
- Moderate the use of egg yolks and organ meats.

Milk and Milk Products
- Have two or three servings daily. (Count as a serving: 1 cup of milk or yogurt or about 1½ ounces of cheese.)
- Choose skim or lowfat milk and fat-free or lowfat yogurt and cheese most of the time. One cup of skim milk has only a trace of fat, 1 cup of 2-percent-fat milk has 5 grams of fat, and 1 cup of whole milk has 8 grams of fat.

---

encouraged to choose diets that are lower in fat and saturated fat and that provide the calories and nutrients they need for normal growth. Older children and adults with established food habits may need to change their diets gradually toward the goals.

These goals for fats apply to the diet over several days, not to a single meal or food. Some foods that contain fat, saturated fat, and cholesterol, such as meats, milk, cheese, and eggs, also contain high-quality protein and are our best sources of certain vitamins and minerals. Lowfat choices of these foods are lean meat and lowfat milk and cheeses.

Advice for today: Have your blood cholesterol level checked, preferably by a doctor. If it is high, follow the doctor's advice about diet and, if necessary, medication. If it is at the desirable level, help keep it that way with a diet low in fat, saturated fat, and cholesterol: Eat plenty of vegetables, fruits, and grain products; choose lean meats, fish, poultry without skin, and lowfat dairy products most of the time; and use fats and oils sparingly.

Choose a Diet with Plenty of Vegetables, Fruits, and Grain Products

This guideline recommends that adults eat at least three servings of vegetables and two servings of fruits daily. It recommends at least six servings of grain products, such as breads, cereals, pasta, and rice, with an emphasis on whole grains. (See box above for what to count as a serving.) Children should also be encouraged to eat plenty of these foods.

Vegetables, fruits, and grain products are important parts of the varied diet discussed in the first guideline. They are emphasized in this guideline especially for their complex carbohydrates, dietary fiber, and other food components linked to good health.

These foods are generally low in fats. By choosing the suggested amounts of them, you are likely to increase carbohydrates and decrease fats in your diet, as health authorities suggest. You will also get more dietary fiber.

Complex carbohydrates, such as starches, are in breads, cereals, pasta, rice, dry beans and peas, and other vegetables, such as potatoes and corn. Dietary fiber—a part of plant foods—is in whole-grain breads and cereals, dry beans and peas, vegetables, and fruits. It is best to eat a variety of these fiber-rich foods because they differ in the kinds of fiber they contain.

Eating foods with fiber is important for proper bowel function and can reduce symptoms of chronic constipation, diverticular disease, and hemorrhoids. Populations like ours with diets low in dietary fiber and complex carbohydrates and high in fat, especially saturated fat, tend to have more heart disease, obesity, and some cancers. Just how dietary fiber is involved is not yet clear.

Some of the benefit from a higher fiber diet may be from the food that provides the fiber, not from fiber alone. For this reason, it's best to get fiber from foods rather than from supplements. In addition, excessive use of fiber supplements is associated with greater risk for intestinal problems and lower absorption of some minerals.

Advice for today: Eat more vegetables, including dry beans and peas; fruits; and breads, cereals, pasta, and rice. Increase your fiber intake by eating more of a variety of foods that contain fiber naturally.

Use Sugars Only in Moderation

Americans eat sugars in many forms (see box on page 498). Sugars provide calories and most people like their taste. Some serve as natural preservatives, thickeners, and baking aids in foods. This guideline cautions about eating sugars in large amounts and about frequent snacks of foods containing sugars and starches.

What is Meant By "Sugars"?

table sugar (sucrose)	honey
brown sugar	syrup
raw sugar	corn sweetner
glucose (dextrose)	high-fructose corn syrup
fructose	molasses
maltose	fruit juice concentrate
lactose	

Read food labels. A food is likely to be high in sugars if its ingredient list shows one of the above first or second or if it shows several of them.

For Healthier Teeth and Gums—

- Moderate the use of foods containing sugars and starches between meals.
- Brush and floss teeth regularly.
- Use a fluoride toothpaste.
- Ask your dentist or doctor about the need for supplemental fluoride, especially for children.
- Do not use a nursing bottle with any beverage other than water as a pacifier.

Sugars and many foods that contain them in large amounts supply calories but are limited in nutrients. Thus, they should be used in moderation by most healthy people and sparingly by people with low calorie needs. For very active people with high calorie needs, sugars can be an additional source of calories.

Both sugars and starches—which break down into sugars—can contribute to tooth decay. Sugars and starches are in many foods that also supply nutrients—milk; fruits; some vegetables; and breads, cereals, and other foods with sugars and starches as ingredients. The more often these foods—even small amounts—are eaten and the longer they are in the mouth before teeth are brushed, the greater the risk for tooth decay. Thus, eating such foods as frequent between-meal snacks may be more harmful to teeth than having them at meals.

Regular daily brushing with a fluoride toothpaste helps reduce tooth decay by getting fluoride to the teeth. Fluoridated water or other sources of fluoride that a doctor or dentist suggests are especially important for children whose unerupted teeth are forming and growing.

Diets high in sugars have not been shown to cause diabetes. The most common type of diabetes occurs in overweight adults, and avoiding sugars alone will not correct overweight.

Advice for today: Use sugars in moderate amounts—sparingly if your calorie needs are low. Avoid excessive snacking and brush and floss your teeth regularly.

Use Salt and Sodium Only in Moderation

Table salt contains sodium and chloride—both are essential in the diet. However, most Americans eat more salt and sodium than they need. Food and beverages containing salt provide most of the sodium in our diets, much of it added during processing and manufacturing.

In populations with diets low in salt, high blood pressure is less common than in populations with diets high in salt. Other factors that affect blood pressure are heredity, obesity, and excessive drinking of alcoholic beverages.

In the United States, about one in three adults has high blood pressure. If these people restrict their salt and sodium, usually their blood pressure will fall.

Some people who do not have high blood pressure may reduce their risk of getting it by eating a diet with less salt and other sources of sodium. At present there is no way to predict who might develop high blood pressure and who will benefit from reducing dietary salt and sodium. However, it is wise for most people to eat less salt and sodium because they need much less than they eat and reduction will benefit those people whose blood pressure rises with salt intake.

Advice for today: Have your blood pressure checked. If it is high, consult a doctor about diet and medication. If it is normal, help keep it that way: maintain a healthy weight, exercise regularly, and try to use less salt and sodium. (Normal blood pressure for adults: systolic less than 140 mmHg and diastolic less than 85 mmHg.)

If You Drink Alcoholic Beverages, Do So in Moderation

Alcoholic beverages supply calories but little or no nutrients. Drinking them has no net health benefit, is linked with many health problems, is the cause of many accidents, and can lead to addiction. Their consumption is not recommended. If adults elect to drink alcoholic beverages, they should consume them in moderate amounts (see box that follows).

Some people should **not** drink alcoholic beverages:

Women who are pregnant or trying to conceive. Major birth defects have been attributed to heavy drinking by the mother while pregnant. Women who are pregnant or trying to conceive should not drink alcoholic beverages. However, there is no conclusive evidence that an occasional drink is harmful.

Individuals who plan to drive or engage in other activities that require attention or skill. Most people retain some alcohol in the blood 3 to 5 hours after even moderate drinking.

Individuals using medicines, even over-the-counter kinds. Alcohol may affect the benefits or toxicity of medicines. Also, some medicines may increase blood alcohol levels or increase alcohol's adverse effect on the brain.

Individuals who cannot keep their drinking moderate. This is a special concern for recovering alcoholics and people whose family members have alcohol problems.

Children and adolescents. Use of alcoholic beverages by children and adolescents involves risks to health and other serious problems.

Heavy drinkers are often malnourished because of low food intake and poor absorption of nutrients by the body. Too much alcohol may cause cirrhosis of the liver, inflammation of the pancreas, damage to the brain and heart, and increased risk for many cancers.

Some studies have suggested that moderate drinking is linked to lower risk for heart attacks. However, drinking is also linked to higher risk for high blood pressure and hemorrhagic stroke.

Advice for today; If you drink alcoholic beverages, do so in moderation; and don't drive.

Some of the scientific basis for these guidelines:

The Surgeon General's Report on Nutrition and Health. 1988. Public Health Service, U.S. Department of Health and Human Services.

Diet and Health: Implications for Reducing Chronic Disease Risk. 1989. National Research Council, National Academy of Sciences.

Recommended Dietary Allowances, 10th Ed. 1989. National Research Council, National Academy of Sciences.

Information on how to put the guidelines into practice:

Contact the Human Nutrition Information Service, USDA, Room 325–A, 6505 Belcrest Road, Hyattsville, MD 20782, for how to order:
The USDA Food Guide in "Preparing Foods and Planning Menus Using the Dietary Guidelines." HG–232–8, 1989.
"Dietary Guidelines and Your Diet." HG–232–1 through –11, 1986 and 1989. Bulletins on eating right the Dietary Guidelines way.
"Nutritive Value of Foods," HG–72. 1985.

Contact the National Institutes of Health, Room 10 A 24, Building 31, Bethesda, MD 20892, for this and other bulletins: "Eating for Life." NIH Publication No. 88–3000, 1988.
Contact your county extension home economist (Cooperative Extension System) or a nutrition professional in your local Public Health Department, hospital, American Red Cross, dietetic association, diabetes association, heart association, or cancer society.

Acknowledgments: The U.S Department of Agriculture and the U.S. Department of Health and Human Services acknowledge the recommendations of the Dietary Guidelines Advisory Committee—the basis for this edition. The Committee consisted of Malden C. Nesheim, Ph.D. (chairman); Lewis A. Barness, M.D.; Peggy R. Borum, Ph.D.; C. Wayne Callaway, M.D.; John C. LaRosa, M.D.; Charles S. Lieber, M.D.; John A. Milner, Ph.D.; Rebecca M. Mullis, Ph.D., and Barbara O. Schneeman, Ph.D.

H

Chemistry

In order to better understand nutrition, it helps to review concepts in both biology and chemistry. This appendix begins with a look at cell structure, function, and control. It is in the cell that all nutrients are metabolized. Most of the structures and nutrients that are found in the cell are made of organic molecules. The discussion on the chemical composition of the body will take a look at these organic molecules and investigate the reason for their chemical behavior.

The Cell and Control Systems

Under the ordinary light microscope, the cell seems so simple that it is at first difficult to realize the cell is a living entity. However, the cell is far more than an individual living system. Within this structure is the blueprint to organize a complex tissue, an organ, and even a human being. Obviously, cells must be different in shape, structure, and function to create the diversity of tissue that we find in the human body. Although all cells are different, similar characteristics allow us to take a look at the generalized cell structure.

Cell Membrane

The cell membrane holds the contents of the cell together in a compact package. It also controls what enters and leaves the cell and transmits messages from the external environment into the cell so that the cell can appropriately respond. Since the cell membrane is surrounded by a watery medium on the inside and outside, it could not also be made of a water-soluble substance and be effective. Therefore, the cell

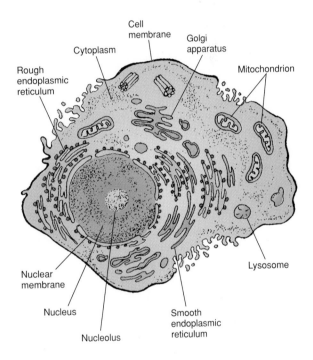

membrane and all the membranes that surround organelles, the structures in the cell, are composed primarily of phospholipids.

Phospholipids are bipolar molecules with a phosphate end and a lipid end. The phosphate (polar) ends extend out toward the aqueous environment on each side of the membrane, whereas the hydrophobic (nonpolar) parts remain together in the middle on the cell membrane. This results in a double layer of phospholipids in the cell membrane. This hydrophobic core tends to restrict the passage of some water-soluble molecules, water, and ions.

Some of the specialized functions of the membrane and its ability to selectively transport molecules is thought to be due to its protein content. Proteins are submerged on each side of the membrane. These proteins found in the cell membrane serve a variety of functions, which include structural support, transport of molecules across the membrane, enzymatic control of reactions, receptors for hormones and other regulatory substances, and recognition markers.

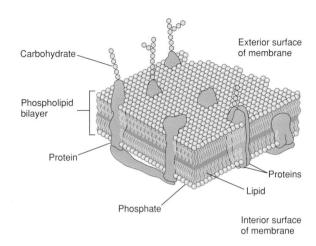

Cytoplasm

Cytoplasm is the jellylike matrix within a cell that provides support for organelles. It is a highly organized structure in which protein fibers are arranged in a latticework.

Nucleus

The nucleus is the control center of the cell and is responsible for its management. Most cells in the body have one nucleus. The nucleus is surrounded by a nuclear membrane that is composed of an inner and outer membrane. These two membranes fuse together at periodic points to form nuclear pores which allow ribonucleic acid (RNA) to leave the nucleus and enter the cytoplasm.

Deoxyribonucleic acid (DNA), the genetic material controlling heredity, is housed in the nucleus. The master plan for all cellular activity is transcribed from DNA to RNA. This messenger RNA leaves the nucleus through the nuclear pores and joins the ribosomes, the organelle where protein synthesis takes place. In the ribosome the messenger RNA is translated into a protein by transfer RNA. Clearly, this is an example of the complexity of the cell's function and the interdependency among components.

Endoplasmic Reticulum

Most cells contain a system of interconnected membrane-forming canals and tubules known as the endoplasmic reticulum. These provide a supporting framework within the cytoplasm. There are two types of endoplasmic reticulum: rough and smooth. The rough endoplasmic reticulum contains ribosomes on its surface and participates in protein synthesis and transport. The smooth endoplasmic reticulum plays a variety of roles in cells. It contains enzymes that inactivate drugs and alcohol, and others that synthesize lipids.

Golgi Apparatus

Proteins that are destined for secretion outside the cell or for incorporation into cellular membranes are transported to the Golgi apparatus. These are flattened sacs that enclose spaces. In the Golgi apparatus, proteins are modified and separated according to their function and destination. These proteins are modified and then released so that they will arrive at their appropriate destination.

Lysosomes

Lysosomes are membrane-enclosed organelles that contain digestive enzymes. These packages destroy old cellular molecules and organelles, as well as particles from outside the cell.

Mitochondria

Mitochondria produce energy for the cell by utilizing oxygen in the combustion of food molecules. They are often called the "powerhouse" of the cell.

These organelles and other structures cooperate to help the cells perform the many functions for which they are specialized. Clearly, from this brief discussion, we recognize that cells possess extraordinary attributes. They are highly organized and complex. In each cell, there is a division of labor among the components, and yet the components work together to perform specific functions. As cells specialize to form cardiac, muscle, liver, and other types of cells, the number and type of organelles a cell contains reflects its function. Last, and perhaps most amazing, most cells are capable of reproducing themselves.

A partial list of the endocrine glands and their hormones.

Endocrine Gland	Major Hormones	Primary Target Organs	Primary Effects
Adrenal cortex	Cortisol Aldosterone	Liver, muscles Kidneys	Glucose metabolism; Na^+ retention, K^+ excretion
Adrenal medulla	Epinephrine	Heart, bronchioles, blood vessels	Adrenergic stimulation
Hypothalamus	Releasing and inhibiting hormones	Anterior pituitary	Regulates secretion of anterior pituitary hormones
Intestine	Secretin and cholecystokinin	Stomach, liver, and pancreas	Inhibits gastric motility; stimulates bile and pancreatic juice secretion
Islets of Langerhans (pancreas)	Insulin Glucagon	Many organs Liver and adipose tissue	Insulin promotes cellular uptake of glucose and formation of glycogen and fat; glucagon stimulates hydrolysis of glycogen and fat
Ovaries	Estradiol-17β and progesterone	Female genital tract and mammary glands	Maintains structure of genital tract; promotes secondary sexual characteristics
Parathyroids	Parathyroid hormone	Bone, intestine, and kidneys	Increases Ca^{++} concentration in blood
Pineal	Melatonin	Hypothalamus and anterior pituitary	Affects secretion of gonadotrophic hormones
Pituitary, anterior	Trophic hormones	Endocrine glands and other organs	Stimulates growth and development of target organs; stimulates secretion of other hormones
Pituitary, posterior	Antidiuretic hormone Oxytocin	Kidneys, blood vessels Uterus, mammary glands	Antidiuretic hormone promotes water retention and vasoconstriction. Oxytocin stimulates contraction of uterus and mammary secretory units
Stomach	Gastrin	Stomach	Stimulates acid secretion
Testes	Testosterone	Prostate, seminal vesicles, other organs	Stimulates secondary sexual development
Thymus	Thymosin	Lymph nodes	Stimulates white blood cell production
Thyroid	Thyroxine (T_4) and triiodothyronine (T_3)	Most organs	Growth and development; stimulates basal rate of cell respiration (basal metabolic rate or BMR)

When cells combine to form tissues, organs, and systems they must be responsive to the external environment. What keeps the cell informed on how to direct its activity are messages from hormones and nervous tissue. The next two sections will examine how these messages affect the cell and how the cell responds to them.

The Endocrine System

Hormones are like a wireless system of communication for the body. They ensure that there is harmony in the goals of the cells, tissues, and organs so that the body functions optimally. Hormones are chemical messengers that are made in a variety of endocrine glands throughout the body. These messengers are released into the bloodstream to influence the behavior of their target cells.

Hormones are able to recognize their target cells by attaching to the appropriate receptor on the target cell membrane. Once the hormone has attached to the cell membrane, it transmits the message for the cell to act or perform differently. For instance, insulin is secreted from the pancreas and released in an inactive form into the bloodstream. When it reaches a target cell, it binds to the receptor on the cell membrane and is changed into the active form of insulin. The cell responds to the presence of insulin by increasing its uptake of glucose into the cell and by stimulating the metabolic pathway that lead to the storage of glucose as glycogen or fat.

The Nervous System

The nervous system is considered the primary communication system in the body. It can not only receive messages to assess the status of body cells and tissues, but the nervous system can also interpret information and respond by transmitting messages back to the body cells. The main control system that decides how to respond to messages is called the central nervous system. This consists of the brain and spinal cord. The "wiring" that transmits the messages throughout the body is known as the peripheral nervous system.

The two control systems, the endocrine and the nervous, coordinate their functionings to maintain homeostasis, a constant internal condition. Homeostasis involves tolerable fluctuations within the body that are compatible with survival. A well-understood example of this coordination is the body's response to stress. The stress response begins when the brain perceives a threat to the body's equilibrium. For instance, a dog charges out from behind a bush right in front of you. Immediately, the brain decides that this dog is protecting his yard and may bite. The brain signals the rest of the body to prepare to defend itself or run. This alarm signal is sent to various cells and organs through the nerves and hormones.

When the cells receive the alarm message, they cause the pupils to dilate, the muscles to tense, the blood glucose level to rise, the heart to beat faster, the blood pressure to rise, and so on. As the owner appears and takes hold of the dog's collar, the brain's perception of the situation changes. The response of the nervous system will rapidly return to normal, but although no further hormone will be released, the effects will still be felt for quite a while until the circulating hormones are inactivated.

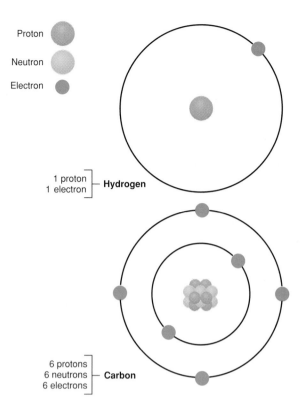

The Chemical Composition of the Body

Atoms, Elements, and Compounds

The complex structure and processes that occur in the cell and the body are based largely on the interaction of atoms, ions, and molecules. Although atoms are too small to be seen under a microscope, scientists have spent great effort to understand their structure. The nucleus of the atom contains two types of particles: protons, which have a positive charge, and neutrons, which are noncharged. Orbiting the positively charged nucleus are electrons, which are negatively charged particles.

The number of positively charged protons equals the number of negatively charged electrons so that the net charge of the atom is zero. The number of protons in an atom is called its atomic number. The protons and neutrons in the nucleus are of equal weight, and their sum gives the atom its atomic weight.

Electrons rotate around the nucleus of an atom in orbitals. The first orbital closest to the nucleus contains only two atoms. If an atom has more than two electrons, the additional electrons must be placed in orbitals further from the

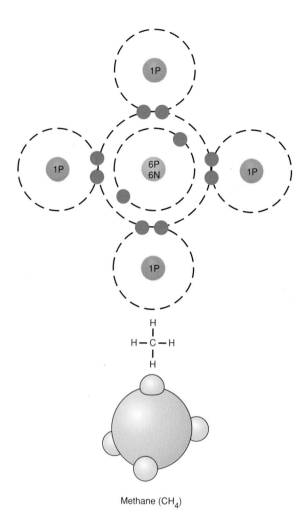

Methane (CH₄)

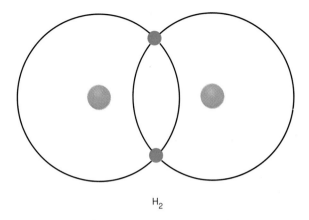

H_2

nucleus. All outer orbitals can contain as many as eight electrons each. The number of atoms in the outer shell determines the chemical behavior of an atom because they are the ones that participate in chemical bonding. Carbon is an atom with six electrons, two in the innermost orbital and four in the second orbital.

Atoms are stable when their outer orbital is full with eight electrons. This can be achieved by sharing their electrons in chemical bonding, or by gaining or losing electrons from their outer shell so that it will either be full or be empty. In the case of carbon, the four electrons in its outer shell could be shared with four hydrogen atoms that have one electron each. This would give the molecule stability because there would be eight electrons in the outer orbit and it would be full.

If a substance is composed of all the same atoms, it is considered an element. There are more than 100 elements, such as hydrogen, oxygen, carbon, iron, and nitrogen. Compounds are substances that are composed of two or more **different atoms or elements. Water (hydrogen and oxygen), and salt (sodium and chloride) are two examples of compounds.**

Chemical Bonds

Molecules are formed when two or more different atoms are joined together by the interaction of electrons in their outer orbits. This interaction is known as chemical bonding.

Covalent Bonds

Covalent bonds occur when electrons are shared between atoms. When the two atoms that join are identical, such as two hydrogen molecules, the electrons are shared equally. This is the strongest type of covalent bonding and is called nonpolar.

Many compounds are formed when two or more nonidentical atoms share their electrons. Water is a good example of this type of polar covalent bond. The oxygen atom in water pulls the electrons from the two hydrogen atoms closer to its side. This unequal sharing causes oxygen to be more electrically negative and the hydrogens to be more electrically positive. Water uses this polar nature to act as a solvent for the body.

Ionic Bonds

Ionic bonds are another type of chemical bond in which the electrons are not shared, but are actually transferred from one atom to another. Common table salt is a good example. Sodium, with eleven electrons, has two electrons in the first orbit, eight in the second, but only one in the outer orbit. This makes it very difficult for

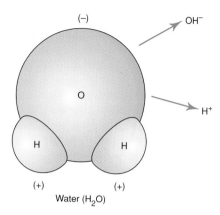

Water (H_2O)

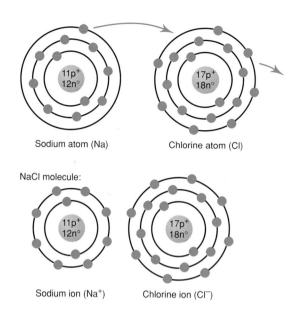

Sodium atom (Na)   Chlorine atom (Cl)

NaCl molecule:

Sodium ion (Na^+)   Chlorine ion (Cl^-)

sodium to share its electrons because it would need seven additional electrons. On the other hand, chlorine is one short of completing its outer orbit of eight. The electron from sodium is attracted to the outer orbit of chlorine. This creates a chlorine ion, a chlorine atom that is negatively charged with one extra electron. There is no additional proton in its nucleus that can neutralize the negative charge. Sodium being short one electron and still having the proton in the nucleus to balance it, becomes positively charged.

Ionic bonds are weak, and when a substance like salt is dissolved in water, they break apart into ions. The positively charged sodium ion and the negatively charged chloride ion are actually more water-soluble as they attract to the opposite charges that can be found in water. This is also true for polar covalent bonds. Molecules composed of mostly nonpolar covalent bonds with few charges cannot attract water molecules and are not soluble. Fat, with its long chains of hydrocarbons, are composed primarily of nonpolar covalent bonds and are therefore not water-soluble.

Hydrogen Bonds

Hydrogen bonds are weak bonds that form in substances like water. As hydrogen forms a polar covalent bond with oxygen, the oxygen pulls the electron closer to its nucleus. The hydrogen will then carry a slightly more positive charge. Since the hydrogen has a slight positive charge, it will have a weak attraction for another electronegative atom. This weak attraction is called a hydrogen bond. Water is held together in its liquid form by just such hydrogen bonds. This allows water to be poured in a stream from one container to another.

Acids, Bases, and the pH Scale

Occasionally, some of the strong polar covalent bonds in water break apart or dissociate. This occurs when one of the hydrogen atoms completely loses its electron to the oxygen atom. This results in the release of a hydrogen ion (H^+) and a hydroxyl ion (OH^-). Very few water molecules dissociate, but those that do produce equal amounts of H^+ and OH^-. The concentration of each in water would equal 10^{-7} molar. Molar is a unit of concentration. This solution would be neutral.

A solution that contains more H^+ ions than OH^- ions is called acidic, and a solution with less H^+ ions than OH^- ions is called basic. A molecule that releases H^+ ions into a solution is an acid. A base is a molecule that lowers the H^+ concentration of a solution. Most bases release OH^- into a solution. This combines with H^+ to form water and thus lowers the H^+ concentration of the solution.

The H^+ concentration of a solution is measured in pH units that range on a pH scale from zero to 14. Pure water has a pH of 7 (neutral), while acidic solutions will have a pH less than 7 and basic solutions will have a pH greater than 7.

Buffers are a system of molecules and ions that prevent changes in H^+ concentration and thus stabilize a solution. For instance, in the bloodstream the pH is stabilized by a reversible reaction involving the bicarbonate ion (HCO_3^-) and carbonic acid (H_2CO_3):

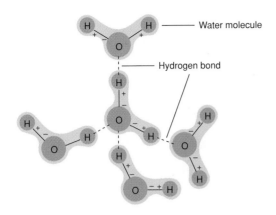

H —— Water molecule

Hydrogen bond

$$HCO_3^- + H^+ \rightleftharpoons H_2CO_3$$

The double arrows indicate that the reaction can go in either direction, depending on the concentration of ions and molecules on either side. For example, if lactic acid was released into the bloodstream it would push the reaction in the direction of the carbonic acid.

$$HCO_3^- + H^+ \rightarrow H_2CO_3$$

Conversely, if the concentration of H^+ is falling in the blood, the opposite reaction would occur.

$$HCO_3^- + H^+ \leftarrow H_2CO_3$$

Bicarbonate ions act to decrease pH while carbonic acid acts to increase pH in the bloodstream, an efficient buffering pair. This buffering system normally maintains the blood pH at a very stable 7.40 ± 0.05.

Organic Molecules

Organic molecules are those that contain the carbon atom. The carbon atom has four electrons in its outer orbit and must therefore share four electrons from another atom to stabilize. This unique bonding requirement allows carbon to bond to other carbons in chains and still allows room for other atoms to also bond to the same carbon. Since each carbon has four available sites for binding, two carbon atoms will bind together and still have room for six hydrogen atoms, three around each of the carbons.

The body is made up of many organic molecules, including carbohydrates, lipids, and proteins. In a carbon chain or ring, the carbon atoms may share one pair of electrons (a single covalent bond) or two pairs of electrons (a double covalent bond).

The hydrocarbon (carbons and hydrogens bonded) chain or ring of many organic

The pH scale		
	H⁺ Concentration (molar)	pH
Acids	1.0	0
	0.1	1
	0.01	2
	0.001	3
	0.0001	4
	10^{-5}	5
	10^{-6}	6
Neutral	10^{-7}	7
Bases	10^{-8}	8
	10^{-9}	9
	10^{-10}	10
	10^{-11}	11
	10^{-12}	12
	10^{-13}	13
	10^{-14}	14

From Stuart Ira Fox, *Human Physiology*, 3d ed. Copyright © 1990 Wm. C. Brown Publishers, Dubuque, Iowa. All Rights Reserved. Reprinted by permission.

molecules is largely unreactive. However, functional groups of oxygen, phosphorus, nitrogen, or sulfer are attached to the hydrocarbon chains and serve as functional groups. These functional groups are chemically reactive and provide the unique chemical properties of organic molecules. The nitrogen (amino group) in amino acids, for instance, is the functional group that makes protein uniquely different from fat or carbohydrate.

Biochemical Structures and Pathways of Important Nutrients

Although some of the biochemical structures for carbohydrates, lipids, and proteins have been pictured in chapters 5, 6, and 7, a more complete diagram listing is given in this appendix. In addition, biochemical structures for each of the important vitamins are depicted.

Following the diagrams of the carbohydrates, lipids, proteins, and vitamins, a summary of the major metabolic pathways is presented. Emphasis is placed on carbohydrate metabolism, with a general overview of acetyl-CoA metabolism. Acetyl-CoA is the confluence of the major metabolic pathways for nearly all carbohydrate and lipid molecules, as well as some amino acids.

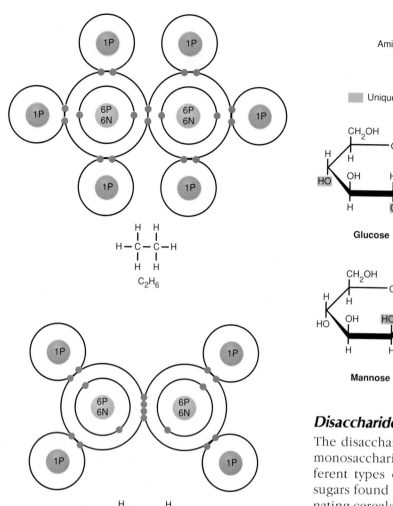

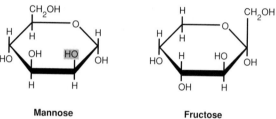

$$\text{Amino (NH}_2) - \overset{|}{\underset{|}{C}} - \overset{|}{\underset{|}{C}} - \overset{|}{\underset{|}{C}} - \overset{\overset{NH_2}{|}}{\underset{|}{C}} - \overset{|}{\underset{|}{C}} -$$

▨ Unique position of the "–OH" on carbon atoms.

Glucose

Galactose

Mannose

Fructose

$$H - \overset{\overset{\displaystyle H}{|}}{\underset{\underset{\displaystyle H}{|}}{C}} - \overset{\overset{\displaystyle H}{|}}{\underset{\underset{\displaystyle H}{|}}{C}} - H$$

C_2H_6

$$\overset{H}{\underset{H}{}} C = C \overset{H}{\underset{H}{}}$$

C_2H_4

Carbohydrates

Carbohydrates are widely distributed both in animal and plant foods. There are three basic classifications of carbohydrates: monosaccharides (cannot be broken down or hydrolyzed into simpler forms), disaccharides (yield two molecules of monosaccarides when hydrolyzed), and polysaccharides (yield more than six molecules of monosaccharides on hydrolysis). The Haworth structures for the various carbohydrates are pictured (D forms).

Monosaccharides

There are many different types of monosaccharides. Of the six carbon monosaccharides, the four most important are glucose, galactose, mannose, and fructose.

Disaccharides

The disaccharides are sugars composed of two monosaccharide molecules. There are many different types of disaccharides. Three common sugars found in foods are maltose (from germinating cereals and malt, or hydrolysis of starch), lactose (from milk), and sucrose (cane and beet sugar, or from many fruits and some vegetables).

Polysaccharides

Two important polysaccharides are starch and glycogen. Starch is formed of a long chain of glucose molecules, and is the most important food source of carbohydrate. Starch is found in cereals, potatoes, legumes, and vegetables. The two chief constituents of starch are amylose (15–20%), which is a nonbranching helical structure, and amylopectin (80–85%) which consists of branched chains. Glycogen is the storage polysaccharide found in animal tissue (animal starch). It is a more highly branched structure than amylopectin.

Protein: Amino Acids

Both animal and plant proteins are made up of 22 common amino acids. The proportion of these amino acids varies from protein to protein, but

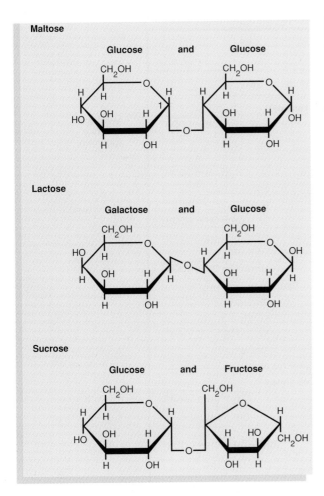

Maltose

Glucose   and   Glucose

Lactose

Galactose   and   Glucose

Sucrose

Glucose   and   Fructose

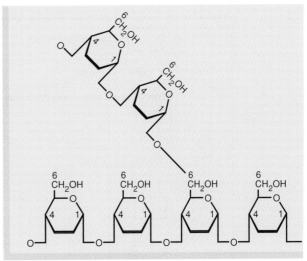

all food proteins (except for gelatin), contain some of each. Nine amino acids—histidine, isoleucine, leucine, lysine, methionine, phenylalanine, threonine, tryptophan, and valine—are not synthesized by humans and are therefore called "essential" because they must come from the diet. Histidine is an essential amino acid for infants, but was not shown to be required by adults until recently.

Amino acids have both an amino (NH_2) and a carboxylic acid (COOH) attached to the same carbon atom. It is convenient to subdivide the amino acids in proteins into seven classes as shown on pages 510–11. The essential amino acids are highlighted.

Lipids

Lipids, which are relatively insoluble in water, are important components of the diet. They have a high energy value and contain fat-soluble vitamins and the essential fatty acids. Dietary lipids

consist mainly of triglycerides, which are compounds of three fatty acids with a molecule of glycerol.

The chemical and physiological properties of lipids are in general related to the kind of fatty acids they contain. Fatty acids vary in the number of carbon atoms in the chain, and the number of double bonds in the carbon chain (or degree of unsaturation). Fatty acids can be classified into two types: saturated and unsaturated. Saturated fatty acids have no double bonds; unsaturated fatty acids contain one or more double bonds and are referred to as monounsaturated or polyunsaturated, respectively. The common names and composition of the more common fatty acids are shown in the chart on page 512.

The presence of a double bond in the fatty acid molecule gives rise to what are called "*cis*" and "*trans*" configurations. In the *cis*-form, the molecule is folded back on itself about each double bond; in the *trans*-form, the molecule is extended to maximum length (see p. 512). Most unsaturated fatty acids occur in the *cis*-form in nature. Fatty acids on the *trans*-form are found only in small amounts in natural fats but occur in large quantities after polyunsaturated fats are

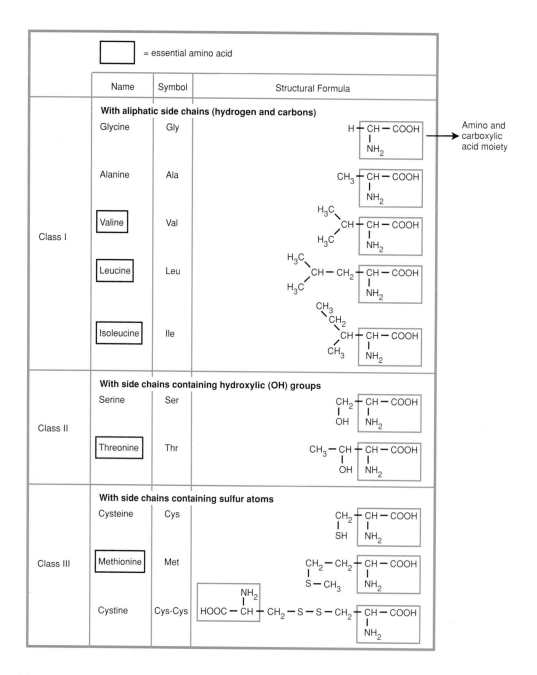

	Name	Symbol	Structural Formula

☐ = essential amino acid

With aliphatic side chains (hydrogen and carbons)

Class I

Glycine — Gly — $H-CH-COOH$, NH_2 → Amino and carboxylic acid moiety

Alanine — Ala — $CH_3-CH-COOH$, NH_2

Valine — Val — $(H_3C)_2CH-CH-COOH$, NH_2

Leucine — Leu — $(H_3C)_2CH-CH_2-CH-COOH$, NH_2

Isoleucine — Ile — $CH_3-CH_2-CH(CH_3)-CH-COOH$, NH_2

With side chains containing hydroxylic (OH) groups

Class II

Serine — Ser — $CH_2(OH)-CH-COOH$, NH_2

Threonine — Thr — $CH_3-CH(OH)-CH-COOH$, NH_2

With side chains containing sulfur atoms

Class III

Cysteine — Cys — $CH_2(SH)-CH-COOH$, NH_2

Methionine — Met — $CH_2-CH_2(S-CH_3)-CH-COOH$, NH_2

Cystine — Cys-Cys — $HOOC-CH(NH_2)-CH_2-S-S-CH_2-CH-COOH$, NH_2

hydrogenated (e.g., the manufacture of shortening and margarines). *Trans*-fatty acids behave like saturated fatty acids, tending to raise serum cholesterol levels.

Sterols, which are fat-soluble alcohols, are present in natural fats and in body tissue fats. Cholesterol is one of the most common naturally occurring sterols and is present in all animal foods. The structure of cholesterol is shown on page 512.

Vitamins

Water-Soluble Vitamins

The water-soluble vitamins have chemical structures that are remarkably varied, but they do share one common trait—they are all soluble in water. Of the water-soluble vitamins, all but one—cobalamin, or vitamin B_{12}—can be synthesized by plants. All of the water-soluble vitamins except vitamin C also serve as coenzymes or cofactors in reactions involving enzymes.

	With side chains containing acidic groups or their amides		
Class IV	Aspartic acid	Asp	$HOOC-CH_2-CH-COOH$ with NH_2
	Asparagine	Asn	$H_2N-\underset{\underset{O}{\|\|}}{C}-CH_2-CH-COOH$ with NH_2
	Glutamic acid	Glu	$HOOC-CH_2-CH_2-CH-COOH$ with NH_2
	Glutamine	Gln	$H_2N-\underset{\underset{O}{\|\|}}{C}-CH_2-CH_2-CH-COOH$ with NH_2
	With side chains containing basic groups		
Class V	Arginine	Arg	$H-N-CH_2-CH_2-CH_2-CH-COOH$ with $C=NH$, NH_2 and NH_2
	Lysine	Lys	$CH_2-CH_2-CH_2-CH_2-CH-COOH$ with NH_2 and NH_2
	Histidine	His	imidazole ring $-CH_2-CH-COOH$ with NH_2
	Ornithine	Orn	$CH_2-CH_2-CH_2-CH-COOH$ with NH_2 and NH_2
	Containing aromatic rings		
Class VI	Histidine (see above)		
	Phenylalanine	Phe	benzene ring $-CH_2-CH-COOH$ with NH_2
	Tyrosine	Tyr	$HO-$ benzene ring $-CH_2-CH-COOH$ with NH_2
	Tryptophan	Trp	indole ring $-CH_2-CH-COOH$ with NH_2
	Imino acids		
Class VII	Proline	Pro	pyrrolidine ring with $N-H$ and $COOH$

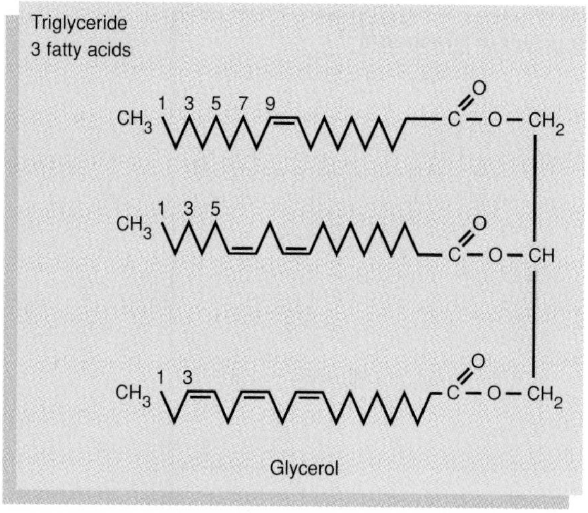

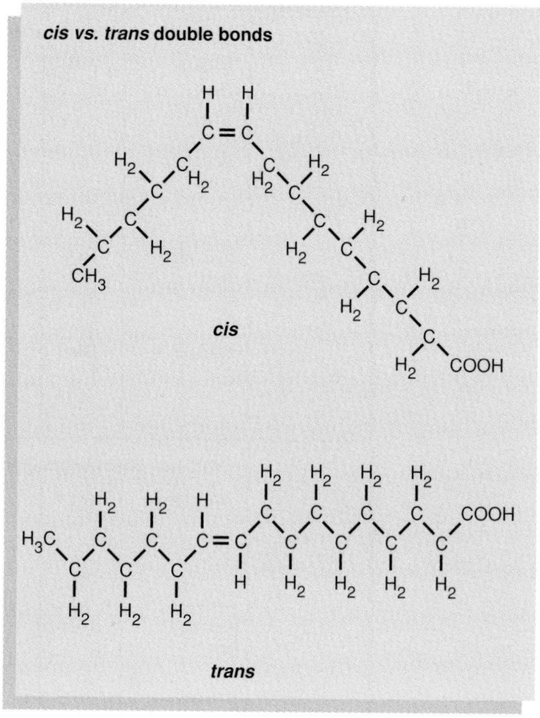

Triglyceride
3 fatty acids

CH_3 ... 1 3 5 7 9 ... C=O O—CH_2

CH_3 ... 1 3 5 ... C=O O—CH

CH_3 ... 1 3 ... C=O O—CH_2

Glycerol

Cholesterol

HO

cis vs. trans **double bonds**

cis

trans

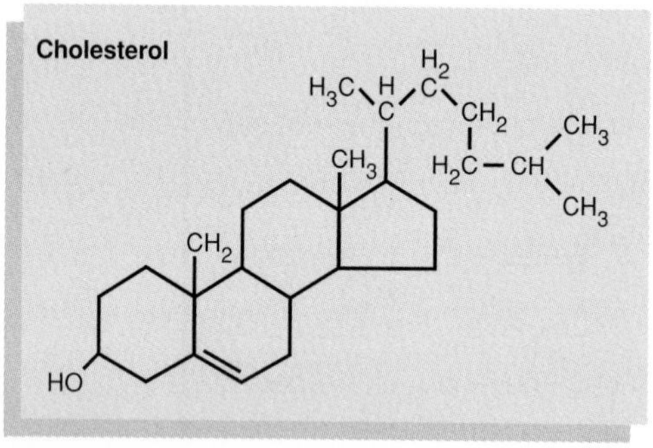

Common Name	Number of Carbon Atoms per Molecule	Number of Double Bonds per Molecule
Saturated fatty acids		
Butyric acid	4	0
Caproic acid	6	0
Caprylic acid	8	0
Capric acid	10	0
Lauric acid	12	0
Myristic acid	14	0
Palmitic acid	16	0
Stearic acid	18	0
Arachidic acid	20	0
Monounsaturated fatty acids		
Palmitoleic acid	16	1
Oleic acid	18	1
Elaidic acid	18	1
(*trans*-form of oleic acid)		
Polyunsaturated fatty acids		
Linoleic acid	18	2
Linolenic acid	18	3
Arachidonic acid	20	4
Eicosapentaenoic acid	20	5
Docosahexaenoic acid	22	6

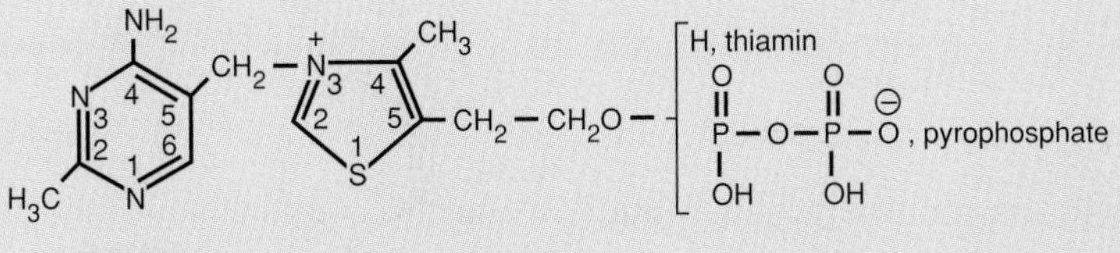

Thiamin

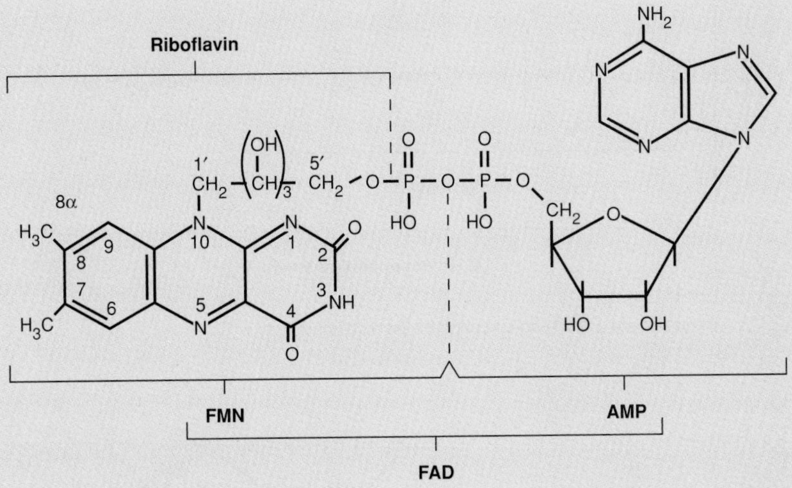

Riboflavin and FMN as components of FAD.

Niacin

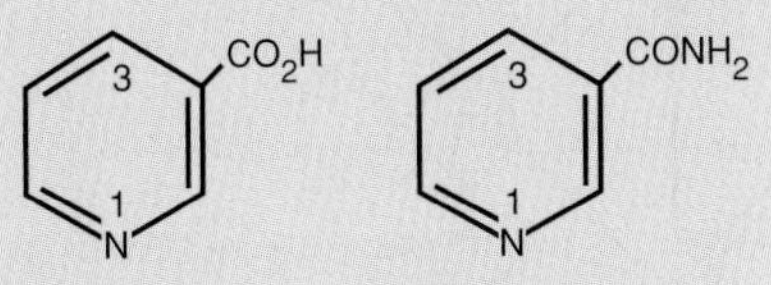

Nicotinic acid   Nicotinamide

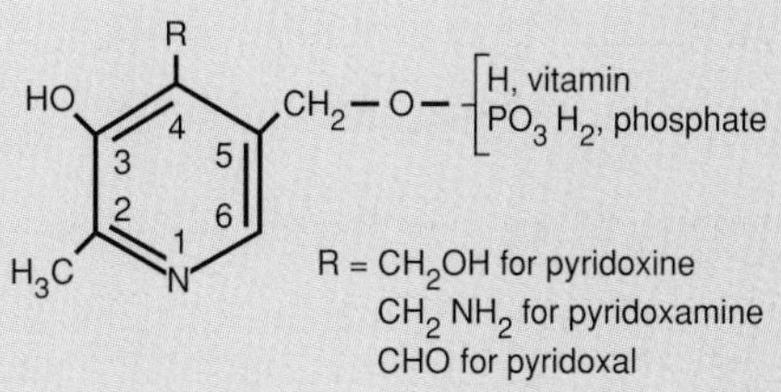

R = CH₂OH for pyridoxine
CH₂ NH₂ for pyridoxamine
CHO for pyridoxal

Free and phosphorylated forms of vitamin B₆.

Thiamin

Thiamin's active form is thiamin pyrophosphate, which serves as a coenzyme.

Riboflavin

Riboflavin is a component of what are called flavin nucleotides—flavin mononucleotide (FMN) and flavin adenine dinucleotide (FAD)—which serve as coenzymes.

Niacin

Niacin—nicotinic acid and nicotinamide—is a part of two coenyzmes.

Vitamin B₆

Vitamin B_6 consists of three closely related, naturally occurring molecules—pyridoxine, pyridoxal, and pyridoxamine.

Pantothenic Acid

Pantothenic acid is an amide of pantoic acid and β-alanine, and is an essential component of coenzyme A.

Pantothenate and 4'-phosphopantetheine as components of CoA.

Cyanocobalamin; vitamin B_{12}

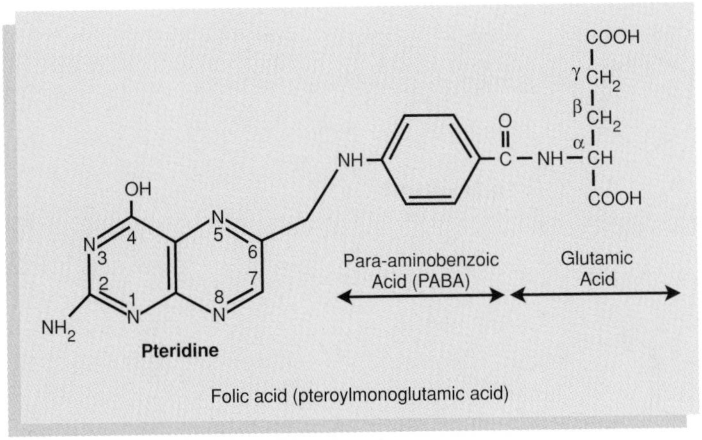

Folic acid (pteroylmonoglutamic acid)

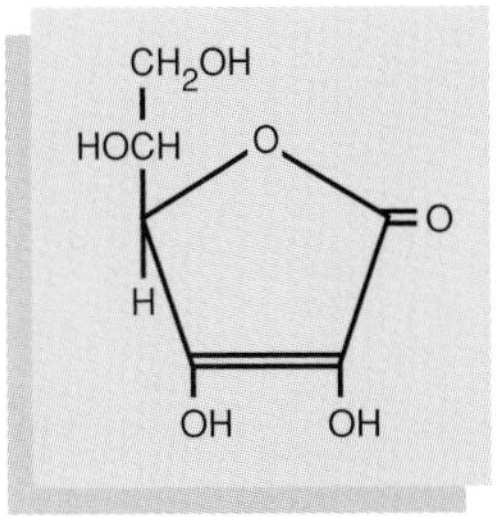

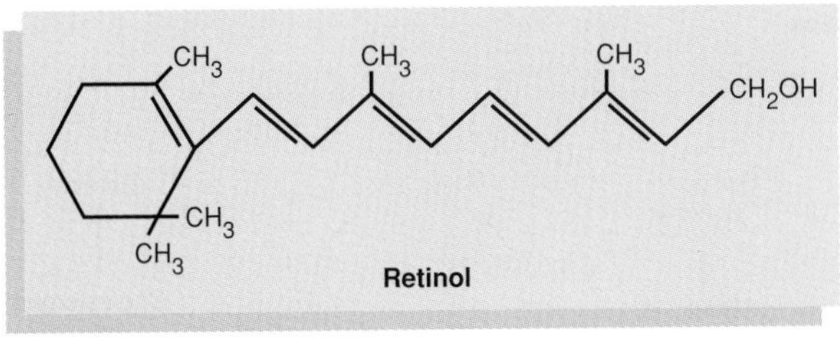

Retinol

Cholecalciferol

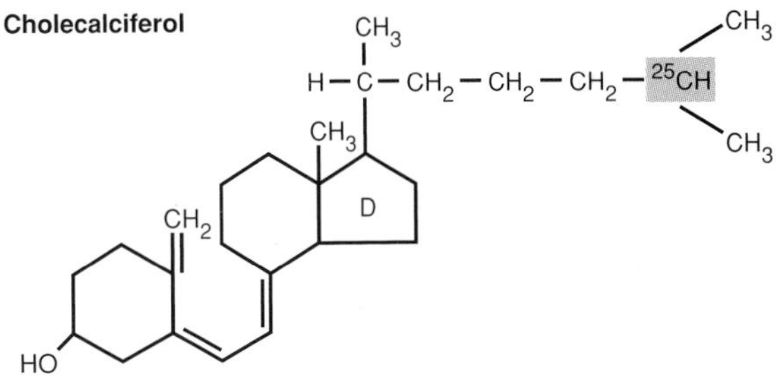

Biotin

Biotin is an imidazole derivative found in a wide variety of foods, and also supplied by intestinal bacteria. Biotin functions as a component of several enzymes.

Vitamin B₁₂

Vitamin B_{12} consists of a corrin ring that includes a cobalt ion at its center. There are several forms of vitamin B_{12}; cyanocobalamin depicted on page 514 is the most stable form.

Folate

Chemically, folate consists of pteridine, para-aminobenzoic acid (PABA), and glutamic acid.

Vitamin C

The structure of vitamin C resembles that of a monosaccharide, but contains an enediol group. (See figure at top right.)

Fat-Soluble Vitamins

The four fat-soluble vitamins—A, D, E, and K—are handled by the gastrointestinal system in the same manner as dietary fat. Thus the fat-soluble vitamins require normal fat absorption to be absorbed themselves.

Vitamin A

Vitamin A is a generic name for retinoids, a class of several types of compounds that exhibit the biologic activity of retinol, which is depicted above (left).

Vitamin D

Vitamin D is the term used as the generic descriptor of all steroids exhibiting the biologic activity of cholecalciferol, depicted above.

Vitamin E

Vitamin E is the generic term used for all tocol and tocotrienol derivatives exhibiting the biological activity of alpha-tocopherol, shown on page 516 (top).

Vitamin K

The term vitamin K is used as the generic descriptor for 2-methyl-1,4-naphthoquinone and all derivatives exhibiting the biological activity of phylloquinone shown on page 516 (middle).

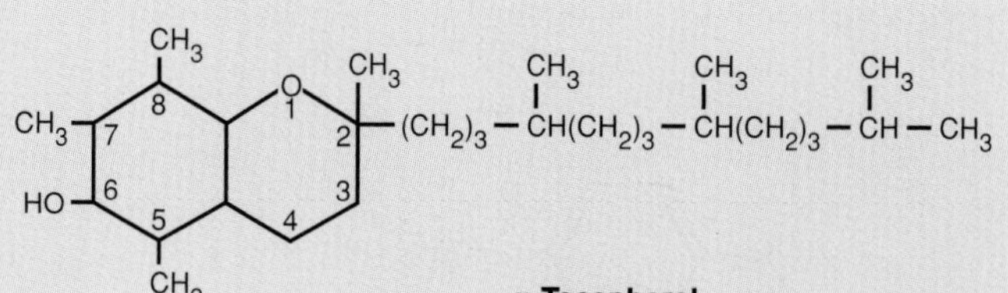

α-Tocopherol

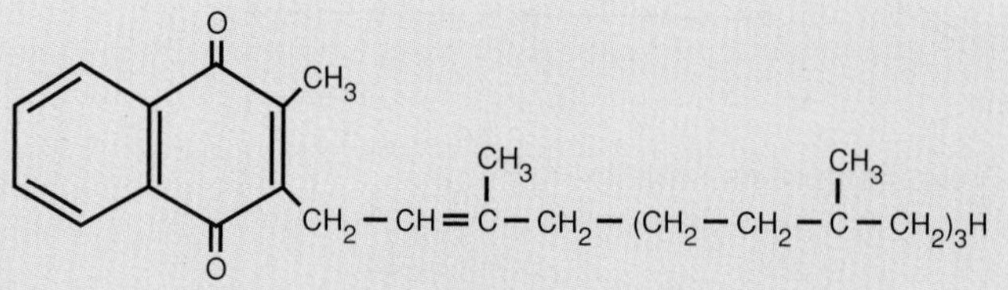

Phylloquinone

Biochemical Pathways

Acetyl-CoA Metabolism

Acetyl-CoA is at the hub of the major metabolic pathways. Nearly all carbohydrate and fat molecules form acetyl-CoA during their breakdown (or catabolism), as do many amino acids. The major function of the citric acid cycle is to act as the final common pathway for the oxidation of carbohydrate, lipids, and protein. Reducing equivalents in the form of hydrogen or electrons are formed during this oxidation, and then pass to the respiratory chain where large amounts of high-energy phosphates (ATP) are generated, supplying energy for the body. The enzymes of the citric acid cycle and the respiratory chain are found within the mitochondria, the power units of the cell.

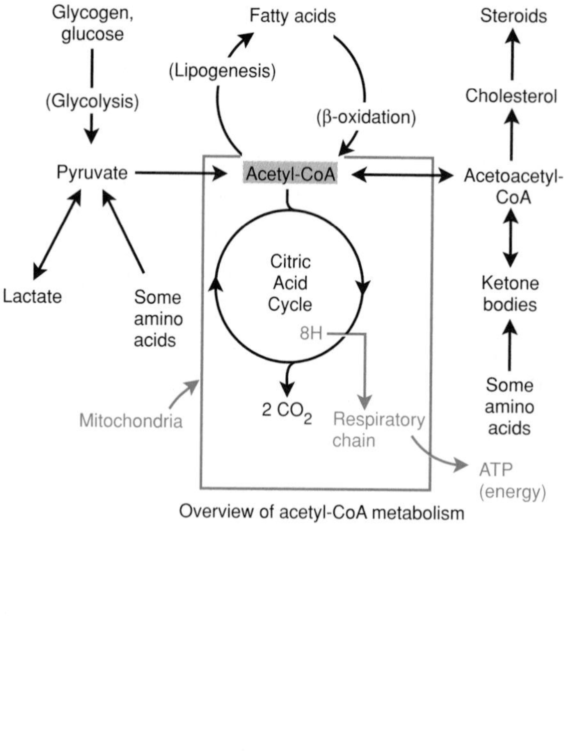

Overview of acetyl-CoA metabolism

Carbohydrate Metabolism

There are four major subdivisions of carbohydrate metabolism:

1. Glycolysis—the oxidation of glucose or glycogen to pyruvate and lactate.
2. Glycogenesis—the synthesis of glycogen from glucose.
3. Glycogenolysis—the breakdown of glycogen to glucose, and pyruvate and lactate.
4. Gluconeogenesis—the formation of glucose or glycogen from amino acids, lactate, and glycerol.

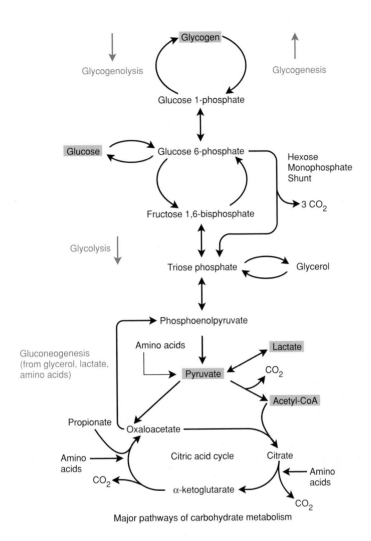

Major pathways of carbohydrate metabolism

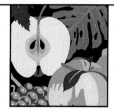

A

adipose tissue Fat tissue.

adolescence The period of life from the beginning of puberty (ages 13 to 15 for boys, 9 to 16 for girls) until maturity. The beginning of puberty and maturity is a gradual process and varies widely among individuals.

aerobic activities Physical activities that use large muscle groups in continuous exercise for long periods of times. These may include jogging, bicycling, aerobic dancing, and cross-country skiing.

aerobic glycolysis The conversion of glucose to pyruvate in preparation to enter Krebs cycle.

aerobic system A major metabolic pathway to produce energy from glucose, amino acids, and fatty acids. It involves both aerobic glycolysis, Krebs cycle, and electron transport system. Also called oxygen system.

alcoholism A chronic, progressive, and potentially fatal disease characterized by tolerance (brain adaptation to the presence of alcohol) and physical dependency (withdrawal symptoms occur when consumption of alcohol is decreased). Alcohol-related problems may include symptoms of alcohol dependence such as memory loss, inability to stop drinking until intoxicated, inability to cut down on drinking, binge drinking, and withdrawal symptoms.

allergic reaction A specific set of symptoms resulting from contact with a substance (antigen) to which the body has become sensitized (antibody). The result of the body initiating a defensive attack on a substance because the body believes that it is foreign and harmful.

amino acid An organic compound that makes up protein. Twenty amino acids are necessary for metabolism and growth, but only 11 are "essential" in that they must be obtained from food. Some proteins contain all the essential amino acids in the correct proportions and are called complete proteins. Examples are dairy products and animal products. Proteins that do not contain all the essential amino acids are called incomplete proteins (plant products).

amniotic fluid Fluid that surrounds the fetus in utero.

amphetamines Synthetic central nervous system stimulants, commonly called "uppers."

amylase An enzyme secreted by the salivary glands and the pancreas, and is responsible for breaking down long chains of glucose molecules in starches.

anaerobic The ability to live or function without oxygen. For example, some bacteria in the colon can break down dietary fiber without using oxygen. During exercise, energy for muscular activity can be produced by certain enzymes in the cell without the presence of oxygen.

anaerobic glycolysis *See* glycolysis.

anaerobic system *See* glycolysis.

anaphylactic shock The most dangerous type of allergic reaction, this can occur within minutes to hours after eating a food to which one is allergic. Symptoms include abdominal pain, nausea, a drop in blood pressure, chest pain, diarrhea, and shock. If untreated, death can occur.

anemia Severe iron deficiency or anemia is characterized by low levels of blood hemoglobin (a protein molecule in red blood cells that contains iron). Anemia is diagnosed when hemoglobin levels in the blood fall below 13 g/dL for men and below 12 g/dL for women.

anorexia nervosa An eating disorder characterized by an intense fear of becoming obese, even when underweight, with a disturbance in the way in which one's body weight, size, or shape is perceived. There is a refusal to maintain body weight over a minimal normal weight for age and height. With females, there is an absence of at least three consecutive menstrual cycles when otherwise expected to occur. This is called amenorrhea.

antibodies Proteins in the body that recognize and attack foreign proteins (bacteria, viruses) that enter the body.

anticoagulant A substance that prevents or delays blood clotting (coagulation).

antidiuretic hormone (ADH) A hormone secreted by the pituitary gland that signals the kidney to preserve water.

antimicrobial agents Substances that inhibit the growth of bacteria in food.

antioxidants The group of additives that retard rancidity (partial decomposition of fats) in foods.

atherosclerosis A type of blood-vessel disease characterized by buildup of lipid, calcium, and fibrous tissue deposits in the wall of the artery. As this plaque material grows, it can eventually close the blood vessel, leading to a coronary heart attack or a stroke.

adenosine triphosphate (ATP) The form of energy in the body that is available for immediate use.

B

basal metabolic rate (BMR) Represents the energy expended by the body to maintain normal body functions.

behavioral modification One of the most widely used treatments for obesity. Behavior modification considers in great detail the eating behavior to be changed, events that trigger the eating, and its consequences (feelings, procedures to provide rewards). The primary behavior to be changed is eating, and a number of exercises are designed to slow the rate of eating and allow body signals indicating satisfaction to exert their effect.

benzocaine A local anesthetic (partial or complete loss of sensation).

beriberi A disease caused by deficiency of thiamin in the diet, characterized by problems with nerves, the brain, and the heart and blood vessel system. Early symptoms include fatigue, irritation, poor memory, sleep disturbances, loss of appetite, and constipation.

bile Substance that is produced by the liver, stored in the gallbladder, and released into the intestine when foods containing fat are eaten. Bile acts as an emulsifier to assist in the absorption of lipid material. It is composed of cholesterol, lecithin, and bile salts.

binge eating Defined as the consumption of large quantities of rich foods within short periods of time.

biological value A measure of how well amino acids in a particular food are incorporated into new protein in the body.

biotin A vitamin widely present in many foods, especially vegetables, legumes, meats, whole grains, fruits, and milk. In addition to dietary sources, biotin is also produced in the intestines. Biotin is very active in many of the body's enzyme systems, especially those involving carbohydrate and fat metabolism. The symptoms of biotin deficiency include skin rash, fatigue, paleness, muscle pains, nausea, hair loss, and increased serum cholesterol.

body mass index (BMI) A ratio of body weight in kilograms divided by height in meters squared.

botulism The most serious type of foodborne bacterial poisoning, caused by toxins produced under anaerobic (no oxygen) conditions. Symptoms occur within 12 to 48 hours and include distress of the stomach and intestines, neurological problems, and paralysis of breathing leading to death. Prompt medical attention is essential.

bulimia Characterized by recurrent episodes of binge eating (at least two per week). During the eating binges there is a feeling of lack of control. The individual regularly engages in either self-induced vomiting, use of laxatives, or rigorous dieting or fasting in order to counteract the effects of the binge eating.

bulk producers These are dietary fiber substances that absorb liquid in the stomach, creating a feeling of fullness. The fibers absorb water, forming a high-fiber gel that produces a feeling of fullness to help switch off the hunger drive.

C

caffeine A chemical found in coffee, tea, and other foods. The brain is stimulated, and urination is increased.

caffeinism A condition caused by regular and excessive use of foods or drinks containing caffeine. Symptoms include flushing of the face, irregular and fast heartbeats, trembling, general depression and anxiety, inability to sleep, and nervousness.

calcium The most abundant mineral in the human body. Ninety-nine percent of body calcium is stored in the bones and skeleton. The Recommended Dietary Allowance (RDA) for adults has been set at 800 mg/day. The small amount of calcium outside the bones plays a vital role in nerve and muscle function. Calcium is also important for blood clotting, normal functioning of heart muscle cells, activation of certain enzymes and hormone secretion, and for the integrity of cell substances.

Calorie The amount of heat needed to change the temperature of one liter of water from $14.5°$ C to $15.5°$ C. Also called kilocalorie.

cancer A group of diseases in which abnormal cells grow out of control and can spread throughout the body. Normally, the cells of the body reproduce themselves in an orderly manner so that regular body functions can continue. Occasionally, certain cells undergo an abnormal change and begin a process of uncontrolled growth.

carbohydrate A group of chemical substances, including sugars and starches, that contain only carbon, oxygen, and hydrogen. Carbohydrate is one of these classes of nutrients (including fats and proteins), and are a basic source of energy.

carbohydrate loading A regimen to increase the amount of muscular carbohydrate (glycogen) stores. The recommended scheme utilizes a slow tapering of execise over a six-day period, with a 70 percent carbohydrate diet consumed during the last three days.

carcinogenic Capable of producing cancer.

carotene A yellow pigment found in various plants and animal tissues. It is abundant in yellow vegetables and is a precursor of vitamin A.

cellulite The term used to describe unsightly fat tissue that causes the overlying skin to appear dimpled like an orange peel. Most medical and nutrition authorities contend that cellulite is simply subcutaneous fat, packaged somewhat differently in normal connective tissue.

cerebrovascular accident A stroke.

chloride A negatively charged electrolyte. Sodium chloride or table salt is 60 percent chloride and 40 percent sodium.

cholecalciferol (vitamin D_3) Vitamin D_3 is a natural substance occurring in animal cells and formed by the action of sunlight on a cholesterol derivative in the skin. The activity of vitamin D_3 is actually similar to that of a hormone because it is formed in the skin and then travels through the blood to act on a target organ.

cholecystokinin (CCK) CCK is a hormone involved in digestion (especially of fat). CCK is sold by some companies for treatment of obesity, claiming that this substance will reduce hunger and cause sudden and dramatic weight loss. No CCK product has been approved by the FDA for public sale for any purpose.

cholesterol A sterol found in animal tissues, eggs, and dairy products. It can be made by the liver and is a normal part of bile.

chromium This mineral is believed to be important in maintaining normal blood glucose levels. The Food and Nutrition Board has estimated that the safe and adequate dietary intake is .05–0.20 mg per day. Peanuts, prunes, oils, various vegetables, whole-wheat bread, and chicken are good sources of chromium.

chylomicron The principle lipoproteins that are made in the intestinal wall. They deliver triglycerides that have recently been digested to the muscle, liver, or adipose tissue.

cobalt An essential nutrient for which no recommended dietary allowance has been established. Cobalt is an essential component of vitamin B_{12} (cobalamin). When vitamin B_{12} from animal foods is consumed, cobalt is also ingested. Although no vitamin B_{12} is found in plant foods, cobalt by itself is found in green leafy vegetables.

cocaine The major psychoactive ingredient extracted from the leaves of the coca plant; the most powerful central nervous system stimulant of natural origin.

copper This mineral is part of several important enzymes that are needed for proper utilization of iron and for the manufacture of hemoglobin and red blood cells in the bone marrow. The integrity of connective tissues, bones, nerves, the cardiovascular system, the immune system, and the blood clotting system are all in part dependent on copper. The estimated safe and adequate daily dietary intake is two to three mg. Seeds and nuts, seafood, dried fruits, legumes, and whole-grain cereals are good sources of copper.

crack A form of smokable cocaine; one of the most addictive substances ever known.

cruciferous vegetables Vegetables belonging to the mustard family, whose plants have flowers with four leaves in the pattern of a cross. These include cabbage, broccoli, Brussels sprouts, kohlrabi, and cauliflower. Some studies have suggested that consumption of these vegetables may reduce the risk of cancer, particularly of the gastrointestinal and respiratory tracts.

cytoplasm The fluid interior of a cell.

D

Daily Food Guides Foods can be grouped into major and minor food groups. In an attempt to translate nutritional information in easy-to-understand terms, the United States Department of Agriculture (USDA) has been publishing Daily Food Guides since 1917. The Daily Food Guide suggests food combinations that together supply nutrients in the amounts needed.

dehydration A condition resulting from excessive loss of body water (loss of body exceeds water intake).

deoxyribonucleic acid (DNA) Genetic material located in each cell's nucleus.

DHEA This unapproved drug (dehydroepiandrosterone or dehydroandrosterone) is derived from human urine and other sources. Manufacturers tout DHEA as a ''natural'' weight-loss product, but this has not been substantiated.

diabetes mellitus A group of disorders that have glucose intolerance (high serum levels of glucose) in common. There are two common types: Type I, insulin-dependent diabetes mellitus (IDDM); and Type II, non-insulin-dependent diabetes mellitus (NIDDM). IDDM can occur at any age, but especially in the young, and is characterized by an abrupt onset of symptoms and a need for insulin to sustain life. NIDDM is most common, usually occurring in people who are obese and over age 40.

dietary fiber Complex plant cell wall materials that cannot be digested by the enzymes in the human small intestine. Examples from plants include cellulose, hemicellulose, pectin, mucilages, and lignin.

Dietary Goals for the United States In February 1977, the U.S. Senate Select Committee on Nutrition and Human Needs issued the *Dietary Goals for the United States*. This was the first of several government reports setting prudent dietary guidelines for Americans as a reaction to the negative changes occurring in the U.S. diet. The committee submitted seven dietary goals, which included specific guidelines for improving the quality of the American diet.

Dietary Guidelines for Americans Guidelines promoted by the United States Department of Agriculture (USDA) to improve the quality of the American diet. The *1985 Dietary Guidelines for Americans* focused on seven guidelines.

dietary history One of several methods used to measure the diets of Americans. In this method, an individual, with the help of a trained nutritionist, fills out a form concerning the usual intake of different types of foods for a given period of time (usually the previous three months or year). The diet history interview reveals long-range dietary practices, and this is the major benefit of this technique.

dietary recall One of several methods used to measure the diets of Americans. In this method, food consumption for a specified period of time is recalled in as much detail as possible. The recall period may vary from one day to several weeks.

diet record One of several methods used to measure the diets of Americans. In this method, the individual records all foods and beverages consumed over a three- to seven-day period. Often the person carries a diet record throughout the day to record every mouthful consumed.

disaccharides A simple sugar that is the combination of two monosaccharides. Sucrose, lactose, and maltose are examples.

diuretics Various medications used for increasing urination and loss of body water. Diuretics are commonly used for controlling high blood pressure.

diverticulim Sacs or pouches in the wall of the colon. Inflammation can occur, causing pain and constipation. Some researchers have reported that a low-fiber diet increases the risk of these colon outpouchings.

E

Economic Research Service (ERS) The United States Department of Agriculture's ERS supplies ''food disappearance'' data (quantities of 350 foods that ''disappear'' into the food distribution system) to measure dietary trends by Americans.

edema The swelling of body tissues due to the accumulation of water outside the blood vessels.

elderly Individuals who reach or pass the age of 65. This group of Americans now represents the fastest-growing minority in the United States.

electrical muscle stimulators (EMS) EMS devices give a painless electrical stimulation to the muscle. Manufacturers claim that muscles are toned without exercise. Other benefits include facelifts without surgery, slimming and trimming, weight loss, bust development, spot reducing, and removal of cellulite. The Food and Drug Administration considers claims for EMS devices promoted for such purposes to be misbranded and fraudulent.

electrolyte Scientists call minerals like sodium, chloride, and potassium "electrolytes" because in water they can conduct electrical currents. Sodium and potassium ions carry positive charges, whereas chloride ions are negatively charged.

electron transport system An additional metabolic pathway from which the products of Krebs cycle enter and yield ATP. This cycle requires oxygen.

elimination diet A diet excluding foods suspected of causing food allergy.

embolus A blood clot that breaks loose and travels to smaller arterial vessels, where it may lodge and block the blood flow.

emulsifier Substances that have the property of mixing well with both fats and water. These may be used in the food industry to keep salad dressings from separating. Bile is an emulsifier.

enrichment The addition of nutrients to food, enriching the amount of vitamins or minerals normally found in the food.

enterotoxin A poison of the intestinal tract produced by foodborne bacteria.

enzyme Complex proteins that induce and accelerate the speed of chemical reactions without being changed themselves. Enzymes are present in digestive juices, where they act on food substances, causing them to break down into simpler molecules.

epinephrine A hormone primarily excreted from the adrenal medulla. This hormone is also called a catecholamine and is involved in many important body functions, including the elevation of blood glucose levels during exercise or stress.

epithelial tissue Those cells which form the outer surface of the body and line the body cavities (stomach and intestines), blood vessels, and ducts from glands.

ergocalciferol (vitamin D_2) Vitamin D occurs in two major forms, vitamin D_2 (ergocalciferol) and vitamin D_3 (cholecalciferol). Synthetic vitamin D_2 is formed when ergosterol found in plants is exposed to ultraviolet light.

essential amino acids Nine amino acids that cannot be manufactured by the body and must be included in the diet.

essential fatty acids Fatty acids that are not manufactured by the body. These include linolenic and linoleic acids.

estrogen replacement One of the mainstays of prevention and management of osteoporosis is estrogen replacement. Women who are past menopause and who are at high risk for osteoporosis are often given estrogen replacements by physicians, and it is highly effective.

ethyl alcohol (ethanol) Grain alcohol. Ethyl alcohol is a social drug that is called a "sedative-hypnotic" because of its dramatic effects on the brain. Ethanol (CH_3CH_2OH) is a small, water-soluble molecule that is absorbed rapidly and completely from the stomach and small intestine.

expiration date The last date often marked on the food package, indicating when the food can be safely consumed.

extracellular Outside of the body cell.

F

fats Fats serve as a source of energy. In food, the fat molecule is formed from one molecule of glycerol combined with three molecules of fatty acids. Fats have a high caloric value, yielding about nine Calories per gram, as compared with four Calories per gram for carbohydrate and proteins. Saturated fats have no double bonds, are generally hard at room temperature, and have been associated with increased risk of heart disease. Monounsaturated fats and polyunsaturated fats have one or two double bonds, respectively, are generally liquid at room temperature, and have been associated with decreased risk of heart disease.

fat cell theory One of the many theories explaining obesity. Fat cell number can increase two to three times normal if an individual ingests too many Calories. And once formed, the extra fat cells cannot be removed by the body. This can happen anytime during the life span of an individual but appears to be particularly important during infancy, when fat cells are still dividing.

fat-soluble vitamins One of two types of vitamins (water-soluble being the other). There are four fat-soluble vitamins: A, D, E, and K.

fetal alcohol syndrome (FAS) Heavy use of alcohol by pregnant women may result in FAS in their offspring. The effects of FAS may include growth retardation with decreased weight, height, and head circumference; impairment of intellectual and motor functions; and head abnormalities.

fluoride A mineral present in nearly all soils, water supplies, plants, and animals. However, because the concentration of fluoride varies considerably, drinking water is the most reliable and consistent source. Dental caries are reduced dramatically when fluoride is used regularly. The Food and Nutrition Board in 1980 estimated that the safe and adequate intake for adults is 1.5 to 4.0 mg per day, a range easily obtained in communities whose water supplies contain 1 mg per liter.

folate (folic acid) A water-soluble vitamin that is used to build a family of coenzymes that work closely with vitamin B_{12}. DNA and RNA synthesis, blood cell synthesis and maturation, and rapid cell division are vital functions dependent on folate and vitamin B_{12}. The RDA for folate for both men and women is 400 mcg.

food additives Any substance that becomes a part of a food product or that otherwise affects the characteristics of any food, directly, or indirectly through producing, processing, treating, packaging, transporting, or storing of food.

Food and Drug Administration (FDA)
An agency of the government that is responsible for the safety of our food and drug supply. Resource people in the FDA can help answer questions about food, drugs, medical devices, cosmetics, products that emit radiation, animal feed, regulatory requirements, sanitation standards, and good manufacturing practices. For answers to your questions, telephone or write to the Consumer Affairs Office located nearest you.

food challenge A method to measure which foods are causing food allergies. After implementing an elimination diet of suspected food allergens, if two to four weeks have passed without symptoms, suspected foods are added back to the diet one at a time to check for allergic reactions.

food composition tables Food composition tables give the average energy, protein, fat, carbohydrate, mineral, and vitamin content of a defined amount of food. Commonly used food consumption tables include the USDA Handbook No. 8, USDA Handbook No. 456, USDA Bulletin No. 72, and Food Values of Portions Commonly Used.

food disappearance studies The measure of approximately 350 foods that "disappear" into the civilian food distribution system. Sometimes referred to as the U.S. per capita food supply. The data are collected annually by the Economic Research Service of the United States Department of Agriculture (USDA). Although these figures are good for year-to-year comparisons, they tend to overestimate the actual food eaten by people.

food enhancers Substances that modify the taste of food without contributing a flavor of their own.

food exchange system Many weight-management programs and diabetic diet plans are based on the Exchange System because it makes the task of counting Calories much simpler. This system gives values that are averages of the nutrient values of the foods in a group, with more weight given to foods that are used more often.

food fortification Food is fortified when minerals and vitamins not normally found in the food are added by food manufacturers. For example, breakfast cereals are fortified with vitamin C, which is not normally found in cereal products.

food supplements Substances or pills that are added to the diet. Most reputable nutritionists state that vitamin or mineral supplementation is unwarranted for people eating a balanced diet.

Food Values of Portions Commonly Used A book containing food composition tables. Food items are listed by groups, for example, breads, cereals, and cereal products. In addition, the household measure, as well as the gram weights, is given and brand names are used for some items.

foodborne infections Illnesses caused by eating foods that are contaminated by large numbers of living organisms.

freshness date A date on the label of baked products that indicates the last day the product is considered fresh. After this date the product may taste stale.

G

genetic factors One of the several theories advanced to explain the high prevalence of obesity in Western countries. Some studies have demonstrated that certain people are more prone to obesity than others due to genetic factors. Such people have to be unusually careful in their dietary and exercise habits to counteract these inherited tendencies.

geophagia A condition in which a person eats inedible substances such as chalk, clay, earth, or laundry soap.

glucagon A hormone that is secreted by the pancreas and helps to raise blood glucose levels by stimulating the breakdown of liver glycogen.

glycogen Body stores of carbohydrate. Glycogen is often called "animal starch" because it is found in animal muscle and liver.

glycolysis A metabolic pathway that converts glucose to lactic acid (anaerobic glycolysis) to produce energy in the form of ATP, or to pyruvate (aerobic glycolysis) to be shuttled to the mitochondria for oxidation.

goiter An enlargement of the thyroid gland due to lack of iodine in the diet.

grapefruit pills For several decades, grapefruit has been promoted by various people as having special fat-burning properties. This myth has been spread far and wide. Grapefruit pills contain grapefruit extract, diuretics, and bulk-forming agents. Some contain phenylpropanolamine (PPA), along with herbs or other ingredients.

GRAS list A list of over 600 additives in common use before the Food, Drug, and Cosmetics Act of 1958. These additives were exempt from the requirement to prove they were harmless and were thus given the title of the "generally recognized as safe" list.

growth hormone A hormone released from the pituitary that elevates blood glucose. As its name indicates, this hormone also helps in the regulation of growth.

growth hormone releasers Various products that are sold with the claim that if they are taken before retiring, weight loss will occur overnight due to the increased release of growth hormone from the amino acids arginine and ornithine contained in the products. This is an erroneous concept.

H

half-life The time required by the body, organ, or tissue to metabolize or inactivate half the amount of a substance taken in.

health The World Health Organization has defined health as a state of complete physical, mental, and social well-being, and not merely the absence of disease.

health promotion The science and art of helping people change their life-style to move toward optimal health.

heartburn A feeling of pressure and burning in the chest due to a reflux of the acidic stomach contents into the esophagus.

heme iron Forty percent of the iron in animal products is called heme iron. The remaining 60 percent of the iron in animal products and all the iron in vegetable products are called nonheme iron. Heme iron is more easily absorbed by the body.

hemoglobin The iron-containing pigment of the red blood cells. Its function is to carry oxygen from the lungs to the tissues. Having low levels of hemoglobin is called anemia.

Herbalife International A company that sells items described as ''herbal-based'' health, nutrition, weight-control, and skin-care products, marketing them through a multilevel program.

heroin A semisynthetic, narcotic drug derived indirectly from a natural narcotic by modifying chemicals contained in opium.

high density lipoprotein cholesterol (HDL-C) Cholesterol is carried by the high density lipoprotein to the liver. The liver then uses the cholesterol to form bile acids, which are finally excreted in the stool. Thus, high levels of HDL-C have been associated with low cardiovascular disease risk.

high fructose corn syrup (HFCS) This is a special sugar that is commercially produced from cornstarch. Certain enzymes are used to convert the starch into fructose. The high fructose corn syrup (HFCS) can be used in slightly smaller amounts to produce the same sweetness as sugar, while costing less. Most soft-drink companies now use HFCS as the major sweetener in soft drinks.

homeostasis State of equilibrium of the internal environment of the body.

hormone A substance secreted from an organ or gland which is transported by the blood to another part of the body.

household consumption studies Some researchers go to the homes of Americans and measure what they are actually consuming. There are two large-scale national surveys of the food consumption of individuals. These are the Nationwide Food Consumption Survey (NFCS) conducted by the United States Department of Agriculture (USDA), and the National Health and Nutrition Examination Survey (NHANES), conducted by the United States Department of Health and Human Services (HHS).

hydrochloric acid A constituent of the gastric juice produced by glands in the wall of the stomach. It assists in the digestion of protein.

hydrogenation A process that breaks the double bond in an unsaturated fat in order to add hydrogen atoms. This creates a hydrogenated or saturated fat.

hyperactivity A cluster of symptoms that include a short attention span, impulsiveness, excitability, and general behavior problems in children.

hypercalcemia An excessive amount of calcium in the blood.

hypertension High blood pressure, defined as higher than 140/90 mm Hg.

hyperthermia High body temperature.

hypothalamus A portion of the brain located below the thalamus. Secretions from the hypothalamus are necessary in the control of important body functions, including the regulation of water balance, appetite, and body temperature.

I

immune system The human body has an amazing array of internal bodyguards called the immune system to counter the vast army of invisible enemies that continually besiege the system. Specialized white blood cells cleanse the lungs of foreign particles, rid the bloodstream of infectious bacteria and viruses, and destroy cancer cells.

insulin A hormone secreted by special cells (beta cells) in the pancreas. Insulin is essential for the maintenance of blood glucose levels.

insulin-dependent diabetes mellitus (IDDM) The form of diabetes mellitus in which the pancreas does not make or secrete insulin. The patient must use an external source of insulin to sustain life. This type of diabetes mellitus is also called Type I, or juvenile-onset diabetes.

international units (I.U.) An internationally accepted amount of a substance. Usually this is used for fat-soluble vitamins and some other substances, such as hormones and enzymes. Vitamin A is an example. The recommended dietary allowance (RDA) of vitamin A is now given in retinol equivalents (R.E.). Previously, vitamin-A content in foods was expressed in international units (I.U.). Both measurements for vitamin A are still widely found today in charts, graphs, and food labels. To convert, one retinol equivalent equals 3.33 I.U. of retinol, or 10 I.U. of carotene.

intracellular Inside the cell.

intrinsic factor (IF) A substance in the gastric digestive juices of humans that makes absorption of vitamin B_{12} possible. Absence of IF leads to vitamin B_{12} deficiency and pernicious anemia.

iodine Approximately three-fourths of the body's store of the mineral iodine is concentrated in the thyroid gland and is an important component of thyroid hormones. Iodine deficiency decreases production of thyroid hormones, resulting in weight gain, lack of energy, low blood pressure, slow resting heart rate, and decreased muscle strength. The RDA of iodine for adults is 0.15 mg/day. In many sections of the world, including parts of the U.S. formerly known as ''goiter belts,'' the amount of iodine in the water and land is too low. Before the modern era, when iodine was supplemented in table salt and other products, some people living in iodine-deficient areas developed simple goiter. Simple goiter is defined as an enlargement of the thyroid gland.

iron Iron is one of the major minerals and is an important component of hemoglobin, myoglobin (a muscle protein molecule that contains iron), and a number of enzymes. Iron deficiency is the most common single nutritional deficiency in the world today. The RDA for men and women is 10 mg/day and 18 mg/day, respectively. Lean meats, fish, and seafood are good sources of iron. Many plant foods such as molasses, fortified breakfast cereals, seeds and nuts, dried fruits, and legumes are also high in iron. There are two basic types of iron-deficiency states. Mild iron deficiency, or iron depletion, is characterized by low iron stores in the body. Severe iron deficiency, or anemia, is characterized by low blood hemoglobin.

K

keratin A tough protein substance in hair, nails, and horny tissues.

Keshan disease A disease state related to selenium deficiency, first noted in China. Some children living in a wide area across China have developed this fatal disease of the heart muscle. The disease can be reduced 80 percent by giving selenium to the children. Symptoms of Keshan disease included racing heart rates, large hearts, abnormal heart electrical patterns, and low blood selenium levels.

ketoacidosis A serious metabolic condition resulting from the buildup of ketones in the blood supply. Ketoacidosis results from the incomplete metabolism in fatty acids and is commonly observed in starvation, a high-fat diet, pregnancy, and untreated diabetics.

ketones Substances produced during the oxidation of fatty acids.

kilocalorie *See* Calorie.

Krebs cycle Final common metabolic pathway for fats, proteins, and carbohydrate that yields additional ATP. Carbon dioxide and water are produced.

kwashiorkor A disease resulting from a deficiency of protein in the presence of adequate Calories.

L

lactase An enzyme in the small intestine that splits the milk sugar called lactose into glucose and galactose. Deficiency of this enzyme results in lactose intolerance.

lactose The milk sugar, a disaccharide made up of glucose and galactose.

lactose intolerance Some people do not have sufficient amounts of the enzyme lactose to metabolize some or all of the lactose in food, resulting in bloating, cramping, gassiness, and diarrhea. This problem is common among American Indians, American Blacks, Asians/Orientals, and Mexican Americans.

lecithin A common phospholipid that may act as an emulsifier.

lead toxicity Occurs frequently in children who ingest lead by chewing on painted surfaces and in adults who are exposed to lead-containing substances and fumes. Symptoms include loss of appetite, nausea, vomiting, salivation, anemia, abdominal pains, muscle cramps, and pains in the joints.

lean body mass The nonfat tissue of the body, which includes muscle and other protein tissues, bone, and water.

life expectancy The average number of years of life expected in a population at a specific age, usually at birth.

life span The maximal obtainable age by a particular member of the species, which is primarily related to one's genetic makeup.

lipases Digestive enzymes produced in the pancreas and small intestine. They break down triglycerides into glycerol, fatty acids, and monoglycerides.

lipid A general term used for several different compounds, including both solid fats and liquid oils. There are three major classes of lipids: triglycerides, phospholipids, and sterols.

Lipid Research Center Program (LRCP) A study providing information on food and nutrient intake and blood lipid profiles of Americans. The LRCP is a program of the National Health, Lung, and Blood Institute (NHLBI) of the National Institutes of Health (NIH).

lipoprotein A soluble aggregate of cholesterol, phospholipids, triglycerides, and protein. This package allows for easy transport through the blood. There are four types of lipoproteins: chylomicrons, low density lipoprotein (LDL), very low density lipoprotein (VLDL), and high density lipoprotein (HDL).

low-birth-weight infant An infant who weighs less than 5.5 pounds at birth. This is associated with increased mortality during the first year of life.

low density lipoprotein (LDL) Transports cholesterol from the liver to other body cells. LDL is often referred to as "bad" cholesterol because it may be taken up by muscle cells in arteries, and it has been implicated in the development of atherosclerosis.

LSD Lysergic acid diethylamide. A hallucinogenic drug that causes changes in perception, thinking, emotions, and self-image.

M

magnesium One of the major minerals of the human body. Magnesium is required for more than 300 different enzyme systems of the body and is therefore involved in many important activities. In particular, magnesium is indispensable in the formation and use of high energy phosphate bonds (ATP). The use and storage of carbohydrate, fat, and protein in the body involves many reactions that are magnesium-dependent. It is also essential in nerve and muscle activity. The RDA for men and women is 350 and 300 mg/day, respectively. Magnesium-rich foods include seeds and nuts, whole-grain cereals, dark green vegetables, legumes, and dried fruits. Magnesium deficiency is very rare.

major minerals These are minerals needed in amounts greater than 100 mg/day and include calcium, phosphorus, magnesium, sodium, chloride, potassium, and sulfur. Three of these — sodium, chloride, and potassium — are also known as the three body electrolytes.

manganese The mineral manganese is a key part of a large number of enzyme systems. Manganese appears to be important for reproduction, skeletal development, and proper functioning of the brain and spinal cord. Humans need 2.5–5.0 mg/day, as estimated by the Food and Nutrition Board as the safe and adequate daily dietary intake. Nuts and seeds, whole grains, and various fruits and vegetables are good sources of manganese. Very little is present in animal products. Manganese deficiency is rare in humans.

marasmus A disease state caused by the lack of sufficient Calories, starvation.

marijuana A psychoactive drug; a prepared mixture of the crushed leaves, flowers, stems, and seeds of the hemp plant that is usually smoked.

megadoses Extremely high intakes of vitamins or minerals that may lead to health problems and toxicity.

megaloblastic anemia A type of anemia related to folate and vitamin B_{12} deficiency. Large, abnormal red blood cells are present in the blood.

micelle The package that contains the products of lipid digestion.

mild obesity Defined as being 20 to 40 percent overweight.

mineral Of the nearly 45 dietary nutrients known to be necessary for human life, 17 are minerals. Although mineral elements represent only a very small fraction of human body weight, they play very important roles throughout the body. They help form hard tissues such as bones and teeth, aid in normal muscle and nerve activity, act as catalysts in many enzyme systems, help control your body water levels, and are integral parts of organic compounds in the body, like hemoglobin and the hormone thyroxine. Evidence is growing that certain minerals are related to prevention of disease and proper immune-system function.

minor minerals These are trace elements needed in amounts no more than a few mg/day, and include iron, zinc, iodine, fluoride, copper, selenium, chromium, cobalt, manganese, and molybdenum. Of these, only three — iron, zinc, and iodine — have been studied sufficiently to establish required dietary amounts (RDA). For six of the other seven (all except cobalt), "safe and adequate" daily ranges have been estimated by the Food and Nutrition Board of the National Academy of Sciences.

mitochondria The slender filaments or rods inside of cells that are the source of energy. Enzymes important to producing energy from fat and carbohydrate are found inside the mitochondria.

moderate obesity Defined as being 40 to 100 percent overweight.

molybdenum A key part of the enzyme xanthine oxidase, which is needed by animals, humans, and many forms of plant life. Although deficiency can be produced in animals, molybdenum deficiency in humans has not been observed. The Food and Nutrition Board has estimated that the safe and adequate daily dietary intake of molybdenum is 0.14–0.50 mg for adults. Lean meats, legumes, whole grains, and various fruits and vegetables are good sources of molybdenum.

monosaccharides The simplest carbohydrate, containing only one molecule of sugar. Glucose, fructose, and galactose are the primary monosaccharides.

monounsaturated fatty acids *See* fats.

myocardial infarction A heart attack.

myoglobin A muscle protein molecule that contains iron. Myoglobin carries oxygen from the blood to the muscle cell.

N

National Health and Nutrition Examination Survey (NHANES) A periodic survey administered by the National Center for Health Statistics. These surveys provide a wealth of information about dietary patterns and practices of representative samples of the U.S. population.

Nationwide Food Consumption Survey (NFCS) A national food consumption survey administered by the United States Department of Agriculture (USDA). This periodic survey provides information about dietary patterns and practices of Americans.

net protein utilization A method to measure protein quality. Amino acid composition and digestibility of a particular protein are considered.

niacin Niacin is a vital part of coenzymes needed to release energy from carbohydrate, protein, and fat. Niacin is essential for growth, the production of energy in cells, and hormone synthesis. There are two ways to acquire niacin: by eating foods rich in niacin, such as lean meat, poultry, fish, nuts, whole grains, and enriched cereal products; and by consuming foods rich in tryptophan, an amino acid that can be converted into niacin. The RDA for niacin is 18 niacin equivalent (N.E.) and 13 N.E. for adult men and women, respectively. The disease pellagra results from a deficiency of niacin.

night blindness This problem occurs if there is insufficient vitamin A available to resupply the visual pigment, rhodopsin. In dimly lit settings (night driving, movie theaters, etc.), night vision is decreased.

nitrogen balance study A method to measure the utilization of protein in the body.

nitrosamines These are potential carcinogens resulting from metabolic reactions in the human digestive tract of nitrates, nitrites, and substances readily found in foods (especially processed or smoked meats, and nitrate salts used in food processing). Nitrates react with amines or amides in the digestive tract to form nitrosamines and nitrosamides, respectively. Vitamins C and E compete with the amine or amide for the nitrosating agent.

nonessential amino acids Thirteen amino acids that can be manufactured by the body if the nine essential amino acids are present in the diet.

nonheme iron Iron from plant foods, which is less available to the body.

non-insulin-dependent diabetes mellitus (NIDDM) *See* diabetes mellitus.

nutrient density An approach to evaluating the quality of diet in which nutrients are expressed on a per 1,000 Calories basis. Despite the sex or age of a person, nutrient requirements per 1,000 kcal are remarkably constant.

Nutrition Education and Training (NET) One of several government programs that use the RDA as their standard for education. This program complements the school lunch program in providing public school students with adequate nutrition knowledge.

O

obesity An excess of body fat.

Olestra A synthetic fat that is made from a combination of sucrose and fatty acids. It is not digestible.

omega-3-fatty acids A type of fat found in fish oils and associated with lower blood-cholesterol levels, lower blood pressure, and reduced blood clotting.

osmosis The passage of water through a membrane that separates solutions of different concentrations. The water passes through the membrane from the solution of lower concentration of solute to that of a higher concentration of solute, thus tending to equalize the concentrations of the two solutions.

osteomalacia The adult form of rickets in which the bones soften, causing deformities.

osteoporosis Defined as an age-related disorder, characterized by decreased bone mineral content and increased risk of fractures.

oxygen system *See* aerobic system.

P

pack date The day a product was manufactured.

pantothenic acid This vitamin is found throughout the body as part of an enzyme essential to fat, carbohydrate, and protein metabolism. Pantothenic acid deficiency is virtually unknown, except in combination with other B-vitamin deficiencies. Some researchers suggest that symptoms unique to pantothenic acid deficiency may include weakness, cramping, vomiting, insomnia, and a prickling numbness of the extremities, all of which quickly disappear when pantothenic acid intake is normalized. Pantothenic acid is in legumes, nuts, many vegetables, poultry, dried fruits, whole grains, yogurt, and many fresh fruits. The safe and adequate daily intake is 4 to 7 mg for adults.

PCP Phencyclidine. A unique, synthetic drug with stimulant, depressant, psychedelic, hallucinogenic, analgesic, and anaesthetic properties, all of which are dose-dependent.

pellagra A niacin deficiency disease resulting in skin eruptions, digestive and nervous system disturbances, and mental deterioration.

percentage of total Calories Nutritionists use this concept when representing the percentage of protein, carbohydrate, and fat Calories present in the diet. This is a useful skill to know and is calculated based on the fact that one gram each of carbohydrate, protein, and fat equals four Calories, four Calories, and nine Calories, respectively.

pernicious anemia This anemia is characterized by the release of large immature red blood cells from the bone marrow into the bloodstream. The symptoms include weakness, paleness, loss of appetite, shortness of breath, weight loss, depression, confusion, and unsteadiness. Inability to produce the intrinsic factor, which enables vitamin B_{12} absorption, is the cause of pernicious anemia in most instances.

phenylpropanolamine (PPA) This is the active ingredient in most nonprescription weight-control products. PPA is related to amphetamines and has similar side effects, such as nervousness, insomnia, headaches, nausea, tinnitus (ringing in the ears), and elevated blood pressure.

phospholipids Substances found in all body cells. They are similar to lipids but contain only two fatty acids and one phosphorus-containing substance.

phosphorus Phosphorus teams up with calcium in forming bones and teeth. Most of the body's phosphorus, 85 percent, is in the skeleton. Phosphate is involved in the metabolism of carbohydrate, lipids, and protein; helps to regulate the acid-base balance in the body; and functions as a cofactor in many enzyme systems. Phosphorus also enters into all of the high-energy systems that possess very high-energy phosphate bonds. The RDA for phosphorus is 800 mg/day and is found in many dairy products, cereals, and meats.

physical activity Any form of muscular movement.

pica Cravings for non-nutritive materials such as clay or starch.

platelets The clotting material in the blood.

polysaccharides These are known as "complex carbohydrate" because they are made up of many monosaccharides. They include starch and dietary fiber.

polyunsaturated fatty acids *See* fats.

potassium One of three minerals (along with sodium and chloride) that is called an electrolyte. No RDA for the three electrolytes has been established because all three are plentiful and widespread in the American diet. The Food and Nutrition Board has established a safe and adequate daily dietary intake for potassium as 1,875–5,625 mg. Potassium is found widely in fruits and vegetables and nuts. *See also* electrolyte.

pregnancy-induced hypertension A serious complication of pregnancy that is characterized by edema, high blood pressure, and kidney damage.

premenstrual syndrome A syndrome that can occur several days prior to the onset of menstruation. Symptoms include irritability, emotional tension, anxiety, mood changes, headache, breast tenderness, and water retention.

preservatives A group of additives that prevent food spoilage.

progesterone A hormone present in high levels to maintain pregnancy.

prostaglandins A group of hormonelike substances that seem to have a regulatory role in the body.

proteases Protein-digesting enzymes that are secreted into the small intestine.

protein A complex, nitrogen-carrying compound that occurs naturally in plants and animals and yields amino acids when broken down. The amino acids are essential for the growth and repair of living tissue. Proteins are also a source of heat and energy for the body. Protein is found widely in both animal and plant products.

protein Calorie malnutrition A disease state resulting from a deficiency of both Calories and protein.

protein efficiency ratio A method to measure protein quality. This standard looks at how well a particular protein supports growth.

prothrombin A chemical substance in the blood that, after interacting with calcium, produces thrombin, which is important in the clotting process.

puberty The period in life when one becomes functionally capable of reproduction.

pull or sell date The last date a product should be sold.

pyridoxine *See* vitamin B_6.

pyridoxal *See* vitamin B_6.

pyridoxamine *See* vitamin B_6.

Q

quinones There are several related forms of vitamin K known as quinones. Each form originates from a different source, such as alfalfa, fishmeal, and bacteria.

R

reactive hypoglycemia A condition in which abnormally low blood sugar results from an overproduction of insulin from the pancreas. Symptoms include sweating, hunger, weakness, anxiety, lack of ability to concentrate, and rapid and irregular heart beats.

Recommended Dietary Allowances (RDA) The RDA, established by the National Research Council of the National Academy of Sciences, have become the premier nutrient standard in both the U.S. and the world. The RDA are technical standards used for nutrition policies and decision making. The RDA today are used for a wide variety of purposes, ranging from development of new food products to being the standard for federal nutrition assistance programs.

refinement A process that extracts the starch or endosperm of grains, discarding the other cereal parts (the germ and bran).

resting metabolic rate (RMR) This represents the energy expended by the body to maintain life and normal body functions, such as respiration and circulation.

restoration The addition of nutrients to food to compensate for their losses during processing.

retinol Active, preformed vitamin A. The precursor form is called carotene, or provitamin A. Carotene, which is found in plant foods, converts to active vitamin A in the intestinal wall.

retinol equivalents (R.E.) The recommended dietary allowance (RDA) of vitamin A is now given in R.E. Previously, vitamin-A content in foods was expressed in international units (I.U.). Both measurements are widely found today in charts, graphs, and foods labels. To convert, one retinol equivalent equals 3.33 I.U. of retinol, or 10 I.U. of carotene. The adult RDA is 1,000 R.E. for men and 800 R.E. for women.

retinopathy Hemorrhage in the capillaries of the retina of the eye.

rhodopsin Visual purple, which is a pigment in the retina of the eye.

riboflavin This vitamin is a component of two vital coenzymes that help release energy from food. Tissue repair, cellular respiration, fatty acid oxidation, and amino acid breakdown are all dependent on riboflavin. Milk and milk products are the most abundant sources of riboflavin, providing almost half of daily needs. The RDA for men is 1.6 mg and for women is 1.2 mg. Tissue damage, growth failure, and eye problems occur when riboflavin is lacking in the diet. Skin inflammation near the nose and eyes, cracks on the lips and corners of the mouth, swelling of the tongue, eye strain, and headaches are among the symptoms reported. Riboflavin deficiency often accompanies other B-complex vitamin deficiencies.

rickets This disease is a deficiency condition in children that results in inadequate storage of calcium in the bones, causing bone structure abnormalities. The disease is due primarily to vitamin-D deficiency, which affects the absorption of calcium and phosphorus from the small intestine.

risk factors Characteristics that are associated with higher risk of developing a specific health problem.

S

satiety The feeling of fullness and satisfaction.

saturated fatty acids *See* fats.

scurvy This disease results from a deficiency of vitamin C. Symptoms include loss of energy; pains in legs, limbs, and joints; anemia; spongy and bleeding gums; and hemorrhage of small blood vessels in the skin and mucous membranes.

selenium Selenium is part of an important red blood cell enzyme called erythrocyte gluthathione perioxidase. This enzyme helps to destroy chemicals that damage cell membranes. For this reason, some researchers have shown that selenium may play a role in preventing cancer. The estimated safe and adequate daily dietary intake for selenium is 0.05–0.20 for adults. Seafood, nuts, dairy products, and whole-wheat products contain good amounts of selenium. In certain parts of the world where selenium is low in the soil and foods from other areas are not imported, a sickness called Keshan disease can occur.

senile dementia A form of organic brain syndrome; a mental disorder associated with impaired brain function in the elderly.

severe obesity More than 100 percent overweight.

Simplesse An artificial fat manufactured from protein.

smokeless tobacco Use of smokeless tobacco takes two forms. Dipping involves placing a pinch of moist or dry powdered tobacco (snuff) between the cheek or lip and the lower gum. Chewing involves placing a golfball-sized amount of loose leaf tobacco between the cheek and lower gum, where it is sucked and chewed.

sodium This electrolyte is the major cation (positive ion) of fluids outside the body cells. Sodium and chloride ions tend to concentrate outside of body cell walls (extracellular), whereas potassium tends to concentrate inside of body cell walls (intracellular). This arrangement is essential in maintaining the balance of tissue fluids inside and outside of cells. Sodium, potassium, and chloride work with bicarbonate in regulating the acid-base balance of the body. Sodium has an important role in regulating normal muscle tone. The Food and Nutrition Board has established safe and adequate daily dietary intakes for sodium, which is 1,100–3,300 mg.

spirulina This is a dark green powder or pill derived from algae that has been promoted as a weight-loss product.

standards of identity Based on the 1938 Federal Food, Drug, and Cosmetic Act, 200 separate foods are defined according to what ingredients they must contain. Foods that have standards of identity do not have to list their ingredients on the label.

starch A polysaccharide made up of glucose monosaccharides.

starch blockers This enzyme inhibitor is supposed to block the digestion and absorption of ingested carbohydrate. Several studies have now shown these not only to be ineffective, but also a possible risk to health.

sterols A type of lipid such as cholesterol, estrogen, testosterone, and vitamin D.

sugars Monosaccharides (glucose, fructose, galactose) and disaccharides (lactose, mannose, sucrose).

sulfites A group of sulfur-based substances that have widespread use in the food industry as preservatives and antioxidants.

supplementation Use of vitamin or mineral pills to supplement the regular diet.

sweeteners Caloric sugars (see sugars) and noncaloric sweetening agents (e.g., saccharin) that provide sweetness to the diet.

systolic blood pressure The pressure of the blood upon the walls of the blood vessels when the heart is contracting. A normal systolic blood pressure ranges between 90 and 139 mm Hg. When the systolic blood pressure is measured on more than one occasion to be more than 140 mm Hg, high blood pressure is diagnosed.

T

thermic effect of food (TEF) The increase in energy expenditure above the resting metabolic rate that can be measured for several hours after a meal.

thiamin Thiamin is an essential part of a coenzyme, thiamin pyrophosphate, that releases energy from carbohydrate. Thiamin is also needed for nerve transmission and heart muscle tone. Deficiency of thiamin affects the nervous system, cardiovascular system, and gastrointestinal function. Initial deficiency symptoms include fatigue, loss of appetite, nausea, irritability, depression, constipation, indigestion, headaches, and insomnia. As the severity of symptoms from thiamin deficiency increases, the disease beriberi occurs. The best sources of thiamin include seeds, nuts, pork (preferably lean, to reduce saturated fat intake), whole and enriched grains, legumes, wheat germ, and fish. The RDA for average adult males is 1.4 mg, and for females, 1.0 mg.

thrombus A blood clot that forms on top of plaque.

thymus An organ of the immune system that is essential to the maturation of T cells.

tocopherol *See* vitamin E.

tocotrienol *See* vitamin E.

tofu The curd from soy milk.

Total Diet Study A national diet study conducted by the Food and Drug Administration (FDA). This study has provided much-needed information on the mineral intake of Americans.

toxemia *See* pregnancy-induced hypertension.

transit time The time it takes for food to move from the mouth, through the gastrointestinal tract, and out the anus as stool.

triglyceride A type of fat made of glycerol with three fatty acids. Most animal and vegetable fats are triglycerides.

tryptophan An essential amino acid. This amino acid is a precursor for the neurotransmitter, serotonin.

U

urinary incontinence Inability to retain urine in the bladder through loss of control of the sphincter muscle that normally keeps urine from passing.

USDA Bulletin No. 72 This bulletin, published by the USDA for consumers, contains food values for over 730 foods based on average servings or common household units. The figures are derived from Handbook No. 8, 1963 edition.

USDA Handbook No. 8 Since its original publication in 1950, USDA Handbook No. 8 has been the most widely used food composition table. It was revised in 1963. Currently, the latest revision is being published in separate books, each of which contains a table of nutrient data for a major food group.

USDA Handbook No. 456 The figures in USDA Handbook 456 are calculated from the 1963 edition of Handbook No. 8, with a limited amount of updating for some nutrients. This handbook is unique because it uses volume measurements of food, with weight of food in grams given for the various measurements.

U.S. RDA A set of standards developed by the Food and Drug Administration (FDA) for use in regulating nutrition labeling. Although these standards were taken from the RDA, they are based on very few categories, and only 19 vitamins and minerals were included.

V

vegan A vegetarian who avoids use of all animal products, including dairy products and all forms of animal flesh.

vegetarian An individual who does not use any form of animal flesh. There are several types of vegetarians, including lacto-vegetarians (use of milk and milk products), and lacto-ovo-vegetarians (use of milk and eggs).

very-low-Calorie diets (VLCD) Also called the protein-sparing modified fast. The VLCD provides 400–700 Calories per day for people trying to lose weight. Protein is emphasized to help avoid loss of muscle tissue. Patients can use either special formula beverages or natural foods such as fish, fowl, or lean meat (along with mineral and vitamin supplements).

very low density lipoproteins (VLDL) Transport triglycerides to body tissues.

vitamin Vitamins are nutrients which are essential for life itself. The body uses these organic substances to accomplish much of its work. Vitamins do not supply energy, but they do help release energy from carbohydrate, fats, and proteins. They also play a vital role in chemical reactions throughout the body. There are two types of vitamins: fat soluble (A,D,E, and K), and water soluble (eight B-complex and vitamin C). Thirteen vitamins have been discovered, the most recent in 1948.

vitamin A *See also* retinol. The role of vitamin A in the body is to help the eyes readjust to light changes, prevent thickening of the cornea, keep the skin and mucosal linings healthy, aid in bone and teeth formation, and assist in the reproductive process. Carotene may inhibit certain types of cancers. Active, preformed vitamin A is called retinol, and the precursor form is called carotene, or provitamin A. Sources of carotene include fruits and vegetables that are yellow-orange and dark green. Animal foods contain vitamin A in the form of retinol rather than carotene. Primary sources include fish liver oil, liver, egg yolk, milk, cheese, fish, and ice cream. The adult RDA is 1,000 R.E. for men and 800 R.E. for women. Low intakes have been associated with night blindness, xerophthalmia, keratinization of the epithelial tissues, and impaired bone and tooth development. Vitamin A is stored in the liver and released into the body at a steady level for use by the body tissues. When excessive amounts are consumed, beyond the liver's capacity for storage, blood levels dramatically increase. *See also* carotene *and* retinol.

vitamin B₆ Vitamin B_6 comes in three forms: pyridoxine, pyridoxal, and pyridoxamine. Vitamin B_6, in its various forms, works in enzyme systems to build and dismantle proteins. It is also an important participant in the conversion process of tryptophan to niacin, the manufacture of hormones and bile acids, central nervous system control, and the synthesis of hemoglobin. Small quantities of vitamin B_6 are in a wide variety of food. Legumes, dried fruit, seeds and nuts, bananas, rice, and many vegetables are good sources of vitamin B_6. For men and women, the RDA is 2.2 mg and 2.0 mg, respectively. For adults, deficiency symptoms include muscular weakness, nervousness, insomnia, and a facial skin disorder. A type of anemia may also develop.

vitamin B$_{12}$ Coenzymes with vitamin B$_{12}$ are essential for the formation of DNA, maintenance of the protective myelin sheath surrounding nerves, and the production of red blood cells. Vitamin B$_{12}$ works closely with folate in these functions. Vitamin B$_{12}$ has the distinction of being present only in foods of animal origin—none is found in plant foods. All meat and dairy products contain vitamin B$_{12}$, and it is often added to breakfast cereals, soy milk, and meat substitute preparations (meat analogs). Vitamin B$_{12}$ is the most potent vitamin known; therefore, the RDA is quite low. For all adults, the RDA is 3 mcg. Deficiency can lead to pernicious anemia. *See also* intrinsic factor *and* pernicious anemia.

vitamin C Vitamin C has multiple roles in the body. Important functions include synthesis of collagen in the connective tissues of bones, teeth, and tendons; synthesis of hormones; wound healing; promotion of iron absorption; protection of vitamins A and E from oxidation; and protection against injury and infection. The fruit and vegetable group supplies the highest concentration of vitamin C. The RDA for men and women is 60 mg. Although rarely seen today, occasional cases of vitamin-C deficiency or scurvy occur in infants, alcoholics, and the elderly.

vitamin D Vitamin D occurs in two major forms, vitamin D$_2$ (ergocalciferol) and vitamin D$_3$ (cholecalciferol). Vitamin D is needed for bone growth and regulation of blood calcium and phosphorus levels. Active vitamin D functions at three major sites, controlling blood calcium and phosphorus levels. Sunlight exposure is an important means of obtaining sufficient vitamin D. High levels of vitamin D do not naturally occur in foods, and none is found in plant foods. Egg yolks, liver, fatty fish (herring, sardines, tuna, salmon), cream, and butter contain small quantities of vitamin D. Vitamin D is also added to milk. Adults have an RDA of 5 mcg (200 I.U.). Vitamin-D deficiency in children is called rickets, and in adults, osteomalacia.

vitamin E In humans, the principle role of vitamin E seems to be as an antioxidant, preventing oxidation of unsaturated fatty acids, phospholipids, and vitamins A and C by accepting the oxygen that would damage them. Vitamin E is a family of eight naturally occurring compounds called tocopherols and tocotrienols. The most active form of vitamin E is alpha-tocopherol. All other forms are expressed as alpha-tocopherol equivalents. The major food sources of vitamin E are vegetable oils, especially wheat germ oil. Margarine, whole grains, dark green leafy vegetables, nuts, seeds, and legumes also contribute to vitamin E intake. The RDA, as expressed in alpha-tocopherol equivalents (a-TE), is 10 mg a-TE for boys and men, 8 mg a-TE for girls and women.

vitamin K Vitamin K is essential for the production of several protein factors involved in the clotting process. Without vitamin K, normal clotting ability is altered, and bleeding cannot be stopped. There are several related forms of vitamin K, known as quinones. Each form originates from a different source, such as alfalfa, fishmeal, and bacteria. Small amounts of vitamin K are found in a wide variety of foods. Dark green and deep yellow vegetables are the richest sources. Vitamin K is also synthesized in the human intestinal tract. Studies show that approximately 50 percent of the daily requirement for vitamin K is supplied by intestinal bacteria. An estimated safe and adequate daily dietary range of 70–140 mcg per day is suggested.

W

water-insoluble fibers These dietary fibers, including cellulose, hemicellulose, and lignin, are insoluble in water and form the cell walls of many plants.

water-soluble fibers Pectin, mucilages, some types of hemicellulose, gums, and algal polysaccharides are soluble in water, forming a gel.

Wernicke-Korsokoff syndrome In alcoholics, thiamin deficiency may lead to this syndrome. Excessive alcohol consumption increases thiamin requirements and often leads people to eat less food than normal, decreasing thiamin intake. This syndrome is characterized by weakness of eye movements, poor muscle coordination, memory loss, confusion, and short attention span. Immediate treatment is essential to prevent brain damage and heart failure.

white blood cells Special immune system cells that circulate in the blood. These include monocytes, neutrophils, basophils, eosinophils, and lymphocytes.

Wilson's disease A hereditary disease in which copper accumulates in body tissues, causing toxicity.

Women, Infants, and Children (WIC) Government programs such as WIC provide supplemental food and nutrition classes for low-income families. WIC provides vouchers or coupons for high-nutrient foods such as dairy products, infant formulas, baby cereals, juice, peanut butter, and dried beans. In addition to these food supplements, parents attend brief nutrition education classes.

X

xerophthalmia A disease of the eye, proceeding through different stages. With severe vitamin-A deficiency, xerosis, or drying of the conjunctiva and cornea, occurs. Proper treatment, including vitamin-A supplementation, is urgently needed to prevent the advanced state of keratomalacia (softening of the cornea) and subsequent blindness. Young, malnourished children are at high risk for rapid onset of this devastating disease.

xerosis Drying of the conjunctiva and/or cornea from vitamin-A deficiency. In this serious development, the cornea becomes opaque and distorted.

Z

zinc The mineral zinc is a part of more than 70 major enzyme systems of the body. Zinc is important for synthesis of key tissue proteins and for the synthesis and repair of the basic genetic controllers of life, the nucleic acids, DNA and RNA. These control growth, sexual maturation, wound healing, and the maintenance of skin, hair, nails, and the mucous membranes of the mouth, throat, stomach, and intestines. The RDA for adult men and women was set at 15 mg/day. Seeds and nuts, legumes, whole-grain cereals, dairy products, and lean meats are important sources of zinc.

CREDITS

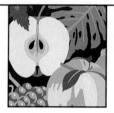

Line Art

Chapter 1
Figure 1.1 and Figure 1.3: Data from National Center for Health Statistics. **Figure 1.4:** From A. H. Maslow, *Motivation and Personality*, 2d ed., 1970. **Figure 1.5:** From L. W. Greene et al., *Health Education Planning: A Diagnostic Approach.* © 1980. Mayfield Publishing Co., Mountain View, CA. Reprinted by permission.

Chapter 2
Figure 2.1: Data from Statistical Abstract of the United States, 1987. **Figure 2.2:** Data from U.S. Department of Agriculture, Economic Research Service. **Figures 2.3–2.10:** Data from U.S. Department of Agriculture, Economic Research Service. **Figures 2.11–2.13:** Data from National Center for Health Statistics. **Figure 2.16:** From *Nutrition and Your Health: Dietary Guidelines for Americans*, 2d ed., 1985. U.S. Department of Agriculture/U.S. Department of Health and Human Services. **Figure 2.17:** Data from Louis Harris and Associates, 1986.

Chapter 3
Figure 3.1: Data from National Center for Health Statistics. **Figure 3.5:** From M. E. Shils and V. E. Young. *Modern Nutrition in Health and Disease*, 7th ed. Philadelphia: Lea & Febiger, 1988. **Health-Promotion Activity 3.1:** From "A How-To Guide to a Balanced Diet," *FDA Consumer*, October 1986, p. 25. **Health-Promotion Activity 3.2:** © 1985 by D. R. Hall, Wellsource, Inc., P.O. Box 569, Clackamas, OR. Used with permission.

Chapter 4
Figure 4.1: From C. W. Lecos, "Shopping for the Second 50 Years," *FDA Consumer*, July-August 1986, p. 31. **Figure 4.2:** From *Safe Food to Go*, Bulletin No. 242, November 1985. U.S. Department of Agriculture. **Figure 4.3:** From *The Safe Food Book*, Bulletin No. 241, 1985. U.S. Department of Agriculture. **Figure 4.4:** From J. Heenan, "Can Your Kitchen Pass the Food Storage Test?" *FDA Consumer*, March, 1974.

Chapter 5
Figure 5.4: From John W. Hole, Jr., *Human Anatomy and Physiology*, 3d ed. Copyright © 1984 Wm. C. Brown Publishers, Dubuque, Iowa. All Rights Reserved. Reprinted by

permission. **Figure 5.7:** From U.S. Senate Select Committee on Nutrition and Human Needs. *Dietary Goals for the United States*, 2d ed., 1977.

Chapter 6
Figure 6.7: From U.S. Senate Committee on Nutrition and Human Needs. *Dietary Goals for the United States*, 2d ed., 1977. **Figure 6.12:** From The Framingham, Massachusetts, Heart Study. **Health-Promotion Activity 6.3:** From J. W. Farquhar, *American Way of Life Need Not Be Hazardous to Your Health*, © 1987 by Stanford Alumni Association. Pages 38–41. Reprinted with permission of Addison-Wesley Publishing Co., Inc., Reading, MA.

Chapter 7
Figure 7.12: Data from R. L. Phillips and D. A. Snowdon. Mortality among Seventh-day Adventists in Relation to Dietary Habits and Lifestyle. Evaluation of Plant Proteins: Application, Biologic Effect, Composition/Chemistry. American Chemical Society. 1986.

Chapter 8
Figure 8.6: From F. Katch and W. D. McArdle, *Nutrition, Weight Control, and Exercise*. © 1988. Lea and Febiger, Philadelphia. Reprinted by permission. **Figure 8.7:** Basic data from 1983 Metropolitan height and weight tables. Courtesy of the Metropolitan Life Insurance Co.

Chapter 9
Figure 9.1: Data from National Center for Health Statistics. **Figure 9.3:** From W. J. Millar and T. Stephens, "The Prevalence of Overweight and Obesity in Britain, Canada, and the United States," *American Journal of Public Health*, 77:38–41, 1987. Used with permission. **Figure 9.4:** From S. L. Gortmaker and W. H. Dietz, Increasing Pediatric Obesity in the United States. *American Journal of Diseases in Children*, 141:535–40, 1987. **Figure 9.9:** Data from W. H. Dietz and S. L. Gortmaker, "Do We Fatten Our Children at the Television Set? Obesity and Television Viewing in Children and Adolescents," *Pediatrics*, 75:807, © 1985. Reproduced by permission of *Pediatrics*. **Figure 9.13:** Data from R. D. Hagan et al., "The Effects of Aerobic Conditioning and/or Caloric Restriction in Overweight Men and Women," *Medicine and Science in Sports and Exercise*, 18:87–94.

© American College of Sports Medicine, 1986. Used with permission. **Figure 9.14:** Data from J. O. Hill et al., "Effects of Exercise and Food Restriction on Body Composition and Metabolic Rate in Obese Women," *American Journal of Clinical Nutrition*, 46:622-30, 1987. © American Society for Clinical Nutrition. Used with permission.

Chapter 10
Figure 10.9: From B. L. Carlson, "Loss of Vitamin C in Vegetables During the Foodservice Cycle." *Journal of the American Dietetic Association*, 88:65-67, 1988. **Figures 10.11 and 10.12:** From *Cancer Facts and Figures—1988*, American Cancer Society. Used with permission.

Chapter 11
Figure 11.1: Data from J. A. T. Pennington et al., "Mineral Content of Foods and Total Diets." *Journal of the American Dietetic Association*, 86:876-91, 1986. **Figure 11.4:** Data from G. Block et al., "Nutrient Sources in the American Diet: Quantitative Data from the NHANES II Survey." *American Journal of Epidemiology*, 122:13-26, 1985. **Figure 11.6:** Data from G. Block et al., "Nutrient Sources in the American Diet: Quantitative Data from the NHANES II Survey." *American Journal of Epidemiology*, 122:13-26, 1985. **Figure 11.7:** From "Salt Heads Health Concerns," *FDA Consumer*, December 1984-January 1985, p. 3. **Figure 11.8:** Data from G. Block et al., "Nutrient Sources in the American Diet: Quantitative Data from the NHANES II Survey." *American Journal of Epidemiology*, 122:13-26, 1985. **Figure 11.9:** Data from G. Block et al., "Nutrient Sources in the American Diet: Quantitative Data from the NHANES II Survey." *American Journal of Epidemiology*, 122:13-26, 1985. **Figure 11.10:** Data from National Center for Health Statistics.

Chapter 12
Figure 12.6: Data from National Center for Health Statistics. **Figures 12.7 and 12.8:** Data from National Institute on Alcohol Abuse and Alcoholism. **Figure 12.9:** From D. L. Costill and J. M. Miller, "Nutrition for Endurance Sports: Carbohydrate and Fluid Balance," *International Journal of Sports Medicine*, 1:2-14, 1980. Used with permission from Georg Thieme Verlag, Publishers, Stuttgart, West Germany.

Chapter 13

Figure 13.1: From John W. Hole, Jr., *Human Anatomy and Physiology*, 3d ed. Copyright © 1984 Wm. C. Brown Publishers, Dubuque, Iowa. All Rights Reserved. Reprinted by permission. **Figure 13.3:** Adapted from K. L. Moore, *The Developing Human.* © 1988. W. B. Saunders, Philadelphia. Used with permission. **Figure 13.6:** Data from National Center for Health Statistics. **Health-Promotion Activity 13.1:** Food Group Chart © 1983, 1984. Dairy Council of California. Reprinted with permission.

Chapter 14

Figure 14.1: From P. V. V. Hamill et al., "Physical Growth: National Center for Health Statistics Percentiles." *American Journal of Clinical Nutrition*, 32:607-629, 1979 © American Society for Clinical Nutrition. Used with permission. **Figures 14.2-14.4:** From *Women, Infants, Children* (Supplemental Food Section). California Department of Health Services, Sacramento. Used with permission. **Figure 14.5:** From *High School Seniors Survey.* National Institute on Drug Abuse. **Figure 14.6:** From John W. Hole, Jr., ESSENTIALS OF HUMAN ANATOMY AND PHYSIOLOGY, 3d ed. Copyright © 1989 Wm. C. Brown Publishers, Dubuque, Iowa. All Rights Reserved. Reprinted by permission. **Figure 14.7:** From John W. Hole, Jr., *Human Anatomy and Physiology*, 4th ed. Copyright © 1987 Wm. C. Brown Publishers, Dubuque, Iowa. All Rights Reserved. Reprinted by permission.

Chapter 15

Figure 15.1: Data from U.S. Bureau of the Census. **Figures 15.2 through 15.5:** Data from National Center for Health Statistics. **Figure 15.6:** Data from U.S. Bureau of the Census projections and National Institute on Aging prevalence estimates. **Figure 15.9:** Data from U.S. Bureau of the Census projections and National Center for Health Statistics. **Figure 15.10:** From a report of the Consensus Development Conference on Osteoporosis convened by the National Institutes of Health. Free single copies of the report are available from the U.S. Department of Health and Human Services, NIH, Office of Medical Applications of Research, Building 216, Bethesda, MD 20205. **Figure 15.11:** From P. Jaret, "Our Immune System: The Wars Within," *National Geographic*, June 1986, pp. 702-734. Used with permission.

Hans & Cassady, Inc. provided computer-generated art for the following figures: Figures 1.1-1.5, 2.1-2.17, 3.1-3.4, 4.1-4.4, 4.7, 5.1, 5.2, 5.3, and 5.6. Art accompanying Table 5.5 on page 118. Art for Health-Promotion Activity 5.3 on page 131. Figures 5.5, 5.7, 5.8, 6.1, 6.2, 6.4-6.13, 7.1-7.8, 7.10-7.12, 8.1-8.8. Art for Health-Promotion Activity 8.1 on page 199. Art for Health-Promotion Activity 8.2 on page 200. Figures 8.10, 8.11, 9.1, 9.3-9.6, 9.8-9.14, 10.1, 10.4, 10.6, 10.9, 10.11, 11.1-11.10, 12.1-12.9, 13.2, 13.3, 13.5, 13.6, 14.2-14.5. Art for Sidebar 14.1 on page 379. Art for Sidebar 14.2 on page 383. Figures 15.1-15.7, 15.9-15.11.

Photos

Chapter 1

Page 6: © Mark Antman/The Image Works; **page 10 top:** © Mark E. Gibson; **middle:** © George Gardner/The Image Works; **bottom:** © Photri/Marilyn Gartman Agency; **page 11:** © Mark Antman/The Image Works; **page 12 top:** © Wayne Floyd/Unicorn Stock Photos; **page 14 bottom:** © Patrick James Watson.

Chapter 2

Page 23 top: © Tom Firak/Marilyn Gartman Agency; **bottom:** © Mary Stadtfeld/Unicorn Stock Photos; **page 24 top:** © 1989 Lee Balterman/Marilyn Gartman Agency; **bottom:** © 1989 Martin R. Jones/Unicorn Stock Photos; **pages 25, 26 both:** Mary Stadtfeld/Unicorn Stock Photos; **page 27:** © Len Berger/Berg and Associates; **page 30:** Bob Daemmrich; **page 31:** © 1989 Martin R. Jones/Unicorn Stock Photos; **page 37:** © Bob Daemmrich/The Image Works; **page 39:** © Ellis Herwig/Marilyn Gartman Agency.

Chapter 3

Page 48: © 1988 John Bird; **page 53:** © Bob Daemmrich/The Image Works; **page 57 top left:** © Mary Stadtfeld/Unicorn Stock Photos; **bottom left:** © Jeffery W. Myers/Stock, Boston; **top right:** © Mike and Carol Werner/Comstock Photos; **bottom right:** © M. Stuckey/Comstock Photos; **page 58 all:** © James L. Shaffer; **page 70:** © Judy White/Berg and Associates.

Chapter 4

Page 80: © Eastcott/Homatiuk/The Image Works; **page 82:** © James L. Shaffer; **pages 83, 86:** © Wayne Floyd/Unicorn Stock Photos; **page 87:** © Herwig/Marilyn Gartman Agency; **4.5:** © Bob Daemmrich/The Image Works; **4.6:** © Greg Greer/Unicorn Stock Photos.

Chapter 5

Page 110: © Wayne Floyd/Unicorn Stock Photos; **page 116:** © Martha McBride/Unicorn Stock Photos; **5.9:** © MacDonald/Photri/Marilyn Gartman Agency.

Chapter 6

6.3: © Greg Greer/Unicorn Stock Photos; **page 143 both:** Wayne Floyd/Unicorn Stock Photos.

Chapter 7

Page 164: © Wayne Floyd/Unicorn Stock Photos; **page 165:** © Margaret C. Berg/Berg and Associates; **page 166:** © James G. White; **page 168:** © James L. Shaffer; **7.9A:** © Photri/Marilyn Gartman Agency; **7.9B:** © Tim Gibson/Envision.

Chapter 8

Page 182: © John Bird; **page 186:** © Peter Menzel/Stock, Boston; **page 187:** © Wayne Floyd/Unicorn Stock Photos; **page 188:** © Patrick James Watson; **8.8:** © Joan Sloane/Berg and Associates; **8.9:** © Fitness Research Center/University of Michigan, Photo by Gary Helfand; **page 195:** © Chuck Nacke/Picture Group.

Chapter 9

9.2: © James L. Shaffer; **page 203 bottom:** © Karen Holsinger Mullen/Unicorn Stock Photos; **page 204:** © Catherine Ursello/Photo Researchers, Inc.; **9.7 both:** © James L. Shaffer; **page 210 left:** © Simon Feldman/Envision; **top right:** © Herb Snitzer/Stock, Boston; **bottom right:** © Arnold J. Kaplan/Berg and Associates; **page 212:** © James L. Shaffer; **page 215:** © Bob Coyle; **page 217:** © Greg Greer/Unicorn Stock Photos; **page 220:** © Bob Coyle; **page 223:** © Russ Kinne/Comstock.

Chapter 10

Page 237: © Greg Greer/Unicorn Stock Photos; **10.2 all:** © David J. Farr/ImageSmythe, Inc.; **10.3A:** © Victoria M. Shellfield/Helen Keller International; **10.3B:** © Alfred Sommer, M.D., Director, International Center for Epidemiological and Preventive Ophthalmology at John Hopkins University Medical Center; **page 244:** © Bob Daemmrich/The Image Works; **10.5:** © Biophoto Associates/Science Source/Photo Researchers, Inc.; **page 246:** © Margaret C. Berg/Berg and Associates; **page 250:** © Mary Stadtfeld/Unicorn Stock Photos; **10.7:** Center for Disease Control, Atlanta, GA; **10.8:** WHO Photo; **page 261:** © Mary Statdfeld/Unicorn Stock Photos; **10.10:** © Lester V. Bergman and Associates, Inc.

Chapter 11

Page 279: © Greg Greer/Unicorn Stock Photos; **page 281:** © Richard Hutchings/Photo Researchers, Inc.; **page 285:** © Bob Daemmrich; **page 292:** © Robert Frerck/Odyssey Productions; **page 296 left:** © Davies/Pashko/Envision; **right:** © Addison Geary/Stock, Boston; **page 299:** © James L. Shaffer; **page 300:** © Daniel E. Wray; **page 303:** © Norman Prince, San Francisco, CA; **page 308:** © Art Brackley/Berg and Associates.

Chapter 12

Page 320: © Steven Mark Needham/Envision; **page 323:** © Kathy Hamer/Unicorn Stock Photos; **page 325:** © Wayne Floyd/Unicorn Stock Photos; **page 334:** © Comstock.

Chapter 13

Page 347: © Mark E. Gibson; **page 351 left:** © Photri/Marilyn Gartman Agency; **right:** © Elizabeth Crews/The Image Works; **13.4:** Fetal Alcohol Research, University of Washington; **page 358:** © Betts Anderson/Unicorn Stock Photos; **page 360:** courtesy of Diane Butterworth; **page 361 left:** © Patrick James Watson; **right:** courtesy of Diane Butterworth.

Chapter 14

Page 370: © Tom McCarthy/Marilyn Gartman Agency; **page 371:** © Michael Plack/Berg and Associates; **page 376:** © Richard Pasley/Stock, Boston; **page 378:** © William Hopkins; **pages 382, 385:** © Robert Frerck/Odyssey Productions; **page 387:** © Bob Daemmrich.

Chapter 15

Page 402: courtesy of David and Catherine Nieman; **page 407:** © Bob Daemmrich; **pages 408, 410:** © James L. Shaffer; **page 412:** © Lorraine Rorke/The Image Works; **page 415:** © Charles Gupton/Stock, Boston; **fig. 15.8:** © Carolina Biological Supply; **page 421 both:** courtesy of David and Catherine Nieman.

I N D E X

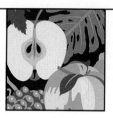

Religion, and eating behaviors, 11
Restaurants
    in dietary trends, 30–31, 32, 39
    fast-food, 30, 31, 32, 39, 390,
        436–39
Resting metabolic rate (RMR), 209, 221
Restoration, 89, 97
Retinol, 237, 515. *See also* Vitamin A
Retinol equivalents (R.E.), 239
Retinopathy, 125
Rhodopsin, 241
Riboflavin, 238, 251–52, 513. *See also*
        Vitamins
Ribonucleic acid (RNA), 158, 159, 502
Rickets, 245–46
RMR, 209, 221
RNA (ribonucleic acid), 158, 159, 502
Saccharin, 94–95
Safety
    allergies, 98–101, 359–60
    checklist for, 105–6
    food faddism and, 101–4
    food handling for, 82–84
    labeling and, 96–98, 99
    vegetarian diet and, 175
    of vitamins, 50, 265
    of water, 319
    See also Health hazards; Poisoning
Salad dressing, composition of, 440–41
Salazar, Alberto, 332
Saliva, 484
Salmonellosis, 80, 81
Salt
    chemical bonds in, 505–6
    composition of, 454–55
    in dietary guidelines, 33
    in dietary trends, 28
    high blood pressure and, 149, 308,
        498–99
    reducing in recipes, 36
    sources of, 42
    See also Sodium
Salt substitutes, 293, 454–55
Sandwiches, composition of, 438–41
Satiety, 186
Saturated fat, 139, 140–41, 142, 495–97
Saturated fatty acid (SFA), 134, 509, 512
Sauces, composition of, 466–67
School-age children, 384–87
    diet of, 384–87
    physical growth of, 384
School lunches, 386–87
Scurvy, 261, 262
Seeds
    composition of, 456–57
    as food group, 56, 57, 59
Selenium, 275, 302–3. *See also* Minerals
Self-responsibility, for eating habits, 12
Sell date, 97
Senile dementia, 404–5, 406, 408
Serotonin, 396
Severe obesity, 213
Sexual performance, and vitamin E,
    247–48

Shellfish poisoning, 85
Simplesse, 145
Sinclair, Upton, 87
Single-value nutrient allowances, 52
Skinfold measurements, 193, 194
Skin-prick test, 99
Small intestine, 484, 485, 487
    alcohol and, 329
    digestion of carbohydrates in, 113
    digestion of lipids in, 135–36
    digestion of protein in, 162
Smoking. *See* Cigarette smoking;
        Tobacco
Snacks
    cholesterol in, 141
    composition of, 452–53
    in dietary trends, 30
    fats in, 141
    for preschool children, 381, 382
Sodium, 275, 286–94
    blood pressure and, 149, 308, 498,
        499
    in cereals, 289
    in cheese, 290
    chemical bonds in, 505–6
    estimated minimum requirements for,
        51
    foods high in, 287
    foods low in, 287
    in mineral water, 288
    moderating intake of, 291, 498–99
    in one-cup portions of food, 286
    substitutes for, 292–93, 454–55
    See also Salt
Sodium Reeducation Campaign, 55
Soft drinks
    caffeine in, 320, 321
    composition of, 430–33
    consumption of, 117, 320, 321
    diet, 39
    sugar in, 117
Soups, composition of, 468–69
Soybean, protein in, 169–70
Spices and herbs, 292–93, 452–55
Spirulina, 219
Sports nutrition, 332–37. *See also*
        Athletes
Spot reducing, 223
Spreads, composition of, 466–67
Stabilizers, 92
Standards of identity, 87
Staphylococcus aureus, 81
Starch, 111, 498
    in dietary trends, 21
    in Food Exchange System, 61
    sources of, 118–19
    See also Carbohydrates
Starch blockers, 219
Sterols, 134, 510
Stomach
    alcohol and, 329
    digestion in, 113, 162, 484, 485, 487
    stapling of, 213, 214

Stomatitis, 251
Stroke, 147
    alcohol and, 330
    risk factors of, 148
    test for risk of, 155–56
    See also Cardiovascular diseases
Sucrose, 110, 111
Sudden infant death syndrome, 351
Sugars
    consumption of, 116, 117
    in dietary guidelines, 31, 33, 497–98
    in dietary trends, 21–22, 26, 27
    as food group, 56, 57, 58
    reactive hypoglycemia and, 122–23
    reducing in recipes, 36
    sources of, 42, 117–18
    tooth decay and, 122
    See also Carbohydrates
Sulfites, 100, 101
Supplementation, 263–65, 349, 354, 411,
        493
Surgeon General's Report on Nutrition
        and Health, 33, 34, 499
Sweat, 332
Sweeteners
    behavior and, 397
    in dietary trends, 21–22, 26, 27
    food additives as, 94–96
Sweets, composition of, 470–75
Systolic blood pressure, 306
Tape measurements, of body fat, 193
Tea
    caffeine in, 319–20
    composition of, 432–33
    consumption of, 321
Teenagers. *See* Adolescents
Teeth
    care of, 498
    decay in, 122, 300
    of elderly, 407
    vitamin A and, 242
Temperature
    body, 315
    conversion of, 488
Teratogens, 345, 351–52
Texturizers, 92
Thermic effect of food (TEF), 187,
        212–13
Thermogenesis, 187–88
Thiamin, 89, 238, 249–51, 513. *See also*
        Vitamins
Thickeners, 92
Thirst, 316, 317
Thrombus, 147
Thymus, 422
Tobacco
    adolescents and, 390–91
    effects of, 115
    smokeless, 391
    See also Cigarette smoking
Tocopherols, 246, 515, 516. *See also*
        Vitamin E